FITNESS AND LIFESTYLE MANAGEMENT FOR LAW ENFORCEMENT

FIFTH EDITION

NANCY WAGNER WISOTZKI

REBECCA FINLAY

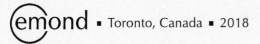 ▪ Toronto, Canada ▪ 2018

Emond Montgomery Publications Limited
60 Shaftesbury Avenue
Toronto ON M4T 1A3
http://www.emond.ca/highered

Reprinted April 2020. Printed in Canada.

We acknowledge the financial support of the Government of Canada. **Canadä**

Emond Montgomery Publications has no responsibility for the persistence or accuracy of URLs for external or third-party Internet websites referred to in this publication, and does not guarantee that any content on such websites is, or will remain, accurate or appropriate.

Vice president, publishing: Anthony Rezek
Publisher: Lindsay Sutherland
Director, development and production: Kelly Dickson
Developmental editor: Katherine Goodes
Production supervisor: Laura Bast
Copy editor: Lila Campbell
Typesetter: Tom Dart
Text designer: Sharon Lucas
Permissions editor: Lisa Brant
Proofreader: Erin Moore
Indexer: Marnie Lamb
Cover image: Uber Images/Shutterstock

Library and Archives Canada Cataloguing in Publication

Wagner Wisotzki, Nancy, 1959-, author
    Fitness and lifestyle management for law enforcement / Nancy Wagner Wisotzki, Rebecca Finlay. — Fifth edition.

Includes index.
ISBN 978-1-77255-061-0 (softcover)

    1. Police—Health and hygiene.   2. Police—Physical training.   I. Finlay, Rebecca, author   II. Title.

HV7936.H4W33 2018   613.02'43632   C2017-904257-2

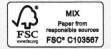

To Tim,
Your love and support is beyond words.
I could not have done this without you.

Love, Rebecca

To Larry, Alexandra, and Christine,
I am eternally grateful for your love, laughter, patience, guidance,
and believing in me as I continue pursuing my dreams.

Nancy (Mom) xo

To the students, graduates, and law enforcement officers
who continue to touch our lives and hearts:
Thank you for your inspiration and your zest for life which continues to
keep health and fitness so important to us.

Nancy and Rebecca

BRIEF CONTENTS

CONTENTS vii

PREFACE xiii

ACKNOWLEDGMENTS xv

ABOUT THE AUTHORS xvi

PART 1 GETTING STARTED TOWARD A HEALTHY LIFESTYLE

CHAPTER 1   Are You Fit for Your Career? 3
CHAPTER 2   Goal Setting 31
CHAPTER 3   Time Management 49

PART 2 PLANNING AND MAINTAINING A FITNESS PROGRAM

CHAPTER 4   Principles of Exercise 69
CHAPTER 5   Cardiorespiratory Fitness 111
CHAPTER 6   Resistance Training 137

PART 3 BODY COMPOSITION AND NUTRITION

CHAPTER 7   Body Composition 171
CHAPTER 8   Nutrition 195

PART 4 UNDERSTANDING AND MANAGING POTENTIAL HEALTH PROBLEMS

CHAPTER 9   Diabetes 243
CHAPTER 10   Cardiovascular Disease 263
CHAPTER 11   Back Health 293
CHAPTER 12   Stress 325
CHAPTER 13   Shift Work and Sleep 363
CHAPTER 14   Common Injuries 389

APPENDIX   BFOR Protocols and Fitness Standards 419

Glossary 453
Index 461
Credits 469

CONTENTS

BRIEF CONTENTS v

PREFACE xiii

ACKNOWLEDGMENTS xv

ABOUT THE AUTHORS xvi

PART 1
GETTING STARTED TOWARD A HEALTHY LIFESTYLE

CHAPTER 1 Are You Fit for Your Career?

Learning Outcomes 3

Health and Wellness 4

A Wellness Profile 5

The Seven Dimensions of Health 6

What Are Law Enforcement Agencies Looking For? 7

Fitness Requirements for Law Enforcement 8

Being Physically Active 8

Importance of Fitness in Law Enforcement 10

Preparing for Fitness 11

Physical Testing Within Law Enforcement 13

Law Enforcement Hiring Information 19

Essential and Developmental Competencies 19

Law Enforcement Selection Processes 21

A Final Thought 25

Key Terms 26

Exercises 26

References 28

CHAPTER 2 Goal Setting

Learning Outcomes 31

The Stages of Behavioural Change 32

Factors That Affect Participation in Physical Activity 36

Self-Management Behavioural Strategies 37

Understanding Your Goals 38

Short- and Long-Term Goals 38

Choosing Effective Goals—Make a SMART plan 39

Staying on Track 41

Rewarding Yourself 42

Your Mission Statement 43

Being Fit and Well for Life 44

Final Thoughts 44

Key Terms 45

Exercises 45

References 47

CHAPTER 3 Time Management

Learning Outcomes 49

The Benefits of Time Management 50

The Stages of Time Management 52

Prioritizing Your Activities 52

Scheduling Your Activities 53

Implementing Your Activities 55

Time Management Strategies for Students 57

Organize Your Workspace to Manage Distractions 57

Organize Your Assignments and Prepare for Tests 57

Create an Exam Study Schedule 59

Tips for Effective Group Work 62

Final Thoughts on Time Management 63

Key Terms 64

Exercises 64

References 65

PART 2
PLANNING AND MAINTAINING A FITNESS PROGRAM

CHAPTER 4 Principles of Exercise

Learning Outcomes 69

Introduction to Anatomy and Physiology 70

Cells, Tissues, and Organs 71

Bones and Muscles 72

How Do Muscles Work? 74

What Is Training? 80

Health-Related Fitness 82

    Cardiorespiratory Endurance 82

    Muscular Strength 82

    Muscular Endurance 83

    Flexibility 83

    Body Composition 84

Performance/Skill-Related Fitness 84

    Speed 84

    Coordination 84

    Reaction Time 84

    Agility 85

    Balance 85

    Power 85

The Health Benefits of Physical Activity 85

The Principles of Exercise 88

The Principles of Physical Training 88

    The Principle of Progressive Overload 88

    The Principle of Specificity 89

    The Principle of Individuality 90

    The Principle of Reversibility 90

    The Principle of Diminishing Returns 91

    The Principle of Recovery 92

Training Methods 92

    Functional Training 92

    Resistance Training 93

    Interval Training 93

    High-Intensity Interval Training 94

    Plyometric Training 94

    Concurrent Training 94

    Periodization 95

Guidelines for Starting a Fitness Program 95

Flexibility and Stretching 97

    The Benefits of Stretching 97

    Stretching Techniques 98

    Safe and Effective Stretching 100

Final Thoughts 102

Key Terms 103

Exercises 104

References 107

CHAPTER 5 Cardiorespiratory Fitness

Learning Outcomes 111

The Importance of Cardiorespiratory Fitness
   in Law Enforcement 112

The Benefits of Cardiorespiratory Fitness 112

Assessing Cardiorespiratory Fitness 113

    Central Cardiorespiratory Fitness 113

    Peripheral Cardiorespiratory Fitness 114

    Maximum Aerobic Capacity 114

Determining Your Cardiovascular Training
   Intensity 116

    Understanding Heart Rates 116

    Heart Rate Monitoring 117

    The Borg Scale 119

    The Talk Test 120

    Understanding METs 120

Creating a Cardiorespiratory Fitness Program 121

    Guidelines for Cardiorespiratory Fitness
      Training 122

    Training for Running 123

    The Basics on Running Mechanics 123

    Training to Your Upper Limit 126

    Training for the Shuttle Run 127

Weather and Your Fitness Program 128

    Preparing to Participate in Outdoor
      Activities 128

Final Thoughts 130

Key Terms 131

Exercises 131

References 133

CHAPTER 6 Resistance Training

Learning Outcomes 137

The Importance of Resistance Training 138

    Bona Fide Occupational Requirements
      (BFORs) 139

    The Benefits of Resistance Training 140

The Basics of Resistance Training 141

    Basic Principles of Resistance Training 142

Basic Guidelines for Resistance Training 146

    Getting Started and Setting Goals 146

    Designing a Program 147

    Training Methods 152

Law Enforcement Resistance Training Programs 154

    PREP Test/A-PREP 155

PARE Test 155
FITCO Test 157
FORCE Workout 157
Other Considerations 158
Fuelling Your Body 158
Performance-Enhancing Substances 159
Women and Strength Training 160
First Time in the Weight Room 161
Final Thoughts 162
Key Terms 163
Exercises 163
References 166

PART 3
BODY COMPOSITION AND NUTRITION

CHAPTER 7 Body Composition

Learning Outcomes 171
Understanding Chronic Disease 172
Misguided Views of the Body 173
Body Composition 175
Somatotypes 176
Metabolism 177
Basal Metabolism 177
Measuring Body Composition 178
Body Mass Index (BMI) 178
Edmonton Obesity Staging System 179
Waist Circumference 179
Waist-to-Hip Ratio Measurement 180
Health Risk Classification 181
Skinfold Measurement 181
Bioelectric Impedance 182
Bodpod 182
Hydrostatic Weighing 183
Eating Disorders 183
Anorexia Nervosa 185
Bulimia Nervosa 185
Body Dysmorphic Disorder 186
Binge Eating Disorder 186
Female Athlete Triad 187
Final Thoughts 188
Key Terms 189

Exercises 189
References 191

CHAPTER 8 Nutrition

Learning Outcomes 195
Maintaining a Healthy Weight 196
Impact of Diet, Nutrition, and Physical Activity
on Cancer 198
Function of Food 199
Basic Nutrients 200
Water 200
Carbohydrates 201
Protein 208
Fats 210
Vitamins and Minerals 215
Calories 220
Nutrition Facts and Labelling 221
Nutrient Content Claims 223
Eating Well for Life 225
Canada's Food Guide 225
Serving Sizes and Recommended Servings 225
Grocery Shopping 101 226
The Benefits Of Other Nutrients In
Your Diet 228
Snacking 229
Caffeinated Drinks 230
Wellness Initiatives 232
Final Thoughts 232
Appendix: Further Information on Nutrition 233
Key Terms 234
Exercises 235
References 237

PART 4
UNDERSTANDING AND MANAGING POTENTIAL HEALTH PROBLEMS

CHAPTER 9 Diabetes

Learning Outcomes 243
Types of Diabetes 244
Symptoms of Diabetes 247
What Happens When You Are Hypoglycemic or
Hyperglycemic? 247

Risk Factors Associated with Diabetes 248
The Changing Face of Diabetes in Canada 250
 What Does the Future Hold? 250
Complications Associated with Diabetes 251
Living with Diabetes and Shift Work 253
Final Thoughts 256
Key Terms 257
Exercises 257
References 259

CHAPTER 10 Cardiovascular Disease

Learning Outcomes 263
The Impact on Our Health-Care System 264
The Demographics of Those with
 Cardiovascular Disease 265
Anatomy of the Heart 267
 How the Heart Functions 267
Types of Cardiovascular Disease 268
 Arteriosclerosis/Atherosclerosis 269
 Coronary Heart Disease 269
 Stroke 277
 Hypertension 282
Reducing the Risks of a Cardiovascular Event 284
Final Thoughts 286
Key Terms 287
Exercises 287
References 289

CHAPTER 11 Back Health

Learning Outcomes 293
The Spine 296
The Causes of Back Pain 297
Risk Factors for Back Pain 298
Etiology of Back Pain 300
 Degenerative Disc Disease 300
 Arthritis 302
 Osteoporosis 303
 Repetitive Strain Injury 305
Treating Back Injuries 307
Preventing Back Pain 307
 Exercises for a Healthy Back 309
Tips on Proper Posture 315
 Proper Sitting in a Vehicle 315
 Proper Sitting at a Desk 316
 Proper Standing Posture 317

Nutritional Considerations for a Healthier Back 317
Final Thoughts 318
Key Terms 319
Exercises 319
References 321

CHAPTER 12 Stress

Learning Outcomes 325
Defining Stress 326
Types of Stress 326
The Stress Response 327
Stressors 328
 Stressors in Daily Life 328
 Stressors Faced by Law Enforcement 330
 Stressors from Workplace Health and
  Safety Hazards 334
 Impact of Stress on the Family 334
The Effects of Stress 335
 Short- and Long-Term Effects of Stress 335
 Chronic Stress 336
Critical Incidents 337
 Types of Critical Incidents 338
 Factors Affecting Responses to
  Critical Incidents 338
 Symptoms of Stress Arising out of
  Critical Incidents 339
 Suicide 343
Coping with Stress 345
 After a Critical Incident 345
 Resiliency and Mindfulness 347
 Strategies for Coping with Stress 348
 Relaxation Techniques 349
Final Thoughts 353
Key Terms 354
Exercises 354
References 356

CHAPTER 13 Shift Work and Sleep

Learning Outcomes 363
Understanding the Importance of Sleep 365
 How Does the Sleep Cycle Work? 368
The Effects of Shift Work on Sleep 369
 Physiological and Psychological Effects 369
 Shift Schedules 372
 Social Effects 372

Medical Conditions Associated with Shift Work 374
    Sleep Disorders 374
    Cancer and Shift Work 376
    Diabetes and Shift Work 377
Coping Strategies for Shift Work 377
    Eating Nutritious Food 377
    The Role of Light 378
    Importance of Breaks While on Duty 379
    Physical Activity 379
    Keeping Healthy Relationships 380
    Healthy Sleep Tips 381
Final Thoughts 382
Key Terms 383
Exercises 383
References 385

CHAPTER 14 Common Injuries

Learning Outcomes 389
Musculoskeletal Injuries 390
    Musculoskeletal Injury Risk Factors 391
    General Treatments for Musculoskeletal
        Injuries 391
    Sorting Out Muscle Soreness 393
Common Sport-Related Musculoskeletal Injuries 394
    Sprain 394
    Strain 395
    Tendinitis 396
    Dislocated Shoulder 399
    Patello-Femoral Syndrome (Chondromalacia
        Patella) 400
    Shin Splints (Tibial Stress Syndrome) 401
    Plantar Fasciitis 402
    Osgood-Schlatter Disease 403
    Iliotibial Band Syndrome 404
    Ligament Sprains to the Knee 404
    Injuries to the Meniscus 405
Concussions 406
    Syndromes Associated with a Concussion 408
    Diagnosis of a Concussion 408
    Treatment 408
Heat- and Cold-Related Injuries and Illnesses 409
    Heat-Related Injuries 409
    Cold-Related Injuries and Illnesses 411

Biological and Chemical Hazards in Law
    Enforcement 413
Final Thoughts 414
Key Terms 415
Exercises 415
References 417

APPENDIX BFOR Protocols and Fitness Standards

Bona Fide Occupational Requirement (BFOR) 419
Physical Readiness Evaluation for Police
    (PREP) Test 419
    Pursuit/Restraint Circuit 420
    Aerobic Fitness Test: Léger 20-Metre
        Shuttle Run 420
Alberta Physical Readiness Evaluation for
    Police (A-PREP) 422
    Pursuit/Restraint Circuit 422
    Aerobic Fitness Test: Léger 20-Metre
        Shuttle Run 424
    Further Resources 424
Physical Abilities Requirement Evaluation
    (PARE) Test 424
    Obstacle Course Section 424
    Push/Pull Section 424
    Weight Carry Section 425
    Further Resources 426
Police Officers Physical Abilities Test (POPAT) 426
    Station 1: 390-Metre (426-Yard) Run 426
    Station 2A: Physical Control Simulator 426
    Station 2B: Vault Rail 428
    Station 3: Torso Bag Carry 428
    Further Resources 428
Fitness Test for Ontario Correctional Officer
    (FITCO) 428
    Cell Search 428
    Emergency Response Circuit 429
    Aerobic Fitness Test: Léger 20-Metre
        Shuttle Run 430
Correctional Officers' Physical Abilities Test
    (COPAT) 431
    Station 1: STAIR RUN 431
    Station 2: Physical-Control Simulator 431
    Station 3: Vault Rail 431
    Station 4: Torso Bag Carry 432

Further Resources 433
Fitness for Operational Requirements of Canadian
Armed Forces Employment (FORCE) 433
20-Metre Rushes 433
Sandbag Lift 434
Intermittent Loaded Shuttles 434
Sandbag Drag 435
Further Resources 435
Ontario Police Fitness Award (OPFA) Standards 436
Push-ups 437
Core Endurance Test 439
Trunk Forward Flexion
(Sit and Reach) 441
1.5-Mile (2.4-Km) Run 442

Maximal Léger 20-Metre Shuttle Run 443
Additional Fitness Standards 444
Bench Press 444
Chin-ups 447
Leg Press 449
Physical Fitness Log 449
Final Thoughts 450
References 451

GLOSSARY 453
INDEX 461
CREDITS 469

PREFACE

There is arguably no more stressful and difficult a career than that of those who choose law enforcement. Depending on the path you choose, you will be faced with a unique set of stressors on your body and your mind.

- In policing, new officers will need to be prepared for periods of heightened activity such as running, lifting, use of force, or self-defence, as well as periods of inactivity such as standing in one spot or sitting in a police cruiser for an entire shift. You will need to have a plan in place on how you will deal with the stressors of the job mentally, physically, and emotionally.

- In corrections, new officers will confront emergency responses, inmate disturbances, and potentially violent situations which will require you to have a high level of fitness, alertness, and ability to handle stress and fatigue appropriately.

- In security, new officers will be required to stand and walk/run for entire shifts and demonstrate the ability to protect people, property, or locations. You may also be tasked with responding to emergencies and have to be prepared to deal with potential physical confrontations in a safe and effective manner.

- In customs, new officers may be required to cover widespread territory and have extensive bouts of standing and walking. Officers will need to be prepared for any situation that may occur while searching persons and vehicles, such as exposure to hazardous materials and weapons, and confrontations with individuals crossing the border.

This fifth edition of *Fitness and Lifestyle Management for Law Enforcement* offers the latest information and advice on becoming and staying fit and healthy for a future career in law enforcement. The resource is divided into to four parts.

- Part 1 is an introduction to the role of fitness in law enforcement, how to create personal goals, modify behaviours, and develop good time-management skills.

- Part 2 provides information on the basics of fitness training, particularly cardiovascular fitness, resistance training, and specific job-related fitness training programs.

- Part 3 delivers effective motivation for healthy eating and body composition.

- Part 4 allows readers to learn how to make healthy choices with respect to heart disease, diabetes, shift work, stress, back health, and preventing injuries.

- The Appendix provides descriptions and diagrams of all of the various law enforcement Bona Fide Occupational Requirement (BFOR) fitness tests in Canada.

Aside from updating to current information throughout the text, you will discover:

- Additional Ontario and Canadian Bona Fide Occupational Requirements (BFOR) protocols and resources (including Canadian Armed Forces, Corrections, Customs, Public and Private Policing and Security)

- Revised *Fit for Duty, Fit for Life* training guide, and aerobic and resistance training programs; all designed specifically to assist meeting BFOR requirements

- Updated physical and mental health issues faced by various law enforcement officers and additional information on PTSD, suicide, nutrition, shift work, and concussions

- Updated Ontario Police Fitness Award Standards.

To accompany the fifth edition, our *Fit for Duty, Fit for Life* training guide provides you with the BFOR protocols for various law enforcement agencies and provides you with ideas for training programs, including pictures to assist you as you create your programs that are suitable for your fitness level. The guidebook provides you with the OPFA standards to use as a guide to determine where you are in terms of fitness training. Included are fitness training logs and scoring sheets to track your progress.

ACKNOWLEDGMENTS

The authors would like to thank the editors who have contributed to reviewing drafts, editing, and offering advice and critiquing our new edition: Lindsay Sutherland, Laura Bast, Katherine Goodes, Lila Campbell, and Lisa Brant. A special thank you to Heather Gough for using her photography skills to add value to our descriptions. We would like to thank the members of PFPO, and Dr. Robert Seguin, of the RCMP, for their continual support in providing research and suggestions to improve the textbook. A special thanks goes out to Tim Finlay for obtaining permission to access his fitness centre and for being our model. The authors and the publisher would like to thank the reviewers of the 4th edition: Julie Rissler, Algonquin; Maria Iannuzziello, Durham; and Jessica McLean, Sherdian.

From Nancy: On a personal note, I would like to thank Janice Pepe, Barb Moore, and Heather White for their input, encouragement, and laughs throughout this entire process. I would especially like to thank Rebecca Finlay for agreeing to take on the task as a new author. I know at times our tasks have seemed daunting, but you have pushed us to produce a relevant and practical updated book that all law enforcement students will benefit from.

From Rebecca: A big thank you to Nancy and the team from Emond for inviting me on board with this book. It has been quite a journey for me from start to finish: mentally, emotionally, and even physically. I could have never imagined what this year would bring to me and my family, and the personal growth that I have had along the way. Thank you for all of your guidance, patience, and support.

Good luck as you begin your journey to an exciting career that will challenge you both mentally and physically.

Be fit and stay healthy.

ABOUT THE AUTHORS

Nancy Wagner Wisotzki's 35-year career has included being a college professor and coordinator for several programs, including Law and Security, Police Foundations, Bachelor of Human Services (Police Studies), Community and Justice Services, and the Pre-Service Firefighter Education and Training Programs, as well as being a qualified appraiser and trainer for PARE, FITCO, PREP, and COPAT protocols. As a Registered Kinesiologist (HBSc Kin), Certified Exercise Physiologist (CSEP), and EIMC-Recognized Exercise Professional Level 2, her focus is on fitness training and Bona Fide Occupational Requirements (BFOR). She has been a member and on the executive of the Police Fitness Personnel of Ontario for over 25 years. Presently, Nancy is a course conductor for the Ontario Police Fitness Pin Appraisers and continues to work part-time at Georgian College teaching, and conducting BFOR appraisals.

Rebecca Finlay received her Bachelor of Science degree in Kinesiology from the University of Waterloo and is a Certified Exercise Physiologist with the Canadian Society of Exercise Physiology. She currently teaches Fitness and Lifestyle Management at Humber College. She has been involved in police, military, and correctional officer fitness training and testing for over 15 years.

PART ❶

GETTING STARTED TOWARD A HEALTHY LIFESTYLE

CHAPTER 1   Are You Fit for Your Career?

CHAPTER 2   Goal Setting

CHAPTER 3   Time Management

ARE YOU FIT FOR YOUR CAREER?

LEARNING OUTCOMES

After completing this chapter, you should be able to:

- Understand the difference between health-related and performance-related fitness.

- Describe the importance of looking after all aspects of your health.

- Review the Bona Fide Occupational Requirements (BFOR) for various law enforcement agencies.

- Identify the Bona Fide Occupational Requirements necessary to meet the minimal requirements of the law enforcement career you have chosen.

- Evaluate the competencies required to apply for a career in law enforcement.

- Understand the physical demands in law enforcement and what requirements organizations expect you to meet in order to be considered for a position.

The 21st century has brought many more demands to a career in law enforcement. Organizations are asking their employees to do more with less and to be prepared to deal with a wide variety of people, circumstances, and accountabilities. It is a job that can be sedentary (for example, sitting in a cruiser, writing out reports), require moderate activity (for example, foot patrol or bike unit), and require maximal effort (for example, apprehending a violent suspect, racing to an emergency). Being fit and mentally prepared helps officers deal with the physical demands of the job.

As a nation with poor nutrition, inactivity, sedentary behaviour, childhood obesity, and declining fitness levels, Canadians have seen the prevalence of obesity nearly triple over the last 25 years: up to 26 percent of young people (2 to 17 years) and one in four adults—roughly 5.3 million people over the age of 18 years—are considered obese (Katzmarzyk, 2008; Public Health Agency of Canada, 2011; Shields, 2006). The First Nations Regional Longitudinal Health Survey (2007) and the Obesity in Canada Snapshot (Public Health Agency of Canada, 2011) reported that off-reserve Indigenous people have an obesity prevalence rate of 25.7 percent compared to on-reserve groups, which have as high as 36 percent, or one in three being obese. As of 2013, less than 20 percent of Canadians meet the minimum guidelines for moderate to vigorous activity per week (Statistics Canada, 2015). This means that, for many Canadians, they are not prepared to take on the physical demands of law enforcement careers.

Most law enforcement officers begin their careers fit and slim. Within 10 to 15 years of service, however, 30 to 40 percent of them become obese and less fit than the general population (Girard, 2013). For many of them, shift work, physical inactivity, nutritional habits, stress, sleep, and commuting are contributing factors. Health conditions like high blood pressure, dyslipidemia (high cholesterol), back pain, and diabetes are also linked to obesity in this population. Helping officers to stay fit and at a healthy weight is a key component of officer and public safety.

Law enforcement students enter college at every level of fitness. Their instructors teach basic concepts in health as well as basic fitness training that will lead students to a lifelong commitment to staying healthy and fit. This basic training includes information on cardiovascular exercise, strength, flexibility, and endurance to help students work toward meeting the fitness requirements laid out by various law enforcement careers. It is up to each individual to decide how to acquire the adequate fitness level to be hired and how to maintain it throughout their life. A negative side of optional and online fitness courses is the number of students who quickly lose interest in maintaining a healthy weight and lifestyle once the course is completed (Basch, 2011). It becomes an issue of extrinsic motivation (surviving fitness) rather than an intrinsic commitment to themselves (keeping active throughout their lives for a personal reason).

HEALTH AND WELLNESS

We continue to see epidemic numbers of Canadians being physically inactive, the rate of obesity rapidly increasing, and the numbers of those suffering from cardiovascular and diabetes growing at alarming rates. In light of this situation, wellness and fitness professionals are well aware that we need to re-evaluate how we entice and encourage others to participate in some kind of activity on a daily basis. Although athleisure clothing is a fashion trend making billions of dollars, it has not assisted in encouraging people into participating in athletic activities. In the past, larger brand names focused on performance and competition. Unfortunately, most people don't see themselves as athletes and so there has been a shift of focus to being active in a more inclusive way. Many facilities have more than workout centres; they are providing meditation spaces, spas, wellness events, and specialty cafés. Wellness is evolving into finding a balance between work and leisure time. As this decade continues to include mindfulness, empathy, exercise, and diet, there will be a shift from the historical "optional" wellness to a "mandatory" wellness, which includes medical research between the brain, skin, and muscles, workplace wellness, ingestibles, and health-tracking nanotechnology.

Many law enforcement services are beginning to see the value of wellness programs. For example, since 2011 the Ottawa Police Service has offered a holistic program that provides activities and support to empower their employees to improve their health and wellness (Ottawa Police Service, 2016). The goal of these programs is to help participants reduce their risk of developing chronic diseases and enjoy a higher quality of life with the unique support of a multi-disciplinary health team. Programs including screening for various cardiovascular diseases, cancer, diabetes, and sleep disorders, providing tools to balance work, family, and personal life, weight-loss programs, as well as stress and anxiety reduction programs. We will look at these topics in later chapters.

A WELLNESS PROFILE

When considering a career in law enforcement, you need to determine how healthy you are and whether you are ready for the demands of shift work, lack of sleep, altercations with individuals, extended periods of inactivity, and being able to respond quickly to critical situations. In this section, you will look at what being healthy may look like.

WHAT DOES HEALTHY LOOK LIKE?

Originally, health was defined as the absence of disease. Many exercise physiologists, kinesiologists, and health educators concluded that this definition was too restrictive. They decided that good health should be defined as wellness and equated with "healthy living." According to the Physical Activity, Fitness, and Health Consensus Statement (Quinney, Gauvine, & Wall, 1994), health has physical, social, and psychological dimensions, each of which lies along a continuum. Positive health is associated with a capacity to enjoy life and to withstand challenges; it is not merely the absence of disease. It moves the definition of health from the mindset based in the management of disease and into areas of prevention and proactive strategies.

Health and wellness are related concepts. Good health means being able to function independently in a constantly changing environment. Wellness can be defined as a way of life in which you make decisions and choices to enjoy the highest level of health and well-being possible. Wellness includes the idea that life is a journey that must be enjoyed and continually fine-tuned in order to benefit as much as possible from all aspects of your life. This means taking the appropriate steps to prevent illness and to lead a richer, more balanced, and satisfying life. By embracing small, positive changes in your lifestyle habits, you empower yourself through self-esteem and self-worth to ensure you have a healthy attitude and lifestyle.

An individual's lifestyle and behaviour clearly affect his or her health. Here is a list of behaviours and habits necessary for wellness:

- taking responsibility for your own health (including research on health issues, regular checkups, and asking questions) and taking an active role in the decisions you make about your life
- learning to manage stress effectively
- maintaining high self-esteem and being able to interact successfully with others
- understanding your sexuality and having satisfying intimate relationships
- developing healthy relationships with spouses, partners, family, friends, and colleagues
- avoiding tobacco and other drugs; using alcohol wisely, if at all
- eating well, exercising, and maintaining a healthy weight
- understanding the Ontario health-care system and the health benefits to which your employment entitles you
- knowing the facts about cardiovascular (heart and blood vessel) disease, diabetes, cancer, sexually transmitted diseases and other infections, and injuries, and using your knowledge to protect yourself against them
- understanding how the environment affects your health and taking appropriate action to protect yourself against environmental hazards
- having a sense of satisfaction with life and appreciating life's different stages
- developing a sense of humour, the ability to express yourself and share feelings, empathy with others, and a tolerance of others' opinions
- achieving a balance in all dimensions of health

THE SEVEN DIMENSIONS OF HEALTH

There are seven dimensions to good health. It is an integrated approach that empowers individuals to make positive choices, focusing away from ideals and specific body types and focusing on healthy eating and participating in physical activity and a variety of exercises to promote overall personal well-being, enhanced quality of life, and better choices in terms of nutrition to maintain a healthy weight. One weak dimension can affect all the others. The seven dimensions of health are as follows:

1. *Physical*—Physical health involves looking after your body as best you can. This means eating properly, exercising, avoiding unhealthy behaviours and substances, making responsible decisions about sex, being aware of the symptoms of disease, having regular checkups, and taking steps to prevent injuries.

2. *Emotional and psychological*—Emotional and psychological health involves maintaining a positive self-concept; dealing constructively with feelings; developing such qualities as optimism, trust, self-confidence, and humour/laughter; and being able to cope with the challenges of daily stressors.

3. *Intellectual*—Intellectual health involves valuing lifelong learning and challenging yourself while searching for answers and solutions. It also involves being able to analyze and evaluate a situation and proposing alternatives or solutions. As well, intellectual health includes self-awareness and learning from life experiences.

4. *Spiritual*—Spiritual health involves searching for meaning and purpose in your life. It also involves coming to terms with what is right and wrong, whether through religion, meditation, art, or some other practice. Spiritual health may involve developing faith in a being or power beyond yourself, as well as the capacity for compassion, altruism, joy, and forgiveness. Research has found that "intrinsic religiosity" plays a role in speedier recovery from depression, anxiety, and illness, and can contribute to a longer life expectancy (Hummer, Rogers, Nam, & Ellison, 1999).

5. *Social and interpersonal*—Social and interpersonal health involves being able to develop meaningful relationships, cultivating a network of supportive friends and family members, and contributing to the community. It also includes valuing diversity—accepting people for who they are. Statistics show that people who are socially isolated are at higher risk of developing illness and even dying (Cacioppo et al., 2002).

6. *Environmental*—Environmental health involves respecting and protecting the environment at the local level and beyond, protecting yourself from environmental hazards, and minimizing the negative impact of your behaviour on the environment.

7. *Occupational*—Occupational health involves deriving satisfaction from the accomplishments and challenges of your job while maintaining a balance between work and the rest of your life. It can also mean contributing through volunteering as experienced professionals, caregivers, mentors, teachers, and volunteers in your community.

WHAT ARE LAW ENFORCEMENT AGENCIES LOOKING FOR?

Law enforcement agencies look for well-rounded healthy individuals to hire. It is crucial when entering a public safety career that you can pass tests in all the different aspects of health. Table 1.1 shows how each of the seven dimensions of health is related to law enforcement, what is required to meet employment requirements, and what will need to be shown to the hiring board.

TABLE 1.1 The Seven Dimensions of Wellness

DIMENSION	REQUIRED TO PASS	WILL NEED TO DEMONSTRATE
Physical	• PAR-Q, blood pressure, and heart rate requirements • fitness test (including job specific and cardiovascular test) • vision and hearing requirements	• proper hygiene • professional appearance • commitment to health and fitness • regular medical checkups
Emotional and Psychological	• a psychological exam	• good self-esteem • being able to control your emotions and self-talk • understanding what causes stress and being able to manage it • knowing when to seek support from friends, family, or professionals
Intellectual	• a general aptitude test (e.g., PATI) • written communication test (e.g., WCT) • a behavioural test (e.g., B-PAD)	• logic • reasoning • problem-solving skills • commitment to lifelong learning
Spiritual	• a comprehensive psychological assessment	• the ability to cope with stress by demonstrating various methods for coping and resiliency
Social and Interpersonal	• a behavioural test (e.g., B-PAD)	• communication and problem-solving techniques • the ability to effectively express oneself
Environmental	• a behavioural test (e.g., B-PAD)	• the ability to make sound and safe judgment calls under varying circumstances • the ability to make safe and sound decisions when faced with critical issues
Occupational	• interviews done by recruiters and employment boards	• the ability to communicate both on a private and public level • the ability to know what the career is about

FITNESS REQUIREMENTS FOR LAW ENFORCEMENT

Students face a great responsibility to meet the fitness requirements of the career they have chosen. Fitness standards now exist for all law enforcement agencies. The onus is not only to pass the Bona Fide Occupational Requirements (BFOR) standards, but to stay fit throughout their careers. Note that being fit is not necessarily the same as meeting the minimum requirements of the various law enforcement agencies' standards. Students who are fit, however, are easily meeting the required standards when they apply for a career in law enforcement

BEING PHYSICALLY ACTIVE

Being physically active plays an important role in the health, well-being, and quality of life of Canadians. People who are physically active live longer, healthier lives. Those that are active are usually more productive, and more likely to avoid illness and injury. A study done by Peter Shipley (2000) found that those OPP officers who were more fit took less sick days.

Physical activity is considered any body movement that works muscles using more than resting energy. It can include free play, structured activities, or activities of daily living. This can include activities like organized sports, walking stairs at work, or doing foot patrol. It includes moderate to vigorous aerobic activities that increase the heart rate and improve cardiovascular endurance, increase muscle/joint range of motion to improve flexibility, high impact weight bearing exercises that promote bone health, and resistance training that improves muscular strength and endurance. In Part 2 of the textbook, we will look at the specifics of fitness training.

Physical fitness is planned, structured, and repetitive physical activity used to condition any part of the body. Physical fitness refers to a physiologic state of well-being that allows one to meet the demands of daily living or that provides the basis for sport performance, physically demanding careers, or all of the above. This can mean anything from playing competitive sports to running after an assailant to confronting an individual who is resisting arrest.

TABLE 1.2 Benefits of Regular Physical Activity and Physical Fitness

- Positive mental aspects (e.g., better academic performance and reduced mental fatigue)
- Prevent or manage cardiovascular and metabolic health (e.g., lower blood pressure, cholesterol levels, insulin levels [diabetes] and waist circumference)
- Reduce the incidence of certain types of cancer (breast and colon)
- Improve or maintain functional health and prevention of falls
- Positive emotional aspects (e.g., improved anxiety and depression symptoms, stress management)
- Positive social health aspects (e.g., improve social skills, self-confidence, self-efficacy)
- Improved sleep
- Reduce and/or control diabetes and cardiovascular disease
- Being prepared to handle disturbances and assaults
- Improved psychological fitness (e.g., stress-buffering, protection against depression and anxiety, increased self-esteem), and behavioural fitness (e.g., good sleep practices, sleep quality)

SOURCES: Basch, 2011; Rasberry et al., 2011; Carson et al., 2013; Carson et al., 2014; Warburton, Katzmarzyk, Rhodes, & Shephard, 2007; McTiernan, 2008; Wolin, Carson, & Colditz, 2010; Janssen & LeBlanc, 2010; Mammen & Faulkner, 2013; Joseph, Royse, Benitez, & Pekmezi, 2014; Gerber, Brand, Holsboer-Trachsler, & Pühse, 2010; van Dijk, Tummers, Stehouwer, Hartgens, & van Loon, 2012; Sheets, 2012; Robson, 2013, p. 23.

COMPONENTS OF FITNESS

Health-related fitness involves aspects of fitness that are linked to a person's health. For example, people who perform weight-bearing exercises in their middle years are less likely to be afflicted with decreasing bone density in their later years. In law enforcement, this may help in a situation where you must physically respond to the demands of a chase or an altercation.

Performance/skill-related fitness is the degree of fitness required to perform a particular job or sport. A person who exercises regularly will likely develop better motor skills (including coordination, agility, speed, and reaction time) and the endurance, muscular strength, and cardiorespiratory power and capacity necessary for peak performance. Law enforcement officers must respond to emergency situations all the time. Impaired speed and reaction time can cost them their lives or the lives of others who depend on them.

Musculoskeletal fitness has been positively associated with functional independence, mobility, glucose homeostasis, bone health, psychological well-being, and overall quality of life. It is negatively associated with the risk of fall, illness, disability, and premature death (Warburton, Gledhill, & Quinney, 2001a, 2001b). It is important then that those involved in law enforcement maintain both the cardio and musculoskeletal components of training to deal with the various situations that they face.

Regular physical activity/fitness should include activities most days of the week, preferably each day. Five or more days of the week should include at least 30 minutes (which can be done in 10-minute increments) of moderate to vigorous intensity activities (Tremblay et al., 2011; CSEP, 2012; Pescatello, Arena, Riebe, & Thompson, 2014). Research has shown a direct relationship between metabolic and cardiorespiratory health and participating in at least 150 minutes of moderate intensity activities per week (Warburton, Charlesworth, Ivey, Nettlefold, & Bredin, 2010). However, if you want to be fitter and excel at the demands of the job, you need to ensure that you are engaging in enough activities at a high enough intensity level that you will see improvements.

IMPORTANCE OF FITNESS IN LAW ENFORCEMENT

When the Bona Fide Occupational Requirements (BFOR) were introduced, there were concerns about the number of women who were not meeting the BFOR's minimum standards. There is a definite learning curve for these machines, but upper-body strength and aerobic conditioning are also important. However, if people are physically motivated, as well as educated about the requirements, they should have no difficulty passing by the time they graduate from their law enforcement program. The keys to success lie in familiarity with the equipment and a commitment to a personal fitness program designed to meet the standards, including a strong aerobic and strength-training program. Today, most students are able to get through the pursuit and restraint component; however, a greater percentage of individuals find it aerobically challenging to meet the various shuttle run requirements for different BFORs and to continue to maintain or improve above that level. It is important that individuals train above the accepted standard in order to achieve the standard on the day of testing.

How can law enforcement officers be convinced to integrate physical fitness into their lives? Simply telling people that physical activity is good for them is not sufficient motivation. There must be some intrinsic or extrinsic motivation for becoming and remaining fit (see the box below). A commitment to lifelong wellness and fitness is an integral part of achieving your career goals.

Ultimately, it is the individual's responsibility to meet competencies in knowledge, skills, and abilities required of their prospective employer. Individuals sometimes self-select into different careers based on their ability or inability to meet the standards in various policing, corrections, customs, and security fields. For many individuals, this was the first exposure to a demanding regime to be mentally and physically fit enough to do a job. Recent evidence has demonstrated convincingly that familiarization opportunities, motivational feedback/coaching during test performance, and participation in a six-week job-specific physical fitness training program can overcome the adverse impact of physiological employment standards on a sub-group of participants, thereby providing "de facto" accommodation (Jamnik, Gumienak, & Gledhill, 2013). It's up to the individual to take advantage of training to meet those standards.

WHAT MOTIVATES YOU TO BE PHYSICALLY ACTIVE?

It will be up to you to determine what will motivate you to become fit and stay fit, in order to meet or exceed the requirements of the career you have chosen and lifestyle you will lead.

There are two general types of motivation. Intrinsic motivation is when you do something because you enjoy it or find it interesting. It comes from within. Examples include:

- Participating in sports because you find it enjoyable.
- Running because you find the challenge fun and exciting.
- Participating in an activity because you want to become more skilled.

Extrinsic motivation is when you do something for external rewards or to avoid negative consequences. Examples include:

- Studying to get a better grade.
- Participating in a sport to win awards.
- Running the BFOR you require for your chosen career to pass your fitness course.

INTRINSIC VERSUS EXTRINSIC MOTIVATION: WHICH IS BEST?

- Intrinsic rewards are great when you already enjoy doing the activity and it is more like play than work. However, they can decrease when completion of a task only requires the minimum work.

- Extrinsic rewards can be used to motivate people to acquire the skill but not to continue the activity. They are not great when you are trying to get people to commit to lifelong fitness.

- Extrinsic rewards can be a source of feedback and reinforcement when a person's performance has achieved a desired standard (for example, meeting the minimum standards of a BFOR assessment).

PREPARING FOR FITNESS
PAR-Q+ / GAQ

The PAR-Q+, ePARmed-X+, and Get Active Questionnaire (GAQ) were developed to enhance the risk stratification process and reduce the barriers to becoming more physically active for all individuals. The health benefits of regular physical activity are clear; more people should engage in physical activity every day of the week. Participating in physical activity is very safe for MOST people. However, some should check with their doctor, another health-care practitioner who is licensed to diagnose, or a qualified exercise professional before they start becoming much more physically active. The PAR-Q+ and GAQ questionnaires will tell you whether it is necessary for you to seek further advice before becoming more physically active or engaging in a fitness appraisal. Go to http://eparmedx.com/?page_id=79 to complete the PAR-Q+ Physical Activity Readiness Questionnaire for Everyone and fill out the ePARmed-X+ Physician Clearance Form if necessary. Go to http://www.csep.ca/en/publications/get-active-questionnaire to complete the GAQ and access the Reference Document if necessary.

PERSONAL PERSPECTIVE

PETE TUCKER

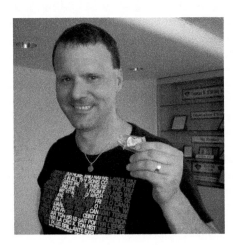

Pete Tucker is a constable with the OPP and was a long-time member of the OPP Golden Helmets precision motorcycle team. In June of 2014, the OPP Golden Helmets were conducting a VIP escort training exercise in preparation for the upcoming Pan Am Games. The group was travelling southbound on Highway 11, just north of Barrie, when a Canada goose flew up from a marsh and struck Constable Pete Tucker in the head while he was driving his police Harley-Davidson. This impact knocked Pete out and rendered him incapable of controlling his bike. His bike veered toward the centre median, where the bike struck the centre box beam.

Pete's left leg got tangled up in the box beam, severing it. Members of the team were able to save Pete's life by applying a tourniquet to stop the bleeding. Gord Keen was the first OPP unit (other than those involved in the training exercise) to arrive on scene. He had never met Pete Tucker prior to that day. Pete was transported to hospital in Toronto in critical condition. After an extended hospital stay and extensive rehabilitation, Pete was able to return home. He continued in rehab and worked vigorously to maintain his fitness.

In June of 2015, the Golden Helmets had arranged to hold their annual requalifications at OPP General Headquarters in Orillia. Gord Keen was asked to conduct their fitness pin testing and was advised that Pete Tucker would be attending with the team and that he wanted to attempt the fitness test. Not only was this a great opportunity for Gord to finally meet Pete, it was an opportunity to promote the fitness pin program, showing others that anything is possible. Fitted with a "high tech" prosthetic leg, Pete completed the Astrand Cycle Test and, almost exactly one year to the day following his life changing collision, Pete attempted and successfully passed his fitness pin test with other members of the Golden Helmets.

Although Pete can no longer ride with the Golden Helmets team, he now participates in their shows as the announcer and is proud to wear his Ontario Police Fitness Award pin.

Story shared by Gord Keen.

INFORMED CONSENT FOR FITNESS TESTING

Part of the requirement prior to testing for law enforcement services is to ensure that you are medically safe to do the testing. By completing the Physical Activity Readiness Questionnaire for Everyone (PAR-Q+), you will assure the assessor that you are physically able to do the test without limitations. Informed consent takes that process one step further in addressing due diligence to ensure that you know about the test protocols and are aware of the stress that they may put you under. Informed consent also ensures that you have followed appropriate guidelines to affirm that you are able to perform the tasks safely.

PHYSICAL FITNESS LOG

As part of your physical fitness training goals, you should chart your progress throughout the course of your study. Depending on the college and semester you are in, you will have certain standards to meet. By charting your results, you will know where you stand and the areas that you should address each semester. Ultimately, it is your responsibility to know where you stand with your goals.

To record the results of your running and workouts over time, see the running and daily workout logs in the *Fit for Duty, Fit for Life* training guide that accompanies this textbook. If you want, you can print off the log so that you can use it in your fitness class and weight room workouts.

PHYSICAL TESTING WITHIN LAW ENFORCEMENT
HISTORY BEHIND FITNESS TESTING AND BFOR PROTOCOLS FOR LAW ENFORCEMENT

In Canada, pre-employment fitness screening can be mandated for physically demanding public safety occupations in which "ineffective or inefficient job performance is a threat to the safety of self, co-workers, the public or property" (*Employment Equity Act*, 1995; Supreme Court of Canada, 1999; *Criminal Code*, 1985; *Canadian Charter of Rights and Freedoms*, 1982; Canadian Human Rights Commission, 2007). As a result, job-specific physical fitness protocols (JSPFPs) have been constructed to satisfy the legal obligations to qualify as a bona fide occupational requirement (BFOR) for physically demanding public safety occupations. This means that police, corrections, military, and security agencies can make a fitness screening an integral part of the hiring process (Jamnik et al., 2013). The focus of a BFOR is to determine if the applicant or incumbent has the necessary physical capabilities to safely and efficiently perform the critical on-the-job tasks encountered in a physically demanding occupation (Gumieniak, Jamnik, & Gledhill, 2013). It ensures that individuals have the necessary attributes to efficiently and safely perform the job tasks that are most important and those that are the most frequently physically required.

 FACTS TO THINK ABOUT

BONA FIDE OCCUPATIONAL REQUIREMENTS (BFORs)

A BFOR for a physically demanding job must meet the following criteria:
- Have a purpose or goal that is rationally connected to performing the job
- Be adopted in good faith, with the belief that it was necessary to fulfill a legitimate work-related purpose
- Be reasonably necessary to accomplish the work-related purpose and not cause undue hardship on the employer. Thus, services have designed employment standards that meet the physical demands of the job and qualify as a bona fide occupational requirement.

Table 1.3 provides a summary of the fitness and BFOR timelines for Canada.

TABLE 1.3 Timeline of Major BFORs in Canada

TIMELINE	EVENTS
1970	• Many police services based hiring on height and weight criteria • Fitness tests at Ontario Police College (OPC) based on fitness levels of the general Canadian population (excluding stats for women and minorities)
1980	• OPC develops fitness standards based on the Canada Fitness Test • 1986—Farenholtz and Rhodes develop the first BFOR Peace Officer's Physical Ability Test (POPAT) in British Columbia • 1987—OPC develop fitness standards based on Canadian Society of Exercise Science to create the Ontario Police Fitness Award (OPFA) program and the creation of the Police Fitness Personnel Ontario (PFPO) • 1989—Bonneau develops PARE (Physical Readiness Evaluation for Police) after POPAT study demonstrates 65% failure rate for females (Bonneau, 1994)
1990	• 1991—RCMP start using the PARE for recruiting process • 1995—Canadian Employment Equity Act and 1999 Supreme Court of Canada deem pre-employment fitness screening can be mandated for physically demanding public safety occupations (followed up the Criminal Code of Canada [2004], Canadian Charter of Rights and Freedoms [2007], and the Canadian Human Rights Commission [2007]) • 1999—Based on the Meiorin decision, the Supreme Court of Canada provides a framework for BFOR standards for testing. These standards had to be rationally connected to the job, reasonably necessary to accomplish the job without undue hardship upon the employer, and reasonably necessary for the safe and efficient performance of the job. • 1999—PREP (Physical Readiness Evaluation for Police in Ontario) was commissioned by the OACP
2000	• 2001—Anderson, Plecas, and Segger (2001) revalidates PARE test and core movements • 2002—Corrections Canada adopts the Correctional Officers Physical Abilities Test (COPAT) • 2005—Following an investigation by the Canadian Human Rights Commission, COPAT is eliminated nationally as a barrier to employability for women, Indigenous persons, and members of visible and other minorities. It is then updated and used by Alberta, British Columbia, Nova Scotia, Prince Edward Island, and Yukon. • 2009—Alberta develops A-PREP (Alberta's Physical Readiness Evaluation for Policing)
2010	• 2010—Ontario Corrections develops FITCO (Fitness Test for Correctional Officers) • 2012—PREP is reassessed and updated • 2015—Canadian Border Security Agency adopts PARE as their BFOR • 2016—RCMP moves PARE testing into recruit training and out of recruiting • 2017—PFPO celebrate 30 years of the Ontario Police Fitness Award program

SOURCES: Anderson & Plecas, 2008; Eid, 2001; Farenholtz & Rhodes, 1986; Jamnik, Gumienak, & Gledhill, 2013; Jamnik, Thomas, Shaw, & Gledhill, 2010; Ministry of Community Safety and Correctional Services, 2014; Ministry of Community Safety and Correctional Services, 2016; OACP, 2016; PFPO, 2017; RCMP, 2005, updated 2011; RCMP, 2013; Reilly, 2013.

THE ONTARIO POLICE FITNESS AWARD (OPFA)

The Ontario Police Fitness Award (OPFA) is a provincial incentive program developed to motivate Ontario police officers and police service employees to remain physically fit throughout their entire careers. The OPFA program is sanctioned by the policing services division of the Ministry of the Solicitor General and the Ontario Association of Chiefs of Police. The testing includes: push-ups, core endurance (modified back extension), sit and reach, and the 1.5-mile run or the shuttle run. The OPFA program is designed and implemented by the Police Fitness Personnel of Ontario (PFPO) executive and delivered through its membership throughout Ontario. The OPFA, developed in the 1980s, is used to assess the fitness level of police officers. The standard of comparison is the general population of Canada. Whereas BFOR standards are for assessing one's physical readiness for the job, the OPFA fitness standards are for assessing one's general fitness level. Those individuals who achieve a 75 percent grade are awarded the OPFA pin. It is exciting to note that there were seven officers who received their 30-year pin in 2017. This is a true testament to those who have valued fitness throughout their careers.

FIGURE 1.1 OPP Auxiliary Officers Earn Their Ontario Police Fitness Award Pin

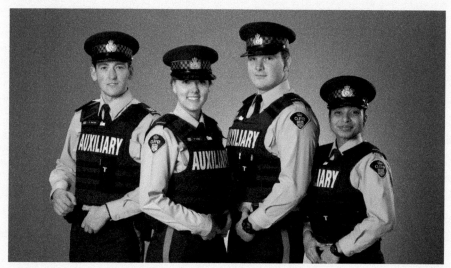

Over a three-year period (March 1996 to March 1999), Mr. Peter Shipley, Physiological Health Science Coordinator at the Provincial Police Academy, conducted a cost–benefit analysis within the Ontario Provincial Police (Shipley, 2000). His research indicated that OPP officers who had earned their five-year OPFA pin used, on average, 4.24 less sick days per year than the average OPP officer. With all these benefits in mind, it is felt that police services should be concerned about their officers' physical fitness levels, not just during the initial hiring phase but throughout their careers. The Ontario Police Fitness Award program was designed to assist police services in monitoring and motivating their officers' physical health.

In the Appendix, you will find testing protocols for the OPFA as well as standards for various Canadian BFORs. Many services use the OPFA standards as benchmarks in hiring of cadets, special constables, recruit training, and promotions. Since the inception of the OPFA pin program, corrections, private police services (for example, Bruce Nuclear, Ontario Power [Pickering Station]), Ministry of Natural Resources, and various emergency response teams have used the pin standards for their own awards.

WHAT ARE THE IMPORTANT, PHYSICALLY DEMANDING, AND FREQUENTLY OCCURRING TASKS IN LAW ENFORCEMENT?

Table 1.4 summarizes the quantitative and qualitative tasks required to do various jobs in law enforcement. From these tasks, BFORs are created.

TABLE 1.4 The Tasks That Are Used to Create a BFOR

BFOR TEST	QUALITATIVE AND QUANTITATIVE TASKS THAT WERE DEEMED NECESSARY
Physical Readiness Evaluation for Policing (PREP) (Ministry of Community Safety and Correctional Services, 2015)	While wearing restrictive vest, belt, and equipment: 1. Pursue a suspect on foot, running a short distance (50–100 m) while negotiating obstacles to apprehend a resisting suspect. 2. Separate, restrain, and remove a disorderly and/or mentally ill person(s) from others at the scene of a disturbance to a vehicle. 3. Conduct an extended search, first aid or CPR, and removal of a missing person in a rural setting. 4. Stand in a static line for an extended period of time (2–4 hours) with the ability to separate, restrain, and remove disorderly persons.
Physical Abilities Readiness Evaluation (PARE) (Bonneau, 2001; Anderson & Plecas, 2007)	Bonneau (2001) reported 11 core movements in the RCMP task analysis including: 1. walking, 2. running, 3. climbing and descending stairs or hills, 4. jumping, 5. vaulting, 6. lifting, 7. carrying, 8. pushing, 9. pulling, 10. dragging, and 11. balancing.
Fitness Test for Ontario Correctional Officers (FITCO) (Jamnik, Thomas, Shaw, & Gladhill, 2010)	While wearing soft body armour and equipment belt: • Relocate and respond to a fight or riot using force to restrain offenders on arrival (separate, control, apply restraints). • Act as a first responder to a partner CO being attacked by inmate. • Control and apply restraints on an inmate who shows aggression toward the CO. • Separate and restrain two or more inmates fighting in the washroom, recreation, cell, or common day areas (intervene, control, and apply restraints). • Conduct strip search of a non-compliant inmate. • Use force to put a non-compliant inmate in restraints (take-down, hand restraints, leg irons, and restraint belt). • Put a non-compliant inmate in restraints into and out of a vehicle, in or out of a cell, or through Admitting and Discharge. • Lift, carry, or transfer a non-compliant inmate (>55 kg) in full restraints from living unit to segregation. • Conduct the search of a cell or living unit looking for contraband or a missing utensil taking up to 10 minutes (enter cell, physically handle all cell items by lifting, shaking, or moving, and examine all surfaces).

WHICH SERVICES ARE USING THESE VARIOUS BFOR TESTS?

From various task analyses like the ones above, the following BFOR tests were created (see Table 1.5). You can determine which test(s) you may want to train for in order to meet the requirements for that service.

TABLE 1.5 BFORs and the Services That Are Using Them

BFOR	WHO IS USING THE TEST	ADDITIONAL INFORMATION
PREP Physical Readiness Evaluation for Policing (PREP), which the Ontario Association of Police Chiefs created as a test for all Ontario police officers	As of 2019, you will have to check each service regarding their Requirements for Fitness. Some will continue to use the PREP while others (like the OPP) have chosen a different requirement. In some Ontario police services. CP Police Service*	Go to http://www.applicanttesting .com/images/stories/pdf/ FittoServe2015Final.pdf for more information on the PREP To see the PREP test, go to https://www.youtube.com/ watch?v=zWBPodHpieQ *CP Police Service requires all candidates to complete either the PARE, PREP, or POPAT
Police Fitness Personnel of Ontario (PFPO) **Ontario Police Fitness Award (OPFA) Standards** Known as the FIT Pin	Ontario Provincial Police (OPP) Individuals must pass the FIT Pin at 75 percent during the first week of training.	Go to https://www.opp.ca/index.ph p?id=115&entryid=56b7c5868f94ac af5c28d17d for more information regarding qualifications and the PFPO Website for explanations and scoring matrix go to http://www. pfpo.org
PARE The Physical Ability Requirement Evaluation (for Policing) (PARE) was designed from research derived from the POPAT	Royal Canadian Mounted Police (RCMP) The RCMP protects all Canadians by enforcing federal, provincial, First Nations, and municipal laws. They have detachments in every province and territory. The PARE is tested on RCMP candidates within two weeks of arrival at depot training.	Go to http://www.rcmp-grc.gc.ca/ en/prepare-for-pare for information on the PARE and the RCMP 12-week training program To see a PARE demonstration, go to http://www.rcmp-grc.gc.ca/en/ pare-demonstration
	Federal, provincial, First Nations, and municipal law enforcement in the provinces/territories of: Prince Edward Island (*6)—e.g., Souris Police Service, Montoague Nova Scotia (*53)—e.g., Halifax Police Service New Brunswick (*44)—e.g., Fredericton Police Service Newfoundland and Labrador (*22)—e.g., Royal Newfoundland Constabulary Quebec (*14)—only does federal enforcement Ontario (*16)—only does federal enforcement Manitoba (*88)—e.g., Little Grande Rapids, Brandon Saskatchewan (*113)—e.g., Swift Current, Moose Jaw Alberta (*116)—e.g., Grande Prairie, Lloydminster, Red Deer, Medicine Hat British Columbia (*151)—e.g., Kelowna, Prince George Nunavut (*26)—e.g., Artic Bay Northwest Territories (*22)—e.g., Fort Resolution, Yellowknife Yukon (*14)—e.g., Dawson Creek, Whitehorse Municipal services in the eastern provinces of Canada—e.g., Charlottetown, Halifax, Fredericton, Moncton, St. John's, St. John, Truro **Specialized Services** Canada Border Services Agency Alberta Sheriffs Alberta Parks Service	PARE (Reference: Find a Detachment at http://www.rcmp-grc.gc.ca/detach/en/d) *designates the number of detachments/services in that province that use **CP Police Service requires all candidates to complete either the PARE, PREP, or POPAT

BFOR	WHO IS USING THE TEST	ADDITIONAL INFORMATION
	Alberta Fish and Wildlife BC Conservation Officers Canada Parks Service Saskatchewan NAIT Protective Services and Special Constables/Community Safety UN Missions CP Police Service** Provincial Corrections in New Brunswick and Newfoundland & Labrador	
A-PREP The Alberta Physical Abilities Requirement (A-PREP) was designed to reflect the job requirements of police officers in the province of Alberta	Used by larger municipal services in the province of Alberta such as Calgary, Edmonton, Lethbridge, Lakeshore Regional, and Camrose.	Go to the Fit to Serve brochure at http://www.calgary.ca/cps/Documents/application-forms/fit-to-serve.pdf?noredirect=1 for more information on the A-PREP
POPAT The Police Officer Physical Abilities Test (POPAT), originally designed for use by the Justice Institute of British Columbia in conjunction with the University of British Columbia	In British Columbia, municipal police services including Abbotsford, Central Saanich, Delta, Vancouver, New Westminster, Nelson, Oak Bay, Port Moody, Saanich, Stl'atl'imx, Vancouver, West Vancouver, and Victoria. BC Sheriffs Service BC Corrections South Coast British Columbia Transportation—Transit Police In Saskatchewan, municipal police services such as Regina, Saskatoon, Moose Jaw, Prince Albert, Estevan, Weyburn, and File Hills. In Manitoba, some municipalities such as Brandon Police Service. Manitoba Conservation Officers CP Police Service*	Go to https://deltapolice.ca/peace-officers-physical-abilities-test-popat for more information on the POPAT and http://www.jibc.ca/programs-courses/schools-departments/school-criminal-justice-security/police-academy/resources/municipal-police-departments for recruiting information *CP Police Service requires all candidates to complete either the PARE, PREP, or POPAT
SPAT-ENPQ SPAT-ENPQ was developed by the University of Montreal to reflect the minimum physical requirements of police officers in the province of Quebec	All Quebec municipal police services, the Sûreté du Québec (SQ)—provincial police, the SPVM (Montreal Police Service), the Groupe tactique d'intervention (GTI)—emergency response team, and CN police inspectors of the STM (Montreal Transit Corporation).	Go to https://bit.ly/2liajNT for more information on the SPAT-ENPQ
WPS-PAT Winnipeg Police Service Physical Abilities Test (WPS-PAT) was designed to reflect the physical demands of the Winnipeg Police Service	Winnipeg Police Service	Go to http://www.winnipeg.ca/police/policerecruiting/officer/physical.aspx for more information on the WPS-PAT
FITCO The Fitness Test for Ontario Corrections Officers (FITCO) was developed by the Ministry of Community Safety and Correctional Services	Ontario Correctional Officer Applicants	Go to http://www.mcscs.jus.gov.on.ca/english/corr_serv/careers_in_corr/become_corr_off/FITCO/cs_FITCO.html for more information on the FITCO

BFOR	WHO IS USING THE TEST	ADDITIONAL INFORMATION
COPAT The Corrections Officers' Physical Abilities Test (COPAT) established by Corrections Canada	Prince Edward Island, Nova Scotia, British Columbia, Saskatchewan, and Yukon Correctional Officers Government of Alberta Enforcement Branches, including Alberta Sheriffs Branch, Alberta Fish and Wildlife Enforcement Branch, Commercial Vehicle Enforcement Branch, and the Alberta Parks Enforcement Branch.	For more information, go to https://www.solgps.alberta.ca/careers/Publications/COPAT%20Requirements.pdf The Appendix provides specifics on the different times required based on the specific service that you are applying to.
MPFS The Minimum Physical Fitness Standard (MPFS) designed by the Canadian Armed Forces as part of FORCE EXPRESS Evaluation	The Minimum Physical Fitness Standard (MPFS) was developed for all military personnel, regardless of trade, classification, age, or gender. Some unique CF occupations have specific job requirements, which demand a higher level of physical fitness than the MPFS; therefore, the Environmental, Military Occupation, and Operational Deployment Standards were developed.	For more information go to https://www.cafconnection.ca/National/Programs-Services/For-Military-Personnel/Military-Fitness/FORCE-Program/Frequently-Asked-Questions/FORCE-Evaluation-FAQs.aspx
CNSFT Canadian Nuclear Security Fitness Test	Used by Canadian National Nuclear Security Officers.	For more information, go to http://nuclearsafety.gc.ca/eng/resources/research/technical-papers-and-articles/2018/fitness-for-duty-nuclear-security.cfm and http://www.nuclearsafety.gc.ca/pubs_catalogue/uploads/REGDOC-2-2-4-Fitness-for-Duty-Vol-III-Nuclear-Security-Officer-Medical-eng.pdf for the fitness protocol

LAW ENFORCEMENT HIRING INFORMATION

The remaining information is about what the services are looking for in potential candidates and the hiring processes. Ultimately, is up to you to meet those requirements. It may take you a couple of years to develop skill sets that services are looking for. Researching them now will give you a direction to follow. In Chapter 2, you may decide that pursuing one of these careers should be added to your goal setting. The one thing that you have total control over is your fitness level. Make sure that you don't let that slide as you work toward realizing your goals.

ESSENTIAL AND DEVELOPMENTAL COMPETENCIES

Competencies are not about duties, they are about people. Competencies focus on the characteristics of people who will be successful performing their job. While developmental competencies can be learnt on the job, services are also looking for essential competencies—the knowledge, skills, and attitudes necessary to make individuals successful and productive in their job.

ESSENTIAL COMPETENCIES

Law enforcement essential competencies are knowledge, skills, and abilities that are being assessed during the entire selection process; they must be demonstrated for the applicant to be considered for the position. The following list of eight competencies have been identified as essential:

1. *Analytical Thinking* The ability to analyze situations and events in a logical way, and to organize the parts of a problem in a systematic way.

2. *Self Confidence* A belief in your own abilities and judgments, and a recognition of personal limitations and development needs.

3. *Communication* The ability to demonstrate effective listening, verbal, and written communication skills.

4. *Flexibility/Valuing Diversity* The ability to adapt your approach in a variety of situations, and to work effectively with a wide cross-section of the community representing diverse backgrounds, cultures, and socio-economic circumstances.

5. *Self-Control* The ability to keep your own emotions under control and to restrain negative actions when provoked or when working under stressful conditions.

6. *Relationship Building* The ability to develop and maintain a network of contacts, both inside and outside the law enforcement service.

7. *Achievement Orientation* The desire for continuous improvement in service or accomplishments.

8. *Medical/Physical Skills and Abilities* Job-related medical/physical skills and abilities, including vision, hearing, motor skills, cardiovascular endurance, and upper-body strength. (OACP, 2016)

DEVELOPMENTAL COMPETENCIES

As the name implies, law enforcement developmental competencies can be acquired through training after a person has been hired as a law enforcement officer. However, some law enforcement services may have an immediate need for specific developmental skills and abilities, and may choose to include these in the hiring process. The following list of 11 competencies have been identified as developmental:

1. *Information Seeking* The ability to seek out information from various sources before making decisions.

2. *Concern for Safety* The ability to exercise caution in hazardous situations in order to ensure safety to self and others.

3. *Assertiveness* The ability to use authority confidently and to set and enforce rules appropriately.

4. *Initiative* Demonstrated ability to be self-motivated and self-directed in identifying and addressing important issues.

5. *Cooperation* The ability to collaborate with others by seeking their input, encouraging their participation, and sharing information.

6. *Negotiation/Facilitation* The ability to influence or persuade others by anticipating and addressing their interests and perspectives.

7. *Work Organization* The ability to develop and maintain systems for organizing information and activities.

8. *Community-Service Orientation* Proven commitment to helping or serving others.

9. *Commitment to Learning* Demonstrated pattern of activities, which contribute to personal and professional growth.

10. *Organizational Awareness* Understanding of the dynamics of organizations, including the formal and informal cultures and decision-making processes.

11. *Developing Others* Commitment to helping others improve their skills.

LAW ENFORCEMENT SELECTION PROCESSES

Take time to do extensive research to know what the service wants and ensure you have the skills that they are looking for. Below is specific information regarding various law enforcement selection processes:

ONTARIO POLICE SELECTION PROCESS

As part of the police selection process you are required to fill out an Applicant Registration form and go through a pre-interview assessment where you are required to:

1. Complete an *aptitude test* (PATI) designed to measure:

   a. Deductive Reasoning: The ability to draw appropriate conclusions from information provided. This is tested through the Syllogism and Travel Time tasks.

   b. Inductive Reasoning: The ability to identify trends or common characteristics in a series of objects or information presented. This is tested through the Classification and Series completion tasks.

   c. Quantitative Reasoning: The ability to apply basic arithmetic operations like addition, subtraction, multiplication, division, and fractions to solve Word problems and Arithmetic tasks.

2. Complete a *written communication test* (WCT) after reading a scenario and organizing important facts to reconstruct what happened in a clear, coherent, and comprehensive manner.

3. Engage in a *medical/physical skills and abilities test*. Specific standards are outlined below:

   a. PAR-Q+ and blood pressure requirements.

   b. Physical Fitness: Pass all components of BFOR standards—PREP test, including completing a pursuit/restraint circuit in 157 seconds or less and running to stage 7.0 on the 20-m Leger Shuttle Run (information regarding protocol is found in the Appendix).

c. Vision: Uncorrected visual acuity should be at least 6/12 (20/40) binocularly (both eyes open). Corrected visual acuity should at least be 6/6 (20/20) binocularly. There are additional minimum requirements regarding refractive surgery farsightedness (hyperopia), colour vision, depth perception, and peripheral vision.

d. Hearing Standards: Normal hearing at frequencies of 500 to 4000 Hz measured by an audiometer.

4. Complete a *behavioural personnel assessment device* (B-PAD) where you will view video-based simulations and you must respond appropriately.

If you are successful with your pre-interview assessment, you can apply to any police agency that is hiring. The service would then contact you to complete a pre-background questionnaire and come in to

a. be interviewed

b. complete a psychological test, and be interviewed by a psychologist

c. If successful in both, you may be called in for an in-depth interview/review and, conditional on a background check and a medical clearance, you may be offered a job.

For more information on the Ontario constable selection process and the Certificate of Results (COR), go to http://www.applicanttesting.com/career-paths/police-constable/testing-information.html.

For medical requirements for candidates, go to http://www.mcscs.jus.gov.on.ca/english/police_serv/const_select_sys/Self-Assess-MedicalRequirementsfor Candidates/Self_Assess.html. For an example of a Self-Assessment Medical Questionnaire, go to https://www.opp.ca/index.php?&lng=en&id=115&entryid=56b7c0938f94ace65c28d17c.

For other provinces, go to the service you are interested in and see their specific requirements (many are similar to the Ontario process but have a different BFOR requirement (information regarding protocol is found in the Appendix)).

RCMP SELECTION PROCESS

For the RCMP, you are required to:

1. Complete an online application.

2. Write the RCMP Entrance Exam.

3. Complete forms including driving record, fingerprinting, education documentation, etc.

4. Complete the Pre-Employment Polygraph exam.

5. Successfully pass a medical and psychological exam.

6. Pass a field investigation and security clearance.

In addition to meeting these basic requirements, individuals must successfully complete the Cadet Training Program, which includes passing the RCMP's BFOR PARE (information regarding protocol is found in the Appendix). For more information regarding the RCMP hiring process, refer to the RCMP How to Apply website at http://www.rcmp-grc.gc.ca/en/how-to-apply.

ONTARIO CORRECTIONAL SERVICES SELECTION PROCESS

In Ontario Corrections, the following are the basic requirements for becoming a correctional service officer:

1. Meet the basic requirements (age, eligibility to work in Canada, education, First Aid and AED requirements).

2. Successful completion of the Fitness Test for Ontario Correctional Officer Applicants (FITCO) (information regarding protocol is found in the Appendix).

3. Successful completion of the Correctional Officer Enhanced Security Clearance process.

4. Successful completion of the correctional officer pre-employment medical exam.

5. Successful completion of Correctional Officer Training and Assessment (COTA) program.

For more information, refer to Careers at Ministry of Community Safety & Correctional Services at http://www.mcscs.jus.gov.on.ca/english/corr_serv/careers_in_corr/become_corr_off/careers_corr_become_off.html.

FEDERAL CORRECTIONS SELECTION PROCESS

For Canadian Federal Corrections, the following are the basic requirements for becoming a federal correctional officer:

1. Apply online.

2. Meet the basic requirements of screening (citizenship, education, experience).

3. Successfully meet the Enhanced Suitability Screening based on suitability, honesty, integrity, and ethics.

4. Successfully pass the written exams (reasoning and problem solving, and communications skills).

5. Successfully pass the interview and reference check.

6. Successfully pass the psychological assessment.

7. Successfully pass the Correctional Training Program.

For Federal Corrections, refer to Before You Apply, Application Process, and Training and Appointment at Correctional Services Canada at http://www.csc-scc.gc.ca/careers/003001-3001-eng.shtml.

In Alberta, British Columbia, and Nova Scotia, they are using the COPAT BFOR. For more information regarding the COPAT test, go to http://www2.gov.bc.ca/gov/content/careers-myhr/job-seekers/featured-careers/bc-corrections/apply.

CANADA BORDER SERVICES AGENCY PROCESS

The application and selection process to become a border services officer trainee involves ten steps:

1. Meet basic requirements (including successful completion of the Canadian Firearms Safety Course [CFSC] and the Canadian Restricted Firearms Safety Course [CRFSC]).

2. Apply online.

3. Write required standardized tests (recognized university and college graduates are no longer required to write the two standardized tests).

4. Complete Second Language Evaluation, if required.

5. Participate in an interview.

6. Meet the physical abilities standard—PARE BFOR.

7. Secret security clearance and personnel security screening.

8. Meet and maintain psychological requirements.

9. Undergo a medical exam.

10. Meet and maintain all conditions of employment.

For more information, go the CBSA website at http://www.cbsa-asfc.gc.ca/job-emploi/bso-asf/req-exig-eng.html.

NATIONAL DEFENCE AND CANADIAN ARMED FORCES

As a member of the Forces you can choose to work full-time in the Regular Force or part-time in the Reserve Force. You also have the option of becoming an officer or a non-commissioned member (NCM), depending on the job you choose.

Officers are trained to be leaders in the Forces and are responsible for the soldiers, sailors, air men, and air women in their command. To become an officer, you will need a university education and leadership training.

Non-commissioned members (NCMs) are skilled personnel who provide operational and support services in the Forces. Some NCMs are trained as operators or technicians, while others may work in the administrative or health services fields. To find out more about the various careers and the specific requirements for the jobs go to http://www.forces.ca/en/page/careeroptions-123.

For more information on the FORCE Evaluation fitness test to assess your level of physical fitness, go to http://www.forces.ca/en/page/training-90.

SPECIAL CONSTABLES

Police special constables, court security, prisoner transport, Special Constable for Queen's Park, TTC, GO Transit, YRT/VIVA Special Constable, and Toronto parking enforcement officers must meet specific requirements. The process to apply for one of these careers involves a series of four or five tests including:

1. General Aptitude Test Battery (GATB) (not used by all).

2. Written Process Test (WPT).

3. The physical test which includes OPFA standards on push-ups, flexibility, back extension (core endurance), and shuttle run. Actual fitness requirements and standards can be found in the Appendix.

4. Vision Screening.

5. Hearing Screening.

For more information, go to Applicant Testing Service (ATS) at http://www.applicanttesting.com/career-paths.html.

For university campus police, the applicant must obtain the COR Certificate from ATS with the PREP as their physical test.

For examples of requirements and hiring processes, see Windsor University Campus Police at http://www1.uwindsor.ca/campuspolice/recruiting-information, University of Waterloo at http://www.hr.uwaterloo.ca/.jd/00001136.html, or University of Western Ontario at http://www.uwo.ca/police/about/recruitment .html.

CANADIAN NUCLEAR SECURITY

Similar to a police constable process, the applicant must complete the following:

1. Written test.
2. Job-specific fitness test.
3. Interview.
4. Psychological assessment.
5. Background check.
6. Level II security clearance check.

For more information about the nuclear security officer fitness requirements, go to http://mypowercareer.com/career-profiles/security/.

SECURITY GUARDS AND PRIVATE INVESTIGATORS

In order to apply to a company, an individual must have their Security Guard and/or Private Investigator's Security Licence (under the Private Security and Investigative Services Act [Ontario Government, 2005], mandated in 2010).

Most application processes involve:

1. Written test—general aptitude/security knowledge.
2. Interview—security knowledge/behavioural based.
3. Background check.
4. Depending on the company, they may require a physical component (for example, Canadian Nuclear Security). (Holden, C., Director of Security, Royal Victoria Hospital, personal communication, November 2, 2016)

For more information, go to http://www.mcscs.jus.gov.on.ca/english/PSIS/ ApplyforaLicence/PSIS_apply.html.

Refer to assignment 1.1, available at www.emond.ca/fitness5e, under the "Assignments" tab. This assignment is designed to self-assess whether you have the medical/visual standards and basic skills/expectations required to apply for a job in law enforcement. Ensure that you have completed the PAR-Q+ and informed consent form (found in the Appendix) and returned them to your instructor.

A FINAL THOUGHT

Most students in their late teens or early twenties do not have enough experience and life skills for services to hire them. Remember that it may take three to five years to earn the opportunity for an interview. Don't be discouraged and remember that what you do and the contributions you make to society matter. It is important that you don't let your fitness level depreciate and that you keep honing your skills in order to achieve the goals that you set for yourself.

KEY TERMS

aerobic conditioning
an exercise program that incorporates activities that are rhythmic in nature, using large muscle groups at moderate intensities for four to seven days per week

Bona Fide Occupational Requirement (BFOR)
pre-employment fitness screening based on the quantitative (most frequent) and qualitative (most important) physical demands of the job

extrinsic motivation
motivation to perform a task or goal based on external rewards to avoid negative consequences

health
the ability of an individual to function independently in a constantly changing environment

health-related fitness
the components of physical fitness that are related to health status, including cardiovascular fitness, musculoskeletal fitness, body composition, and metabolism

informed consent
a legal document that ensures that you know about the test protocols and are aware of the stress that they may put you under while ensuring that you have followed appropriate guidelines to affirm that you are able to perform the tasks safely

intrinsic motivation
motivation to perform a task or goal based on enjoyment of doing the task itself

law enforcement developmental competencies
competencies that can be acquired through training after a person has been hired as a law enforcement officer

law enforcement essential competencies
knowledge, skills, and abilities that are being assessed during the entire selection process; they must be demonstrated to be considered for the position

musculoskeletal fitness
a combined measure of muscular strength, flexibility, and muscular endurance to provide a measure of health

Ontario Police Fitness Award (OPFA)
a provincial incentive program developed to motivate Ontario police officers and police service employees to remain physically fit throughout their entire careers

PAR-Q+
the Physical Activity Readiness Questionnaire for Everyone (PAR-Q+), developed to enhance the risk stratification process and reduce the barriers to becoming more physically active for all individuals

performance/skill-related fitness
the degree of fitness required to perform a particular job or sport

physical activity
all leisure and non-leisure body movement that results in an expenditure of energy

physical fitness
the ability to carry out daily tasks with alertness and vigour, without undue fatigue, and with enough reserve to meet emergencies or to enjoy leisure time pursuits (Maud & Foster, 2006)

seven dimensions of health
an integrated approach that empowers individuals to make positive choices focusing away from ideals and specific body types and focusing on healthy eating and participating in physical activity and a variety of exercises to promote overall personal well-being, enhanced quality of life, and better choices in terms of nutrition to maintain a healthy weight

wellness
a way of life in which you make decisions and choices to enjoy the highest level of health and well-being possible

EXERCISES

MULTIPLE CHOICE

1. Physical inactivity is associated with
   a. occupational sitting, TV watching, eating, and moderate physical activity
   b. occupational sitting, TV watching, eating, and vigorous physical activity
   c. TV watching, eating, occupational sitting, and computer game activity
   d. TV watching, eating, occupational sitting, and low physical activity
   e. eating, TV watching, occupational sitting, and dancing

2. It is important that we encourage children and youth to become moderately physically active to prevent
   a. high blood pressure
   b. obesity
   c. diabetes
   d. depression
   e. all of the above

3. The 2010 *Canadian Guidelines for Physical Activity* for adults recommend
   a. 150 minutes per week of moderate to vigorous physical activity accumulating in bouts of at least 10 minutes each
   b. 150 minutes per week of moderate to vigorous physical activity accumulating in bouts of at least 20 minutes each
   c. 150 minutes per day of moderate to vigorous physical activity accumulating in bouts of at least 10 minutes each
   d. 120 minutes per week of moderate to vigorous physical activity accumulating in bouts of at least 10 minutes each
   e. 120 minutes per day of moderate to vigorous physical activity accumulating in bouts of at least 20 minutes each

4. The wellness concept emphasizes which of the following?
   a. reliance on the health-care system
   b. personal responsibility for well-being
   c. a complete absence of disease
   d. adequate medical insurance coverage
   e. exercising to maximum heart rate every day

5. Which of the following is one of the seven dimensions of health?
   a. wellness
   b. sexual health
   c. environmental health
   d. cardiovascular health
   e. nuclear health

6. Which of these statements about a wellness lifestyle is true?
   a. the rewards of wellness are delayed
   b. living to an old age is a benefit to living a wellness lifestyle
   c. college is a time to think about wellness
   d. wellness involves gaining control of your life
   e. all of these choices are true

7. Wellness includes concepts such as
   a. embracing big, positive changes in order to get fit
   b. taking steps to ensure your wealth when you can finally retire
   c. compromising lifestyle habits to enjoy yearly vacations
   d. allowing someone to dictate how your leisure time is spent
   e. embracing small, positive changes in order to have a healthy attitude and lifestyle

8. The practice of "learning a new skill/language" is an example of which dimension of health?
   a. social
   b. spiritual
   c. occupational
   d. emotional
   e. intellectual

9. Dealing effectively with a stressful situation is an example of which dimension of health?
   a. social
   b. spiritual
   c. occupational
   d. emotional
   e. intellectual

10. Developing a good network of friends both within and outside your career is an example of which dimension of health?
    a. social
    b. spiritual
    c. occupational
    d. emotional
    e. intellectual

11. Finding a rewarding career in law enforcement is an example of which dimension of health?
    a. social
    b. spiritual
    c. occupational
    d. emotional
    e. intellectual

12. Which of the following is a benefit of regular physical activity?
    a. greater resistance to mental fatigue
    b. reduced risk of heart disease
    c. better stress management
    d. improved agility
    e. all of these

13. Physical fitness involves
    a. free play
    b. walking to school while bouncing a ball
    c. structured and repetitive activities
    d. increased risk of bone loss due to activity
    e. decreased flexibility due to movement

14. Health benefits of regular physical activity and fitness do not include
    a. increased risk of cancer
    b. positive mental health
    c. increased functional health
    d. decreased blood pressure
    e. decreased blood glucose levels

15. A BFOR is associated with what type of fitness?
    a. health-related fitness
    b. performance/skill-related fitness
    c. musculoskeletal fitness
    d. sports-related fitness
    e. game-related fitness

16. Based on the Meiorin decision, a framework for BFOR standards testing that reflected the job became mandatory in Canada in
    a. 1970
    b. 1987
    c. 1995
    d. 1999
    e. 2002

SHORT ANSWER

1. Define "healthy living."

2. What are the seven dimensions of good health?

3. Why is it important to put equal emphasis on each dimension of good health?

4. How does wellness apply to law enforcement?

5. What does physical fitness mean to you?

6. What is the difference between health-related and performance/skill-related fitness?

7. Describe the difference between active living and physical inactivity/sedentary behaviour.

8. List some of the ways you can improve your health based on the information in this chapter.

9. Which of the eight essential and 11 developmental competencies required of Ontario law enforcement officers do you possess? Which ones do you need to work on?

10. What are some of the concerns that law enforcement officers have when dealing with issues around being overweight or obese?

11. What are some of the benefits of reducing weight?

REFERENCES

Anderson, G.S., Plecas, D.B., & Segger, T. (2001). Police officer physical abilities testing: Re-validating a selection criterion. *Policing: An International Journal of Police Strategies & Management, 24*(1), 8–31.

Anderson, G.S., & Plecas, D.B. (2007). *Physical Abilities Requirement Evaluation (PARE) Phase 1: Task Analysis.* Retrieved from http://www.ufv.ca/media/assets/ccjr/reports-and-publications/pare_phase_1.pdf

Anderson, G.S., & Plecas, D.B. (2008). *Physical Abilities Requirement Evaluation (PARE) Phase 2: Discrete Item Analysis.* Retrieved from https://www.publicsafety.gc.ca/lbrr/archives/cnmcs-plcng/cn79122656-eng.pdf

Basch C. (2011). Healthier children are better learners: A missing link in school reforms to close the achievement gap. *Journal of School Health,* 81, 593–598. Retrieved from http://www.rmc.org/wpdev/wp-content/uploads/2012/12/A-Missing-Link-in-School-Reforms-to-Close-the-Achievement-Gap1.pdf

Bonneau, J. (1994). Occupational Fitness. In A. Trottier & J. Brown (Eds.), *Police Health: A Physician's Guide for the Assessment of Police Officers.* Canada Communication Group.

Bonneau, J. (2001). Evaluating Physical Competencies Fitness Related Tests Task Simulation or Hybrid. Objectives, process and consensus summary of the National Forum on Bona Fide Occupational Requirements. In N. Gledhill, J. Bonneau, & A. Salmon (Eds.), *Proceedings of the Consensus Forum on Establishing BONA FIDE Requirements for Physically Demanding Occupations* (pp. 23–33). Toronto, ON: York University.

Cacioppo, J.T., Hawkley, L.C., Crawford, L.E., Ernst, J.M., Burleson, M.H., Kowalewski, R.B., et al. (2002). Loneliness and health: Potential mechanisms. *Psychosomatic Medicine, 64,* 407–417.

Canada Border Service Agency. (2016). *Become a CBSA officer.* Retrieved from http://www.cbsa-asfc.gc.ca/job-emploi/menu-eng.html

Canadian Charter of Rights and Freedoms, Part I of the *Constitution Act, 1982,* being Schedule B to the *Canada Act 1982* (UK), 1982, c 11.

Canadian Human Rights Commission. (2007). Bona fide occupational requirements and bona fide justification under the Canadian Human Rights Act:

The implications of Meiorin and Grismer. Cat. no. HR21–53/2007. Ministry of Public Works and Government Services. Retrieved from http://www.chrc-ccdp.ca

Canadian Nuclear Safety Commission. (2018). Fitness for Duty, Volume III: Nuclear Security Officer Medical, Physical and Psychological Fitness. Regulatory document REGDOC-2.2.4. Ottawa, Canada. ISBN 978-0-660-27458-4. Retrieved from http://www.nuclearsafety.gc.ca/pubs_catalogue/uploads/REGDOC-2-2-4-Fitness-for-Duty-Vol-III-Nuclear-Security-Officer-Medical-eng.pdf

Canadian Society for Exercise Physiology (CSEP). (2012). *Canadian physical activity and sedentary behaviour guideline handbook*. Retrieved from http://www.csep.ca/guidelines

Carson V., Ridgers N.D., Howard B.J., Winkler E.A., Healy G.N., Owen N., … Salmon J. (2013). Light-intensity physical activity and cardiometabolic biomarkers in US adolescents. *PLoS One, 8*(8), e71417.

Carson V., Rinaldi R.L., Torrance B., Maximova K., Ball G.D., Majumdar S.R., … McGavock J. (2014). Vigorous physical activity and longitudinal associations with cardiometabolic risk factors in youth. *International Journal of Obesity, 38*(1), 16–21.

Correctional Services Canada. (2014). *Careers at Correctional Services Canada (CSC)*. Retrieved from http://www.csc-scc.gc.ca/careers/index-eng.shtml

Criminal Code, RSC 1985, c C-46. Retrieved from http://laws-lois.justice.gc.ca/eng/acts/C-46/

Eid, E. (2001). Challenges posed by the Supreme Court of Canada in the Meiorin decision to employers in physically demanding occupations. In N. Gledhill, J. Bonneau, & A. Salmon (Eds.), *Proceedings of the National Forum on Bona Fide Occupational Requirements*. Toronto, ON.

Employment Equity Act, SC 1995, c 44. Retrieved from http://laws.justice.gc.ca/eng/acts/e-5.401/

Farenholtz, D.W., & Rhodes, E.C. (1986). Development of physical abilities test for municipal police officers in British Columbia. *Canadian Journal of Applied Sport Sciences, 11*(3), abstract.

First Nations Regional Longitudinal Health Survey (RHS) 2002/03. (March 2007). *Results for Adults, Youth and Children Living in First Nations Communities*. Assembly of First Nations/First National Information Governance Committee. Ottawa, ON.

Gendron A., Poirier S. and Lajoie C. (2017). Standardized Physical Abilities Test Development Project (2017 POLICE SPAT-ENPQ)—Summary. École nationale de police du Québec, 6 pages. Retrieved from https://bit.ly/2IiajNT

Gerber, M., Brand, S., Holsboer-Trachsler, E., & Pühse, U. (2010). Fitness and exercise as correlates of sleep complaints: Is it all in our minds? *Medicine & Science in Sports & Exercise, 42*(5), 893–901.

Girard, G. (2013). Obesity in law enforcement. *Canadian Journal of Diabetes, 37*(2), S243.

Gumieniak, R.J., Jamnik, V.K., & Gledhill, N. (2013) Catalog of Canadian Fitness Screening Protocols for Public Safety Occupations That Qualify as a Bona Fide Occupational Requirement. *Journal of Strength & Conditioning Research, 27*(4), 1168–1173.

Hummer, R.A., Rogers, R.G., Nam, C.B., & Ellison, C.G. (1999). Religious participation and U.S. adult mortality. *Demography, 30*(2), 273–285.

Janssen I., & LeBlanc A.G. (2010). Systematic review of the health benefits of physical activity and fitness in school-aged children and youth. *International Journal of Behavioral Nutrition and Physical Activity, 7*, 40.

Jamnik, V.K., Thomas, S.G., Shaw, J.A., & Gledhill, N. (2010). Identification and characterization of the critical physically demanding tasks encountered by correctional officers. *Applied Physiology, Nutrition, and Metabolism*, 35, 45–58. doi:10.1139/H09-121

Jamnik, V., Gumienak, R., & Gledhill, N. (2013). Developing legally defensible physiological employment standards for prominent physically demanding public safety occupations: A Canadian perspective. *European Journal of Applied Physiology, 113*(10), 2447–2457.

Joseph, R.P., Royse, K.E., Benitez, T.J., & Pekmezi, D.W. (2014). Physical activity and quality of life among university students: Exploring self-efficacy, self-esteem, and affect as potential mediators. *Quality of Life Research, 23*(2), 659–667. doi:10.1007/s11136-013-0492-8

Katzmarzyk, P.T. (2008). Obesity and physical activity among Aboriginal Canadians. *Obesity, 16*(1), 184–190.

Maud, P.J. & Foster, C. (2006). Physiological Assessment of Human Fitness. *Human Kinetics*, 1.

Mammen, G., & Faulkner, G. (2013). Physical activity and the prevention of depression: A systematic review of prospective studies. *American Journal of Preventative Medicine, 45*(5), 649–657. doi:10.1016/j.amepre.2013.08.001

McTiernan, A. Mechanisms linking physical activity with cancer. (2008). *Nature Reviews Cancer, 8*(3), 205–211.

Ministry of Community Safety and Correctional Services. (2015). *PREP. Fit to Serve. Preparing for the PREP—the Physical Readiness Evaluation for Police*. Retrieved from http://www.applicanttesting.com/images/stories/pdf/FittoServe2015Final.pdf

Ministry of Community Safety & Correctional Services (2016). *Careers in Corrections*. Retrieved from http://www.mcscs.jus.gov.on.ca/english/corr_serv/careers_in_corr/careers_corr_about.html

OACP. (2016). *Constable Selection System*. Retrieved from http://www.oacp.on.ca/programs-courses/constable-selection-system

Ontario Government. (2005) Private Security and Investigative Services Act, 2005, S.O. 2005, c. 34. Retrieved from https://www.ontario.ca/laws/statute/05p34

Ottawa Police Service. (2016). *Employee health and wellness*. Retrieved from http://www.ottawapolice.ca/en/annual-report-2014/Employee-health-and-wellness.asp

Pescatello, L.S., Arena, R., Riebe, D., & Thompson, P.D. (Eds). (2014). *ACSM's guidelines for exercise testing and prescription*. Philadelphia, PA: Wolters Kluwer/Lippincott Williams & Wilkins.

Police Fitness Personnel of Ontario. (2017). *Ontario Police Fitness Standards*. Retrieved from http://www.pfpo.org

Public Health Agency of Canada. (2011). *Obesity in Canada. A joint report from the Public Health Agency of Canada and the Canadian Institute for Health Information*. Cat.: HP5-107/2011 E-PDF. Retrieved from https://secure.cihi.ca/free_products/Obesity_in_canada_2011_en.pdf

Quinney, H.A., Gauvine, L., & Wall, A.E.T. (Eds.). (1994). *Toward active living: Proceedings of the International Conference on Physical Activity, Fitness and Health*. Champaign, IL: Human Kinetics.

Rasberry, C.N., Lee, S.M., Robin, L., Laris, B.A., Russell, L.A., Coyle, K.K., & Nihiser, A.J. (2011). The association between school-based physical activity, including physical education, and academic performance: A systematic review of the literature. *Preventative Medicine, 52*(1), S10–20.

RCMP. (2005, updated 2011). *The Royal Canadian Mounted Police Physical Abilities Requirement Evaluation (PARE) protocol*. Ottawa: Author.

RCMP. (2013). *The RCMP PARE Administrator Manual and Forms*. Ottawa: Author

Reilly, T. (2013). Phase II Report. Physical Demands of Common, Essential, Physically Demanding Tasks in the CF. *Fitness for Operational Requirements of CF Employment*. Retrieved from https://www.cfmws.com/en/AboutUs/PSP/DFIT/Fitness/Documents/Phase II Final Report Jun 7 2013.pdf?Mobile=1&Source=%2Fen%2FAboutUs%2FPSP%2FDFIT%2FFitness%2F_layouts%2Fmobile%2Fview.aspx%3FList=f2f67371-9d24-4d91-b191-625c38a5d35b%26View=6b3b

Robson, S. (2013). Physical Fitness and Resilience: A Review of Relevant Constructs. *RAND Project AIR FORCE Series on Resiliency*. Washington, DC: RAND Corporation.

Sheets, S, (2012). Fitness and the police officer. *The Journal of Law Enforcement, 2*(3).

Shields, M. (2006). Overweight and obesity among children and youth. *Health Report,17*(3), 27–42.

Shipley, P. (2000). *Cost-Benefit Analysis of Ontario Provincial Police, OPFA*. Toronto, ON: Queen's Printer for Ontario.

Statistics Canada. (2015). *Directly Measured Physical Activity of Canadian Adults, 2012 and 2013*. Ottawa: Statistics Canada. Retrieved from http://www.statcan.gc.ca/pub/82-625-x/2015001/article/14135-eng.htm

Supreme Court of Canada. (1999). British Columbia (Public Service Employee Relations Commission v. BCGSEU), 3 S.C.R. 3 (Meiorin Decision). Retrieved from https://scc-csc.lexum.com/scc-csc/scc-csc/en/item/1724/index.do

Tremblay, M.S., Warburton, D.E.R., Janssen, I., Paterson, D.H., Latimer, A.E., Rhodes, R.E., et al. (2011). New Canadian Physical Activity Guidelines review. *Applied Physiology, Nutrition and Metabolism, 36*, 36–46.

van Dijk, J.W., Tummers, K., Stehouwer, C.D., Hartgens, F., & van Loon, L.J. (2012). Exercise therapy in type 2 diabetes: Is daily exercise required to optimize glycemic control? *Diabetes Care, 35*(5), 948–954

Warburton, D., Katzmarzyk, P., Rhodes, R., & Shephard, R. (2007). Evidence informed physical activity guidelines for Canadian adults. *Applied Physiology, Nutrition and Metabolism, 32*, 17–74.

Warburton, D.E., Gledhill, N., & Quinney, A. (2001a). Musculoskeletal fitness and health. *Canadian Journal of Applied Physiology, 26*, 217–237.

Warburton, D.E., Gledhill, N., & Quinney, A. (2001b). The effects of changes in musculoskeletal fitness on health. *Canadian Journal of Applied Physiology, 26*, 161–216.

Warburton, D.E.R., Charlesworth, S., Ivey, A., Nettlefold, L., & Bredin, S.S.D. (2010). A systematic review of the evidence for Canada's Physical Activity Guidelines for adults. *International Journal of Behavioral Nutrition and Physical Activity, 7*, 39.

Wolin, K.Y., Carson, K., & Colditz, G.A. (2010). Obesity and cancer. *Oncologist, 15*(6), 556–565.

GOAL
SETTING

LEARNING OUTCOMES

After completing this chapter, you should be able to:

- Understand how self-esteem, self-efficacy, attitude, and intentions play a role in participation in physical activity.

- Understand the process of setting short- and long-term goals that are specific, measurable, attainable, relevant and realistic, and timed (SMART).

- Assess your values and formulate goals that reflect those values.

- Identify and develop strategies to change and maintain lifestyle behaviours that promote health.

- Create a mission statement that will give direction to the decisions you make throughout the course of your life.

As a law enforcement student, you are working toward various goals. Your first goal was achieved when you were admitted into your law enforcement program. To achieve your other goals, you must set up pathways to success. In this chapter, you will assess your values, set short- and long-term goals for yourself, devise strategies for adopting and maintaining healthy behaviours, and create a mission statement. These steps will help you find more meaning and direction in your life.

Increasingly, there is a push for more effective and efficient employees in law enforcement. There is an expectation to do more with less and to do it in a shorter period of time. The expectation to effectively deal with each call, do the necessary paperwork, and move on to the next call is critical for cost effectiveness. You must be able to demonstrate that you have the required knowledge for the job, make use of the resources available to you, and adapt to changing demands, including acquiring knowledge of the ever-changing technologies, databases, and forms. The process alone to apply for a career in law enforcement can be daunting. It is important that before you submit your forms, you have all necessary qualifications and documents that the employer is looking for. Failure to provide these documents means your application will not be looked at. It is important as you proceed with this journey that you obtain the necessary skills and abilities that they are looking for. Start setting goals now to ensure you will be ready when you apply.

Research suggests that 50 percent of individuals starting an exercise program will drop out within the first six months (Kravitz, 2011; Wilson & Brookfield, 2009). Although research (Seguin et al., 2010) shows that affirmative health-related outcomes from an exercise program are a principal catalyst to continuing exercise, outcomes may take months to realize after the initiation of the fitness program. Although feeling good and improving your quality of life is a major motivating factor, setting goals, assessing those goals periodically, and recording improvements can be critical to continuing exercise (Weinberg, 2013). Creating solid goals and steps to achieve these goals will be key to your fitness and wellness. Goals make the person aware of the actual fitness gains they are achieving, and can increase their competence and exercise adherence (Kravitz, 2011).

THE STAGES OF BEHAVIOURAL CHANGE

As the demands of law enforcement change, employers are looking for people with both academic training and practical life experience gained through paid or volunteer work. Law enforcement agencies want independent decision-makers and self-directed learners who have a positive attitude toward work. Candidates need a well-rounded education (including math and computer literacy), communication skills (including a good command of vocabulary and grammar), interpersonal and time-management skills, flexibility, dependability, and a lifelong commitment to physical activity. To be successful, people in law enforcement must be able to adapt to the changing demands of their field and set their goals accordingly.

Behavioural psychologists have undertaken a great deal of research to understand why people find it difficult to follow through on major lifestyle changes or goals. Lifestyle behaviours can have a negative effect on people's ability to stay healthy and free from disease or disability. Unfortunately, many people succumb to behaviours that lead to illness, including alcohol and drug abuse, smoking, inappropriate dieting, and insufficient physical fitness.

The Health Belief Model relates to making key decisions to influence health behaviours (e.g., making healthier food choices to control my diabetes). It centres around six constructs to predict health behaviour: *perceived susceptibility* (perception that you can't get fit), *risk severity* (what are the consequences of not getting fit), *benefits to actions* (perceived benefits of working out), *barriers to action* (obstacles or feelings that get in the way of being successful), *cue to action* (internal and external motivation), and *self-efficacy* (confidence to exercise) (Becker, 1974; Sharma and Romas, 2012). What it can't account for is the attitudes, beliefs, and behaviours of individuals regarding the decision-making process (e.g., you don't believe you need to train to meet the fitness requirements).

According to social cognitive theory (Bandura, 1977, 1986), social influences affect behavioural change using external and internal social reinforcement and past experiences, which can influence reinforcement, expectations, and hopes. The theory focuses on six constructs: *reciprocal determinism* (learned experiences, the environment, and responses decide whether you want to work out), *behavioural capacity* (having the knowledge and skills to work out), *observational learning* (by modelling others or participating in fitness classes you complete the behaviour change), *reinforcements* (internal and external motivation), *expectations* (knowing that engaging in a weight training program will help you pass your BFOR test), and *self-efficacy* (confidence in your ability to succeed).

After studying people who committed themselves to health-related behavioural changes, Prochaska, Norcross, and DiClemente (1994) created the Transtheoretical Model, which shows that people pass through five distinct stages of change: *pre-contemplation* (not ready to exercise), *contemplation* (thinking about exercise), *preparation* (getting ready to exercise), *action* (participating), and *maintenance* (tweaking lifestyle to fit fitness in). Some people pass through all five stages in sequence, whereas others bounce back and forth between stages or get stuck at one stage.

The Transtheoretical Model assumes that people make coherent and logical plans in their decision-making process and this is not always true. What happens is that some people set unrealistic goals that are impossible to achieve. Prochaska and Velicer (1997) conceptualized this termination or relapse not so much as a stage but as a "return from Action or Maintenance to an earlier stage." Individuals revert back to old behaviours and thus relapse out of the action or maintenance stage. At this point, he or she must re-evaluate the triggers for relapse, reassess motivation and barriers, and plan stronger coping strategies for success. Approximately 15 percent of relapsers regressed to the pre-contemplation stage and then most (85 percent) were able to return to the contemplation stage and eventually back into preparation and action with re-evaluation (Nocross, Krebs, & Prochaska, 2011).

One of the most common relapses in fitness training occurs when students go home for Christmas holidays or the summer and diverge from their normal workout routines. It is important to find ways to continue to work out when you are away from your usual surroundings and familiar workout facilities, and to resist the tendency to fall back into old habits.

Some people easily meet the goals they set for themselves while others never achieve their goals. Behavioural change is largely a matter of self-management. It is important, therefore, to recognize barriers and move toward ideas, feelings, and actions that support change. Table 2.1 describes the processes that people go through while trying to change their fitness behaviours in order to exercise.

TABLE 2.1 Applying Stages of Behavioural Changes to Exercise

PROCESS	DESCRIPTION	EXAMPLES
Pre-contemplation	• You do not believe that a problem exists and resist changing that behaviour • Changing external and internal reinforcements influence your decision to participate	• I don't have the time to workout • I don't see the value in working that hard • I don't need to lose weight • People around me are encouraging me to work out with them
Contemplation	• Based on your knowledge, values, and beliefs decide if exercise is valuable enough to be incorporated into your daily routine • Contemplate benefits and types of exercises you are interested in trying • Develop positive intrinsic motivation to help you succeed	• I want to look better • I want that career in law enforcement • I want to reduce the risk of developing diabetes • I have my family supporting me to exercise • I want to pass my fitness class • I will look for a facility to work out in
Preparation	• Develop your plan: where, when, and how you will workout • Reinforce the behaviour to change by positively responding to barriers, external environment stimuli, and following through on your expected outcome • Incorporate your hopes, expectations, and positive behaviours to help you make those changes	• I have found a facility and signed up • I'm going to exercise 5 or 6 days a week • I will sign up for a BFOR practice session • I will sign up for boot camp classes • I know I need external reinforcement to get me to the gym (e.g., call from a friend)
Action (6 months)	• Take action on your plans/goals • Track your progress so you can modify if needed • Develop strategies to deal with barriers like lack of support or goals not being met • Model positive behaviours • Reward yourself for positive changes	• I've got this! I'm going to pass the BFOR requirements • I am attending all my gym classes • I will record my weights, sets, and reps every workout • I set my goals higher than I can accomplish this semester, so I need to ask my instructor/trainer for help • I have the ability to do as well as other classmates on tests
Maintenance (6 months to 5 years)	• Create challenges to keep you motivated to participate • Continue to develop confidence in your success (self-efficacy) by improving on coping skills through new challenges • Continue to reassess goals at regular intervals	• I like where I am at in terms of fitness • I need to find a workout partner that works as hard as I do to improve physical gains, positive reinforcement, and appropriate remodelling • I want to keep improving and setting higher goals • My reward is shopping for new workout clothes
Termination/Relapse	• Sometimes we are faced with setbacks due to injury, personal issues, setting our expectations too high, etc., and we have to quit or take a break	• I will reassess my social influences and internal or external reinforcements/motivators to find ways to get back into the gym

SOURCES: Bandura, 1977; Becker, 1974; Norcross, Krebs, & Prochaska, 2011; Prochaska, Norcross, & DiClemente, 1994; Prochaska & Velicer, 1997; Sharma and Romas, 2012; White 2010.

One factor that affects the likelihood of relapse is whether the individual is intrinsically or extrinsically motivated. Extrinsic motivation depends on an external reward or outcome, such as losing weight, quitting smoking, being physically fit, and being less prone to disease. Unfortunately, this kind of motivation does not keep people participating in exercise programs for long. They can become so focused on the outcome that they ignore the process (why they are exercising). In contrast, those who are intrinsically motivated to exercise regularly or lose weight are motivated by the activity itself—that is, they exercise because they enjoy it. This is why most people lose interest in participating in regular physical activity or sticking to a smoking cessation program within the first six months of trying: they quickly lose their motivation when they are not reaching their goals. Those individuals who successfully adopt attitudes and behaviours for a healthy lifestyle usually have a positive attitude toward themselves and others, as well as a zest for life. They enjoy physical activity as part of their daily routine.

Prochaska, DiClemente, and Norcross (1992) have identified ten processes of change that affect a person's ability to progress through the five stages of change. They include:

- being aware of what and where you are in terms of realizing a goal;

- knowing how emotionally tied you are to achieving that goal;

- being able to implement alternatives to ensure success;

- being able to weigh the benefits and drawbacks of trying to achieve the goal;

- assuming responsibility for the change in behaviour to realize the goal;

- having the ability to counter negative or problem behaviours that are standing in your way to achieve your goal;

- having the ability to change your environment to avoid negative triggers while stimulating positive cues;

- rewarding yourself for changing the target behaviour or realizing your goals;

- surrounding yourself with family or friends who encourage and support your change in behaviour or goals; and

- having the belief, commitment, and recommitment to act on that belief (willpower) using multiple options.

These processes of change include both obvious and non-obvious activities, events, and experiences that affect individuals who are attempting to change their behaviour. This means that you have to be doing the right things at the right time and at the right stage in order to see positive change. Unless you are ready to embrace the steps necessary for success, the change will not happen. Are you ready to see your efforts through to completion?

We know that lifestyle behaviours are affected by an individual's thoughts and feelings and the impact of family, friends, and colleagues. Self-esteem (how one feels about oneself and one's characteristics) is at the centre of personal success. If an

COMMON EXCUSES

What kind of situations and obstacles get in the way of participation in physical activity?

- holidays

- lack of consistent routine

- lack of planning—didn't schedule it in

- time management issues—"no time"

- lack of workout partner

- forgot workout clothes, towel, equipment, etc.

- lack of motivation

- too tired

- body is sore, injured, healing, etc.

- just showered/washed hair and don't want to get sweaty

individual has negative feelings including depression, helplessness, and loneliness, he or she may be unable to develop positive lifestyle behaviours. We know that those who succeed in developing and maintaining healthy behaviours have high self-esteem. They regularly engage in physical activities and maintain good dietary practices.

PERSONAL PERSPECTIVE

NANCY: INTRINSIC MOTIVATION

A few years ago, I had an opportunity to talk to a grad who was doing background checks for her police service. After our interview, she shared with me something that I have been keenly aware of in my students for years. She told me that although she had hated fitness classes when I "made her" run, she really enjoyed running now and could see why I had advised her to make fitness part of her everyday life. In fact, she had just completed her first half-marathon, and she wanted me to know what a difference doing fitness for personal reasons had made in her life.

I realized two things: first, that students often believe it is someone else's responsibility to make them successful (or not). Second, rewarding students extrinsically through marks is less effective than helping them to see the intrinsic rewards of fitness. This principle can apply to just about anything, from success in fitness, to academics, to goals in everyday life. We need to identify the values that are important to us and shift from extrinsic motivation (outcomes) to intrinsic motivation (process for its own sake) if achieving our goals is to become part of our daily life. So, where does *your* motivation come from?

Several dimensions help to determine a person's self-esteem. Intellectual, social, emotional, and physical dimensions combine to affect behaviour, and our perception of this behaviour will influence a healthy lifestyle. People who have a positive perception of themselves (that is, a higher level of self-esteem), even if they are not in great shape, will still have positive outcomes from their physical activity. However, people who possess a negative perception (that is, a poor self-image due to unrealistic cultural, media, and peer pressure) may have unrealistic expectations and, as a result, may make poor lifestyle choices.

Confidence in your ability to take action and perform a specific behaviour is known as **self-efficacy**. Those who are successful have the confidence to believe that they have internal control over their behaviour. They believe in themselves and do not allow external influences to sabotage their efforts toward change. They have the ability to visualize the success they will achieve, and reinforce that success with positive self-talk (such as, "I am a strong person who is committed to seeing these changes in myself"). Those who have strong self-efficacy also surround themselves with people who support these changes, encourage their attempts, and revel in their successes.

FACTORS THAT AFFECT PARTICIPATION IN PHYSICAL ACTIVITY

Ultimately, there are three main reasons why people participate in physical activity. These include health benefits (for example, preventing a heart attack), enjoyment, and self-image (for example, losing weight).

Below are examples of how to apply these factors to motivate you to participate in physical activity. Remember, it helps to find your reason:

- **Health benefits** are easy to recognize—"I want to get in shape," "I want to be able to see my child graduate," "I want to feel better." Many people are looking for improved strength and stamina, stress reduction, or reduced risk of certain diseases. Often this motivation comes when someone experiences a serious illness or health problem.

- **Belief** that physical activity will lead to this success is key. Through personal experience, observation, and education, those who commit to physical activity have determined expected outcomes and believe they will succeed (self-efficacy). This leads to enjoyment of the exercises or activities.

- Having the right **attitude** (value added to one's beliefs) when starting a fitness program is also a key to success. Going into any activity with a positive attitude will help the success of the outcome. This leads to positive self-image and can be a positive intrinsic and extrinsic motivator.

- The right **intention** is important, too. Those who have made informed decisions, designed a plan of action, and made a commitment are more likely to stick with a fitness program. For such intentions to work, the plan must be realistic. Individuals need to be aware of the obstacles they may face (for example, shift work, which does not allow them to work out at the same time each day), and should determine success markers, sources of support, and rewards for their successes. People must also enjoy the physical activity they are doing—very few people who hate running, for example, will ever complete a marathon.

> ## WHAT THE RESEARCH SAYS...
>
> People are motivated to participate in exercise and continue to exercise for three main reasons:
>
> 1. health benefits—reducing the risk of serious diseases (for example, cardiovascular disease, diabetes, cancer, hypertension, obesity, depression, and osteoporosis) and premature death.
>
> 2. enjoyment—Huberty, et al. (2008) found that the more people think they can successfully do exercise, the more they are likely to adhere to an exercise program.
>
> 3. self-image—improved health outcomes and quality of life with exercise (and not just appearance and weight loss results).
>
> SOURCES: Bherer, Erickson, & Liu-Ambrose, 2013; Huberty, et al., 2008; Warburton, Nicol, & Bredin, 2006.

SELF-MANAGEMENT BEHAVIOURAL STRATEGIES

In order to be successful, individuals need to shift their attention from barriers toward ideas, feelings, and actions that support change. The following self-management behavioural strategies will help increase participation in any activity and lead to change:

- *Self-monitoring*—It is important to keep track of what you are doing and how you feel (both when making a change and when avoiding it).

- *Goal setting*—Set realistic daily, specific, and achievable goals (small baby steps rather than leaps). Once you have set some goals, put them into manageable steps or sub-goals. This may help you tackle one small step at a time and reduce procrastination.

- *Cognitive change technique*—This involves changing your mind, attitudes, and feelings. Take negative behaviours such as stress, loss of confidence, and disappointment from not seeing instant gains and turn them into positive attitudes. For example, develop strategies to deal with stress, surround yourself with people who make you feel more confident, and ensure that your goals are realistic.

- *Corrective feedback*—Consciously exchange unhealthy behaviours for healthier ones. For example, instead of stopping off for fast food after work, pack some fruit for the ride home to tide you over till you can make supper.

> 66 If you raise your standards but don't really believe you can meet them then you've already sabotaged yourself. You won't even try; you'll be lacking the sense of certainty that allows you to tap the deepest capacity that's within you... Our beliefs are like unquestioned commands, telling us how things are, what's possible and impossible and what we can and cannot do. They shape every action, every thought and every feeling that we experience. As a result, changing our belief systems is central to making any real and lasting change in our lives. 99
>
> —Anthony Robbins

UNDERSTANDING YOUR GOALS

Once you are able to make positive changes in your behaviour, you will have a greater chance of achieving your goals. To achieve your goals, you must understand what they are and why they are important to you. Take, for example, your long-term goal of a career in law enforcement. One possible reason you are attracted to this field is that you like the physical challenges it presents. You know you can meet these challenges because you value physical fitness and have made it a part of your life. Therefore, what you value is reflected in your goal. **Values** are the things that matter most to us and guide our daily behaviour, activities, and decisions.

Assignment 2.1 begins the process by asking you to assess your values. Refer to it now at www.emond.ca/fitness5e.

SHORT- AND LONG-TERM GOALS

Clear and compelling goals are important to the success of your personal development. Values define what you are about. Simply put, we need to know who we are and where we want to go in order for our goals to become reality.

In setting your goals, you need to look at short-term goals (for example, goals for next semester, next year, or the next two years) and long-term goals (goals for five and ten years down the road). Short-term goals are as simple as passing the test on Thursday, meeting fitness requirements for the semester, or earning a 3.4 grade-point average for the year. Short-term goals are smaller and more manageable than long-term goals and exist within limited time frames. Long-term goals can last a lifetime and are a better reflection of who you are as a person and where your interests lie. Long-term goals may have to be adjusted due to changing circumstances in one's life (for example, adjusting when you will take time off to travel for a job opportunity).

Five kinds of goals (both short- and long-term) drive your life:

1. *Personal goals*—These reflect your personality—who you are, how you think, and how you look. Are you prepared to make fitness a lifelong commitment? Do you value your health? Do you have short- or long-term goals that include overcoming personal obstacles?

2. *Family and relationship goals*—Have you thought about relationships? What kind of lifestyle are you interested in? Will it involve a significant other or children? Do you get on well with your family? What does "family" mean to you? Are your goals the same as those of your significant other (if you have one)?

3. *Professional goals*—These reflect your career aspirations. What career would you like to pursue? Do you have the academic background and basic skills that law enforcement requires? Are you prepared to do whatever your course of study demands to achieve your career goals? Do you have the basic skills to successfully pass the law enforcement agencies' selection process? Do you have the medical clearance that agencies require (that is, have you had a full medical examination, had your eyes tested for vision and colour-blindness, and so on)?

4. *Financial goals*—Are you choosing a career that will financially support the lifestyle you want? Can you handle loans, credit cards, and other financial obligations? Have you demonstrated a good credit rating?

5. *Lifestyle goals*—Do you want to travel before getting a full-time job? Where do you want to live? Are you prepared to move anywhere in the province or country to have the career of your choice? Will you commit some of your leisure time to volunteer work with the Girl Guides, the Scouts, sports teams, Neighbourhood Watch, a crisis-intervention team, or similar groups?

Refer to **assignment 2.2** at www.emond.ca/fitness5e and begin to determine which goals are important to you and what being successful means to you.

CHOOSING EFFECTIVE GOALS—MAKE A SMART PLAN

Understanding our values makes us aware of why we choose certain goals and prepares us to make more effective decisions about our lives. According to the Canadian Society for Exercise Physiology (2003) and Meyer (2003), effective goals are specific, measurable, attainable, relevant and realistic, and timed (SMART goals). See Table 2.2.

TABLE 2.2 SMART Goals

SMART	DEFINITION	EXAMPLE
Specific	Goals are clearly formulated. You can answer what, when, where, and how you wish to accomplish your goal.	"I want to be able to run to stage 7.0 by the end of the semester."
Measurable	You know when a goal has been accomplished because you can measure it. Measuring progress will help you stay on track.	"In September I was only able to run 3 km. By November I could run 5 km. My goal for April is to run a 10-km race."
Attainable	The goal is possible for you to achieve in terms of your current abilities. You may need to stretch to achieve them, but they are not completely out of reach.	If you are sedentary, an attainable training goal might be to start strength training three days a week, as opposed to every day.
Relevant & **R**ealistic	The goal is important and meaningful to you. It is realistic in terms of your life, budget, and tools available to you.	In order to train for an Ironman triathlon you would need to have access to a pool, a bike, have unlimited training time, as well as the discipline for such a strenuous event.
Time-Oriented	Setting a time frame for achieving your goal. This will help keep you on track and help ensure success.	"I would like to be able to bench press my weight by December 31."

Now that you know something about choosing effective goals, refer to **assignment 2.3** at www.emond.ca/fitness5e to see whether your prioritized goals meet the criteria of effectiveness. Use the chart "SMART Goal-Setting and Action Planner" to develop your action plan. You will determine what steps to take to work toward your goals and what indicators will show you that you have succeeded. Also determine some rewards to keep yourself motivated.

The first time most people set goals, they usually do not succeed in listing all of them. Some people have difficulty thinking beyond the next semester. If you are having trouble setting goals, simply take a break and return to this task when you feel fresher. Setting goals is an important step in the process of developing an effective action plan. If you can break down a goal into sub-goals, you have more chance of succeeding.

As you work on your goals, focus on the effects that are most meaningful to you. Remember that in order for these goals to be successful, they must be tied to your values of success. Expect and anticipate obstacles. Make sure that you acknowledge the challenges that you face and assess your readiness for change. Build and maintain rapport with individuals who will help support your goals. Finally, re-evaluate your goals on a regular basis to ensure that you have the appropriate behavioural strategies in place to succeed.

Table 2.3 may help you develop strategies to ensure effectiveness in changing your behaviours.

DID YOU KNOW?

Fifty percent of people who start a fitness program are no longer participating in it six months later (Gledhill, 2001). How can you ensure that you do not become one of those statistics?

TABLE 2.3 Strategies to Change Behaviour When Participating in Fitness

	STRATEGIES TO CHANGE BEHAVIOUR
Beginning a Program	• Use SMART (Specific, Measurable, Attainable, Relevant and Realistic, Timely) goals when first starting out (e.g., I will do a 1.5-mile run two times per week for the next four weeks) • Self-determine your intention to exercise (e.g., intrinsic motivation to lose weight, get fit, etc.) and list ways to cope with barriers that you might face • Find a workout that you like and put it into your schedule in order to make it a lasting behavioural change; choose self-compassionate activities (i.e., ones that are enjoyable and make you feel good at the level of exertion that is comfortable to maintain) • Find different activities to participate in that will move your fitness level forward (walking, running, cycling classes to build your cardio) • Start off doing longer duration of less intense physical activity; research shows beginners have more positive benefits in the beginning rather than participating in HIIT • If you are not comfortable working out on your own, find a partner who can be there to encourage you
Action Stage	• Re-assess your goals to ensure that you're on the right track (are they realistic and attainable or do you need to adjust them?) • Look at your barriers to see if you can create some different rewards to help you overcome those challenges • Determine if you need to redesign your program to get a better workout (e.g., start incorporating a HIIT workout two times per week) • Keep a positive attitude and focus on what you can do rather than on what you can't • Think of fitness as an activity in your daily routine (e.g., make a habit of climbing stairs rather than taking the elevator) • If you are having difficulty working out alone then join a fitness class to get that support
Maintenance Phase	• Rethink your goals to challenge yourself more by going for performance rather than participation (e.g., achieve 7 on the shuttle run for the PREP test, run a 1.5-mile run in 11 minutes) • Find a person who is supportive; camaraderie can offer some competitive aspiration • Focus on the self-efficacy of health outcomes and physical changes to your exercise adherence

SOURCES: Carraro and Gaudrea, 2013; Casiro, Rhodes, Naylor, & McKay, 2011; Deci and Ryan, 1985; Fortier, Duda, Guerin &Teixeria, 2012; Kilpatrick, Kraemer, Bartholomew, Acevedo, Jarreau, 2007; Seguin et al, 2010; Sirosis, Kitner &Hirsch, 2015; Zhang, Brackbill, Yang, Becker, Herbert, & Centola, 2016.

STAYING ON TRACK

We inevitably put up obstacles and resistance when we are trying to change. Here are some suggestions to help you deal with this problem.

- When your desire to continue a negative behaviour is stronger than the motivation and commitment to change, remember that *change does not happen overnight*. In fact, the behaviour may have to become more annoying or a greater health risk before you are able to change. Smokers, for example, usually make three or four attempts to break their habit. Don't be too hard on yourself.

- Be aware that *making lifestyle changes carries costs* as well as benefits. For example, the time commitment to physical activity may require you to reschedule or even abandon other activities. You will need to weigh the short-term costs against the long-term gains, such as decreased risk of cardiovascular diseases, cancers, diabetes, and premature death.

- *Be accountable*. Tell someone your goal!!! You are five to ten times more likely to achieve your goals if you share them with a friend, family member, or mentor. It is too easy to blow off a goal if you keep it a secret, but you are much more likely to be consistent if you have someone checking in on you.

- *Social involvement* is a key component in achieving goals. Many people, especially young people, pursue activities based more on whom they do them with rather than the activity itself. In this case, the buddy system keeps people involved in the activity. If you have the support of family and friends in the early stages of a fitness program, you will be more likely to succeed in making behavioural changes and to have continued commitment to maintaining them. Find the support you need. If your family or close friends cannot offer you support, find a support group that will.

- *Make small changes*. It is actually easier to stick to a plan if the behaviour change is small. For example, instead of saying "I am going to cut out eating sugar," you can try "I will eat one big salad every day." When changing a behaviour, ask yourself "Out of 10, what are the chances that I can commit to this for 30 days?" If the score you give yourself is 9 or 10, then it is a realistic change. But if not, then you need to start with a smaller, simpler goal.

- If an activity is just not for you, *try something else*. People who have been turned off by aerobics classes, for example, can get the same benefits from a program that incorporates martial arts into the exercises.

- Although physical activities can reduce stress, you may have to take time out from one if you feel it is adding stress to your life. Try something new, or *take a small break* and then approach the activity again from a different angle.

- Focus on the real problem. Some people blame others for their inability to change, making excuses and putting things off. *Accepting responsibility* for your actions and refocusing on the goal may help you succeed.

- *Track your efforts* in your chosen activity so that you can review your action plan for the goals you have set to ensure that you are monitoring the small gains.

REWARDING YOURSELF

Behaviours that are rewarded tend to be repeated. Building in different types of rewards to reinforce your efforts will increase your chances of success. Rewards can include treats, breaks from other tasks, monetary rewards (such as a new outfit), and special activities (such as a movie). Remember that everyone has setbacks. Learn from each experience, and try to avoid negative thoughts and comments. Focus on the positive, and move on from there.

WHAT MAKES PHYSICAL ACTIVITIES ENJOYABLE AND ACHIEVABLE?

Consider the "Five C's":

1. **Competence:** People are more likely to engage and maintain participation in a program that makes them feel competent while they learn new skills.

2. **Challenge:** The skill being learned needs to match the ability of the individual. If the challenges are too hard, most people will give up quickly. Conversely, to keep motivation up, the skill must constantly become more challenging.

3. **Control:** A sense of personal control leads to higher motivation. This goes back to intrinsic motivation (for example, improving one's time in the 1.5-mile [2.4-km] run) rather than extrinsic motivation (for example, passing the requirements of a course).

4. **Choice:** By choosing a variety of activities to achieve a goal, people have a greater chance of accomplishing it.

5. **Commitment:** People who have sufficient competence and are involved in a challenging situation that they choose are more likely to stay motivated and committed to the activity.

SOURCE: Canadian Society for Exercise Physiology, 2003.

YOUR MISSION STATEMENT

Having assessed your values, priorities, and long-term goals, you might be ready to begin creating your own mission statement. Your mission statement will reflect your values and goals and be a road map that guides you through life for the next five years.

It may take a few attempts to create a mission statement that accurately reflects your values and goals. A mission statement is a very personal document about what you want out of life and what you are striving to achieve. Make sure that your mission statement is dynamic—that is, flexible enough to respond to changes in your life. As your life progresses, so will your goals and mission statement. Remember to think in terms of both professional and personal priorities.

The following is an example of a mission statement:

My mission is to help educate, motivate, and support students and individuals who work in the law enforcement field with a positive attitude to help them plan and attain measurable and realistic goals. I aim to help them optimize a successful experience in planning and implementing a valuable fitness and nutrition program as part of their overall lifestyle that will assist them in realizing their dreams. I will work toward inspiring people to be more physically active and committed to being lifelong learners in the areas of fitness and nutrition. I will strive to balance work with family time, physical activity, and independent growth, while remembering that my family and friends are my first priority.

Remember that your mission statement is exclusively yours. It empowers you to have control over the decisions you must make. The mission statement must truly reflect your goals and guide your everyday decisions.

BEING FIT AND WELL FOR LIFE

Your first attempts at behavioural change may take a bumpy road. For some people, staying at the maintenance stage will be difficult the first time. To stay fit and be ready for a career in law enforcement takes a great deal of determination and work. When you are able to maintain your healthy behavioural changes, you will realize that this empowerment will lead you forward to achieve new goals. Maintenance takes effort, and your goals will constantly change as new information and circumstances affect your choices.

66 Stay focused, go after your dreams and keep moving toward your goals. 99

—LL Cool J

FINAL THOUGHTS

Some of you may need two years to meet the standards of the various BFOR tests (for more information on these tests, see the Appendix). Others will need to learn only the specific skills involved and then refine their ability to improve their results; if you are one of those people, you will need to focus on challenging yourself to continue to maintain and improve your fitness level.

Although you do not have total control over every aspect of your life, especially your health, you do have the ability to create a lifestyle that minimizes your health risks and improves your fitness level while maximizing your well-being and enjoyment of life.

Good luck!

KEY TERMS

attitude
value added to one's beliefs

belief
acceptance of an idea on the basis of knowledge and conviction

extrinsic motivation
motivation to perform a task or goal based on external rewards to avoid negative consequences

health benefits
improvements to physical, mental, and psychological health

intention
a determination to achieve an aim

intrinsic motivation
motivation to perform a task or goal based on enjoyment of doing the task itself

mission statement
a concise statement of major values and goals that is meant to give direction to the decisions a person will make throughout his or her life

self-efficacy
one's ability to take action and perform a specific behaviour

self-esteem
how one feels about oneself and one's characteristics

self-management behavioural strategies
strategies that shift their attention from barriers toward ideas, feelings, and actions that support change

SMART goals
goals that are specific, measurable, attainable, relevant and realistic, and time-oriented

social involvement
the support of other people to assist you in achieving your goals

values
the things that matter most to us and guide our daily behaviour, activities, and decisions

EXERCISES

MULTIPLE CHOICE

1. Prochaska and colleagues' five stages of change include pre-contemplation, contemplation, preparation, _____, and _____.
   a. goal setting; behavioural change
   b. consciousness raising; social liberation
   c. commitment; behavioural change
   d. motivation; support
   e. action; maintenance/termination

2. The stage of change where people acknowledge that they have a problem and are considering doing something about it is the _____ stage.
   a. pre-contemplation
   b. contemplation
   c. preparation
   d. action
   e. there is no such stage

3. The stage of change in which a person is actively participating in a fitness program for two years is an example of the _____ stage.
   a. pre-contemplation
   b. contemplation
   c. preparation
   d. action, maintenance
   e. there is no such stage

4. People who deny that they need to practise for law enforcement evaluation tests or stop smoking to make the tests easier are in the _____ stage.
   a. pre-contemplation
   b. contemplation
   c. preparation
   d. action
   e. there is no such stage

5. At the maintenance stage of making changes in your lifestyle, which behavioural change should you have already completed?
   a. continue to challenge yourself with different exercise programs
   b. set goals to focus on performance
   c. develop different ways to overcome barriers and prevent relapse
   d. continue to seek support to help you stay on track
   e. set goals toward becoming active

6. The key to effective behavioural change is
   a. writing a goal statement and posting it in a prominent place
   b. enlisting the help of those around you
   c. identifying the stage of change you are in and using the correct strategies for that stage
   d. setting up a reward system for each process
   e. having a lot of desire and willpower

7. Self-efficacy refers to
   a. rewarding yourself for making changes in your life
   b. one's judgment of self-worth
   c. confidence in another's ability to help organize and execute the course of action for you to perform a specific behaviour
   d. confidence in your ability to take action and perform a specific behaviour
   e. confidence in your ability to master avoidance rather than execute a specific action to arrive at an appropriate behaviour

8. A cognitive change technique that would elicit a positive behavioural change is
   a. setting realistic goals
   b. changing your mind, intentions, and feelings to reflect positive attitudes
   c. rewarding yourself for not meeting your goals that week
   d. setting goals that overestimate your physical ability
   e. drawing on negative experiences to change your behaviour

9. Self-esteem
   a. is dependent on what people think about you
   b. is dependent on social behaviours and physical attributes
   c. is how you look at your emotional status
   d. is how you feel about yourself and your characteristics
   e. is not taken into consideration when someone tries to help motivate someone else into participating in fitness

10. The three major reasons why people choose to participate in a fitness program are
    a. health benefits, self-image, and enjoyment
    b. health benefits, self-efficacy, and learning a new skill
    c. self-image, self-efficacy, and self-esteem
    d. self-image, learning a new skill, and determination
    e. to learn a new skill, to master that skill, and to meet people

11. Having the right intentions to participate in a fitness program includes
    a. having extrinsic motivation to keep you going
    b. making an informed decision, designing a program, and making a commitment
    c. designing a program, looking for extrinsic motivation, and setting goals for yourself
    d. having someone design a program that is based on extrinsic motivation with high-expectation goals
    e. designing a program that is based on extrinsic motivation with low-expectation goals

12. When it comes to values around physical activity, the things that matter most to us are based on
    a. attitude, goal setting, and facilities available
    b. daily behaviours, fitness programs available, and physical prowess
    c. daily behaviours, individual decisions, and facilities available
    d. daily behaviours, activities available, and individual decisions
    e. attitude, goals, and physical prowess

13. Staying on track to achieve a goal **does not** involve
    a. making big changes all at once
    b. tracking your progress in your chosen activity
    c. seeking support from friends
    d. understanding that change does not happen over night
    e. commitment and time

14. A 240-lb individual says that they want to lose 20 lbs. Which of the following SMART principles does their goal NOT meet?
    a. specific
    b. measurable
    c. attainable
    d. realistic
    e. time-oriented

15. Striving to be hired by a law enforcement agency in the next five years would be an example of what type of goal?
    a. personal
    b. family and relationship
    c. professional
    d. financial
    e. lifestyle

SHORT ANSWER

1. What are values?

2. What five kinds of goals drive our lives?

3. Describe the five stages of change using an example from your life.

4. Using an example, what is the difference between intrinsic and extrinsic motivation?

5. Why is it important to understand values when choosing goals?

6. Describe the five characteristics that make goals attainable.

7. Define the "SMART" principal and using one of your fitness goals, apply the SMART principal (can be put into a chart form).

8. Define self-efficacy, and describe how you would boost your own.

9. List and give examples of the four self-management behavioural strategies required to be successful in fitness.

10. List and describe the five C's as they relate to making a fitness program achievable and enjoyable.

11. What is a mission statement? How can you apply a mission statement to a career in law enforcement?

REFERENCES

Bandura, A. (1977). *Social learning theory*. Englewood Cliffs, NJ: Prentice Hall.

Bandura, A. (1986). *Social foundations of thought and action: A social cognitive theory*. Englewood Cliffs, NJ: Prentice-Hall.

Becker, M.H. (1974). The Health Belief Model and personal health behavior. *Health Education Monographs, 2,* 324–508.

Bherer, L., Erickson, K.I., & Liu-Ambrose, T.L. (2013). A review of the effects of physical activity and exercise on cognitive and brain functions in older adults. *Journal of Aging Research, 2013*, article ID 657508. doi:10.1155/2013/657508

Canadian Society for Exercise Physiology (CSEP). (2003). *The Canadian physical activity, fitness and lifestyle approach: CSEP—health and fitness program's health-related appraisal and counselling strategy*. Ottawa: Author.

Carraro, N., & Gaudreau, P. (2013). Spontaneous and experimentally induced action planning and coping planning for physical activity: A meta-analysis. *Psychology of Sport Exercise, 14*, 228–248. doi:10.1016/j.psychsport.2012.10.004

Casiro, N., Rhodes, R.E., Naylor, P.J., & McKay, H.A. (2011). Correlates of inter-generational and personal physical activity of parents. *American Journal of Health Behavior, 35*: 81–91. doi:10.5993/AJHB.35.1.8. PMID:20950161

Deci, E.L., & Ryan, R.M. (1985). *Intrinsic motivation and self-determination in human behavior*. New York, NY: Plenum.

Fortier, M.S., Duda, J.L., Guerin, E., & Teixeira, P.J. (2012). Promoting physical activity: Development and testing of self-determination theory-based interventions. *International Journal of Behavioral Nutrition and Physical Activity, 9*(1), 20. doi:10.1186/1479-5868-9-20

Gledhill, N. (2001, October 26). *The latest research*. Paper presented at the OASES 13th Annual Professional Development Day and Internet Conference, Toronto, Ontario.

Huberty, J. L., Ransdell, L.B., Sidman, C., Flohr, J.A., Shultz, B., Grosshans, O., & Durrant, L. (2008). Explaining long-term exercise adherence in women who complete a structured exercise program. *Research Quarterly for Exercise and Sport, 79*(3), 374–384.

Kilpatrick, M., Kraemer, R., Bartholomew, J., Acevedo, E., & Jarreau, D. (2007). Affective responses to exercise are dependent on intensity rather than total work. *Medicine and Science in Sports and Exercise, 39*, 1417–1422. PubMed doi:10.1249/mss.0b013e31806ad73c

Kravitz, L. (2011). What Motivates People to Exercise? Research: Reasons and strategies for Exercise Adherence. *Idea Fitness Journal*. Retrieved from http://www.ideafit.com/fitness-library/what-motivates-people-to-exercise

Meyer, P.J. (2003). What would you do if you knew you couldn't fail? Creating S.M.A.R.T. goals. In *Attitude is everything: If you want to succeed above and beyond.* Scotts Valley, CA: The Meyer Group.

Norcross, J.C., Krebs, P.M., & Prochaska, J.O. (2011). Stages of change. *Journal of Clinical Psychology, 67*, 143–154.

Prochaska, J.O., DiClemente, C.C., & Norcross, J.C. (1992, September). In search of how people change. *American Psychologist, 47*, 1102–1114.

Prochaska, J.O., Norcross, J.C., & DiClemente, C.C. (1994). The five stages of change. In *Changing for good* (pp. 36–50). New York: William Morrow.

Prochaska, J.O., & Velicer, W.F. (1997). The transtheoretical model of health behavior change. *American Journal of Health Promotion, 12*(1), 38–48.

Seguin, R.A., Economos, C.D., Palombo, R., Hyatt, R., Kuder, J., & Nelson, M.E. (2010). Strength training and older women: A cross-sectional study examining factors related to exercise adherence. *Journal of Aging and Physical Activity, 18*(2), 201–218.

Sharma M., & Romas J.A. (2012). *Theoretical foundations of health education and health promotion* (2nd ed.). Sudbury, MA: Jones & Bartlett Learning.

Sirois, F.M., Kitner, R., & Hirsch, J.K. (2015). Self-compassion, affect, and health-promoting behaviors. *Health Psychology, 34*(6), 661–669. doi:10.1037/hea0000158

Warburton D.E.R, Nicol C.W., & Bredin S.S.D. (2006). Health benefits of physical activity: The evidence. *Canadian Medical Association Journal, 174*(6), 801–809.

Weinberg, R.S. (2013). Goal setting in sport and exercise: Research and practical applications. *Revista da Educação Física / UEM, 24*(2), 171–179. doi:10.4025/reveducfis.v24.2.17524

White, S.M., Mailey, E.L., & McAuley, E. (2010). Leading a physically active lifestyle: Effective individual behavior change strategies. *ACSM's Health & Fitness Journal, 14*(1), 8–15.

Wilson, K., & Brookfield, D. (2009). Effect of goal setting on motivation and adherence in a six-week exercise program. *International Journal of Sport and Exercise Physiology, 6*, 89–100.

Zhang, J., Brackbill, D., Yang, S., Becker, J., Herbert, N., & Centola, D. (2016). Support or competition? How online social networks increase physical activity: A randomized controlled trial. *Preventive Medicine Reports*, (4), 453–458.

3

TIME MANAGEMENT

LEARNING OUTCOMES

After completing this chapter, you should be able to:

- Understand the importance of time management.

- Evaluate your time-management skills.

- Demonstrate better time management by prioritizing tasks and creating and using action plans.

- Understand the effectiveness of scheduling with time-management tools.

Are you back at school after a number of years? Do you have one or more part-time jobs? Do you have time-consuming family or volunteer commitments? Are you on your own for the first time? If you answered yes to any of these questions, then as a student, you need to be aware of your time.

While critical thinking and comprehension skills are essential for your education, it is also important to have the ability to manage your time. Many students discover the need to develop or hone their time-management skills when they come to college. Unlike high school, where teachers typically structured your class time and assignments, you will have less in-class time, more outside-class homework, and a great deal of freedom and flexibility. Students who fall behind in their work face the stress of trying to keep up. Many students are not used to 13- to 15-week semesters. In high school, many of you had four courses per semester, but now have six to eight courses per semester. At times you can feel overwhelmed by twice the workload. New experiences both in the academics and in the social life at college lead some students to be caught off guard by how quickly their school work can snowball within the first few weeks. Many get behind and spend the rest of the semester playing "catch-up." If you can keep up, not only will you be able to follow along with more confidence in class, but you will also experience less stress. If you can develop a balance between school, work, and family and social life, you will be successful in your endeavours.

In the previous chapter, you learned about setting short- and long-term goals. In this chapter, you will start to see how your goals can be achieved by managing your time well. Time management is essential for successful people in any line of work. In law enforcement, officers are expected to manage the time demands of shift work, court appearances, and personal life. Many people who do shift work struggle to maintain a normal routine in their personal life. Those who work 12-hour shifts soon realize that their 4-day workweek seems to be consumed by work, commuting, and sleep. If court time is added to workdays or days off, organizing all these activities becomes a struggle. The amount of paperwork has increased exponentially. There is now a requirement to produce more detailed reports, answer emails promptly, and be more accountable for your time

Setting goals, organizing your time, and adhering to a schedule are critical to a less stressful lifestyle. There is no excuse for officers who cannot carry out a job such as responding quickly to a call because they have mismanaged their time. As in any profession, failure to complete a task can have adverse career repercussions. To be effective, officers must be skilled at juggling different duties. Therefore, as someone pursuing a career in law enforcement, you must make a conscientious effort to manage your time effectively.

In order to deal with time management issues we have to identify what we waste our time on. Figure 3.1 is an infograph that identifies some common time wasters. Can you relate to any of them?

THE BENEFITS OF TIME MANAGEMENT

Time management is a way of taking short-term goals and dividing them into manageable daily, weekly, and monthly increments, which in turn makes your long-term goals more achievable. Here are some other benefits of time management:

- Organizing your time gives meaning to daily activities by increasing your productivity, accountability, and commitment to the tasks at hand.
- It gives you a sense of order, progress, and success.
- It gives you a sense of control over your life.
- It distinguishes between priorities and non-priorities.
- It helps you deal with mundane tasks in a more effective manner.
- It helps to improve your relationships both on and off the job.
- It allows you to do the things that have to be done while having time to do the things you want to do.
- It reduces stress and provides more enjoyment of everyday life.

FIGURE 3.1 Twelve Time Wasters

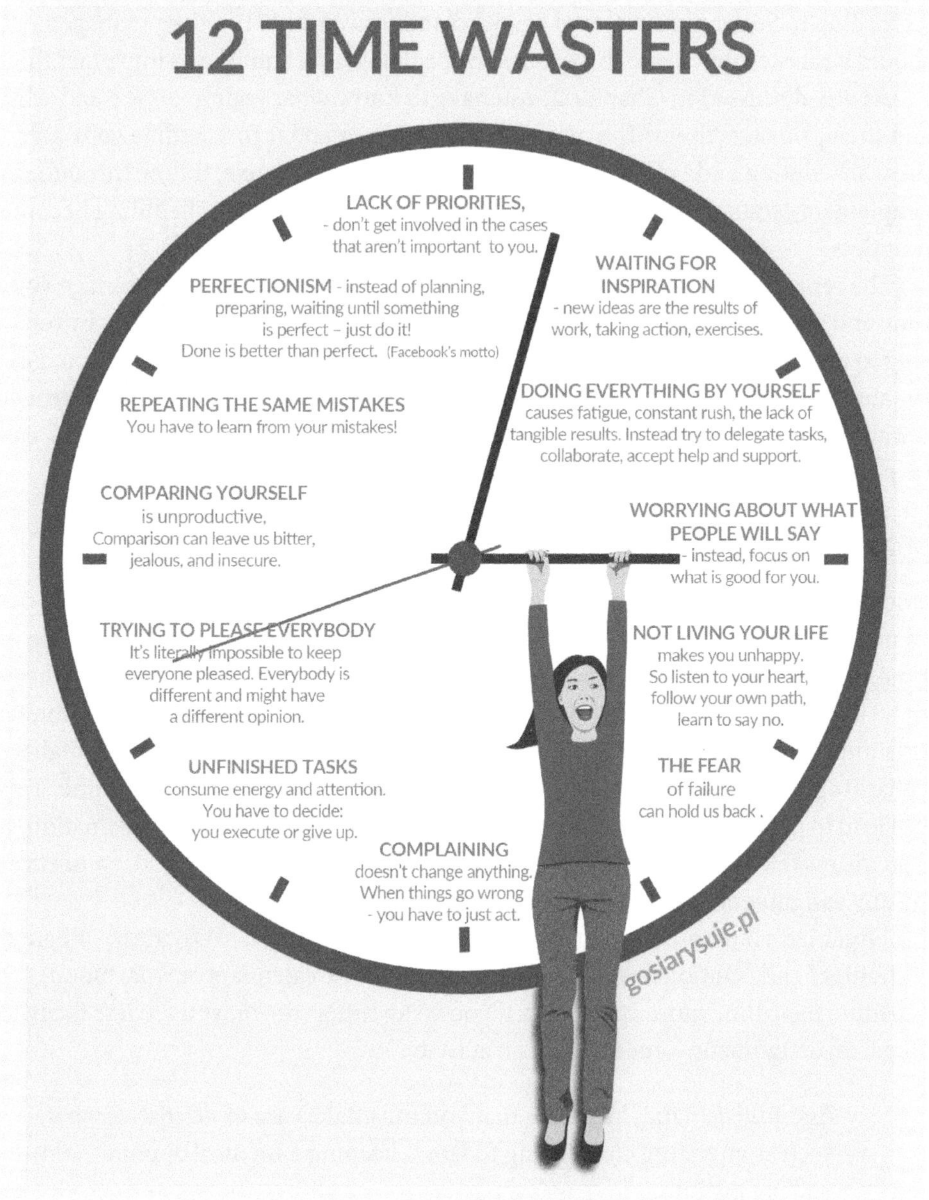

12 TIME WASTERS

LACK OF PRIORITIES,
- don't get involved in the cases that aren't important to you.

WAITING FOR INSPIRATION
- new ideas are the results of work, taking action, exercises.

PERFECTIONISM - instead of planning, preparing, waiting until something is perfect – just do it! Done is better than perfect. (Facebook's motto)

DOING EVERYTHING BY YOURSELF causes fatigue, constant rush, the lack of tangible results. Instead try to delegate tasks, collaborate, accept help and support.

REPEATING THE SAME MISTAKES You have to learn from your mistakes!

COMPARING YOURSELF is unproductive, Comparison can leave us bitter, jealous, and insecure.

WORRYING ABOUT WHAT PEOPLE WILL SAY - instead, focus on what is good for you.

TRYING TO PLEASE EVERYBODY It's literally impossible to keep everyone pleased. Everybody is different and might have a different opinion.

NOT LIVING YOUR LIFE makes you unhappy. So listen to your heart, follow your own path, learn to say no.

UNFINISHED TASKS consume energy and attention. You have to decide: you execute or give up.

THE FEAR of failure can hold us back.

COMPLAINING doesn't change anything. When things go wrong - you have to just act.

gosiarysuje.pl

At the heart of time management is an important shift in focus: you concentrate on results instead of on being busy. Many people spend their days in a frenzy of activity but achieve very little because they are not concentrating on the right things. Often a lack of time leaves us angry and hostile, unable to focus and maintain our productivity. Some people convert wasted time into a dollar amount (number of hours wasted times hourly salary) to see how much money they have "lost." Money lost can speak volumes, and usually helps motivate people to rethink how they use their day.

What remains unseen is the toll on people and organizations in terms of stress and even illness. Ultimately, those who have good time-management skills are those who enjoy their job.

THE STAGES OF TIME MANAGEMENT

According to Seaward (2004) and Seaward and Seaward (2011), time management should be broken down into three stages: prioritizing, scheduling, and implementing.

As was discussed in Chapter 2, you have to know what your goals are and why, and then prioritize them. The next step is to use a calendar to schedule your activities. Scheduling adds clarity to your day. You must, of course, follow through on (implement) your scheduled activities, or your prioritizing and scheduling become pointless.

The remainder of this chapter will help you evaluate how well you manage your time and get you started on developing your time-management skills. Start by referring to **assignment 3.1** (on the Emond website at www.emond.ca/fitness5e) and estimate where your time is spent over the course of a week. Then go on to **assignment 3.2** and actually monitor where you are spending your time. These assignments will help those who need to make better use of their time.

PRIORITIZING YOUR ACTIVITIES

Prioritization can be explained as "ranking responsibilities and tasks in their order of importance" (Seaward & Seaward, 2011, p. 331). To get on track in your use of time, you need to devise an *action plan* or *to-do list* that arranges the tasks that need to be accomplished. You want to avoid getting everything done at the last minute. It is important to avoid working very intensely for the last few days (and nights), collapsing from lack of sleep, and then coasting along until the next deadline. This can lead to periodic bouts of extreme stress, burnout, and chronic procrastination. It also means that, in most cases, you are spending only the minimum time and effort on any assignment, which does not reflect your true abilities.

Organize your to-do list using the headings "Essential Activities," "Regular Activities," and "Optional Activities." Some people use calendars or smartphones to schedule their time more effectively. If you write things down, you are less likely to forget an assignment, a meeting, or an activity.

- *Essential activities* are those that you must take care of no matter what, such as attending class, going to work, keeping a medical appointment, and paying bills.

- *Regular activities* are those that you normally carry out daily or a few days each week, such as grocery shopping, working out, and doing homework. These activities are important but, in terms of scheduling, they offer more flexibility than essential activities.

- *Optional activities* include those you would like to do but can reschedule without much sacrifice, such as a trip to the mall, a social telephone call, or attending a sports event.

Your self-reflection should make you aware of your time-management skills. A helpful place to begin is to make sure that you are prioritizing your tasks for each day/week. If you over- or underestimate your hours, you may be overwhelmed in your attempts to prioritize. There are three common mistakes in setting priorities:

1. *technical errors*, such as tackling major assignments for school too early or too late in the day for your energy levels, answering one more call or email before leaving for appointments or school, and misgauging the time necessary to complete a task

2. *external realities*, including disruptive environments (not studying in a quiet location), unrealistic schedules, or obligations to others (for example, promising you will help someone for an hour and three hours later the task is still not completed)

3. *psychological obstacles*, such as being chronically late because of poor judgment of dressing or driving time, or arriving too early and then sitting around waiting for others. Some people are convinced that they can't creatively think and write unless there is pressure of a deadline and then they become overloaded when they have multiple readings, assignments, and tests all due at the same time.

SCHEDULING YOUR ACTIVITIES

In addition to your priorities or to-do list, your calendar should record the following:

- due dates for papers, projects, presentations, and tests
- birthdays, anniversaries, and other special occasions
- benchmarks for steps toward a goal, such as due dates for sections of a project, a deadline for losing 2 kilograms, or a date on which you need to contact someone
- important meetings, medical appointments, and due dates for bill payments
- your employment schedule (paid and volunteer work)
- your travel time to and from activities
- your workout schedule
- commitments of a personal nature

Refer to **assignment 3.3** at www.emond.ca/fitness5e and determine your to-do list for this week. Figure out, based on importance, what needs to be done, or could be done this week, and then try mapping out the list on the activity chart.

SCHEDULING TIPS

- **Take time to schedule** Spending 10–15 minutes on time-management planning at the beginning of your day can save time later. Many activities must be pared down, eliminated, consolidated, or delegated.

- **Refer to your schedule** Make sure your calendar and to-do list are easily accessible. Keeping a log may help you identify time wasters.

- **Develop a game plan** Decide and schedule beforehand how many hours you will spend studying for a test or working on a project/paper including test/due dates.

- **Recognize the limits on your time** There are only 168 hours in a week. Don't set yourself up for failure by asking too much of yourself.

- **Prioritize activities for the week, month, or semester** By estimating how many hours your important activities will take this week, you will be able to determine how much time you have for other activities. Break assignments into steps and based on the weeks you have, you can estimate the time needed to complete each assignment. With practise and monitoring, you should be able to create enough time on a weekly basis so that you don't have to cram at the last moment. Some of the steps could include:
  - choosing a topic
  - having topic approved by instructor
  - doing the research
  - organizing the research to create an outline
  - writing a rough copy so someone can edit/comment
  - revising the rough copy
  - doing references and footnotes
  - printing the final copy

- **Get in the habit of setting time limits for tasks** Set a limit for each task and stick to it.

- **Delete, delay, delegate, diminish** You may have to decide whether you need to delete some tasks because they are not worth doing, delay them if they are lower-priority tasks (this is not procrastination), delegate them to ease your workload, or diminish the time you spend on them (more is not always better).

- **Take a break when needed** When you need a break, take one. This could mean taking quick stretches or going for a walk to clear your head.

- **Make the most of class** Read the assignment or chapter before class rather than reading just before a test. You will understand lectures better and be able to take better notes. Read your notes at the end of the day or at least at the end of each week.

- **Schedule downtime** Everyone needs time to relax and refresh. Make sure your downtime schedule includes activities you enjoy. Remember to enjoy life.

- **Keep your workspace in order** Spending 10 minutes at the end of the day cleaning up your workspace to get things in order can save valuable time and give you a fresh start on tomorrow.

- **Get plenty of sleep, eat a healthy diet, and exercise regularly** Leading a healthy lifestyle can improve your focus and concentration. This should help you improve your efficiency so that you complete tasks in less time.

- **Reward yourself** Plan rewards for yourself for attempting to keep to a schedule and reducing wasted time.

- **Remember that practise makes perfect** Time management, like any new skill, takes time to perfect. Don't forget to review your overall approach to scheduling once in a while to see whether you need to make any changes.

- **Ask for professional help** If you feel that you are losing control of your time, your school counselling service has people who can assist you. Don't hesitate to use their services.

IMPLEMENTING YOUR ACTIVITIES

After you have scheduled your activities, you must follow through on them. Otherwise, you will find yourself falling behind as new tasks arise.

It is important to develop a big-picture view of your day-to-day life in order to clarify what is driving particular activities and what motivates you to stay engaged with them. You will need to refer back to this overall view on a regular basis to ensure that you are on the right track.

People typically run into implementation problems by failing to prioritize activities or by setting an unreasonable schedule for themselves. You also need to avoid procrastination and other time traps (see Schafer, 1996; Steel, 2007; Wohl, Pychyl, & Bennett, 2010).

PROCRASTINATION AND OTHER TIME TRAPS

Many people fail to achieve their goals because they procrastinate over immediate tasks. Procrastination is postponing unpleasant or burdensome tasks. It happens when individuals *cognitively* focus on their present self as opposed to their future self, and in so doing, sabotage their long-term emotional well-being and success by shifting the behavioural and psychological burden to their future self (Sirois & Pychyl, 2013). Procrastination is often deliberate, especially when you are facing a frightening prospect, such as having to get a major task done in very little time. Some of the most common tasks that people procrastinate over are paying bills, paying taxes, saving for retirement, and starting assignments. This tendency may reflect task aversion, where people dislike the task (such as cleaning the house), or boredom, where individuals are not interested in the task at hand (writing a paper on something that does not interest you). For others, the issue may stem from fear of failure, fear of success, perfectionism, self-consciousness, or evaluation anxiety. These factors all relate to harsh appraisal (Beck, Koons, & Milgrim, 2000; Levinson et al., 2015). Still other reasons people procrastinate include fear of losing autonomy (wanting control over when and how you have to do something instead of following instructions) and fear of being alone (having to do a solitary activity without someone helping or being around). Whatever the reason, such fears can paralyze you and keep you from taking action, until discomfort and anxiety overwhelm you and force you to get the task done or give up (Burka & Yuen, 2004).

Many students report spending nearly a third of their days avoiding important tasks by texting, tweeting, watching TV, or sleeping (Pychyl, Lee, Thibodeau, & Blunt, 2000). Meier, Reinecke, and Meltzer (2016) revealed that "…media use conflicted with other important goals on more than half of all media use occurrences (61.2%), underlining that media use poses a particularly difficult self-regulatory challenge for many people in day-to-day settings" (p. 66). This behaviour is tied to unhealthy sleep, diet, and exercise patterns. It does not indicate laziness or lack of discipline but instead usually results from unproductive, deep-seated habits.

Refer to **assignment 3.4** at www.emond.ca/fitness5e to determine your level of procrastination. If you find yourself with no time left to revise and proofread a paper, feel a rush of adrenaline when you finish a paper ten minutes before it is due, and often pull all-nighters, you may have procrastination issues.

> **DID YOU KNOW?**
>
> It is estimated that about 15–20 percent of the general population and 80–95 percent of college students engage in procrastination.
>
> SOURCE: Steel, 2007.

Here are some strategies for dealing with procrastination. Remember, there are no quick fixes. You are not going to wake up tomorrow and never procrastinate again. However, you might figure out how to do one or two simple tasks that will help you finish a draft a little earlier or reduce your level of stress.

- Weigh the benefits of completing the task against the drawbacks of procrastinating. If you have two assignments that are due the next day, you may not be able to spend the time that you should on each, and will have to determine which one merits greater attention or is more beneficial (in terms of marks).

- Get started—don't make excuses or distract yourself with other tasks simply to avoid the task you don't want to face. Successful, effective people are those who launch directly into their major tasks and then discipline themselves to work steadily and persistently until those tasks are complete.

- Activity does not equal accomplishment. Many people spend all day being "busy"—talking, emailing, having meetings, making plans—but never actually complete a task. Don't waste time doing small, meaningless jobs while avoiding the real tasks that need to be done.

- Eat the frog! Mark Twain once said that if the first thing you do each morning is to eat a live frog, you can go through the day with the satisfaction of knowing that that is probably the worst thing that is going to happen to you all day long. Your "frog" is your biggest, most important task, the one you are most likely to procrastinate on if you don't do something about it. Discipline yourself to begin immediately and then to persist until the task is complete before you go on to something else.

- Reward yourself for completing a task. Punishing yourself every time you put something off will not help you change. Try to be a little less critical of yourself.

- Ask for help with school, work, and domestic tasks. Learn to delegate (but don't dump all the work on someone else).

- Don't expect to be perfect—just do your best.

- Set goals that can realistically be accomplished in the time you have. Connect daily activities to your work and life goals.

- Adopt a positive attitude.

- Analyze a task and break it down into manageable parts. Just as you have scheduled classes on specific days, you need to designate specific days or times to complete your tasks and assignments.

- Make time for exercise and relaxation so that you can rejuvenate and develop a fresh perspective.

- You do not need to answer every call/text/email/message/post right away. If you are already overloaded, tell your friends and family that you are busy and won't be answering their messages immediately. They will understand and respect your decision.

❝ You get to decide where your time goes. You can either spend it moving forward, or you can spend it putting out fires. You decide. And if you don't decide, others will decide for you. ❞

—Tony Morgan

TIME MANAGEMENT STRATEGIES FOR STUDENTS

ORGANIZE YOUR WORKSPACE TO MANAGE DISTRACTIONS

An important first step in efficient time management is organizing your workspace or home. Even if your schedule is well ordered, if your workspace is a disaster, you will waste time trying to work efficiently in a disorderly place. The following are some suggestions to help you set up your workspace to better manage your time:

- Put visual distractions like photos or posters where you can't see them when working at your desk. Instead, put up your calendar schedule, a list of your goals or tasks for that week, or post the amount of time and money you have invested so far in your education to remind you of why you're here.

- Make sure that ergonomically the computer and keyboard are at the right height. (Your desk and chair should allow your elbows to be at a 90-degree angle and your monitor should be set so that the top of it is at eye level.)

- Ensure that you have proper lighting—ambient (room) lighting as well as task (desk) lighting to minimize eye strain and fatigue.

- Ensure the room temperature is warm enough so your hands and feet don't get cold but not so warm that the room gets stuffy and you nod off.

ORGANIZE YOUR ASSIGNMENTS AND PREPARE FOR TESTS

Here are some helpful tips for when you are working on an assignment with a deadline:

- There is no "right" way to break up your work tasks and get started—this depends on your personality.

- You can begin in the middle of the assignment and work outward, or start with the most difficult part, the most important part, or the most profitable part (the part that has the most marks attached to it).

- Nibble at the corners: ease into a tough assignment by doing the simple, routine, or more pleasant parts first.

- Consider the deadline. Make sure you understand the task so that if you need information or equipment it will be there when the deadline looms. There is no excuse for running out of paper or printer ink.

- Some people work in bursts and intersperse other activities, such as a workout, before returning to a project. Others need to stay focused and work continuously to get it done. Schedule your time according to your strengths.

Strategies to help prepare for tests:

- Refer to the course syllabus and pre-read the chapters that are going to be covered in the lecture so that you have some understanding of the material prior to class. This will help you take better notes and prepare questions relating to the material.

- Identify the best time to study, whether it is morning, afternoon, or early evening. If your classes do not start until afternoon, use your free time in the morning to get studying done.

- Find a homework-friendly location away from distractions (roommates, TV, smartphone), where you can focus on your studies.

- Review your notes after class. If they do not make sense, the information will still be fresh in your head to correct them, or to make a note to ask your instructor for clarification.

- Coordinate study time with friends and roommates. Students who coordinate their study times can support each other and work toward finishing assignments. Then, distractions such as watching TV can turn into rewards when the tasks are completed.

- Temporarily de-activate social media sites. If necessary, use free applications that block popular sites and online games for specific periods of time.

- Study the more challenging components first, when you are less fatigued. When you become tired, it is easier to cover the material you enjoy more.

- If you are falling asleep, take a ten-minute nap, but set an alarm. Then come back to the material when you are more refreshed.

- Use waiting time (public transportation, the hour between classes) to learn small pieces of information, or write notes out on cue cards that you can go over to help you memorize facts.

- Treat school as a full-time job. Remember that for every hour you are in class, you probably will be expected to do one to two hours of work outside the classroom. It takes time to read textbooks, attend class, review instructors' notes, and study for tests. If you have to work at a part-time job, know your limits and try to stick to set hours that you can handle.

DID YOU KNOW?

How many times would you estimate that you check your smartphone every day? Thirty, forty, or fifty times? Take whatever number you came up with and double it, and then you might be getting close.

New research conducted by British psychologists shows that young adults use their smartphones roughly twice as much as they estimate that they do. In fact, the small preliminary study found that these young adults used their phones an average of five hours a day—that's roughly one-third of their total waking hours.

SOURCE: Andrews, Ellis, Shaw, & Piwek, 2015.

CREATE AN EXAM STUDY SCHEDULE

One of the most difficult periods in the semester for a student is exam time. It is extremely hard to balance all aspects of life and then, on top of that, study the appropriate amount of time for each exam. Students wind up cramming for exams because of lack of preparation and poor time-management skills, and they often feel unprepared and regret that they didn't spend more time studying.

The following list describes how to create an exam study schedule that will use your time more efficiently and help reduce stress.

1. *Draw a calendar on a large piece of paper* (at least 11" x 14") representing the last 2 to 3 weeks of your semester.

2. *Record each of your exams* on your calendar and block off the appropriate amount of time for each.

3. *Record other mandatory commitments* on your calendar and block off the appropriate amount of time for each (including classes, work, sports practice/games, workouts, volunteer work, group meetings, family commitments). Make sure that you include travel time to and from your commitments if longer than 30 minutes.

4. *Decide how much time you need to study for each exam.* This may differ for each course and will be dependent upon many factors, such as how much the exam is worth, how much material is being covered, the format of the exam, if it is an open book exam. A 3-hour exam covering all the material from the course may require 20 hours of studying, whereas a 1-hour exam made up of a short essay may only require 6 hours.

5. *Starting with the LAST exam on your schedule, use 2- to 3-hour time blocks and block off the full study time you have allotted for this exam.*

6. *Repeat with each course,* working your way from the last exam to the first, until all of your exams have their full study time blocked off. Start as early in the day as you want/need to (recommended start time would be 8 or 9 a.m.) and try to finish by 10 p.m. to leave some time to wind down. You know what time of day you are most alert and effective, so use that time to study for the most important exam in your schedule. You may encounter times when you have to be studying for two exams in one 2- to 3-hour time block, so cut it in half.

7. *Add in due dates for any major assignments* and consider blocking off time to work on these too.

8. *Consider including chapters/concepts to review during each time block.*

Figure 3.2 provides an example of a 5-day exam study schedule. Notice that everything is scheduled, including work, meals, workouts, and even relaxing. This student committed 11 hours of studying to each of their three exams. Had this schedule not been planned out, the student may not have realized that on Monday they needed to already be studying for their Thursday and Friday exams.

FIGURE 3.2 Sample Exam Study Schedule

	Monday	Tuesday	Wednesday	Thursday	Friday
8:00–9:00	Study Provincial Offences	Study Provincial Offences	Study Youth in Conflict with the Law	Study Youth in Conflict with the Law	
9:00–10:00					**Issues in Diversity Exam**
10:00–11:00		Workout/Eat lunch			
11:00–12:00	Basketball/Eat		Basketball/Eat	**Youth in Conflict with the Law Exam**	
12:00–1:00	Study Youth in Conflict with the Law	Study Provincial Offences	Study Issues in Diversity		Finished school!! Eat/Relax/Hang out with friends
1:00–2:00				Eat lunch/Relax	
2:00–3:00	Study Provincial Offences		Relax	Study Issues in Diversity	
3:00–4:00		**Provincial Offences Exam**	Study Youth in Conflict with the Law		
4:00–5:00					
5:00–6:00	Eat dinner/Relax		Eat dinner/Drive	Eat dinner/Workout	
6:00–7:00		Eat/Relax/Visit with friends	Work		
7:00–8:00	Study Issues in Diversity			Study Issues in Diversity	
8:00–9:00					
9:00–10:00					

TIPS IF YOU BECOME OVERWHELMED

Here are some time-management tips that may keep you from becoming overwhelmed in the first place:

- Don't say yes when you really don't have the time. Learn to say no graciously; you will experience less stress and be able to enjoy some time to yourself when you learn to say no to people.

- Limit your social time. Socializing is important, but going out five nights a week is not going to bring you success in school.

- Delegate. Some things you must do for yourself, but there are times when you can ask for a favour (just be sure you do one in return). Be reasonable about how many tasks you can accomplish.

- Don't try to do too much. Many people attempt too much and become stressed or suffer **chronic time urgency**. This occurs when people put pressure on themselves to perform an unreasonable number of tasks in too short a time. Such people often become agitated because they feel that they are always in a hurry and will let others down if they cannot complete everything they set out to do. Leave some time open for unplanned circumstances that are beyond your control.

- Limit use of social media, text messaging, email, and your smartphone. Set aside a specific time frame for these activities, and stick to it even if you are not finished (for example, first thing in the morning, just before lunch, and an hour before shutting down your computer). Sometimes it's better to leave one detailed message explaining exactly what information you require rather than two or three additional messages.

- Do not multitask when on the phone or having face-to-face conversations. Focusing solely on the conversation will ensure that all of the key information is conveyed and keeps the conversation concise.

- Ask for help. There are a multitude of people at your college who are there to assist you, including faculty, counsellors, learning strategists, and librarians. Learn what other resources your college has to offer. Many colleges have writing centres, math labs, and career centres. Some offer e-learning programs, such as SkillSoft E-Learning (Cisco Learning Network, 2012), that are designed to help with basic computer skills, word processing, and web design.

- Ensure to make time for breaks. Breaks give you time to digest and process the information you are learning. They help reduce stress, sustain motivation, and increase concentration and productivity.

- Work at a reasonable pace. Try to realize that you must work at a pace that is conducive to health, and set only realistic goals. Step back now and then to ensure that your priorities are reasonable. Stop hurrying when there is no need to hurry.

- Reward yourself when you finish tasks on time. The reward should reflect the difficulty of the task and the time spent on it. For example, reward yourself with time for social media, or take a break to enjoy a movie or workout.

TIPS FOR EFFECTIVE GROUP WORK

It is important to ensure group work proceeds efficiently from beginning to end. If it is well planned, has a defined purpose, follows an agenda, and proceeds crisply, it will be an effective process. Unfortunately, group work does not always go well—time spent on group meetings may be too long and waste time dealing with extraneous issues (group dynamics, timetable schedules, part-time jobs, people who arrive late and disrupt the flow, and so on). Here are seven tips for having an effective experience:

1. If you are allowed to choose your group, choose people who complement your work methods (not necessarily those who work the same way you do) and who work well in team settings.

2. Create an agenda prior to when you meet, so that it is organized to achieve the purpose and that ensures everyone is "on the same page." Have a purpose that all participants know and understand (for example, to analyze or solve a problem, to achieve a training objective, to reconcile a conflict). Make sure the chairperson keeps people on task.

3. Give people ample notice so that they can prepare based on the agenda sent out, be able to notify you whether they can attend, and arrive on time. Start your meetings at the appointed time. Keep the time limit you have set for the meeting. Restate the relevant points of the agenda when the discussion veers from the objectives.

4. Do not allow small groups to start up separate conversations. Prevent individuals from dominating the discussion by asking them to allow others to speak. Ask open-ended questions to obtain different points of view and to make sure that everyone's point of view is heard.

5. Set goals for different tasks. Start with small projects to ensure that the group is on the right track. Define from the outset how the group wants each task accomplished—what are the criteria for a "good" job? Delegate both popular and unpopular components and try to evenly distribute the workload. Having this discussion will save frustration and time later. Agree on deadlines.

6. Encourage participants to understand their role, come prepared, and make contributions; then stand back and allow individuals to do their jobs. As a group, agree who is in charge of overseeing the project. Plan periodic reviews and schedule them when you first start the assignment.

7. Have a post-meeting follow-up where necessary. Include off-target subjects to be discussed at a later meeting. At the periodic reviews and when the final product is brought together, make sure to review the project as a team before handing it in or presenting it. Hold people accountable for their contribution.

FINAL THOUGHTS ON TIME MANAGEMENT

Remember that the more you use your time-management skills, the closer you will be to achieving your long-term goals. It is very important to follow a schedule. If you fail to keep to your schedule, ask yourself why and attempt to change the behaviours that caused the problem. If you need help, ask for it. Every college campus has counselling services to help you make your academic career a success. A faculty member can point you in the right direction if you are unsure where to turn, such as choosing a topic for a project paper.

Remember that you have to find a balance between work and play.

66 The key is not to prioritize what's on your schedule but to schedule your priorities. 99

—Stephen Covey

KEY TERMS

chronic time urgency
a constant state of stress due to putting pressure on yourself to do too much in too little time

eat the frog
a term that means combatting procrastination by taking on the hardest task first

procrastination
the postponement of unpleasant or burdensome tasks

EXERCISES

MULTIPLE CHOICE

1. Which of the following is a health-related consequence of an unrealistic schedule?
   a. suffering from stress
   b. being late for classes
   c. missing your bus or car pool
   d. failing to return calls
   e. forgetting your textbooks in the cafeteria

2. Travel to and from school and work, household chores, and child care are examples of
   a. essential activities
   b. non-essential activities
   c. regular activities
   d. optional activities
   e. none of the above

3. An example of planning a regular activity would be
   a. attending class
   b. going to work
   c. getting your workout in after class
   d. going to the mall
   e. hanging out with your friends

4. An example of an optional activity would be
   a. paying your monthly phone bill
   b. going to your dentist for a filling
   c. preparing supper
   d. attending the varsity basketball game
   e. getting homework done for class

5. What is the first step to managing time effectively?
   a. analyzing your current time use
   b. establishing priorities
   c. making a schedule
   d. monitoring your current time use
   e. creating a calendar of your monthly events

6. Writing down your goals will help you to
   a. organize them
   b. evaluate them
   c. remember them
   d. publish them
   e. share them with others

7. Managing your time by organizing and scheduling activities will
   a. not make a difference
   b. give you more control over daily stress
   c. give you no more time for other activities
   d. just be a paper exercise
   e. let others see how busy you are

8. The three stages of good time management are
   a. prioritizing, scheduling, and involving
   b. scheduling, implementing, and assessing
   c. scheduling, organizing, and implementing
   d. prioritizing, organizing, and implementing
   e. prioritizing, scheduling, and implementing

9. In recent years, the amount of time the average person spends at work has
   a. decreased
   b. increased
   c. remained the same
   d. fluctuated up and down
   e. depended on each person's needs

10. Which is most likely to suffer due to a lack of time?
    a. work
    b. chores
    c. sleep
    d. relationships
    e. travel time

11. Chronic time urgency refers to
    a. teachers assigning you too much homework
    b. putting too much pressure on yourself to perform a number of tasks
    c. having your family expect you to help clean up around the house before doing your homework
    d. organizing a number of tasks in order to get them done on time
    e. setting realistic goals for yourself

12. What does "eating the frog" mean?
    a. a method to give you more time
    b. actually eating a live frog
    c. a method of cleaning up your workstation
    d. a method to deal with procrastination
    e. a way to justify using time

SHORT ANSWER

1. Why is it important to organize your time?

2. How does time management relate to goal setting?

3. Briefly describe the three headings under which activities can be prioritized.

4. What are some effective methods to assist you with your schedule?

5. What is procrastination? How can it be overcome?

6. What signs may indicate that you are procrastinating?

7. What are some other time traps? How can they be overcome?

8. What can you do to prevent multimedia and electronic devices from monopolizing your time?

9. What can you do to make studying time more effective?

10. How can you organize yourself to ensure that all your assignments are completed and handed in on time?

REFERENCES

Andrews, S., Ellis, D.A., Shaw, H., & Piwek, L. (2015). Beyond Self-Report: Tools to Compare Estimated and Real-World Smartphone Use. *PLoS ONE 10*(10), e0139004. doi:10.1371/journal.pone.0139004

Beck, B.L., Koons, S.R., & Milgrim, D.L. (2000). Correlates and consequences of behavioural procrastination: The effects of academic procrastination, self-consciousness, self-esteem and self-handicapping. *Journal of Social Behaviour and Personality, 15,* 3–13.

Burka, J.B., & Yuen, L.M. (2004). *Procrastination: Why you do it, what to do about it.* New York: Da Capo Press.

Cisco Learning Network. (2012). *SkillSoft E-Learning.* https://learningnetwork.cisco.com/docs/DOC-6622.

Georgian College Corporate Training and Consulting. (2001). *Time management training.* Barrie, ON: Author.

Levinson, C.A., Rodebaugh, T.L., Shumaker, E.A., Menatti, A.R., Weeks, J.W., White, E.K., … Liebowitz, M.R. (2015). Perception matters for clinical perfectionism and social anxiety. *Journal of Anxiety Disorders, 29,* 61–71. http://doi.org/10.1016/j.janxdis.2014.11.002

Meier, A., Reinecke, L., & Meltzer, C.E. (2016). "Facebocrastination"? Predictors of using Facebook for procrastination and its effects on students' well-being. *Computers in Human Behavior, 64,* 65–76.

Pychyl, T.A., Lee, J.M., Thibodeau, R., & Blunt, A. (2000). Five days of emotion: An experience sampling study of undergraduate student procrastination. *Journal of Social Behavior and Personality, 15,* 239–254.

Schafer, W. (1996). *Stress management for wellness* (3rd ed.). Orlando, FL: Holt, Rinehart and Winston.

Seaward, B.L. (2004). *Managing stress: Principles and strategies for health and wellbeing* (4th ed.). Boston: Jones and Bartlett.

Seaward, B.L, & Seaward, B. (2011). *Managing stress: Principles and strategies for health and well-being.* Burlington, MA: Jones and Bartlett Learning.

Sirois, F.M., & Pychyl, T. (2013). Procrastination and the priority of short-term mood regulation: consequences for future self. *Social and Personality Psychology Compass 7,* 115–127. doi:10.1111/spc3.12011

Steel, P. (2007). The nature of procrastination: A meta-analytic and theoretical review of quintessential self-regulatory failure. *Psychological Bulletin, 133*(1), 65–94.

Wohl, M.J.A., Pychyl, T.A., & Bennett, S.H. (2010). I forgive myself, now I can study: How self-forgiveness for procrastinating can reduce future procrastination. *Personality and Individual Differences, 48,* 803–808.

PART 2

PLANNING AND MAINTAINING A FITNESS PROGRAM

CHAPTER 4   Principles of Exercise

CHAPTER 5   Cardiorespiratory Fitness

CHAPTER 6   Resistance Training

PRINCIPLES OF EXERCISE

LEARNING OUTCOMES

After completing this chapter, you should be able to:

- Understand basic concepts of anatomy and physiology and how these apply to exercise.

- Explain how health-related and performance/skill-related fitness are important in law enforcement.

- Describe the physical and psychological benefits of exercise.

- Understand the principles of exercise and how to apply them in your fitness program.

- Explain the benefits of stretching and incorporate safe, effective stretching into your fitness program.

- Describe the proper way to start a fitness program.

The law enforcement communities promote the importance of "fitness for duty, fitness for life," and the health benefits of being physically fit are widely acknowledged. Law enforcement agencies strive to have officers in their best physical condition both when they are hired and throughout their careers, for a variety of reasons. These include maintaining a professional image, improving job performance, having the ability to handle shift work, reducing the likelihood of excessive force, and ensuring the quality of backup. The benefits of fitness for life include preventing health problems, reducing disability, increasing quality of life, and enjoying a longer life.

In general, physical fitness has been defined as the ability to carry out daily tasks with alertness and vigour, without undue fatigue, and with enough reserve to meet emergencies and to enjoy leisure time pursuits (Maud & Foster, 2006). In law enforcement, investing in staying fit throughout your career may prevent injuries, keep you safe, and/or save your life. Specifically, those who choose careers in law enforcement and maintain a high level of fitness have the ability:

- physically deal with altercations while performing examinations, searches, and seizures
- handle, transport, and keep custody of prisoners
- deal with unprovoked attacks by citizens, inmates
- sit or stand for prolonged periods of time
- wear weighted uniforms and gear
- deal with ergonomic issues around workspace, including vehicles and the use of smartphones (neck and eye fatigue)
- reduce the impact of fatigue from shift work
- chase, apprehend, and handcuff an individual who is fleeing
- efficiently search a person, vehicle, or cell
- easily perform body control and restraint activities

  (Adams et al., 2010; Anderson, Plecas, & Seggar, 2001; Bonneau & Brown, 1995; Jamnik et al., 2010)

In this chapter, you will learn about the components of physical fitness, the many benefits of physical activity, and the principles of exercise. As you begin your studies toward a career in law enforcement, you must apply this information by starting a fitness program that will prepare you for the physical challenges of law enforcement. The information in this chapter will serve as an important foundation for this training.

INTRODUCTION TO ANATOMY AND PHYSIOLOGY

Before we look at the principles of exercise and its benefits, it is important to have a basic understanding of how the human body is structured and how it works. Many of the concepts that we will discuss later with respect to fitness standards and leading a healthy lifestyle—in particular, ways to improve our bodies' function and avoid harming them—will build on this knowledge. This section describes the basics of human anatomy and physiology so that you can develop skills to meet the physical demands of daily life, physical activities, sports, and job-related performance.

CELLS, TISSUES, AND ORGANS

The human body is a complex system of parts that work together. The building blocks of all living organisms are cells. There are trillions of cells in the human body and they are grouped together into four basic kinds of tissue, each of which performs a specific function:

1. *Epithelial tissue* is made up of tightly packed cells. One of its most important functions is protection. It covers our whole body in the form of the outer layer of our skin, lines the digestive tract, and surrounds the organs, keeping them separate from one another and holding them in place.

2. *Connective tissue* adds support and structure to the body. There are several types of connective tissue, including tendons, ligaments, cartilage, blood, bone, and fat tissue.

3. *Muscle tissue* is specialized tissue that can contract. Muscle is made up of specialized proteins (actin and myosin) that slide past one another allowing movement.

4. *Nerve tissue* helps coordinate actions of other tissues by generating electrical signals and transmitting them down the spinal cord to the parts of the body.

Organs are structures that perform a function or functions in the body. They are made up of two or more types of tissue. All mammals possess these ten major organ systems:

1. The *circulatory system* transports oxygen, nutrients, and wastes through the body. It includes the heart, blood vessels, and blood.

2. The *lymphatic system* defends against disease by destroying viruses and microbes, and removes excess tissue fluid to the blood. It includes the lymph nodes, lymph, and white blood cells.

3. The *digestive system* breaks down food, absorbs nutrients, and eliminates non-useable materials. It includes the mouth, stomach, and intestines.

4. The *endocrine system* transmits chemical messages through the body, working with the nervous system. It includes the many glands in the body that secrete hormones, such as the thyroid and pituitary glands.

5. The *muscular system* allows us to move voluntarily, and controls involuntary movements in the body such as circulation. It includes the body's skeletal and smooth muscles.

6. The *nervous system* transmits electrical messages through the body to produce movement. It receives, processes, and reacts to stimuli, and with the endocrine system controls processes such as circulation and digestion. It includes the brain and spinal cord.

7. The *reproductive system* produces cells that allow humans to reproduce. It includes the ovaries in females and the testes in males.

8. The *respiratory system* exchanges gas between the blood and the outside environment, absorbing oxygen and expelling carbon dioxide. Among other organs, it involves the lungs and the nose.

9. The *skeletal system* provides structure and support for the body, and protects the organs. With the muscular system, it allows movement. It includes bone, cartilage, and ligaments.

10. The *excretory system* filters out wastes, toxins, and excess water. Among other organs, it involves the kidneys and bladder.

In the next section, we'll look more closely at the skeletal and muscular systems. We will explore the circulatory and respiratory systems in more detail in Chapter 5.

FYI

METABOLISM

Chemical processes happen constantly within our bodies. Our **metabolism** converts the food we eat into the energy our bodies need to function, and also affects how efficiently we use that energy. It is controlled by our nervous system and by hormones secreted by the glands of the endocrine system.

Various factors determine our metabolic rate, or how quickly our metabolism works. These include our body size, age, gender, genes, amount of body fat and lean muscle tissue, level of physical activity, presence of illness, mental state, and drug use. Even though we cannot change some of these factors, we can increase our metabolic rate through exercise. Aerobic workouts can help burn more calories in the short term, and building up muscles through weight training helps increase a person's metabolic rate in the long term.

BONES AND MUSCLES

There are 206 bones in the adult human body, including 29 in the skull, 26 in the spinal column, and 126 in the limbs. Our bones give our bodies form and serve a number of other functions, which help determine their individual sizes and shapes. Long bones in the arms and legs function as levers, while short ones (for example, in the wrist) provide additional flexibility. Other bones protect our organs, such as the sternum, which protects the lungs and heart, and the skull, which protects the brain.

The bones of the human body are shown in Figure 4.1.

Our bones meet at joints and are attached to each other by strong, fibrous connective tissue called ligaments. The end of each bone is covered with resilient and smooth tissue called cartilage. It acts like a rubber-like padding that covers and protects the end of the bone. While some joints do not move (for example, the fixed joints in the skull), the most common kind, called synovial joints, function as pivot points, allowing for varying degrees of bending, twisting, or sliding and thereby permitting us to move. The full movement potential of a joint—that is, the degree to which it can move in each direction—is called its range of motion.

Joints are classified according to the type of movement they allow. In a hinge joint—such as an elbow or a knee joint—the bones are connected in a way that allows movement in one plane only (flexion and extension). But in a ball-and-socket joint—such as a shoulder or a hip joint—the round head of one bone is held in the cup-like cavity of another bone, allowing movement in all directions.

DID YOU KNOW?

The longest bone of your body is the femur, or thigh bone, measuring approximately one-quarter of your height, while the smallest is the staples bone in your ear, measuring just one-quarter of a centimetre.

FIGURE 4.1 Skeletal Front View

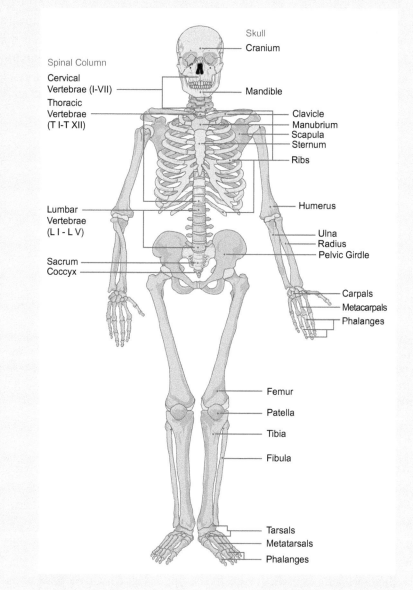

We would not be able to move our bones if not for our muscles, which stretch across joints and attach bone to bone, and **tendons**, the tough cords of tissue that attach our muscles to our bones. However, our muscles do not only allow us to move. They are constantly working to hold us up, to stabilize our joints, and to provide other involuntary movements. Figure 4.2 shows the tendons and ligaments of the lower leg

Humans have three types of muscle tissue, each with a specific function

1. *Cardiac muscle*, also called myocardium, is found only in the heart. Myocardium allows the heart to contract continuously without tiring, in response to nerve signals from the brain.

FIGURE 4.2 Tendons and Ligaments

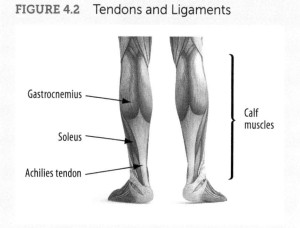

2. *Skeletal muscle* is controlled voluntarily by the nervous system and the brain and allows us to move.

3. *Smooth muscle* is an involuntary muscle that is controlled automatically by signals from the brain and body and plays a key role in functions that happen without our thinking about them. Almost every organ contains smooth muscle including the digestive tract and circulatory, respiratory, and excretory systems.

Figure 4.3 shows the different kinds of muscles in the human body.

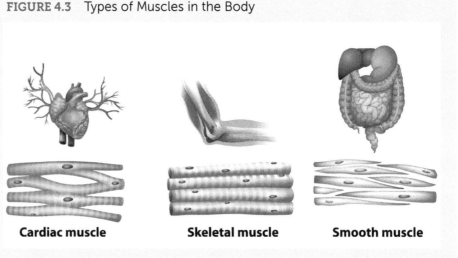

FIGURE 4.3 Types of Muscles in the Body

Cardiac muscle   **Skeletal muscle**   **Smooth muscle**

We have approximately 640 muscles in our bodies, which can make up half of our weight. Like our bones, our muscles come in different sizes and shapes, which determine their functions. You do not need to know the names of all of them, but you should be familiar with the major muscle *groups*. The exercises described in this text, and in the accompanying *Fit for Duty, Fit for Life* training guide, refer to these larger groups to indicate which muscles a particular exercise is training. For example, the two major muscle groups in the upper leg, which we refer to as the hamstrings and the quadriceps, are actually made up of three and four muscles, respectively. The individual muscles within these groups work together to carry out their group's function.

Figure 4.4 shows the major muscle groups.

Refer to **assignment 4.1** at www.emond.ca/fitness5e and see how many of the body's bones and muscles you can identify and name.

HOW DO MUSCLES WORK?

Our skeletal muscles are composed of bundles of cells called *muscle fibres* (Figure 4.5). Each of these long, tube-like cells is packed with hundreds of thinner fibres, made of protein, called *myofibrils*. Myofibrils in turn contain two kinds of *myofilaments*: thin filaments, made of actin proteins, and thick filaments, made of myosin proteins. The thick and thin filaments are organized into bundles called *sarcomeres*.

FIGURE 4.4   The Major Muscle Groups

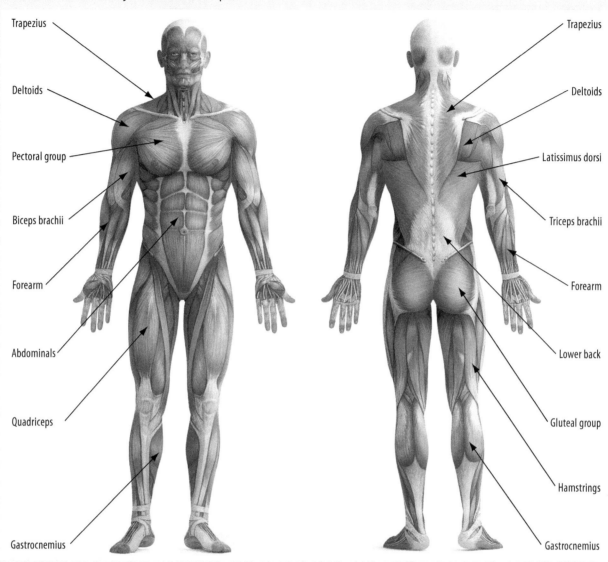

Trapezius

Deltoids

Pectoral group

Biceps brachii

Forearm

Abdominals

Quadriceps

Gastrocnemius

Trapezius

Deltoids

Latissimus dorsi

Triceps brachii

Forearm

Lower back

Gluteal group

Hamstrings

Gastrocnemius

FIGURE 4.5   Muscle Fibre

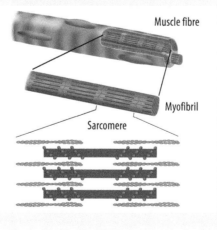

Muscle fibre

Myofibril

Sarcomere

When a muscle is relaxed, the thick and thin filaments within a sarcomere overlap each other slightly. When a nerve impulse tells a muscle fibre to contract, the thick and thin filaments slide past each other until they overlap, shortening the sarcomere (Figure 4.6). The same action happens to every sarcomere within a muscle fibre, causing the muscle fibre to contract. As the load increases, more muscle fibres are recruited by the central nervous system and a stronger force is generated by the muscle.

Conversely, when a muscle stretches, the overlap of the actin and myosin filaments decreases, allowing the muscle fibre to elongate. Once the muscle fibres reach their maximum length, the surrounding connective tissue is stretched. The more fibres that are stretched, the greater the length developed by the stretched muscle.

Because muscle fibres work as a result of electrical impulses, our muscles need to be insulated from one another to prevent the activation of one fibre from activating others—for example, so that we can contract our quadriceps without contracting our glutes. A connective tissue wrapping around individual muscles isolates them from others.

FIGURE 4.6 Relaxed and Contracted Muscle Fibre

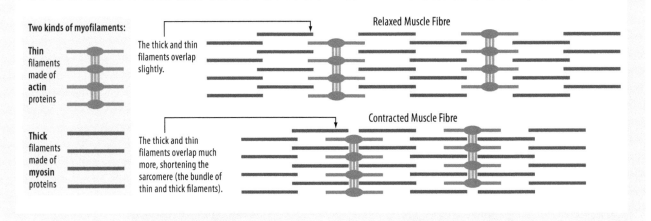

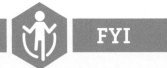

FYI

STRAINS VERSUS SPRAINS

Strains and sprains are two common injuries, but they are not the same thing.

A **strain** refers to a muscle or tendon that has been stretched or torn by applying too much tension or pressure. Strains cause pain in the muscle, tenderness, and sometimes swelling and bruising. Warming up properly, which increases blood circulation to the muscles, can prevent strains.

A **sprain** is an injury in which ligaments are either overstretched or torn. Sprains can be mild, moderate, or severe. Ankles and wrists are the most common joints to be sprained. Because sprains swell and appear bruised, they can be confused with broken bones.

You will learn more about both these common injuries in Chapter 14.

TYPES OF MUSCLE FIBRES

Our muscles contain two different kinds of fibres: fast-twitch and slow-twitch. Most of the muscles in our body contain both types of fibres.

- *Fast-twitch fibres* can contract very quickly, providing powerful acceleration. They build force rapidly but also use up oxygen and muscular energy rapidly (usually in less than 60 seconds, or 1 to 3 reps). This means they can produce small amounts of energy very fast but are easily fatigued.

    Fast-twitch fibres are bigger in diameter and contain fewer mitochondria than slow-twitch fibres. Because they do not use oxygen to produce energy, they do not require a rich supply of blood. For this reason, muscles that contain a lot of fast-twitch fibres are lighter in colour than muscles that contain a lot of slow-twitch muscle fibres.

- *Slow-twitch fibres* produce large amounts of energy slowly. They build force slowly, consume less energy, and use muscular energy more gradually. They are more resistant to fatigue than fast-twitch fibres, so they can work for longer periods without becoming tired.

    Slow-twitch fibres are smaller in diameter than fast-twitch fibres. They contain more mitochondria and require a rich supply of oxygenated blood to produce the energy they need for muscle contraction. Muscles that contain a lot of slow-twitch fibres are red because of the many blood vessels they contain.

The ratio of slow-twitch to fast-twitch fibres in our muscles is determined by our genetics. It is possible to specifically train one fibre type, but you cannot change slow-twitch fibres into fast-twitch fibres and vice versa.

TABLE 4.1 Summary of Muscle Fibre Comparison

FIBRE TYPE	CONTRACTION SPEED	TIME TO PEAK (MILLISECONDS)	RATE OF FATIGUE	MITOCHONDRIA	OXIDATIVE CAPACITY
I (slow-twitch)	Slow	100	Slow	Many	High
IIA (fast-twitch)	Fast	50	Fast	Few	Low
IIB (fast-twitch)	Very fast	25	Fast	Few	Low

Because of these differences, fast-twitch and slow-twitch fibres serve different purposes in the body and are useful for different kinds of activities. Fast-twitch fibres are good for sprinting and for quick movements, like jumping. These kinds of fibres make up the muscles that move the eyes, and are found in large numbers in the muscles of the arms. Slow-twitch fibres, by contrast, are useful in helping maintain posture and in activities that require endurance, like long distance running. The soleus (a muscle in the calf) is made up mainly of slow-twitch fibres, as are the muscles in the back that help keep the spine upright and those in the neck that keep the head upright.

HOW MUSCLES COOPERATE WITH EACH OTHER

Our muscles work both as movers *and* as stabilizers. Certain muscles work primarily as movers (for example, the biceps muscle), while others serve primarily to give stability to the joints (for example, the multifidus, one of the muscles in the back). Depending on the movement involved, many muscles can function as movers *or* stabilizers.

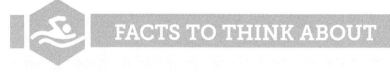

Our muscles move our bones by contracting and relaxing. They are arranged around joints in pairs known as agonists and antagonists (see below). When muscles cause a limb to move through the joint's range of motion, they usually act in cooperating groups composed of the following:

- **Agonists** are muscles that move a bone in one direction. They contract to move a limb through a normal range of motion. Agonists are known as prime movers because they generate movement.

- **Antagonists** are muscles that move a bone in the direction opposite to that of the agonist. They return the limb to the original position. They also stabilize our joints.

- **Synergists** are muscles that assist the agonists indirectly in producing a joint's movement. Because synergists play various roles, several terms are used to describe them, including stabilizer, neutralizer, and fixator.

- **Fixators** are the muscles that provide the support to hold the rest of the body in place while movement occurs.

Muscles are not agonists, antagonists, synergists, or fixators in isolation; they act as such specifically in the context of particular movements. For example, the biceps muscle is not always an agonist, but it is an agonist in elbow flexion, which moves the lower arm toward the shoulder.

Some common agonist/antagonist muscle pairs include:

- biceps/triceps
- quadriceps/hamstrings
- pectorals/latissimus dorsi
- abdominals/spinal erectors

Many people focus on agonists in training sessions, sometimes causing imbalance and dysfunction when these muscles are overtrained at the expense of undertraining antagonists. For example, in seeking to develop their chest muscles, some people over-develop their pectorals (agonists) but do not adequately develop the rhomboids and mid-/lower trapezius in the back (antagonists). This can eventually pull the scapulae out of alignment, causing the shoulders to round forward. For the best possible performance, it is important to achieve a balance between agonists and antagonists.

FYI

DESCRIBING BODY POSITIONS AND MOVEMENTS

There are a number of terms you should be familiar with that relate to the body and its movements, as you will encounter them in the names and descriptions of exercises.

CATEGORY	TERM	DEFINITION
POSITIONS	**Supine**	The position of lying face up (for example, when doing crunches)
	Prone	The position of lying face down (for example, when beginning a push-up)
MOVEMENTS *Note that the following terms always refer to the joints involved in an action, as this is where movement occurs.*	**Extension**	Any movement that moves a limb or body part from a bent to a straight position or opens a joint (for example, a backbend or extending your arm or leg behind the midline of your body).
	Flexion	Any movement that bends a limb or a joint, or brings the bones closer together (for example, elbow flexion occurs in a bicep curl).
	Adduction	This refers to the arms, legs, fingers, or toes moving toward the midline of the body (for example, if you are standing with your legs hip-width apart, adduction at the hip joint will bring your feet closer together; if your arms are above your head, adduction of the shoulder joints will bring them back down to your sides).
	Abduction	This refers to the arms, legs, fingers, or toes moving away from the midline of the body (for example, abduction of the joints at the base of your knuckles will spread your fingers apart; if your arms are down at your sides, abducting the shoulder joints will raise your arms).
	Medial (internal) rotation	This action, which occurs at the shoulder and hip joints, turns a limb in toward the midline of the body (for example, medial or internal rotation of the hip joint occurs when you turn your left leg so that your left toes are pointing toward the right).
	Lateral (external) rotation	This action, which occurs at the shoulder and hip joints, turns a limb away from the midline of the body (for example, if your feet are together, opening your toes out so that your feet form a "V").
	Rotation	This refers to the spinal column and neck twisting either to the right or the left (for example, turning your head to look over your shoulder).
	Circumduction	This action occurs at the shoulder and hip joints and combines flexion, extension, adduction, and abduction to create a circular movement (for example, the action in your shoulder joint when swimming the backstroke).

MUSCULAR CONTRACTIONS

When we speak of a muscle "contracting," this does not necessarily imply that the muscle shortens. Instead, it means only that tension has been generated. Muscles can contract in the following ways:

- In an isotonic contraction, a muscle contracts in response to a constant force or load that is applied to it. There are two types of isotonic contractions:

  — *Concentric contractions* take place when the muscle actively shortens against the opposing load and the ends of the muscle are drawn closer together. A biceps curl on the way up is an example of an exercise that produces a concentric contraction.

  — *Eccentric contractions* take place when the muscle actively lengthens as it resists the load and the ends of the muscle are pulled farther apart. A biceps curl on the way down is an example of an exercise that produces an eccentric contraction.

  Eccentric contractions are much stronger than concentric contractions and therefore can produce greater exercise benefits. However, eccentric contractions cause more muscle soreness and increase the risk of soft tissue damage.

- In an isometric contraction, the muscle is activated but does not lengthen or shorten. There is no movement, and the muscle remains at a fixed length. This kind of muscular action occurs when muscles attempt to push or pull an immovable object—for example, if you were to stand facing a wall, extend your arms out at a 90-degree angle, and push against the wall.

- In an isokinetic contraction, the muscle length changes to contract maximally throughout the full range of movement. Various isokinetic exercise machines are available, which generally involve the use of a wheel, lever, crank, or similar device. The most popular, called the isokinetic dynamometer, provides resistance that matches that of the user as it measures the strength and power of various muscle groups.

Figure 4.7 illustrates the difference between isotonic and isometric contractions. Concentric repetitions in weight training cause muscles to shorten in length. Over time, your muscles can shorten to the point where their range of motion becomes restricted. This can result in a decrease in the amount of force you can generate in the muscle. However, stretching can counter the effects of concentric repetitions so that your elongated muscle can generate more force.

WHAT IS TRAINING?

In the simplest terms, training refers to making your body more efficient. If you can train your body through general fitness activities (for example, running or weight training), you will be able to do parts of your job more efficiently (for example, chasing potential criminals, enduring a physical altercation, or being able to function at 4 a.m. when asked to search for a lost person).

FIGURE 4.7   Difference Between Isotonic and Isometric Contractions

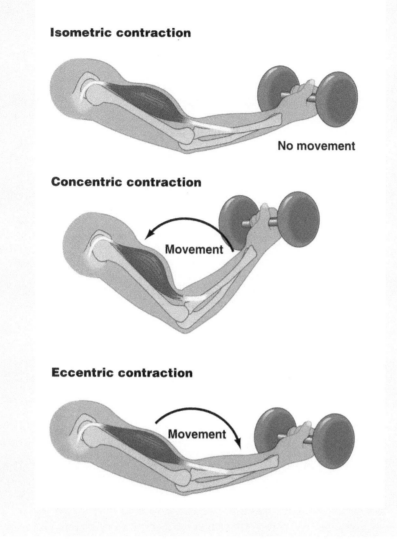

This process and the changes that take place depend on the individual who is training and the goals that he or she has set. The goal may be to gain more muscle, to reduce body fat, to have the best time on the 1.5-mile (2.4-km) run, or to reduce stress.

Training is an individual process. It depends on the objectives of the workout and the attributes of the individual involved. There are a number of ways in which to modify your body's attributes, and each person must understand that there may be a variety of options available to achieve those changes. Finding out which way works best for you will take time and effort. Human performance results cannot be completely standardized. In other words, no one program works the same for each person. It is impossible to expect that a fitness instructor would be able to give your entire class the same program and have the same results for everyone by the end of the course. Ultimately, you will have to do a great deal of training on your own to find a program that works best for you.

FYI

"NO PAIN, NO GAIN"?

It is common to feel varying degrees of soreness in the muscles both during and sometimes for several days following strenuous exercise. The two kinds of pain have different causes.

When we exercise vigorously, we may feel soreness or a burning feeling in an active muscle—for example, during sprints. This soreness results from a buildup of lactic acid, which occurs whenever the muscles are active for more than a minute or two and become fatigued. This usually encourages us to stop the activity. Within a few hours to a day, the lactic acid is cleared away by the body and the burning disappears.

In addition to soreness during strenuous activity, we may also experience **delayed-onset muscle soreness (DOMS)**, particularly after trying a new exercise or suddenly increasing the length or intensity of our workout. DOMS is characterized by severe muscle tenderness, stiffness, decreased strength, and decreased range of motion that usually peaks between 24 and 72 hours after a hard workout. Placing new demands or stresses on a particular muscle can cause microscopic tears in the muscle fibres, which can cause soreness, swelling, and inflammation as the muscle repairs itself. After the rebuilding process—which is one reason why you must give your body sufficient time to recover following a hard workout—the muscle is stronger than before. This means that the next time you do the activity that caused the DOMS, you will likely experience less soreness. To cause the same amount of micro-damage to the muscle fibre the next time, you would need to add more stress to those muscles. This is the principle behind building muscle mass.

Research has shown that eccentric contractions result in more muscle cell damage than concentric contractions, so exercises involving these kinds of contractions—such as downhill running—will result in increased soreness in the days following the exercise.

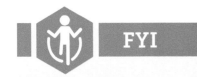

FYI

The Police Fitness Personnel of Ontario (PFPO) has advocated the importance of health-related fitness in policing for over 30 years. It compiles evidence to support the fact that officers who are fit will be able to do their jobs more effectively and safely, and has promoted a lapel-pin fitness award (the Ontario Police Fitness Award (OPFA), discussed in Chapter 1). Ontario Corrections and Bruce Power have adopted similar programs.

HEALTH-RELATED FITNESS

The five components of health-related fitness are cardiorespiratory endurance, muscular strength, muscular endurance, flexibility, and a healthy body composition. Regular physical activity leads to improvements in all five areas.

CARDIORESPIRATORY ENDURANCE

Cardiorespiratory endurance (heart and respiratory system endurance) is the ability of the heart to pump blood throughout the body efficiently. This means your body can perform prolonged large-muscle activities, such as swimming or jogging, at moderate to high intensity. It is probably the most important component of fitness. When you regularly engage in activities that improve cardiorespiratory endurance, you enhance your body's ability to regulate blood flow and use oxygen and other fuels. As a result, you lower your resting heart rate and blood pressure, and your ability to dissipate heat increases. Having the stamina for a foot chase is one example of how cardiorespiratory endurance is important in law enforcement. Cardiorespiratory endurance is dealt with in greater detail in Chapter 5.

MUSCULAR STRENGTH

Muscular strength is the amount of force a muscle can produce with a single maximum effort. Muscular strength can be developed by training with weights, kettlebells, medicine balls, or body based exercises (for example, push-ups or chin-ups). Strong muscles are important for daily activities such as lifting and pulling heavy objects, climbing stairs, vacuuming, and carrying groceries. Abundant musculature provides good structural support for the back and helps prevent back and leg pain. It enhances recreational activities—for example, by helping a player jump higher in volleyball, hit a tennis ball harder, and kick a soccer ball farther.

Muscular strength is also important for overall health. A greater muscle mass increases the body's metabolic rate (the rate at which the body breaks down food, producing energy). Strength training is vital to prevent diseases such as osteoporosis.

Muscular strength is dealt with in greater detail in Chapter 6 and in the *Fit for Duty, Fit for Life* training guide that accompanies this textbook.

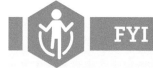

FYI

BLOOD PRESSURE AND RESTING HEART RATE

Among the many benefits of physical activity are lower blood pressure and a lower resting heart rate:

- As blood travels through the body, it exerts a force against the blood vessels. The force is called blood pressure, and it changes over the course of a day. When blood pressure stays high for a longer period of time, it is called high blood pressure, or hypertension, and it poses health risks. Hypertension makes the heart work harder and can cause the walls of the arteries to harden (called arteriosclerosis). Among other medical problems, this increases the risk of heart disease and stroke.

- Our resting heart rate is influenced by factors including our genes, age, and fitness level, as well as medical conditions, medication, and stress. A higher resting heart rate is a risk factor for heart disease, and is correlated with an increased risk for high blood pressure and atherosclerosis. In addition to exercise, you can lower your resting heart rate by using stress-reducing techniques, avoiding tobacco products, and losing weight.

MUSCULAR ENDURANCE

Muscular endurance is the ability of a muscle to sustain a prolonged contraction or to contract over and over again. Muscular endurance is important for injury prevention and proper posture. Without a good back and well-built abdominal muscles, a person's spine is subjected to stress that can result in lower-back pain. For law enforcement officers, who must wear an equipment belt weighing 7 to 9 kilograms, core endurance is important. Muscular endurance can be achieved by exercising with weight-training equipment and body-based activities (see Chapter 6 and Fit for Duty for more information about muscular endurance). In these exercises, light weights are combined with many repetitions.

FLEXIBILITY

Flexibility is the ability to move the joints freely through their full range of motion. As a person ages, lack of flexibility can create poor posture and be debilitating. Stiff joints and a restricted range of motion can lead to lower-back problems, an issue that we will look at in Chapter 11. Without flexibility, it is easier to get hurt when reaching or twisting inappropriately. In particular, lower-back and hamstring inflexibility can be issues when getting in and out of a police cruiser. Greater flexibility leads to muscles that are more supple and less prone to injury. Flexibility can be maintained by following a regular fitness program.

You will read more about flexibility later in this chapter.

BODY COMPOSITION

Body composition (discussed in greater detail in Chapter 7) refers to the proportion of lean tissue (muscle and bone) to fat in the body. A healthy body composition requires a large proportion of lean tissue and a small proportion of fat. Fat is important for organ protection, for control of heat production and heat loss, and as a source of energy that the body can use. However, people with excessive fat are at risk for joint problems, back pain, heart disease, high blood pressure, stroke, gallbladder disease, cancer, and other illnesses. The healthiest way to lose fat is to exercise and to adhere to a sensible diet recommended by your doctor. Weight training is the best way to increase lean tissue mass.

PERFORMANCE/SKILL-RELATED FITNESS

The six components of performance/skill-related fitness are speed, coordination, reaction time, agility, balance, and power. These are greatly enhanced when you exercise regularly. Although not considered essential for a healthy life, the six components are especially important in law enforcement—for example, if you are involved in a foot chase, a physical altercation, or a rescue. All of these situations require you to be in top physical condition and be able to respond to trouble quickly and appropriately. Both health-related and performance/skill-related fitness are evaluated by the Physical Readiness Evaluation for Policing (PREP) test, the Fitness Test for Ontario Correctional Officers (FITCO), the Physical Ability Requirement Evaluation (PARE) test, the Police Officer Physical Abilities Test (POPAT), the Correction Officers Physical Abilities Test (COPAT), the Alberta Physical Readiness Evaluation for Police (A-PREP), the Fitness for Operational Requirements of Canadian Armed Forces Employment (FORCE) for the Canadian Armed Forces, and the Standardized Physical Abilities Test (SPAT) for Quebec police officers. These tests will be discussed in detail in the Appendix.

SPEED

Speed is the ability to move quickly. During a foot chase, for example, a law enforcement officer requires leg and foot speed.

COORDINATION

Coordination involves the mind and body working together to perform motor tasks smoothly and accurately. Good coordination is needed, for example, to jump over obstacles, kick a soccer ball, and hit a golf ball. Using firearms also requires good coordination. Without it, hitting a target is almost impossible.

REACTION TIME

Reaction time is the time that elapses between stimulation and the beginning of a person's reaction to the stimulus. For a law enforcement officer, being able to react quickly to a volatile situation can mean the difference between success and failure and even between staying alive and getting killed.

AGILITY

Agility is the ability to rapidly and accurately change the body's direction of movement. Skiing, mountain biking, and self-defence are examples of activities that require agility.

BALANCE

Balance refers to the body's ability to maintain equilibrium while stationary or moving. Walking across a support beam, performing on a balance beam, and self-defence are activities that require good balance.

POWER

Power is the ability to transform energy into force at a rapid rate. Power is necessary in sports such as discus throwing and the shot put. In law enforcement, power is necessary to move a person out of the way, scale a wall, or jump a railing.

THE HEALTH BENEFITS OF PHYSICAL ACTIVITY

Before reading any further, refer to **assignment 4.2** at www.emond.ca/fitness5e and see if you can list some of the health benefits of physical activity.

Regular physical activity produces long-term improvements in body function. As shown in Table 4.2, these benefits are both physical and psychological.

> **DID YOU KNOW?**
>
> Between 2012 and 2014, we have seen a decline from one in five adults to one in ten adults who achieved the recommended 150 minutes of moderate to vigorous physical activity (in 10-minute periods) per week set out by the *Canadian Physical Activity Guidelines* for adults and for older adults.
>
> SOURCES: Health Canada, 2013; Statistics Canada, 2015.

TABLE 4.2 Physical and Psychological Benefits of Physical Activity

PHYSICAL BENEFITS	• maintenance of healthy weight • improved digestion • improved posture and balance • stronger muscles and bones • increased bone density • better circulation • strengthened heart and lungs • strengthened immune system • prolonged good health in seniors • reduced risk of premature death from heart disease, stroke, and certain types of cancer • reduced risk of developing high blood pressure; lower total blood cholesterol and triglycerides and increased high-density lipoproteins (HDL or "good" cholesterol)
PSYCHOLOGICAL BENEFITS	• reduced stress levels • relief from symptoms of depression and anxiety • increased energy • improved sleep • more confidence and a more positive outlook on life • improved mood • prolonged independence in seniors • better quality of life

SOURCES: Statistics Canada, 2012; Statistics Canada, 2014b; Statistics Canada, 2016.

Refer to **assignment 4.3** at www.emond.ca/fitness5e and list the physical and psychological benefits of physical activity that are most important to you.

We know that fitness is important, but we are learning how important it is to be active throughout the day and to limit the time we are sitting. It is not just about adding a workout to our day but also increasing the amount of time we move throughout the day. Physical activity levels among children and youth are low, with 62 percent of waking hours—or 8.6 hours every day—devoted to sedentary activities (CBC News, 2011). Inactive time increases with age: the same study found that adults were sedentary for 69 percent of their waking hours, or 9.5 to 10 hours per day (Colley et al., 2011a). Sedentary behaviour includes sitting for hours in front of computers or workstations, sitting in classes, and playing on electronic devices. It also refers to sitting in a cruiser or security vehicle, watching security or correctional monitors, writing reports, or sitting in court. Sitting has now become an independent risk factor for increasing your risk for various diseases. Those who sit the most (versus those who sit the least) have 112 percent increased risk of diabetes, 147 percent increased risk of cardiovascular disease, and are 50 percent more likely to die prematurely (of all causes) (Wilmot et al., 2012).

Combining the rates of obese and overweight adults indicates that 62 percent (8.1 million) of Canadian men and 45.1 percent (5.8 million) of Canadian women had an increased health risk because of excess weight (Statistics Canada, 2013; Statistics Canada, 2014a). Approximately one in four adults are obese and this not only has a negative impact on health but the quality of life (Public Health Ontario, 2014).

Some of the physical issues that overweight and obese individuals face when trying to become physically active include lacking the flexibility to move through the entire range of motion of the exercise; stress on bones and joints, especially knees (one third of the injuries); increased risk of back injuries; increased risk of fractures; and osteoarthritis (a degeneration of cartilage and its underlying bone within a joint) (Hootman et al., 2002; Janney & Jakicic, 2010).

> ### DID YOU KNOW?
> Sedentary behaviour is "any waking behaviour characterized by an energy expenditure less than or equal to 1.5 METs while in a sitting or reclining position" (a MET is equivalent to spending about 1.8 calories per minute for a 70-kilogram person).
>
> SOURCE: Jetté, Sidney, & Blümchen, 1990.

FACTS TO THINK ABOUT

CANADIAN YOUTH, PHYSICAL ACTIVITY, AND WEIGHT ISSUES

- Four out of five Canadian adolescents do not participate in the recommended volume of physical activity suggested by the *Canadian Physical Activity Guidelines*.
- Slightly more primary school than secondary school youth are physically active on a daily basis (19 percent versus 17 percent). Only 6 percent of Canadian children take the recommended 12,000 steps per day.
- Only 7 to 10 percent of youth under the age of 19 are meeting the guidelines of at least 60 minutes of moderate-to-vigorous physical activity daily.
- Overweight children experience physical and psychological health problems. They are at increased risk of developing chronic diseases later in life, because they are more likely to become overweight adults.
- The most profound concern has been a progressive increase in the body mass index (BMI) of Canadian youth (aged 7 to 13) noted from 1981 to 1996, with the prevalence of obesity in this age group more than doubling over this period.
- As of 2009, 25 percent of children and youth were overweight or obese.

SOURCES: Active Healthy Kids Canada, 2014; Barnes, Colley, & Tremblay, 2012; Canadian Adolescents at Risk Research Network, 2004; CSEP, 2011a; Colley, Garriguet, Janssen, Craig, Clarke, & Tremblay, 2011b; Hobin, Leatherdale, Manske, Dubin, Elliott, & Veugelers, 2013; Janssen & LeBlanc, 2010; Perez, 2003; Tremblay et al., 2010; Tremblay & Willms, 2000.

FIGURE 4.8   Adults Who Are Obese, 2014, by Province and Territory

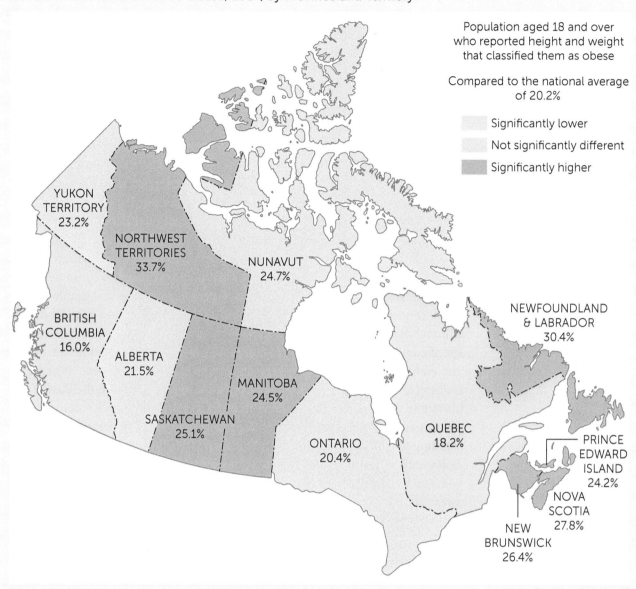

Population aged 18 and over who reported height and weight that classified them as obese

Compared to the national average of 20.2%

Significantly lower
Not significantly different
Significantly higher

YUKON TERRITORY 23.2%

NORTHWEST TERRITORIES 33.7%

NUNAVUT 24.7%

NEWFOUNDLAND & LABRADOR 30.4%

BRITISH COLUMBIA 16.0%

ALBERTA 21.5%

MANITOBA 24.5%

SASKATCHEWAN 25.1%

ONTARIO 20.4%

QUEBEC 18.2%

PRINCE EDWARD ISLAND 24.2%

NOVA SCOTIA 27.8%

NEW BRUNSWICK 26.4%

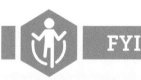

FYI

COSTS OF PHYSICAL INACTIVITY

If the economic burden of inactivity, smoking, and excessive weight continue at the 2012 rates ($50.3 billion) (Janssen, 2012), we will see an increase of at least 4.9 percent annually (Krueger, Krueger, & Koot, 2015; Krueger, Turner, Krueger, & Ready, 2014). The Canadian government has undertaken the development of a healthy living strategy with an emphasis on physical activity, where areas such as healthy body weight, mental health, and injury prevention will be identified (Ministry of Health, 2005). Since 2010, there has been an added focus on preventing weight gain in children and youth as well as getting them to be more physically active (Public Health Agency of Canada, 2010).

The implications of health-related diseases associated with physical inactivity can be reversed if individuals are willing to take ownership of their physical well-being. As you research the components of physical training, remember the goals you set in Chapter 2. They will assist you in determining which goals may be most important.

THE PRINCIPLES OF EXERCISE

The goal of exercise is to bring about some of the physical and psychological benefits discussed above and to improve the body's functioning. Although there is inevitably a limit to the level of fitness and performance you can attain—a limit that varies from person to person—training gives everyone the chance to experience at least some of the physical and psychological benefits of exercise.

Particular fitness outcomes require particular exercises. For example, to conform to the aerobic component of the Bona Fide Occupational Requirements (BFORs) (in the Appendix), you have to be willing to devote some time to running. Léger (1985; Léger & Lambert, 1982) has equated level 7.0 in the shuttle run component of the PREP to running 1.5 miles (2.4 km) in approximately 12 minutes (Public Safety Canada, 2008). The level at which a person completes the shuttle run does not necessarily correlate with the time that it takes the person to run that distance, although results do indicate that those who can successfully run 1.5 miles in the specified time have no difficulty in completing level 7.0 in the shuttle run. Strength and endurance training is also very important in law enforcement. Whether it is training for use of force, walking, foot pursuits, or arresting an individual, it is important to develop muscular balance in order to respond to these emergencies and prevent and/or rehabilitate injuries, especially low-back problems from sitting or standing too long (Anderson, Zutz, & Plecas, 2011; Bullock, 2007). Exercise principles outline the criteria that guide your training. Following these principles well will lead to successful outcomes. Let's look at those principles that you need to be aware of when planning a fitness program.

THE PRINCIPLES OF PHYSICAL TRAINING

The basic principles of physical training are progressive overload, specificity, individuality, reversibility, diminishing returns, and recovery (CSEP, 2003).

THE PRINCIPLE OF PROGRESSIVE OVERLOAD

Progressive overload refers to placing a greater stress or load on the body than it is used to. The body needs to be subjected to increasing gradual demands in order to produce continual improvements. If the body is not worked hard enough or, on the other hand, is worked too hard, physical training will not produce benefits. Excessive exercise may in fact cause detraining and injuries.

The principle of progressive overload takes into account that both the skeletal and cardiac muscles adapt to the overloading. This means that the body becomes more efficient and able to handle greater loads. For example, in order to complete a 1.5-mile run easily, your training has to go from a jog to a run, from running for 20 minutes to 40 minutes, and increasing your pace from about 9 to 12 kilometres per hour. If you decrease your levels of exercise, the gains that you achieved will start to disappear.

Progressive overload is accomplished by gradually increasing the frequency, intensity, time, or type of exercise. This is known as the FITT principle.

THE FITT PRINCIPLE

The FITT principle is a set of guidelines to adhere to in order to benefit from a specific fitness program. It includes:

- F—*Frequency* Most objectives require a training level of three to five times a week. People whose fitness level is low should begin with three times a week, and then gradually build up to five. Remember the *Canadian Physical Activity Guidelines* say at least 150 minutes of moderate- to vigorous-intensity aerobic physical activity per week for cardio, in bouts of 10 minutes or more, and for muscle and bone strengthening activities using major muscle groups, at least two days per week (CSEP, 2011b). Once your goals are reached, physical activity two or three times a week is needed to maintain your fitness level.

- I—*Intensity* To benefit from an exercise, you need to increase the intensity of the exercise gradually over the course of your training program—for example, by slowly increasing the weight pushed or pulled for strength training, gradually raising jogging speed to increase cardiorespiratory intensity, or stretching muscles more and more with each workout to increase flexibility. But increasing the intensity of a workout must be done in small steps to avoid injuries. Also, for beginners, intensity is less important than frequency and duration.

- T—*Time* (duration) Exercise produces benefits only if your exercise sessions last for extended periods of time. As you progress, you should increase the duration of the sessions. A runner who wants to increase cardiorespiratory endurance, for example, may begin with 20-minute sessions and slowly move up to 60-minute sessions (20 to 60 minutes is typical for endurance training).

- T—*Type of exercise* The type of exercises relate to the specific program you are involved in. In aerobic training, they include activities that work large-muscle groups and that can be done in a rhythmic fashion, such as brisk walking, cycling, swimming, and running. In weight training, they include activities that focus on the muscles that you want to strengthen or increase. Bodybuilders tend to isolate a muscle group and work it to exhaustion. Athletes in sports, on the other hand, train movements rather than muscles. It is important to divide your time and energy among various types of movements—endurance, strength and power, speed and agility, and tactical—that mirror the BFOR tests, taking into account the importance of recovery time (see The Principle of Recovery, below).

THE PRINCIPLE OF SPECIFICITY

The principle of specificity refers to the body's ability to adapt to a particular type and amount of stress placed on it. To develop a particular fitness skill, you must choose exercises tailored to that skill. Over the past 20 years, the primary reason many law enforcement students have failed the shuttle run has been their lack of commitment to aerobic training—specifically, running. Although interval training, weight training, and cycling provide some cross-training effects, nothing can take the place of running. Similarly, the demands of the push–pull machine and the arm-restraint device are best met by a strength training program. A commitment to law enforcement requires a well-rounded fitness program with training components tailored to cardiorespiratory endurance, strength, and flexibility.

The specificity principle is sometimes referred to as the SAID (specific adaptation to imposed demand) principle. Muscle adaptation will occur when you place a specific demand for improvement on a specific skill. It is important, then, to train to a high aerobic level to be successful in aerobic training. It is also important to train anaerobically to manoeuvre easily up and down the stairs on all of the BFORs. It is imperative that you have leg strength to use the push–pull machine easily.

THE PRINCIPLE OF INDIVIDUALITY

The principle of individuality suggests that training programs are adjusted for personal differences such as abilities, skills, gender, age, experience, motivation, physical condition, the ability to recover after a workout, and susceptibility to injury.

These factors play a part in designing a program. For example, in weight training, individuals must either change the number of repetitions or sets they are performing, or for a few weeks change their entire program, in order to confuse the muscles into having to work in a different way and cause changes at the cellular level. It also may include how and when you are most motivated to participate in the program; whether you like exercising in the morning or at night, whether you like group activities, how your body responds to certain kinds of workouts. Remember that you can't expect to improve your cardiorespiratory system if you are training more for strength and neglecting the aerobic and anaerobic components.

THE PRINCIPLE OF REVERSIBILITY

According to the principle of reversibility, all the benefits of exercise are lost if you stop training. Atrophy occurs when muscles undergo periods of complete or near-complete inactivity. In fact, up to 20 percent of exercise benefits can be lost in the first two weeks of not training, and as much as 50 percent can be lost in less than two months. Not only do muscles lose strength with disuse, but they also decrease in size. *Detraining* is the term used to describe the time period in which someone who has undergone a significant amount of training either stops completely or to a large extent. This happens for a number of reasons, including the inability to train because of an injury, the lack of an available open gym when an individual is off-shift, a lack of motivation, or the need for family time. One way to prevent much of this loss is to maintain the intensity of your workouts, even if you cannot maintain the frequency and duration.

Equally, by overtraining—when you don't allow sufficient recovery time between workouts—you can hamper your progress. Table 4.3 explains what can happen in the body with overtraining. Overtraining syndrome is the full spectrum of overtraining and can result in hormonal, nutritional, mental/emotional, muscular, neurological, and other imbalances.

TABLE 4.3 Training Effects and Signs of Overtraining Syndrome (OTS)

EFFECTS OF OVERTRAINING	
ACUTE	CHRONIC
• Muscle worked to exhaustion • Muscles always feel sore • Traumatic orthopedic injury • Body exhausted after workout • Glycogen depleted • Sympathetic response elevated • Increased Cortisol levels (stunting or inhibiting adaptation)	• Muscles become weaker over time • Increased risk of orthopedic overuse injury • Lack of ability to concentrate • Disturbances in rhythm and flow of movement • Body becomes weaker • Glycogen depleted • Increased Parasympathetic response • Increased cortisol levels to stress resulting in risk of increased appetite and weight gain, visceral fat, diabetes • Decreased levels of testosterone
SIGNS OF OVERTRAINING RESPONSES	
SYMPATHETIC NERVOUS SYSTEM	PARASYMPATHETIC NERVOUS SYSTEM
Chronic state of "fight or flight" in which the body is under constant stress	Chronically trying to repair the body
• Increased resting heart rate and blood pressure • Decreased sports performance • Decreased maximal blood lactate concentrations • Slower recovery after exercise • Weight loss • Decreased appetite • Decreased desire to exercise • Increased irritability and depression • Increased incidence of injury • Increased incidence of infection and suppression of the immune system	• Decreased resting heart rate • Faster return of heart rate to resting value after exercise • Decreased sports performance • Decreased blood lactate concentrations during submaximal and maximal exercise • Insomnia • Unemotional behaviour

SOURCES: Andrews, Herlihy, Livingstone, Andrew, & Walker, 2002; Bruunsgaard et al., 1997; McKenzie, 1999; Meeusen et. al., 2013.

THE PRINCIPLE OF DIMINISHING RETURNS

The principle of diminishing returns is based on the fact that a person's training gains will reflect his or her prior level of training. People who have had little training make significant gains both in terms of strength and aerobic capacity. Those who are highly trained make relatively small gains. For example, those who start running at the beginning of a course for the first time are able to see significant decreases in their times (sometimes by as much as 3 to 4 minutes), while those who run regularly usually see only small gains (their run time decreases by less than one-half minute). It becomes very important to try new training methods or different equipment in order to see further gains.

Devising an exercise program that is most suited to you depends on your goals, the requirements of the law enforcement community, and your fitness level. Depending on your ability, you may have to spend substantially more time in a program to meet the demands of the BFOR standards and prepare for the demands of the job.

THE PRINCIPLE OF RECOVERY

The principle of recovery is tied to the recuperation time or amount of rest required after a workout. Torn muscle tissue needs time to repair. In cardiorespiratory training, beginners should exercise at least five times a week and leave at least a day to rest. Similarly, in weight training, beginners should allow a day's rest between each day of training. In strength training, beginners may need 48 hours or more between workouts. Also, be aware that more demanding exercise programs typically require more rest between training sessions.

People who do not feel a small increase in strength after each workout, or who experience pain with each workout, may need to reduce the frequency with which they train.

Refer to **assignment 4.4** at www.emond.ca/fitness5e and set your fitness training goals.

TRAINING METHODS

When training for the BFOR tests, it becomes necessary to focus on increasing your speed, endurance, strength, agility, and flexibility. To achieve these goals, a number of training methods have been devised to provide variety and challenge, including functional training, resistance training, interval training, high-intensity interval training (HIIT), plyometric training, concurrent training, and periodization.

FUNCTIONAL TRAINING

Functional fitness involves exercises that train your muscles to preform daily tasks by simulating common movements you do at home, at work, or in sports. It focuses on training a specific task (for example, restraining a non-compliant individual) as opposed to training the muscles that are used in the task (for example, bench press or bicep curl). Functional training includes coordination, different types of muscular contractions (concentric, eccentric, isometric), speed of movement, and range of motion through multiple joints. It can be done in all types of settings, with all types of equipment, and should supplement traditional strength training.

The focus of functional training is around locomotion (running); your ability to level change (for example, having the knee flexion to support the hips when jumping); the ability to push and pull, including throwing, pushing away, and holding objects (for example, the ability to effectively use the body control simulator in the BFOR tests); and the strength to effectively rotate (for example, change direction when running, have the ability to swing a golf club). Programs are centred around body weight exercises and/or equipment such as free weights, pulley and bands, medicine balls, stability balls, and bells. Research indicates that functional training assists muscles to be better stabilizers whereby function of a joint is enhanced.

The three key groups in need of stability training include the deep abdominals (transversus abdominis and internal oblique), hip abductors and rotators, and scapula stabilizers. This means that you first have to train with single-joint exercises to improve a larger area. For example, the Police Fitness Personnel of Ontario have advocated training transversus abdominis and multifidus to improve low-back health and reduce lower back pain. They have moved away from the crunch and curl-up (which compress lower lumbar segments, restrict the excursion of the diaphragm, weaken the pelvic floor, and cause high shearing strains across the high lumbar segments) and advocated other exercises to reduce lower back pain (see Chapter 11 for more information). By coordinating multi-joint and multi-planar (sagittal, frontal, and transverse) movements, the acts of getting in and out of a car or dealing with high-intensity, short-duration confrontations such as taking a non-compliant individual to the ground can be functional in terms of strength and range of motion. See Chapter 6 for more information.

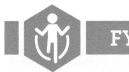

FYI

AEROBIC VERSUS ANAEROBIC EXERCISE

The two basic categories of exercise are aerobic and anaerobic. It is helpful to understand the differences between them, because both should be incorporated into any fitness routine to produce the greatest benefit.

The word "aerobic" means "with oxygen." As the name implies, aerobic exercise uses oxygen to produce the energy necessary for muscle movement, by burning fats and carbohydrates. Aerobic exercise is usually called "cardiovascular exercise," or just "cardio." It includes activities that work large muscle groups and increase the heart rate and respiration during and shortly following the exercise—for example, walking, cycling, swimming, jumping rope, and running. Aerobic exercise builds endurance and strengthens the major muscles, the lungs, and the heart. Among its many benefits are a lower resting heart rate and lower blood pressure, a decreased risk of heart disease, and improved lung function.

In contrast to "aerobic," the term "anaerobic" means "without oxygen." As the name implies, this kind of exercise does not require oxygen to produce energy, and only carbohydrates are burned. When we exercise anaerobically for longer periods of time, lactic acid accumulates and we experience muscle fatigue. Examples of anaerobic exercise include high-intensity activities that expend energy in short bursts, such as weight lifting, interval training, high intensity interval training, and the 100-m sprint. Anaerobic exercise helps increase muscle mass and strength.

RESISTANCE TRAINING

Resistance training (also referred to as weight training) is the use of resistance in performing muscular contractions to increase muscle mass, strength, and endurance, as well as potential for improving flexibility and range of motion. Resistance training is usually associated with a reduced number of injuries. Benefits depend on the number of repetitions and sets, the length of rest periods between exercises, and the intensity and volume of workouts. Individuals can use dumbbells, exercise balls, bands, or machines.

Pilates programs have become a very popular resistance workout. The Pilates system focuses on increasing flexibility and strength without building bulk by doing a series of controlled isometric movements.

INTERVAL TRAINING

Interval training is based on the concept that the body's energy systems can make both aerobic and anaerobic gains by training with relatively intense exercises followed by a period of recovery. Intensity and recovery times depend on the individual's level of fitness. Usually, this approach means alternating short, high-intensity bursts of speed with slower recovery phases throughout a single workout. For example, runners will do intervals of 400 metres to train for 1.5-mile (2.4-km) runs with a rest period of walking 50–100 metres and then repeating the 400-metre run.

By attempting to increase the number of repetitions and varying the speed, many runners are able to reduce their time on the run.

HIGH-INTENSITY INTERVAL TRAINING

High-intensity interval training (HIIT) is a type of interval training that mixes high-intensity bursts of exercise with recovery periods. It can be exhausting but has considerable advantages. It can be the quickest way to lose fat, become fit, and increase sports performance. This type of training is one of the most effective ways to increase your VO_2 max and increase shuttle run performance. An example would be to do five to six all out 30-second sprints with a two-minute slow jog recovery, working to reduce the recovery time to one minute. The goal is to increase your anaerobic threshold. This is the point during the anaerobic exercise when lactic acid starts to build up at a rate greater than it can be removed from the muscle. Based on the individual's speed, anaerobic threshold training typically lasts 20 minutes; the threshold is reached when an athlete attains between 50 and 85 percent of maximum aerobic capacity (the more fit the athlete, the higher the percentage). Because this type of training completely exhausts your muscles of energy, it is important to have a day or two between such workouts. You must do an extensive warm-up to prime your muscles properly, and then cool down and stretch after the workout.

A current program that reflects HIIT is the Tabata® workouts, which are designed to have shorter work periods to rest periods (8 sets of 20 seconds' work; 10 seconds rest). These types of exercise regimes cause a higher heart rate, which ultimately helps to improve VO_2 max.

PLYOMETRIC TRAINING

Plyometric training is a form of resistance training that works on developing strength, power, and agility. Through a series of drills that usually use one's own body weight or medicine balls, exercise bands, stability balls, or weighted vests, individuals develop programs that include exercises that feature explosive movements through counter-movements to build muscular energy and power. These exercises focus not only on the contraction of the muscle but also on how fast it can contract. Examples include squat-jumps, box drills, hopping, jump-rope, and ballistic medicine ball drills. Individuals have to be highly motivated to do this kind of training.

CONCURRENT TRAINING

Concurrent training refers to the principle that you train for either strength or power at the same time you train for cardiovascular endurance. Those who train more generally have leaner muscle mass and lower body-fat composition, which makes the tasks of the job easier to do. This means you are doing your cardiovascular and resistance training workouts during the same training session, or within one hour of each other. The advantage of the concurrent approach is the parallel development of all qualities. The disadvantage is the risk of overtraining and the consequent limits on training effects. Depending on the intensity of the cardiovascular training, there may be some reduction in performance. For example, while doing leg presses after a cycling class, you may see some reduction in strength. For this reason, some individuals train for strength before working the cardiovascular system. The reverse approach is used when weight loss and endurance gains are a priority.

PERIODIZATION

Periodization refers to an overall training plan in which an individual maximizes performances at peak times. This approach reduces the risk of injury and mental burnout. In sports, training periods are separated into off-season, pre-season, and in-season. There is a distinct period during which athletes learn necessary skills and motor development, and then gradually improve in skill, strength, and endurance while competing in their sport. Some of you may want to consider this as a method for reaching your goals.

In order to pass fitness standards, individuals need to set up programs. These should include a brief period in which to become familiar with the BFOR equipment. The preparation period that follows should include a high-volume, low-intensity training program in order to learn the routine. In the preparation period, it is important to ensure that you work on both agonist and antagonist muscle groups, as well as smaller muscle groups to ensure musculoskeletal balance. This should be followed by a strength phase, in which strength is built up to perform a task with ease, and a power phase to address the fact that training intensity increases while volume may be decreasing. Hypertrophy (increased muscle size) and maximal strength usually occur midway through this phase. The competitive or in-season stage usually combines shorter periods of training in specific skills at more intense levels, with tapering or complete rest just prior to a competition.

In terms of meeting BFOR standards, this means that individuals need to train generally toward increasing their level of fitness. Then they are required to train on the equipment needed to practise the push–pull, arm-restraint, shuttle run, and victim relocation components, as well as jumping over objects and interval training on stairs. The final stage is meant to ensure that the individual can easily attain level 7 on the shuttle run, do the equipment movements with ease, and be able to complete the circuit in the required time frame prior to testing. This also refers to training specific muscle fibres. He or she would have maximum strength and power in this maintenance phase. Then less time is required to maintain strength, while more emphasis is placed on tactical and skill-based training.

GUIDELINES FOR STARTING A FITNESS PROGRAM

To ensure that you enjoy exercising and do so safely, here are some guidelines for starting a fitness program:

- *Start slowly* When you begin your program, remember that duration and frequency should take precedence over intensity. If you are experiencing muscle soreness 48 hours after your workout, or are experiencing a lack of energy or decreased physical performance, you are probably suffering from overtraining and are at risk of injury. Remember that you are making a lifelong commitment to fitness, so it is not important to get in shape as fast as possible. Instead, gradually build up to your desired fitness level, and then work on maintaining that level.

- *Train specifically to meet the job demands of law enforcement* Your body will adapt to the demands that you place on it. You need to focus on upper-body strength, cardiorespiratory endurance, and flexibility training to stay as healthy as you can throughout your career.

- *A proper warm-up and cool-down are essential* A warm-up should gradually warm up the muscles, including the heart, so that they can respond to the demands of your physical activity. A warm-up should include exercises that increase your heart rate as well as stretch all muscle groups, and include low-intensity movements similar to the exercises you will be doing. A cool-down should bring the body back to normal through the use of slow and gradual movements to prevent the pooling of blood.

- *Think about the order in which you do your exercises* Start with the large muscle groups and work your way down to the smaller ones. Training large muscle groups (such as thighs, chest, and back) will take most of your energy; therefore, you need to do them when you are at your strongest. Smaller muscles (such as biceps, triceps, and forearms) should be trained after larger muscles because they do not require as much energy to train.

- *Get enough fluids into your system* Two hours before a workout you should have at least half a litre of a cool drink. During a workout, you should have 150 to 225 millilitres of fluid every 15 minutes. After a workout, you should drink about 1 litre for every kilogram of body weight lost. You can determine how much body weight you lose during a workout by weighing yourself before and after the workout. Drinking water is a good way to replenish your fluids. Sports drinks, which help to replace electrolytes lost through sweating, are also acceptable, although many people find them too hard on the digestive system and need to dilute them.

- *Train regularly* Remember that you need a regular workout routine. Three to five times a week is necessary to see results from endurance training and to maintain those results. Intersperse your sessions with weight training or interval training on the other days. People who exceed the recommended number of workouts risk injury.

- *Try one of the different fitness classes offered through your school* You do not have to make a long-term commitment, but you might find them challenging and outside your normal workout practices, which can help improve your skills and level of fitness.

- *Train with a partner* The motivation and encouragement that you get from a fitness partner will help you through the hard times when your fitness routine does not seem to be producing results. A partner is also invaluable in weight training as a spotter and generally to ensure that you are adhering to the proper techniques.

- *Remember that everyone has a unique physical makeup* Everyone progresses at a different rate or experiences different improvements. Fitness is a very personal thing. If you compare yourself to others, you may set yourself up for failure, especially if the others are already at a higher fitness level.

FLEXIBILITY AND STRETCHING

Flexibility—the ability to move joints freely through their full range of motion—is determined by the type of joint being used. The range of motion of most joints can be maintained or increased with proper training, but can decline quickly with disuse.

Flexibility is an important component of a balanced fitness program, but one that is often neglected. It is achieved by incorporating stretching exercises into your fitness program. In this section, we will look at the benefits of stretching and describe a number of stretching techniques. The *Fit for Duty, Fit for Life* training guide that accompanies this textbook includes descriptions and photographs of recommended upper- and lower-body stretching exercises.

THE BENEFITS OF STRETCHING

There are a number of reasons for incorporating stretching into your fitness program (Behm & Chaouachi, 2011; Page, 2012; Plowman & Smith, 2007; Trehearn & Buresh, 2009):

- It enhances your body's ability to perform the exercises in your program.
- Stretching hamstrings, quadriceps, hip flexors, and low-back muscles regularly will help reduce the strain on the back. Flexibility training will improve your posture and help prevent low-back pain.
- It reduces the risk of injury from exercising, including joint sprains and muscle strains.
- It increases your range of motion and helps to keep your body feeling loose and agile.
- It promotes relaxation and helps reduce stress.
- It can enhance physical fitness.
- It increases blood supply and nutrients to joint structures.
- It can reduce the severity of painful menstruation (dysmenorrhea).
- It can reduce resistance and tension in muscles.
- It can optimize the learning, practice, and performance of many types of skilled movements.
- It can promote the development of body awareness.
- Submaximal aerobic activities and dynamic stretching may help our muscles and tendons work more efficiently prior to running and participating in specific activities over static stretching.

Stretching not only helps prevent injury and reduce low-back pain, but it may also help you recover from injury faster (Carragee, 2005). Debate continues regarding the best time to stretch—for example, before, during, or after a workout. According to Shrier (2004), stretching can reduce the risks of sport or workout injury, but it may slow performance if done just prior to the activity.

As noted, muscle tissue is broken down during any weight-bearing activities. Under stress, tiny micro-tears develop in the muscle fibres. This contributes to

> **DID YOU KNOW?**
>
> In general, women tend to be more flexible than men throughout the lifespan. However, a regular, properly designed stretching program can help to close the "gender gap."
>
> SOURCE: Peterson, 2011.

muscle soreness that often accompanies a strenuous workout. Because stretching brings nutrients to the musculoskeletal system, it can help repair fibres and speed up the healing process. As a result, there is less muscle soreness, so you can come back stronger for your next workout.

STRETCHING TECHNIQUES

There are five stretching techniques: static stretching, dynamic stretching, ballistic stretching, proprioceptive neuromuscular facilitation (PNF), and fascial stretching.

STATIC STRETCHING

Static stretching is an effective technique for improving flexibility. It is done after exercise, and involves bringing a muscle to a controlled maximum or near-maximum stretch by contracting the opposing muscle and holding the stretch for at least 20 to 30 seconds (without pain). Each stretch is repeated two or three times. Because static stretching is performed slowly, the strong reflex action that characterizes ballistic stretching (see below) does not occur.

Static stretching was developed to prevent injury, increase flexibility, and enhance performance. Athletes whose sports require an increased range of motion, such as gymnastics, are believed to benefit from static stretching, although some research has questioned this. It also relieves muscle soreness and helps prevent muscle imbalance, knots, and tightness.

DYNAMIC STRETCHING

Dynamic stretching, or functional stretching, consists of exercises that use the specific movements of the tasks or skills you are doing to prepare the body for movement. It involves moving your body and gradually increasing your reach, speed, or both. Dynamic stretching consists of controlled leg and arm swings that gently move you through your range of motion. Kicking an imaginary soccer ball is a dynamic stretch for the hamstrings and groin muscles. Twisting from side to side is a dynamic stretch for the trunk.

Some of the benefits of dynamic exercises include developing balance, "waking up" the muscles by increasing blood flow and nutrients to the tissue, providing specific movements commonly used in a particular skill or sport (Hendrick, 2000), and enhanced performance (Needham, Morse, & Degens, 2009). Dynamic stretching does not seem to elicit the performance reduction effects that static and PNF stretching (see below) do in runners.

BALLISTIC STRETCHING

Ballistic stretching involves quick, well-coordinated action–reaction movements using the momentum of a moving limb to stretch the muscles beyond their normal range of motion, sometimes involving bouncing during a stretch. It is not recommended as it promotes the stretch reflex increasing risk of injury, and many textbooks avoid discussing it (Ethyre & Lee, 1987). An example in law enforcement would be when you are throwing a punch and the elbow joint goes beyond the normal range of motion. Recent research has shown that although ballistic stretching produces less stretch than static stretching, fewer individuals suffer injuries or complications from bouncing to stretch past their normal range of motion than was previously believed (Covert, Alexander, Petronis, & Davis, 2010). Other research has shown some effect in increasing power, suggesting that dynamic stretching may be more productive (Samuel, Holcomb, Guadagnoli, Rubley, & Wallmann, 2008). More research is required before ballistic stretching is adopted for particular activities.

PROPRIOCEPTIVE NEUROMUSCULAR FACILITATION

Proprioceptive neuromuscular facilitation (PNF) involves contracting and relaxing the muscles before stretching. Usually, the exercises require the assistance of a partner (see Figure 4.9). Originally used in physiotherapy, this type of stretching has gained acceptance in the general fitness community. The two common types of PNF are:

- *Contract–relax (C–R) stretching* The muscle you want to stretch is contracted and then relaxed passively first. The now-relaxed muscle is then slowly actively stretched isometrically. This technique requires equipment (a towel or skipping rope) or a partner's assistance.

- *Contract–relax–antagonist–contract (CRAC) stretching* Begin by contracting and relaxing the muscle opposite to the one to be stretched (for example, while grasping a towel under your foot to draw your toes toward your head, first contract the gastrocnemius, then relax and pull on the towel to stretch the gastrocnemius further). Follow this by contracting the muscle to be stretched. The final action is the stretch itself. Contracting the opposite muscle promotes a reflex relaxation of the muscle to be stretched. This technique requires the assistance of a well-trained partner.

FIGURE 4.9   Proprioceptive neuromuscular facilitation (PNF)

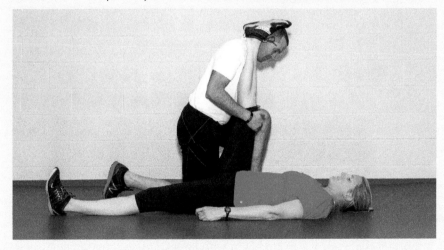

PNF is believed to be the most effective way of enhancing active flexibility, which is the active contraction and relaxation of the muscles that are being stretched (Alter, 1990, p. 10). By relaxing the muscle, PNF allows it to be stretched farther, but PNF presents a higher risk of injury than static stretching and can increase blood pressure to dangerous levels (Alter, 1990). It also has the disadvantage of often requiring a knowledgeable partner's assistance to avoid injury from overstretching.

FASCIAL STRETCHING

Fascia consists of interwoven layers of connective tissue that surrounds all muscles, bones, tendons, joints, and nerves and provides support, protection, and acts as a shock absorber. Fascia is the most energy efficient material in the body and optimizes muscular forces. It has two to eight times the strength and resistive force of the muscle it surrounds. For example, when you stretch your triceps by contracting your biceps, the fascia acts like a rubber band when you stop contracting and return the triceps back to its starting position. Trauma, overuse injuries, and postoperative healing can affect the ability of the fibres to slide over each other and cause adhesions (Pavan, Stecco, Stren, & Stecco, 2014). This increases the density of the fascia reducing circulation, lymphatic flow, and movement. This results in stiffness, chronic pain, loss of strength, and/or loss of mobility and flexibility from the excessive buildup of dense fascia and scar tissue.

Fascial stretching is important to keep fascial tissue pliable so that sticky adhesions don't form. To stretch the fascia as well as the muscle involves positioning multiple joints at different angles and planes of movement. These movements involve slow whole-body stretches. Techniques include self-massage using foam rollers and/or lacrosse balls over parts of the body, and performing various yoga techniques ensuring you hold stretches 30 to 90 seconds.

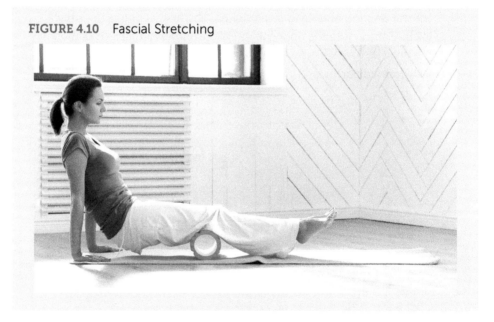

FIGURE 4.10   Fascial Stretching

SAFE AND EFFECTIVE STRETCHING

It is important that your warm-up begin with large-muscle activities such as walking or jogging, which facilitate safe stretching by increasing muscle temperature. A pre-exercise warm-up should consist of at least 5 to 15 minutes of light aerobic exercise followed by stretching exercises for all the major muscle groups. Examples appear in the *Fit for Duty, Fit for Life* training guide that accompanies this textbook. Performing stretching exercises at the end of your workout will increase your flexibility. Whether the workout is aimed at cardiorespiratory or resistance training, your body temperature will be raised, making stretching easier.

The FITT formula introduced earlier in this chapter provides a template for you to devise a stretching routine that meets your needs:

- *Frequency* Daily stretching is the best. You need to stretch before and after a workout. Regular stretching can help prevent tightness, muscle imbalance, and soreness. Stretching after exercises can help return muscles to their normal length, remove waste products that have built up from the workout, and reduce stiffness.

- *Intensity* Stretch to your limit, but avoid painful stretching, holding at least 20 to 30 seconds, and repeating the stretch 2 to 4 times. In dynamic stretching, you should do the exercises at a lower intensity than your workout, repeating 4 to 5 times over an 8- to 10-minute period. A cardiovascular exercise routine should involve at least 8 to 10 minutes of stretching at a low intensity (50 to 60 percent maximum heart rate). Before resistance training, you should do a set of exercises for large- and then small-muscle groups, using lighter weights to warm up.

- *Time* Stretch at least 8 to 10 minutes as part of your warm-up and cool-down (some athletes stretch for as long as an hour).

- *Type* Static and dynamic stretching are great to do with a workout. PNF and fascial stretching are good choices when recovering from an injury or working on increasing range of motion. Based on studies by McNair, Dombroski, Hewson, and Stanley (2000), and Knudson, Bennett, Corn, Leich, and Smith (2001), dynamic stretches involving slow, controlled movements through the full range of motion are considered more appropriate for a warm-up, while static stretches are more appropriate in a cool-down.

Assignment 4.5, available at www.emond.ca/fitness5e, will help you assess your flexibility and then choose specific exercises tailored to your goals. You will have to decide based on trial and error which helps you more while preventing injury.

TOP TIPS ...

FOR SAFE AND EFFECTIVE STRETCHING

- Complete a range of stretching exercises for all the different muscle groups. Pay attention to the muscle groups that are involved most in any sport you participate in.
- Proceed slowly and avoid ballistic stretching by not bouncing.
- Breathe out as you stretch and continue to breathe as you hold the stretch.
- Use the proper movements for each exercise.
- Stretch individual muscle groups one at a time.
- Don't strain to compete with the person next to you.
- When working with a partner, ensure that he or she knows your limits.
- Stop the stretch if you begin to feel pain.

Remember, too, that in order for your exercise program to work effectively, you must make it fit your needs.

FINAL THOUGHTS

Designing your own fitness program with creativity and variety is important for program adherence. Important factors when designing your program include intensity, frequency, and time. Try to incorporate the different principles of exercise based on your needs and abilities to ensure you can meet the requirements of the law enforcement career that you have chosen. In the balance of Part 2 of this book, Chapter 5 will give you more specifics relating to cardiovascular training, while Chapter 6 focuses on resistance training.

> There are really only two requirements when it comes to exercise. One is that you do it. The other is that you continue to do it.
>
> —*The New Glucose Revolution for Diabetes* by Jennie Brand-Miller, Kaye Foster-Powell, Stephen Colagiuri, and Alan W. Barclay

KEY TERMS

aerobic exercise
exercise that uses oxygen to produce the energy necessary for muscle movement, by burning fats and carbohydrates

agonist
a muscle that causes specific movement by contracting

anaerobic exercise
exercise that does not require oxygen to produce energy, and only carbohydrates are burned

anatomy
the study of the structure and parts of the body in relationship to one another

antagonist
a muscle that acts in opposition to the movement caused by the agonist, returning a limb to its initial position

ball-and-socket joint
the round head of one bone is held in the cup-like cavity of another bone, allowing movement in all directions

ballistic stretching
a stretching technique that promotes the stretch reflex but increases the risk of injury to muscles and tendons; it requires quick, well-coordinated action–reaction movements that stretch the muscles beyond their normal range of motion

body composition
the proportion of lean tissue to fat in the body

cardiorespiratory endurance
heart and respiratory system endurance; the ability to perform prolonged large-muscle activities at moderate to high intensity

concentric contraction
takes place when the muscle actively shortens against the opposing load and the ends of the muscle are drawn closer together

concurrent training
training for either strength or power at the same time as training for endurance

delayed onset muscle soreness (DOMS)
severe muscle tenderness, stiffness, decreased strength, and decreased range of motion that usually peaks between 24 and 72 hours after a hard workout

dynamic stretching
a stretching technique that involves performing movements within the full range of motion of the joint; it gradually increases reach and range of motion while the limbs are moving

eccentric contraction
takes place when the muscle actively lengthens as it resists the load and the ends of the muscle are pulled farther apart

fascial stretching
the stretching of the connective tissue that surrounds muscles, bones, joints, and nerves to improve flexibility

FITT principle
a guideline to design a fitness program based on frequency, intensity, time, and type of activity

fixator
a muscle that provides support while movement occurs

flexibility
the ability to move the joints freely through their full range of motion

functional fitness
training with exercises for a specific task

high-intensity interval training (HIIT)
a form of training designed to increase aerobic performance

hinge joint
the bones are connected in a way that allows movement in one plane only (flexion and extension)

interval training
training that is based on the concept that the body's energy systems can make both aerobic and anaerobic gains by training with relatively intense exercises followed by a period of recovery

isokinetic contraction
occurs when muscle length changes, contracting maximally throughout the full range of movement

isometric contraction
occurs when muscle length remains constant, or when contractile force equals resistive force

isotonic contraction
contraction of a muscle in response to a load applied to it; includes concentric and eccentric contractions

ligament
strong, fibrous connective tissue that connects bones at joints

metabolism
the chemical process of converting the food we eat into the energy our bodies need to function

muscular endurance
the ability of a muscle to sustain a prolonged contraction or to contract over and over again

muscular strength
the amount of force a muscle can produce with a single maximum effort

overtraining
the breakdown of the body from training too hard without sufficient rest

periodization
overall training plan where an individual maximizes performances at peak times

physical fitness
the ability to carry out daily tasks with alertness and vigour, without undue fatigue, and with enough reserve to meet emergencies or to enjoy leisure time pursuits (Maud & Foster, 2006)

physiology
the study of function of the human body, or how the parts work and carry out their life-sustaining activities

plyometric training
a form of resistance training that works on developing strength and power

principle of diminishing returns
refers to the fact that a person's training gains will reflect his or her prior level of training; people who have had little training make significant gains both in terms of strength and aerobic capacity while those who are fit must work harder to see results

principle of individuality
refers to training programs that are adjusted for personal differences based on abilities, skills, gender, age, experience, motivation, physical condition, the ability to recover after a workout, and susceptibility to injury

principle of progressive overload
refers to training and overloading the muscles that help the body to adapt to more and more stress

principle of recovery
refers to the recuperation time or amount of rest required after a workout

principle of reversibility
refers to all the benefits of exercise that are lost if you stop training

principle of specificity
refers to the ability of the body to adapt to a particular type and amount of stress placed on it

proprioceptive neuromuscular facilitation (PNF)
a stretching technique that involves contracting and relaxing the muscles before stretching

range of motion
the distance and direction a joint can move to its full potential

resistance training
the most common form of weight training, which incorporates exercises that result in gains to muscle mass and strength as well as the potential for improved flexibility and range of motion

sprain
an injury in which ligaments are either overstretched or torn

static stretching
a stretching technique that involves bringing a muscle to a maximum or near-maximum stretch by contracting the opposing muscle and holding the stretch for 20–30 seconds without pain

strain
refers to a muscle that has been stretched too far by applying too much tension or pressure

synergist
a muscle that assists an agonist indirectly in producing a joint's movement

tendon
fibrous tissue that connects muscles to bones

EXERCISES

MULTIPLE CHOICE

1. The four basic kinds of human tissue include
   a. ligaments, tendons, bones, and muscles
   b. skeletal, smooth, connective, and epithelial
   c. agonists, antagonists, synergists, and fixators
   d. epithelial, connective, muscle, and nerve
   e. bones, muscles, nerves, and organs

2. During which of the following contractions does muscle length remain constant?
   a. concentric
   b. eccentric
   c. isometric
   d. isokinetic
   e. isotonic

3. The warm-up and cool-down components of your workout should each last _____.
   a. 5 minutes
   b. 5–15 minutes
   c. 10–25 minutes
   d. 25–40 minutes
   e. don't need these

4. When speaking about resistance training, which best describes the "F" in the FITT formula?
   a. 1–3 days per week
   b. 3–5 days per week
   c. 2–3 days per week
   d. 5–7 days per week
   e. none of these

5. Intensity, type of exercise, _____, and _____ are the four factors involved in fitness development.
   a. time; speed
   b. frequency; distance
   c. frequency; time
   d. distance; time
   e. none of these

6. The purpose of a warm-up is
   a. to avoid tearing large-muscle groups
   b. to prepare for the workout psychologically
   c. to increase heart rate
   d. to increase internal temperature
   e. all of these

7. The most important health-related component of physical fitness is
   a. body composition
   b. cardiorespiratory endurance
   c. muscular strength
   d. muscular endurance
   e. flexibility

8. The best indicator for measuring the intensity of your workout is
   a. the total time you take to work out
   b. rapid breathing
   c. the amount you sweat
   d. your heart rate
   e. your fatigue level

9. Skill-related fitness components include
   a. aerobic and strength training
   b. speed and endurance training
   c. speed and agility
   d. flexibility and hand–eye coordination
   e. body composition and aerobic training

10. Which of the following terms refers to the ability of a muscle to exert force for only one maximum effort?
    a. muscular atrophy
    b. muscular hypertrophy
    c. muscular overload
    d. muscular strength
    e. muscular endurance

11. The maintenance of equilibrium while stationary or while moving is termed
    a. agility
    b. balance
    c. coordination
    d. poise
    e. reaction time

12. Which should be the primary advantage of good health-related physical fitness?
    a. improved work efficiency
    b. excellence in sports
    c. enjoyment of leisure
    d. prevention of disease
    e. a good appearance

13. _____ training refers to interval training of distances at high intensity levels followed by recovery periods at predetermined intervals of moderate intensity.
    a. periodization
    b. concurrent
    c. HIIT
    d. interval
    e. plyometric

14. The _____ training technique involves training for power or strength at the same time as endurance training.
    a. periodization
    b. concurrent
    c. resistance
    d. interval
    e. plyometric

15. Using your body weight and minimal equipment, _____ training involves a series of drills that involve explosive movements through counter-movements to build muscular energy and power.
    a. periodization
    b. concurrent
    c. resistance
    d. interval
    e. plyometric

16. _____ training is based on the concept that the body's energy systems can make both aerobic and anaerobic gains by training with relatively intense exercises followed by a period of recovery.
    a. Periodization
    b. Concurrent
    c. Resistance
    d. Interval
    e. Plyometric

17. The disadvantage of concurrent training is
    a. you see gains in all areas that you work
    b. you see more gains in aerobic over strength
    c. you see more gains in strength over aerobic
    d. you risk overtraining and limit the gains that can be seen
    e. there are no disadvantages

18. Stretching for flexibility is most effective during which of the following?
    a. the warm-up
    b. the workout
    c. endurance training
    d. the cool-down
    e. doesn't really matter when

19. Dynamic stretching involves
    a. quickly moving a limb to its limits
    b. the full range of motion achieved in a slow, controlled stretch
    c. a natural response that causes a stretched muscle to contract
    d. a stretch–contract–stretch partner-assisted flexibility program
    e. alternating between a slow, controlled stretch and then a few quick stretches

20. Proprioceptive neuromuscular facilitation (PNF) involves
    a. quickly moving a limb to its limits
    b. the full range of motion achieved in a slow, controlled stretch
    c. a natural response that causes a stretched muscle to contract
    d. a stretch–contract–stretch partner-assisted flexibility program

    e. alternating between a slow, controlled stretch and then a few quick stretches

21. Which of the following involves quick, coordinated movements that stretch the muscles while you are moving and incorporates the stretch reflex?
    a. PNF stretching
    b. ballistic stretching
    c. static stretching
    d. concentric stretching
    e. eccentric stretching

22. Match the right stretch with the right definition.
    Dynamic Stretching
    PNF
    Static Stretching
    Fascial Stretching
    Ballistic Stretching
    a. contract and relax muscles as you stretch
    b. quick, well-coordinated action–reaction movements involving bouncing
    c. controlled movements to functionally improve your range of motion
    d. controlled movement to bring the muscle near maximal stretch
    e. techniques that stretch the muscle and connective tissue to improve mobility and flexibility

SHORT ANSWER

1. Describe how isotonic and isometric contractions differ.

2. Identify and distinguish between the two types of muscle fibre.

3. What are the components of health-related fitness?

4. What are the components of performance/skill-related fitness?

5. What are some of the physical benefits of participating in a fitness program?

6. What are some of the psychological benefits of participating in a fitness program?

7. Identify and explain the five principles of physical training.

8. What guidelines should you be aware of when beginning a fitness program?

9. Describe the principle of specificity and give an example.

10. How do you apply the principle of overload? Give an example.

11. How do you counter the principle of reversibility? Give an example.

12. How would you use periodization training to prepare for the shuttle run?

13. Describe HIIT training and how it can apply to training for the BFORs.

14. Describe interval training and how it can improve your 1.5-mile (2.4-km) run.

15. Describe functional training and how it prepares you for a job in law enforcement.

16. Using the plyometric training technique, describe how you could train for the various components of the PREP or PARE BFORs.

17. List four signs of overtraining.

18. What are some of the benefits of stretching?

19. Why is flexibility so important for those in law enforcement?

REFERENCES

Active Healthy Kids Canada. (2014). Is Canada in the running? *The active healthy kids Canada report card on physical activity for children and youth.* Toronto, ON: Author.

Adams, J., Schneider, J., Hubbard, M., McCullough-Shock, T., Cheng, D., Simms, K., … Strauss, D. (2010). Measurement of functional capacity requirements of police officers to aid in development of an occupation-specific cardiac rehabilitation training program. *Proceedings (Baylor University. Medical Center), 23*(1), 7–10.

Alter, M.J. (1990). *Sport stretch.* Champaign, IL: Human Kinetics.

Anderson, G.S., Plecas, D.B., & Segger, T. (2001). Police officer physical abilities testing: Re-validating a selection criterion. *Policing: An International Journal of Police Strategies & Management, 24*(1), 8–31.

Anderson, G., Zutz, A., & Plecas, D. (2011). Police officer back health. *The Journal of Criminal Justice Research, 2*(1), 1–17.

Andrews, R.C., Herlihy, O., Livingstone, D.E.W., Andrew, R., & Walker, B.R. (2002). Abnormal cortisol metabolism and tissue sensitivity to cortisol in patients with glucose intolerance. *Journal of Clinical Endocrinology & Metabolism, 87*(12), 5587–5593.

Barnes, J.D., Colley, R.C., & Tremblay, M.S. (2012). Results from the active healthy kids Canada 2011 report card on physical activity for children and youth. *Applied Physiology, Nutrition & Metabolism, 37*, 793–797.

Behm, D.G., & Chaouachi, A. (2011). A review of the acute effects of static and dynamic stretching on performance. *European Journal of Applied Physiology, 111*, 2633–2651. doi:10.1007/s00421-011-1879-2 .PMID:21373870

Bonneau, J., & Brown, J. (1995). Physical ability, fitness and police work. *Journal of Clinical Forensic Medicine, 2*, 157–164.

Brand-Miller, J., Foster-Powell, K., Colagiuri, S., & Barclay, A.W. (2007). *The new glucose revolution for diabetes.* Cambridge, MA: Da Capo Press.

Bruunsgaard, H., Galbo, H., Halkjaer-Kristensen, J., Johansen, T.L., MacLean, D.A., & Pedersen, B.K. (1997). Exercise-induced increase in serum interleukin-6 in humans is related to muscle damage. *Journal of Physiology, 499*(3), 833–841.

Bullock, T. (2007). Police officer injury study. *VML Insurance Programs Law Enforcement Newsletter, 1*(2).

Canadian Adolescents at Risk Research Network. (2004, February). *Physical activity patterns in Canadian adolescents.* Kingston, ON: Queen's University.

Canadian Society for Exercise Physiology (CSEP). (2003). *The Canadian physical activity, fitness and lifestyle appraisal: CSEP's guide to healthy living.* Ottawa, ON: Author.

Canadian Society for Exercise Physiology (CSEP). (2011a). *Canadian physical activity guidelines.* Retrieved from http://www.csep.ca

Canadian Society for Exercise Physiology (CSEP). (2011b). *Canadian physical activity guidelines for adults 18–64 years.* Retrieved from http://www.csep.ca

Carragee, E.J. (2005). Persistent low back pain. *New England Journal of Medicine, 352*(18), 1891–1898.

CBC News. (2011, January 19). Canadian youth woefully inactive: Report. Retrieved from http://www.cbc.ca/news/health/story/2011/01/19/fitness-canadians-health.html

Colley, R.C., Garriguet, D., Janssen, I., Craig, C.L., Clarke, J., & Tremblay, M.S. (2011a, January). *Physical activity of Canadian adults: Accelerometer results from 2007 to 2009 Canadian health measures survey.* Ottawa, ON: Statistics Canada.

Colley, R.C., Garriguet, D., Janssen, I., Craig, C.L., Clarke, J., & Tremblay, M.S. (2011b, March). Physical activity levels of Canadian children and youth. Research article. *Health Reports, 22*(1). Catalogue no. 82-003-XPE. Ottawa, ON: Statistics Canada.

Covert, C.A., Alexander, M.P., Petronis, J.J., & Davis, D.S. (2010). Comparison of ballistic and static stretching on hamstring muscle length using an equal stretching dose. *Journal of Strength & Conditioning Research, 24*(11), 3008–3014.

Ethyre, B.R., & Lee, E.J. (1987). Comments on proprioceptive neuromuscular facilitation stretching techniques. *Research Quarterly for Exercise and Sport, 58*, 184–188.

Gumieniak, R., Jamnik, V.K., & Gledhill, N. (2011). Physical Fitness Bona Fide Occupational Requirements for Safety-Related Physically Demanding Occupations; Test Development Considerations. *Health & Fitness Journal of Canada, 4*(2), 47–52.

Health Canada. (2013). Directly measured physical activity of adults, 2012 and 2013. *2012–2013 Canadian Health Measures Survey (CHMS).* Statistics Canada. Retrieved from http://www.statcan.gc.ca/pub/82-625-x/2015001/article/14135-eng.htm

Hendrick, A.N. (2000). Dynamic flexibility training. *Strength and Conditioning Journal, 22*(5), 33–38.

Hobin, E.P., Leatherdale, S., Manske, S., Dubin, J.A., Elliott, S., & Veugelers, P. (2013). Are environmental influences of physical activity distinct for urban, suburban, and rural schools? A multilevel study among secondary school students in Ontario, Canada. *Journal of School Health, 83(5),* 357–367.

Hootman, J.M., Macera, C.A., Ainsworth, B.E., Addy, C.L., Martin, M., & Blair, S.N. (2002). Epidemiology of musculoskeletal injuries among sedentary and physically active adults. *Medicine & Science in Sports & Exercise,34*(5), 838_844.

Jamnik, V.K., Thomas, S.G., Shaw, J.A., & Gledhill, N. (2010). Identification and characterization of the critical physically demanding tasks encountered by correctional officers. *Applied Physiology, Nutrition and Metabolism, 35*(1), 45–58.

Janney, C.A., & Jakicic, J.M. (2010). The influence of exercise and BMI on injuries and illnesses in overweight and obese individuals: A randomized control trial. *International Journal of Behavioral Nutrition & Physical Activity, 7*(1). Retrieved from https://www.ncbi.nlm.nih.gov/pmc/articles/PMC2818622/

Janssen, I., & LeBlanc, A.G. (2010). Systematic review of the health benefits of physical activity and fitness in school-aged children and youth. *International Journal of Behavioural Nutrition and Physical Activity, 7*, 40.

Janssen, I. (2012). Health care costs of physical inactivity in Canadian adults. *Applied Physiology, Nutrition, & Metabolism, 37*, 803–806.

Jetté, M., Sidney, K., & G. Blümchen. (1990). Metabolic Equivalents (METs) in exercise testing, exercise prescription, and evaluation of functional capacity. *Clinical Cardiology, 13*(8), 555–565.

Kelly, K.R., & Jameson, J.T. (2016). Preparing for combat readiness for the fight: Physical performance profile of the female U. S. marines. *Journal of Strength & Conditioning Research, 30*(3), 595–604.

Knudson, D., Bennett, K., Corn, R., Leich, D., & Smith, C. (2001). Acute effects of stretching are not evident in kinematics of the vertical jump. *Journal of Strength & Conditioning Research, 15*(1), 98–101.

Krueger, H., Krueger, J., & Koot, J. (2015). Variation across Canada in the economic burden attributable to excess weight, tobacco and physical inactivity. *Canadian Journal of Public Health, 106*(4). Retrieved from http://www.cpha.ca/uploads/e-mail/cjph/v106i4/Volume_106_4_e171-e177.pdf

Krueger, H., Turner, D., Krueger, J., & Ready, A.E. (2014). The economic benefits of risk factor reduction in Canada: Tobacco smoking, excess weight and physical inactivity. *Canadian Journal of Public Health, 105*(1), e69–e78.

Léger, L. (1985). SportMed Technology fitness appraisal kit: 20-metre shuttle run test with one-minute stages. Montreal, QC: SportMed Technology.

Léger, L.A., & Lambert, J. (1982). A maximal multistage 20-m shuttle run test to predict VO$_2$ max. *European Journal of Applied Physiology, 49*, 1–5.

Maud, P.J. & Foster, C. (2006). Physiological assessment of human fitness. *Human Kinetics, 1*.

McKenzie, D.C. (1999). Markers of excessive exercise. *Canadian Journal of Applied Physiology, 24*(1), 66–73.

McNair, P., Dombroski, E., Hewson, D., & Stanley, S. (2000). Stretching at the ankle joint: Viscoelastic responses to holds and continuous passive motion. *Medicine & Science in Sports & Exercise, 33*, 354–358.

Meeusen, R., Duclos, M., Foster, C., Fry, A., Gleeson, M., Nieman, … Urhausen, A. (2013). Prevention, diagnosis, and treatment of overtraining syndrome: Joint consensus statement of the European College of Sport Science and the American College of Sports Medicine. *Medicine & Science in Sports & Exercise, 45*(1), 186–205.

Ministry of Health. (2005). *The Integrated Pan-Canadian Healthy Living Strategy.* The Secretariat for the Intersectional Healthy Living Network, the F/T/P Healthy Living Task Group, and the F/T/P Advisory Committee on Population Health and Health Security. Catalogue no. HP10-1/2005.

Needham, R.A., Morse, C.I., & Degens, H. (2009). The acute effect of different warm-up protocols on anaerobic performance in elite youth soccer players. *Journal of Strength & Conditioning Research, 23*(9), 2614–2620.

Nindl, B.C. (2015). Physical training strategies for military women's performance optimization in combat occupations. *Journal of Strength & Conditioning Research, 29*(11), S101–106.

Nindl, B.C., Jones, B.H., Van Arsdale, S.J., Kelly, K., & Kraemer, W.J. (2016). Operational physical performance and fitness in military women: Physiological musculoskeletal injury, and optimized physical training considerations for successfully integrating women into combat-centric military occupations. *Military Medicine, 181*(1), 50–62.

Page, P. (2012). Current concepts in muscle stretching for exercise and rehabilitation. *International Journal of Sports Physical Therapy, 7*(1): 109–119.

Pavan, P.G., Stecco, A., Stern, R., & Stecco, C. (2014). Painful connections: Densification versus fibrosis of fascia. *Current Pain & Headache Reports, 18*(8), 441.

Perez, C. (2003). Children who become active. *Health Reports (Suppl.), 14*, 17–28.

Peterson, J.A. (2011). Nice-to-know facts about flexibility and stretching. Retrieved from http://www.fitness.com/articles/1354/nice_to_know_facts_about_flexibility_and_stretching.php

Plowman, S.A., & Smith, D.L. (1997). *Exercise physiology for health, fitness, and performance.* Needham Heights, MA: Allyn and Bacon.

Public Health Agency of Canada (2010). The Pan-Canadian healthy living strategy. Strengthened Pan-Canadian healthy living strategy framework -2010. Retrieved from http://www.phac-aspc.gc.ca/hp-ps/hl-mvs/ipchls-spimmvs/ld2-eng.php

Public Health Ontario. (2014). *OBESITY A burden across the life course.* Interactive Web Report. Retrieved from http://www.publichealthontario.ca/en/DataAndAnalytics/OntarioHealthProfile/Pages/OHP-IWR-Obesity.aspx#

Public Safety Canada. (2008). Fit to serve: Preparing for the Alberta PREP: Alberta Physical Readiness Evaluation for Police. Retrieved from https://www.publicsafety.gc.ca/lbrr/archives/cnmcs-plcng/cn31683-eng.pdf

Samuel, M.N., Holcomb, W.R., Guadagnoli, M.A., Rubley, M.D., & Wallmann, H. (2008). Acute effects of static and ballistic stretching on measures of strength and power. *Journal of Strength & Conditioning Research, 22*(5), 1422–1428.

Seguin, R. (2015). Factors associated with success in PARE testing among RCMP officers. Western University Electronic Thesis and Dissertation Repository. Retrieved from http://ir.lib.uwo.ca/cgi/viewcontent.cgi?article=4257&context=etd

Shrier, I. (2004). Does stretching improve performance? A systematic and critical review of the literature. *Clinical Journal of Sports Medicine, 14*(5), 267–273.

Solomonson, A.A., Dicks, N.D., Kerr, W.J., & Pettitt, R.W. (2016). Influence of load carriage on high-intensity running performance estimation. *Journal of Strength & Conditioning Research, 30*(5), 1391–1396.

Statistics Canada. (2012). Health indicator profile, age-standardized rates annual estimates, by sex, Canada, provinces and territories (CANSIM Table 105-0503). Ottawa, ON: Author.

Statistics Canada. (2013). Overweight and obese adults, Health Fact sheets (2013), Canadian Community Health Survey 2007–2013. Retrieved from http://www.statcan.gc.ca/pub/82-625-x/2014001/article/14021-eng.htm

Statistics Canada. (2014a). Overweight and obese adults (self-reported), 2014, Canadian Community Health Survey 2014. 82-625-X. Ottawa, ON: Author. Retrieved from http://www.statcan.gc.ca/pub/82-625-x/2015001/article/14185-eng.htm

Statistics Canada (2014b). Physically active Canadians. Cat. No. 82-003-XWE; Vol. 18, No. 3. Retrieved from http://www.statcan.gc.ca/pub/82-003-x/2006008/article/phys/10307-eng.htm

Statistics Canada. (2015). Comparison of physical activity adult questionnaire results with accelerometer data: Methodological insights. Catalogue no. 82-003-X. *Health Reports, 26*(7), 11–17.

Statistics Canada. (2016). Physical activity during leisure time, by age group and sex (percent) (CANSIM Table 105-0501). Ottawa, ON: Author.

Trehearn, T.L., & Buresh, R.J. (2009). Sit and reach flexibility and running economy of men and women collegiate distance runners. *Journal of Strength & Conditioning Research, 23*(1), 158–162.

Tremblay, M.S., Shields, M., Laviolette, M., Craig, C.L., Janssen, I., & Connor Gorber, S. (2010). Fitness of Canadian children and youth: Results from the 2007–2009 Canadian Health Measures Survey. *Health Reports, 21*, 1–14. Statistics Canada Catalogue no. 82-003. Retrieved from http://www.statcan.gc.ca/pub/82-003-x/2010001/article/11065-eng.pdf

Tremblay, M.S., & Willms, J.D. (2000). Secular trends in the body mass index of Canadian children. *Canadian Medical Association Journal, 163*(11). Retrieved from http://www.ecmaj.ca/content/163/11/1429.full

Wenger, H. A. (2007). *Developing upper body strength for women in the Canadian Forces.* Canadian Forces Morale & Welfare Services. Retrieved from https://www.cfmws.com/en/AboutUs/PSP/DFIT/Documents/Publications%20and%20Reports/Developing%20Upper%20Body%20Strenght%20for%20Women%20in%20the%20Canadian%20Forces.pdf?Mobile=1

Wilmot, E.G., Edwardson, C.L., Achana, F.A., Davies, M.J., Gorely, T., Gray, L.J., ... Biddle, S.J. (2012). Sedentary time in adults and the association with diabetes, cardiovascular disease and death: Systematic review and meta-analysis. *Diabetologia, 55*(11), 2895–2905.

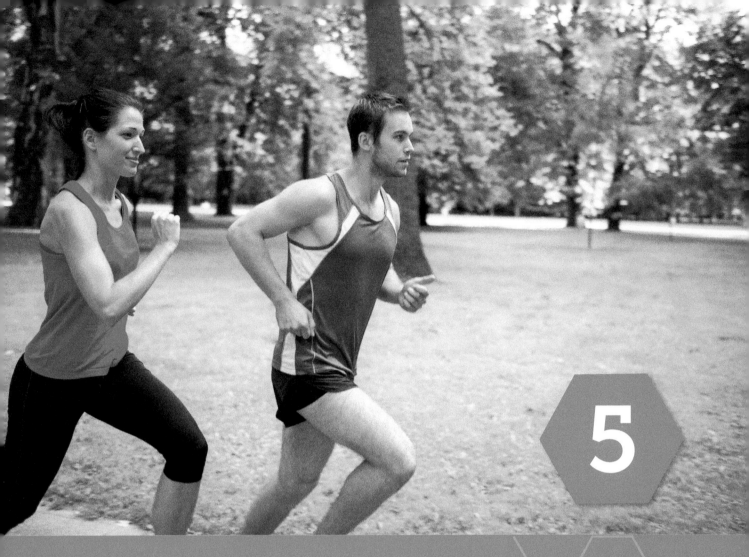

CARDIORESPIRATORY FITNESS

LEARNING OUTCOMES

After completing this chapter, you should be able to:

• Explain why cardiorespiratory fitness is important in law enforcement.

• Understand and monitor your heart rate at rest and during exercise.

• Determine your target heart rate zone for exercise.

• Determine how high-intensity interval training (HIIT) can fit into your cardiorespiratory program to assist you in successfully completing BFOR testing.

• Set up a cardiorespiratory fitness program that is most suited to you.

Cardiorespiratory fitness (endurance), probably the most important component of fitness, is the ability to perform prolonged large-muscle activities at moderate to high intensity. This chapter will examine the importance of cardiorespiratory fitness in law enforcement and provide advice on creating a cardiorespiratory fitness program that will help you meet law enforcement requirements.

THE IMPORTANCE OF CARDIORESPIRATORY FITNESS IN LAW ENFORCEMENT

WHAT WILL BE YOUR MOTIVATION?

"Urbanization, mechanization and an increased use of motorized transport have reduced physical activity levels globally. Canada must resist the decline in habitual movement fueled by these trends—and not just by creating policies, strategies, facilities and bike lanes, but also by encouraging and re-establishing Canadian cultural norms where being physically active all year long, through outdoor play, transportation, recreation and sport are the Canadian standard, not the exception." Dr. Mark Tremblay, Director of the Healthy Active Living and Obesity Research Group comments on the 2016 ParticipACTION Report Card.

Cardiorespiratory fitness makes your body more efficient and helps you cope with the physical demands of your job and everyday life. The key to cardiorespiratory fitness is aerobic exercise—prolonged, rhythmic exercise that uses large-muscle groups. Examples of aerobic exercise include swimming, running, and cycling. Emergency services, including those in law enforcement, experience higher physical demands than workers in more sedentary occupations (Anderson, Plecas, & Segger, 2001). Research by the Ontario government and the RCMP (Canadian Border Services Agency, 2016; Ontario, 2015; RCMP, 2016; Seguin, 2015) has demonstrated the importance of aerobic conditioning in law enforcement. The researchers found that aerobic conditioning not only facilitated foot chases and the effort required to control and restrain an individual but also helped law enforcement officers to cope with long shifts, changing demands of the job, and stress (Gledhill, Jamnik, & Shaw, 2014).

All law enforcement services stress the importance of aerobic conditioning by incorporating a cardiorespiratory component into their BFOR (Bona Fide Occupational Requirement) evaluations (see the Appendix). When Ontario Corrections did an analysis of the most important physically demanding tasks on the job, endurance or cardiovascular fitness was significant when performing various tasks in combination or repeatedly (Jamnik et al., 2010). The RCMP stress training both the aerobic and anaerobic energy systems to be successful at the PARE and to sustain a high level of work, keep up with team members during a chase, or follow a track with a dog handler for extended periods of time (RCMP, 2016). In the task specific BFORs for specialized units, applicants must also carry the additional weight of body armour and various use of force equipment.

THE BENEFITS OF CARDIORESPIRATORY FITNESS

As you have read in Chapter 4, exercise has many benefits. For health benefits, you need to burn at least 1,000 calories per week and at least 2,000 calories to see greater benefits (Bushman, 2012). The following are some of the benefits of cardiorespiratory fitness:

- improved cardiorespiratory functioning, which allows the heart to meet the demands of everyday life more efficiently (blood pressure and the risk of heart disease are also reduced)(Elley & Arroll, 2002; Warburton et al., 2005)

- reduced levels of cholesterol, triglycerides, and other potentially harmful substances in the blood, which in turn reduces the risk of heart disease (Mann, Beedie, & Jimenez, 2014; Varady & Jones, 2005)

- improved metabolism (metabolism is, among other things, the process by which the body converts food into energy) (Bouchard, Shephard, Stephens, Sutton, & McPherson, 1990; Hassinen et al., 2010)

- increased bone density, which reduces the risk of osteoporosis and improves posture, balance, and coordination, and can help reduce the risk of falls (Arnold & Faulkner, 2010; Warburton, Gledhill, & Quinney, 2001a, 2001b)

- improved immune system (excessive training, however, can depress the immune system) (Bouchard et al., 1990; Nieman, Henson, Austin, & Brown, 2005; Shanely et al., 2011)

- reduced risk of developing type 2 diabetes and its associated risks (in conjunction with resistance exercise) (Larose et al., 2011; Sigal et al., 2007)

- reduced risk of some cancers, including those of the colon, breast, and female reproductive organs (Irwin et al., 2008; Smith, Phipps, Thomas, Schmitz, & Kerzer, 2013; Vainio & Bianchini, 2002)

- increased energy, stamina, and resistance to physical fatigue (Bouchard et al., 1990; Gibala et al., 2006)

- ability to fall asleep faster and deeper (Buman & King, 2010)

- improved concentration, productivity, and mood (Buman & King, 2010)

- improved psychological and emotional well-being resulting from improved appearance, enhanced self-image and self-confidence, and decreased stress, anxiety, and depression (Papousek & Schulter, 2008; Shephard, 1997; Stubbs, Rosenbaum, Vancampfort, Ward, & Schuch, 2016)

ASSESSING CARDIORESPIRATORY FITNESS

Your cardiorespiratory fitness affects your body's ability to maintain a level of exertion (exercise) for an extended period of time. The ability to supply energy for activities lasting more than 30 seconds depends on the consumption and use of oxygen (O_2). Most physical activities in daily life and athletics take more than 90 seconds; most BFOR tests last 2 to 5 minutes and may include a maximal aerobic assessment (20-m shuttle run), so O_2 consumption is critical for survival as well as performance.

Aerobic fitness consists of two main components. The first is central cardiorespiratory fitness (heart and lungs). The second, peripheral component is the specific muscles involved in the movement.

CENTRAL CARDIORESPIRATORY FITNESS

The central cardiorespiratory system will improve if you stress your cardiac function and ventilation system (see Figure 5.1). Your improvement is limited by three factors:

1. cardiac output: the amount of blood pumped per minute, which is a function of stroke volume (amount of blood pumped per heartbeat) and heart rate (heartbeats/minute)

> **DID YOU KNOW?**
> Besides its cardiorespiratory benefits, physical activity delivers oxygen and nutrients to your tissues to help you work more efficiently and have energy to do other things that you enjoy. It also stimulates various brain chemicals that leave you feeling happier and more relaxed than you were before your workout.

2. blood volume: dehydration or other factors affecting volume reduce the effectiveness of the cardiovascular system

3. red blood cell count and O_2 carrying capacity

PERIPHERAL CARDIORESPIRATORY FITNESS

The peripheral component of aerobic fitness requires specific training to cause the muscles to adapt to the specific task (that's why cross-training on a bike will help your running but will not replace the need to run). The two biggest limiting factors in peripheral aerobic fitness are:

1. the ability of the muscles to remove CO_2 and use O_2 from the blood

2. the ability of the muscles to maintain a balanced pH (specifically, minimizing the buildup of lactic acid, thus delaying the onset of fatigue)

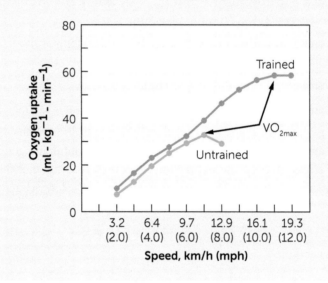

FIGURE 5.1 Comparison of Trained Versus Untrained Aerobic Capacity

MAXIMUM AEROBIC CAPACITY

A person's maximum aerobic capacity (VO_2 max or MVO_2) is a measure of his or her cardiorespiratory fitness. VO_2 max is the maximum volume of oxygen consumed per minute. It is the point at which an individual's O_2 uptake plateaus and does not increase with further increases in workload. Once people reach their maximum aerobic capacity, they cannot continue to work at that intensity for more than a minute or two because their demand for oxygen exceeds their ability to supply it. Figure 5.1 shows the results of two individuals' VO_2 max tests. Notice that the trained individual has a greater oxygen uptake and is able to run to a faster speed.

Proper testing of a person's VO_2 max is costly and requires a controlled laboratory environment (see Figure 5.2). The test is time-consuming, and requires a highly motivated subject if an accurate assessment is to be obtained. It requires specialized equipment and someone trained to measure and record the results. Only one person can be tested at a time.

Less time consuming tests were adopted where multiple individuals could perform the test at the same time. For example, in the late 1970s the Ontario Police College, adopting the standards set by Dr. Kenneth Cooper (1982), implemented a 1.5-mile (2.4-km) run as an indirect measure of cardiorespiratory fitness (see the Appendix for further details). When the Physical Readiness Evaluation for Policing (PREP) was implemented, the 20-metre shuttle run (Léger & Gadoury, 1989; Léger & Lambert, 1982; Léger, Lambert, Goulet, Rowan, & Dinelle, 1984; Léger, Mercier, Gadoury, & Lambert, 1988) replaced the 1.5-mile (2.4-km) run. Other tests of cardiorespiratory fitness include the Astrand-Rhyming bicycle ergometer test, the YMCA bicycle ergometer test, the Rockport Fitness Walking Test, the Ebbeling treadmill test, and the Canadian Physical Fitness and Lifestyle Appraisal (CPFLA) step test.

For law enforcement applicants who do not run on a regular basis, or who are obese or otherwise in poor condition, cardiorespiratory training is of the utmost importance. You need to be physically fit to meet the demands of the 20-m shuttle run and BFOR tests and other tests of occupational skills administered to law enforcement applicants. Conditioning your cardiorespiratory system will help you work toward your goals.

FIGURE 5.2   Running on a Treadmill to Assess Your MVO_2

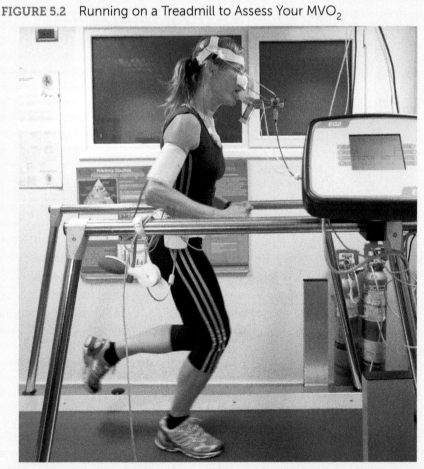

The subject runs on a treadmill and their O_2 and CO_2 are measured while the speed and grade increase until their values plateau and/or they no longer can continue.

A word of caution: those who do not engage in regular physical activity and have joint or obesity problems or high blood pressure (over 144/94 or 160/90, depending on the test protocol) may require medical clearance before taking a cardiorespiratory test. Be sure to fill out the Physical Activity Readiness Questionnaire (PAR-Q+) in **assignment 1.1,** available at www.emond.ca/fitness5e, and talk to your fitness instructor before taking any cardiorespiratory test.

Refer to **assignment 5.1** at www.emond.ca/fitness5e and assess your current cardiorespiratory fitness level.

DETERMINING YOUR CARDIOVASCULAR TRAINING INTENSITY

Before you begin cardiorespiratory training, consider the frequency, intensity, duration, and type of your aerobic exercise sessions. These considerations are addressed by the FITT (frequency, intensity, time, and type) formula below (Table 5.1).

TABLE 5.1 The FITT Formula

FITT	HEALTH-RELATED BENEFITS	PERFORMANCE-RELATED BENEFITS	HIGH-PERFORMANCE-RELATED BENEFITS
Frequency (days/week)	7	3–4	5+
Intensity (% of MHR)	50–60	60–85	70–90*
Time (minutes/day)	60	20–60	30–60
Type	Any rhythmic activity, including walking, cycling, jogging, swimming, and using a stairmill/treadmill/rowing machine		

*At this intensity, there may be risk of overtraining, which can lead to injuries and rhabdomyolysis.

Although all four variables in the FITT formula are important, intensity is the key variable in cardiovascular training. The Canadian Society for Exercise Physiology (2003) identifies four techniques that effectively allow you to judge the intensity of your workout: heart rate monitoring, the Borg scale, METs, and the talk test. Intensity can be checked during and at the end of the workout to determine whether you are at the required target heart rate.

UNDERSTANDING HEART RATES

The first heart rate (HR) that you should be aware of is your resting heart rate, which is ideally taken prior to getting out of bed in the morning. It also can be taken while sitting quietly for at least 5 minutes during the day. Resting heart rates vary between 40 and 100 beats per minute (bpm), with 70 bpm being the average. With exercise, you can decrease your resting HR as your heart and lungs become stronger. The heart is then able to pump more blood (increase *stroke volume* [SV]) throughout the body with less effort. The lungs can take in more oxygen (increase *maximum oxygen uptake* [VO₂ max or MVO₂]) with less effort, which means more blood and oxygen will reach the working muscles. Having enough oxygen going into the blood helps to remove the lactic acid (hydrogen ions) so that you can sustain a prolonged aerobic workout.

Maximal heart rate (MHR) is the rate at which your heart beats at maximal aerobic activity. MHR can be found predictively using the following formula: 220 minus your age. Or, it can be found more precisely by measuring your heart rate at the end of a maximal test. You will normally never work at 100 percent of your maximum unless you are doing a specific program or test in a supervised setting (for example, a maximal treadmill test or 20-m shuttle run).

Exercising heart rate is the rate when your body is in motion during sustained exercise. The goal is to stay within your target heart rate (THR) range, which is normally between 60 and 85 percent of maximal heart rate; the fitter you are the higher the potential to work at a higher percentage.

HEART RATE MONITORING

Heart rate monitoring—the most common technique—is easily learned. You put your index and middle fingers over either the radial artery (located on the wrist just below the base of the thumb) or the carotid artery (located on the left and right sides of the neck). Do not press too hard on the carotid artery, as this may trigger a reflex that slows the heart rate. During exercise, the heart rate is determined by counting the beats for 10 seconds and then multiplying by 6 to get beats per minute. When you are at rest, you should count the beats for 15 seconds and then multiply by 4.

Exercising heart rate = (_____beats in 10 sec) × 6
Resting heart rate = (_____beats in 15 sec) × 4

DETERMINING YOUR TARGET HEART RATE ZONE

To judge whether you are exercising at a benefit-producing intensity, you must determine your target heart rate (THR) zone. First, determine your maximal heart rate by subtracting your age from 220. This gives you your MHR in beats per minute. Next, multiply your MHR by 60 percent and 85 percent. The resulting numbers are the lower and upper limits, respectively, of your THR zone.

Here's how to determine the THR for a 25-year-old:

MHR = 220 − 25
MHR = 195 bpm
THR = 195 × 0.60 = 117 bpm
THR = 195 × 0.85 = 166 bpm

So a person who is 25 years of age exercising between 60 percent and 85 percent of their MHR would keep their heart rate between 117 and 166 beats per minute. Refer to **assignment 5.2** at www.emond.ca/fitness5e and determine your resting heart rate and target heart rate.

To benefit from exercise, you must exercise at an intensity that raises your heart rate into the THR zone for 30 to 60 minutes 3 to 5 times a week. Unfit people who exercise at an intensity just short of the lower limit of their THR zone will obtain some health benefits but will not improve or maintain aerobic fitness. Physical activity should include both moderate activities (such as brisk walking, skating, and bike riding) and vigorous activities (such as running and playing soccer). In fact, Health Canada is encouraging all Canadians to be physically active by increasing their awareness and understanding of the benefits of physical activity and the range of opportunities to be physically active in daily life (Healthy Living Unit, 2008).

In 2016, the Canadian Society for Exercise Physiology (CSEP) released the first *Canadian 24-Hour Movement Guideline for Children and Youth (5 to 17 years)* for physical activity, sedentary behaviour, and sleep, which include:

- an accumulation of at least 60 minutes *per day* of moderate to vigorous physical activity involving a variety of aerobic activities. Vigorous physical activities and muscle and bone strengthening activities should each be incorporated at least three days per week;

- several hours of a variety of structured and unstructured light physical activities (CSEP, 2016).

CSEP (2011) also set guidelines for adults 18 to 64 years, which include:

- accumulating *at least* 150 minutes of moderate to vigorous intensity aerobic physical activity per week, in bouts of 10 minutes or more;

- muscle and bone strengthening activities using major muscle groups, at least two days per week (CSEP, 2011).

Figure 5.3 shows the THR zone for ages 20 to 70. This chart is often posted on gym walls. Table 5.2 lists the effects of training if you are working out at the various target heart rate zones.

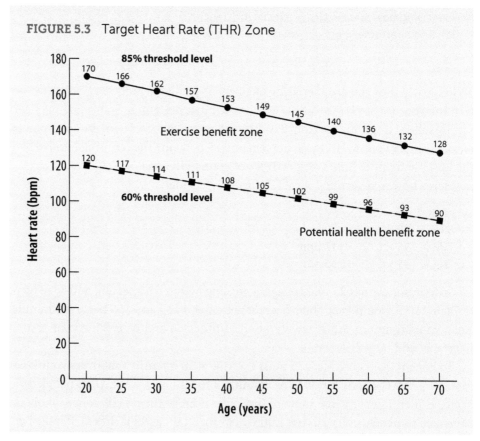

FIGURE 5.3 Target Heart Rate (THR) Zone

TABLE 5.2 Effects of Training at Various Target Heart Rate Zones

TARGET HEART RATE ZONE	EFFECT ON TRAINING: WORKING AT THIS TARGET HEART RATE ZONE
50–60%	• keeps health risks to a minimum • does not produce visible gains, but maintains cardiovascular capacity for daily activities
65–75%	• is the level used by novices starting out and as a warm-up and cool-down for advanced individuals • builds a proper cardiorespiratory base • improves transport of nutrients and oxygen throughout the body • can be sustained for long periods of time
80–85%	• works both aerobic and anaerobic energy systems • burns significant numbers of calories • is used not only to build cardiorespiratory endurance (improving heart and lung capacity) but also to improve leg strength • can be sustained for long periods of time
85–90%	• is used only for interval training (i.e., HIIT training) • is extremely intense and should be used only by highly conditioned individuals; novices need to develop a solid cardiorespiratory base first • is important for improving power (maximal muscular contraction in an explosive movement), speed (how fast you can go), and quickness (ability to change direction very fast) • uses only the anaerobic energy system and thus cannot be sustained for long periods

THE BORG SCALE

Developed by Gunnar A. Borg (1998), a Swedish psychologist, the Borg scale method does not involve counting the number of heartbeats, which can be difficult for some people while they are exercising. The Borg rating of perceived exertion (RPE) is a scale with numbers 6 to 20 and allows you to judge how hard you are working during exercise. It is based on the physical sensations a person experiences during physical activity, including increased heart rate, increased respiration or breathing rate, increased sweating, and muscle fatigue. At 6 there is no exertion at all; at 9 it's very light activity like walking slowly; at 10 to 13 you are working somewhat hard but feel alright (moderate intensity); at 14 to 17 you are pushing yourself strenuously (vigorous intensity); and at 19 to 20 it's extremely strenuous activity that you cannot continue for long (Nelson et al., 2007).

With experience of monitoring how your body feels, it will become easier to know when to adjust your intensity. For example, a walker who wants to engage in moderate-intensity activity would aim for a Borg scale level of "somewhat hard" (12–14). If that person describes his or her muscle fatigue and breathing as "very light" (9 on the Borg scale), then he or she would want to increase intensity. On the other hand, if the walker felt the exertion was "extremely hard" (19 on the Borg scale), he or she would need to slow down to achieve a moderate-intensity range. (See Figure 5.4.)

FIGURE 5.4   The Borg RPE* Scale®

#	LEVEL OF EXERTION
6	No exertion at all
7	
8	
9	Very light
10	
11	Light
12	
13	Somewhat hard
14	
15	Hard (heavy)
16	
17	Very hard
18	
19	Extremely hard
20	Maximal exertion

* Rating of Perceived Exertion

SOURCE: Perceived Exertion (Borg Rating of Perceived Exertion Scale), 2015.

Although this is a subjective measure, a person's exertion rating may provide a good estimate of the actual heart rate during physical activity (Borg, 1998). There is a high correlation between a person's perceived exertion rating multiplied by ten and their actual heart rate during physical activity. For example, if a person's RPE is 12, then $12 \times 10 = 120$; if the person's heart rate were measured, it should be approximately 120 beats per minute. Note that this calculation is only an approximation of heart rate, and the actual heart rate can vary quite a bit depending on age and physical condition.

The disadvantage of using the Borg scale is that some people underestimate or overestimate their level of exertion. Beginners may not be able to tie their intensity to a subjective perception of exertion so it is important for them to check their heart rate regularly to determine whether they are within their THR zone.

THE TALK TEST

The talk test is a handy guide for beginners who are concerned about their exercise intensity. A person who is active at a light intensity level should be able to sing while doing the activity. One who is active at a moderately intense level should be able to carry on a conversation comfortably while engaging in the activity. If a person becomes winded or too out of breath to carry on a conversation, then the activity would be considered vigorous and the person may find it too hard to continue.

UNDERSTANDING METs

Aerobic fitness intensity can be defined in terms of METs. The Metabolic Equivalent of a Task (MET) or simply metabolic equivalent is the physiological measure of the ratio of energy expenditure of a physical activity compared to rest. A 4 MET activity expends four times the amount of energy used by the body at rest.

- Light-intensity activities are defined as 1.1 to 2.9 METs.
- Moderate-intensity activities are defined as 3.0 to 5.9 METs.
- Moderate- to vigorous-intensity activities are defined as 6.0 METs or more.

Canadian Physical Activity Guidelines (Tremblay et al., 2011) point out that doing moderate-intensity or vigorous-intensity physical activity is necessary for substantial health benefits. By doing at least the recommended 150 minutes of moderate-intensity activity per week, adults can achieve 500 to 1,000 MET-minutes per week. This range has been recommended to reduce your risk of premature death and breast cancer (Nelson et al., 2007). A person could do a 4 MET activity for 30 minutes or a 8 MET activity for 15 minutes and both methods would achieve 120 MET-minutes. Table 5.3 is a sample of activities at the various intensity levels.

TABLE 5.3 Various Activities at Different METs Intensities

SEDENTARY TO LIGHT (<3 METs)	MODERATE (3–5.9 METs)	MODERATE TO VIGOROUS (6–10 METs)	VIGOROUS (+10 METs)
• Lying quietly and watching television • Sitting, using phone, computer, or texting • Driving • Walking one flight of stairs • Standing stationary (directing traffic, examining passports, monitoring secured facility)	• Leisure bicycling (5.5 mph/8.85 kmh) • Walking at work (3 mph/4.8 kmh) • Carrying groceries • Resistance training, multiple exercises (8–15 reps) • Calisthenics (e.g., push-ups, pull-ups), moderate effort • Circuit training, moderate effort • Brisk walk to slow jog, 4 mph/6.44 kmh (19.5 minute 1.5-mile run) • Shooting baskets • Making a passive arrest	• Pick-up basketball, soccer, hockey • Calisthenics (e.g., jumping jacks), vigorous effort • Circuit training (e.g., kettlebells with aerobic movement) • Jogging 5 mph/8.05 kmh (18 minute 1.5-mile run) • Cycling 12 mph/19.3 kmh • Rowing stationary, 100–150 watts • Stairmill, eliptical, treadmill, swimming lengths • Shuttle run of 5.5 (MVO$_2$ - 37.1 mL/kg/min) • Cross-country skiing • Altercation with an individual	• Competitive hockey, soccer, rugby • Running 8 mph/12.87 kmh (11.15 minute 1.5-mile run) • Running to level 7 on the shuttle (MVO$_2$ - 41.7 mL/kg/min) • Cycling 200–250 watts • Rope skipping • Running stairs • Running 10 mph/ 16.09 kmh (9 minute 1.5-mile run) • Chasing a suspect, inmate

SOURCES: ACSM, 2013; Fletcher, Froelicher, Hartley, Haskell, & Pollock, 1990; Jamnik, Thomas, Shaw, & Gledhill, 2010; Léger, 1989; MCSCS, 2015; Morris et al., 1993; Ramsbottom, Brewer, & Williams, 1988; Veteran Affairs Canada, 2006.

CREATING A CARDIORESPIRATORY FITNESS PROGRAM

When creating a cardiorespiratory fitness program, you first need to determine your goal. Is it to get healthy (reduce your risk of cardiovascular disease or type 2 diabetes)? Is it to lose weight? Is it to improve your performance on the 20-m shuttle run? Once you have established your goal, you can focus in more clearly on what type of aerobic training you will do.

Many people use aerobic training to help reduce weight. Most research acknowledges that a conventional way to burn body fat effectively is to choose a modality (type of cardiorespiratory exercise) and perform it for at least 30 minutes at a moderate level of intensity. It is also important to understand the benefits of high-intensity cardio exercise. Training at higher levels of intensity allows your metabolism to stay elevated for a longer duration after exercise and therefore burns a greater percentage of calories during the day. Make sure that if weight loss is your goal you are changing your program to include greater intensities and exercises that you enjoy.

Other students train strictly to improve their aerobic performance so that they are able to complete the 20-m shuttle run that accompanies many BFORs. To improve your 20-m shuttle run score you need to incorporate the progressive over-load principle. To use this approach effectively you need to establish a baseline and then gradually increase either speed, incline, resistance, and/or time as you become better conditioned.

A beginner who runs on a treadmill at 8.5 km/h (5.3 mph) for 30 minutes will see caloric expenditure, cardiorespiratory conditioning, and burning of body fat at first. Over time, they will need to increase their speed, increase the incline of the treadmill, or run for longer if continued results are to be achieved.

Another approach to cardiovascular training is doing high-intensity interval training (HIIT), as discussed in Chapter 4. The goal of HIIT is to improve your aerobic capacity by working out at an elevated heart rate (85–95 percent MHR). Because you cannot maintain that intensity for long, you should build recovery stages into your workout. The time frames are usually done minute by minute, while adjusting intensity to affect heart rate and the rating of perceived exertion on the Borg scale. This type of training is geared to those who are in advanced cardiorespiratory shape and do not have any pre-existing conditions that limit their ability to exercise safely as outlined in Chapter 1. Some popular training programs include CrossFit® and Tabata® aerobic programs.

So what program should you follow? Your instructor may have already established a regime that he or she expects you to follow. If not, the following pages offer some simple guidelines for a training program. If your fitness level is poor to fair, ask your instructor to help you establish a program that is safe and effective for you and that he or she can monitor. For those who have already reached an excellent level of fitness, all that is required is maintenance.

GUIDELINES FOR CARDIORESPIRATORY FITNESS TRAINING

This section offers guidelines to help you set up your fitness program. Prior to participating in an aerobic program

1. Make sure you answered "no" to all the questions on the PAR-Q+ questionnaire (in **assignment 1.1** at www.emond.ca/fitness5e) or have been cleared by a medical examination. Check with your instructor if you are unsure about your medical suitability to undertake a fitness program at this time.

2. Begin each session with a proper warm-up and end with a cool-down. It is important to do a warm-up that mimics what you are going to be doing. For example, if you are doing a cycling class, then you should be warming up for at least five minutes (can be on a bike or track) prior to the start of the class. It is also important to include a proper cool-down where you lower your heart rate and stretch your muscles. Examples are included in the *Fit for Duty, Fit for Life* training guide that accompanies this text.

3. Check the intensity of your exercise by monitoring your heart rate, or use the Borg scale or talk test. The optimum cardiovascular training zone is between 60 and 85 percent THR.

4. If you experience aches or pains or suffer an injury, stop exercising or reduce the intensity of your exercise until you are fit to continue or have seen a doctor. Be sure to advise your instructor of the problem.

5. Start out slowly (especially if you are in poor condition) and try to increase your time and/or intensity until you can reach your desired duration or pace (progressive overload principle).

6. Remember that there are many modalities that you can participate in. They include treadmill, bike, elliptical, rowing machine, stairclimber, swimming laps, or playing sports.

TRAINING FOR RUNNING

The value of cardiorespiratory fitness has been validated in many of the BFORs for law enforcement in Canada. For example, the PREP, A-PREP, and FITCO in Ontario have the 20-m shuttle run as their aerobic assessment based on criterion-based on-the-job tasks and aerobic fitness requirements (Gledhill & Jamnik, 2014).

Table 5.4 is an example of a running training program. The focus of this program is on increasing the running time duration rather than the speed. When you complete this program, you can continue to add more running in with less walking until you run the entire time. You can increase time to these runs every week (5 minutes per week), depending on how you feel and how your times are improving. Once you can run without stopping, then you can focus more on speed. Remember that rest days are very important to prevent injuries.

Many running programs that are offered in your community will start at a 3 minute run with a 1 minute walk for beginners. Ultimately, your fitness level and motivation will determine how long you can run and when and if you need to walk. Eventually you should be able to complete a 2.4-km (1.5-mile) run without stopping.

The premise behind programs like this one is that you get used to running farther than you are required to for your fitness tests. For the 20-m shuttle run, you need to go 1220 metres without stopping. The timed run, which is used in the Ontario Police Fitness Award, is twice that distance.

THE BASICS ON RUNNING MECHANICS

Learning to run is more than just putting one foot in front of the other, although for many that is how they start. Here are some common technique suggestions:

1. *Fast Cadence*   Running speed is the result of stride length multiplied by stride frequency. The more you touch the ground the more energy is required to go forward. You can count your steps for 15 seconds and multiply it by 4 to get foot strikes per minute. Optimum is about 180 strikes per minute; if you are slower than that then you might think about increasing your cadence. One way to assist you is to run to songs that are 90 or 180 beats/min, which will help you run at that pace.

2. *Avoid Heel Striking*   You cannot push off your foot when it's in front of your body. Your hips must be over your feet to propel you forward. There has been a trend to wear minimalist running shoes to help with the timing of ground contact. For some individuals, it helps to practise sprinting on grass and working your way up to running longer periods. Make sure your foot strikes under your knee, not in front of it, which can lead to injury, especially shin splints.

TABLE 5.4 Training to Run 5 km

	MONDAY	TUESDAY	WEDNESDAY	THURSDAY	FRIDAY	SATURDAY	SUNDAY
Run for 3 minutes/walk for 1 minute							
Week 1	Run/walk 30 minutes	Walk 30 minutes	Run/walk 30 minutes include HIIT	Walk 30 minutes	Rest	Run/walk 5 km (3.1 miles)	Rest or walk 30 minutes
Sprint Training (HIIT) 3–5 sprints once/week							
Run for 4 minutes/walk for 1 minute							
Week 2	Run/walk 30 minutes	Walk 30 minutes	Run/walk 30 minutes include HIIT	Walk 30 minutes	Rest	Run/walk 5.5 km (3.4 miles)	Rest or walk 30 minutes
Sprint Training (HIIT) 4–6 sprints once/week							
Run for 5 minutes/walk for 1 minute							
Week 3	Run/walk 30 minutes	Cross train 30 minutes	Run/walk 30 minutes include HIIT	Walk 30 minutes	Rest	Run/walk 2.4 km (1.5 mile) Time yourself	Rest or walk 30 minutes
Sprint Training (HIIT) 5–8 sprints (incorporate up to 3 times/week)							
Run for 6 minutes/walk for 1 minute							
Week 4	Run/walk 30 minutes	Cross train 30 minutes	Run/walk 30 minutes include HIIT	Walk 30 minutes include hill work	Rest	Run/walk 6 km (3.7 miles)	Rest or walk 30 minutes
Sprint Training (HIIT) 6–8 sprints, 3 times/week							
Run for 6 minutes/walk for 30 seconds							
Week 5	Run/walk 30 minutes	Cross train 30 minutes	Run/walk 30 minutes include HIIT	Walk 30 minutes	Rest	Run/walk 5.5 km (3.4 miles)	Rest or walk 30 minutes
Sprint Training (HIIT) 7–8 sprints, 3 times/week							
Run for 7 minutes/walk for 30 seconds or less							
Week 6	Run/walk 30 minutes	Cross train 30 minutes	Run/walk 30 minutes include HIIT	Walk 30 minutes	Rest	Run 2.4 km (1.5 mile) Time yourself	Rest or walk 30 minutes
Sprint Training (HIIT) 8 sprints, 3 times/week							
Run for 8 minutes/walk for 30 seconds or less							
Week 7	Run/walk 30 minutes	Cross train 30 minutes	Run/walk 30 minutes include HIIT	Walk 30 minutes	Rest	**Test day Run 5 km (3.1 miles)**	Rest or walk 30 minutes
Sprint Training (HIIT) 8 sprints							
Cross training includes biking, swimming, elliptical trainer. REMEMBER TO DO AT LEAST A 5 MINUTE WARM-UP AND A 5 MINUTE COOL-DOWN. It is important to take a rest day to prevent injuries.							

SOURCES: Denham, Feros, & O'Brien, 2015; Rebecca Finlay, personal communications, 2017; Galloway, 2008; RunningWithUs, n.d.

3. *Work on Muscle Mobility in Your Lower Extremity* Stride length is affected by the range of motion in your lower body, especially around the hips. It is important to lengthen the muscles properly to prevent injury and improve performance. Good momentum has to do with the ability to lean from your ankles to prevent vertical running. Keep your head as level as possible and avoid bouncing up and down as you run forward. It is recommended that you do a dynamic warm-up and save the static stretching for after your run.

4. *Relax Your Upper Body* It is important to keep your upper body relaxed and that your elbows are at 90 degrees so your arms swing properly and your hands are loose. It can help to lift your shoulders toward your ears and then roll your shoulders back and down to a relaxed position. Relax the abdomen as well; keeping abdominal muscles tight can lead to cramps. If you get a cramp, you can look up a bit, hold the arm up on the side that is hurt, and use the other hand to gently push in the area that is affected. Usually it is our lungs hitting our diaphragm causing it to go into spasms.

5. *Practise Running Faster* Although it is important to run for distance, you can only get faster by training in that manner. Whether it is hill training (which helps ensure efficient form) or various speed work on a track or treadmill, to get faster you must train for that speed. This applies to both running the 1.5-mile run, completing a BFOR, or meeting a higher stage on the 20-m shuttle run.

6. *Learn to Breathe Properly* Hyperventilating results in depriving oxygen in your lungs. When you first start out, you should be able to talk while you're running. Some people find that taking a breath in for two steps and then breath out for two steps helps. Other people find that breathing in through their nose and out through their mouth helps when they are learning to run.

TOP TIPS ...

FOR RUNNING HILLS

Going up:

- Don't bend at the waist or hunch over; rather keep your head and chest up and think about the bend coming from the ankles rather than the torso
- Push up and off the hill, springing from your toes while you look straight ahead
- Keep your hands and fists loose while looking straight ahead

Going down:

- Keep your torso upright while looking ahead
- Step softly; don't let your feet slap the pavement while taking quick short steps

Remember that an exercise program can be affected by conditions in the environment in which you exercise. You may need to adjust your running program to compensate for these variables. For example, a run may involve one or more of the following factors:

- topographical features such as hills and sand, or wet surfaces that make for slippery conditions
- obstacles such as ditches, fences, and underbrush
- meteorological and air-quality factors such as heat, humidity, cold, snow, wind, pollution, and thin air at higher altitudes
- bulky clothing or equipment that obstructs movement

TRAINING TO YOUR UPPER LIMIT

There are three energy pathways that we use when exercising. These pathways are intensity and duration dependent (Wells, Selvanduria, & Tien, 2009, p. 83):

1. *ATP-PC Energy System*   High power/short duration (lasting approximately 12 seconds)—used in altercations, use of force, and quick sprints to emergencies.

2. *The Glycolytic System*   Moderate power/moderate duration (lasting approximately 50 seconds until fatigue from lactic acid buildup)—needed for all out sprint or chase, getting to the emergency, running stairs, physical fights.

3. *The Oxidative System*   Low power/long duration (starts at around 45 to 50 seconds and lasts almost indefinitely if substrates are available [O_2 and glucose])—used in runs, security tours, walking or bike patrols, and canine tracking.

Gore (2000) predicted that during BFOR testing, for those who are unfit, that the ATP-PC and glycolytic systems quickly drop as you use up your energy substrates (ATP) (usually happens in the first two laps of a BFOR [Seguin, 2015, p. 127]). Most people do not feel the drop in their performance during the anaerobic alactic dominated period (1 to 30 seconds) but notice it during the lactic range (50 to 240 seconds). This implies that pace training is important to enhance your ability to work at an intense pace throughout the test.

When you work at your upper heart rate limit and over 85 percent MVO_2, you go into what is termed an *anaerobic or lactate threshold*. That is, if you push too hard for too long, your body can no longer meet its demand for oxygen. You start feeling exhausted, you hyperventilate from excess amounts of lactic acid in your body, and your heart can no longer provide enough oxygen to your working muscles to sustain the demands of the task. At this point, you are typically able to continue for only a short period of time, 30 seconds to 1 minute. However, you can increase your anaerobic threshold by implementing high-intensity interval training (HIIT) into your training program. By resting between these high-intensity interval training (HIIT) anaerobic sessions, you enable the oxygen-rich blood to help clean out the lactic acid from your muscles and you can catch your breath before the next set.

 PERSONAL PERSPECTIVE

REBECCA FINLAY

Prior to having my second baby, my aerobic fitness was not that great, and I can remember that my last attempt at the 20-m shuttle run pre-baby was 6.0. After giving birth to Gillian, I was limited to doing workouts in my basement, and was not able to go out running very often. I had two sets of dumbbells (5 and 10 lbs each) and a timer. I focused on interval training, with 30 to 60 second bouts of *max* effort doing all sorts of different exercises. I included functional exercises, strength and endurance exercises with free weights, and lots of body based cardio exercises, like burpees and box jumps, sprawls and high knees. I could sneak in a quick 4 km run maybe once every 2 to 3 weeks, but that was all the running that I did. After 4 to 5 months of training, I ran to 7.5 on the shuttle run.

It is important to realize that improvements in aerobic performance can be made in a small space, with limited equipment, and do not have to be limited to just running. You need to work hard and push your limits to achieve them.

TRAINING FOR THE SHUTTLE RUN

To train to meet an acceptable level on the 20-m shuttle run, an individual must be doing cardiovascular training 3 to 5 times per week working at an intensity of 75 to 85 percent of his or her maximum heart rate. You can use some of the following training regimes to help build up your aerobic capacity and speed required:

1. Train with the Shuttle Run Track

   a. Determine what level you can obtain. When you can no longer run any further, stay in your lane and keep walking. When you feel that you can run again, do another 20 metres or more if possible. This way you will have a better understanding of the speed that you must work toward.

   b. The 20-m shuttle run requires you to run 1220 metres. If you are not running this distance at least three times per week, then you need to start.

   c. When you run the shuttle, make sure you are efficient by pivoting on the 20-metre line. Don't make wide turns and put one foot on or over the line. You do not have to put two feet over the line.

   d. The 20-m shuttle run test starts at 8.5 kph and continues to increase by 0.5 kph every full stage. It is important that if you are practising the actual test that you have measured out the distance using a tape measure so that you are running the 20 metres.

2. Train on a Treadmill

   a. The suggested training regime for the shuttle run (Table 5.5) is an example of continuous increases in intensity. This example of a high-intensity workout includes changes in incline and speed to challenge your cardiorespiratory system, and to push those who are fitter a little further. This chart can also be found in your *Fit for Duty* workbook, so you can use it in the fitness centre on a treadmill. Remember that you need to train to at least 11.5 kph (7.15 mph) to meet the level 7 on the shuttle run. If you are unsure how fast you run, then getting on a treadmill to determine this would give you a starting point.

3. Develop a High Intensity Interval Training (HIIT) Program

   One way to improve your shuttle run performance is to do interval training. A study by Gunnarsson and Bangsbo (2012) showed improved performance and MVO_2 by running intervals, even with a reduction in the amount of training time. Make sure that you start with a 5 to 10 minute dynamic warm-up (like the one included in the *Fit for Duty* book).

TABLE 5.5 Suggested Training Regime for the 20-m Shuttle Run

TIME (MIN)	SPEED (MPH)	INCLINE	RPE (1–20)*
1	4	1	2
2	4.5	1	2
3	5	1	3
4	5.5	2	4
5	6	2	5
6	6.5	2.5	6
7	7	3	8
8	7.5	3	10
9	8	3.5	12
10	8.5	3	14
11	9	1	16
12	5	4	12
13	5	6	14
14	6	8	16
15	6	10	20
16	6	4	14
17	5	3	10
18	5	3	8
19	4	2	6
20	4	1	4

* RPE = Rating of Perceived Exertion

a. An example of a beginner HIIT program is a *30-20-10.* The individual increases their speed as they run for:

    i. 30 seconds at 50 percent MHR followed by

    ii. 20 seconds at 70 percent MHR followed by

    iii. 10 seconds at 90 percent MHR

Each set lasts one minute. Repeat for a minimum of five and maximum of ten sets.

b. An example of an advanced HIIT program (Gibala, Little, MacDonald, & Hawley, 2012; Hood, Little, Tarnopolsky, Myslik, & Gibala, 2011), where constant-load, low-volume HIIT may be a practical, time efficient strategy to induce metabolic adaptations, is running for:

    i. 1 minute at 90 percent MHR followed by

    ii. 1 minute active recovery

Your goal is to repeat this ten times, for a 20-minute workout.

c. You can also add sprint training into a strength workout to save time and induce rapid physiological adaptations (aerobic and anaerobic) (Gibala et al., 2006):

    i. Sprint for 1 to 2 minutes at 90 percent MHR.

    ii. Complete two or three weight exercises.

    iii. Repeat sprints as many times as necessary to accommodate your full strength workout.

Remember that you are increasing intensity to prepare your body for what it will be like when doing the shuttle run. Be aware that the treadmill is not the same as running in the gym or outdoors. In running, you must absorb the pounding of each step while you propel your body forward. There is also an energy cost for accelerating and decelerating the body at each end of the 20 metres. Ultimately, you cannot expect to succeed by practising only on a treadmill.

WEATHER AND YOUR FITNESS PROGRAM

Staying active during the four seasons in Canada can be enjoyable. Whether you head out for a run, a walk, a day of skiing, or a hike on the Bruce Trail, dressing for comfort will increase your enjoyment. A career in law enforcement also means that you will experience various weather conditions throughout the year.

PREPARING TO PARTICIPATE IN OUTDOOR ACTIVITIES

Heat gain or loss is governed by the following physical means

1. Conduction—transfer of heat to or from the body by direct physical contact.

2. Convection—transfer of heat by movement of air or water over the body.

3. Radiation—emission of heat from the body into space and absorption of radiation (sunlight) on the body's surface.

4. Evaporation—loss of heat by the body when converting sweat to vapour.

In a cold or cool environment, conduction and convection, along with some evaporation of sweat, can maintain the heat balance. However, if the person is exposed to a very cold environment (cold temperatures, water, wet clothes), they may not be able to generate enough heat and thus suffer from cold-related illnesses (covered in Chapter 14).

In a warm or hot environment, evaporation of sweat becomes the main way of controlling the rise in core temperature. Evaporation can keep the body's exercising temperature in the normal range of 38.9 to 40.5 °C under normal environmental circumstances. However, if there is high humidity (over 50 percent), lack of air movement, or sunlight adding radiant heat, heat-related illnesses can arise (covered in Chapter 14). Of special concern is rhabdomyolysis, which is a rapid breakdown, rupture, and death of muscle tissue due to heat stress and prolonged physical exertion, causing irregular heart rhythms, seizures, and kidney damage.

Always check the air temperature, humidity, and/or wind chill factor (combined effect of temperature and wind) before exercising in the cold. The Police Fitness Personnel of Ontario use industrial standards established by the National Institute for Occupational Safety and Health (NIOSH) (2016) as the guideline for safe exercise participation in extreme weather conditions.

General guidelines for when you would want to avoid maximal testing/exertion outside include (ACSM, 2013; Armstrong et al., 2007; Castellani et al., 2006):

- days when the temperature is over 28 °C (wet-bulb globe temperature)
- days when the humidity is above 70 percent
- smog alert days (Government of Canada, 2014)
- full sun exposure, which occurs from 11 a.m. to 3 p.m. Consider being outside in the early morning and late in the day, making sure you are properly hydrated and dressed in clothes that allow for maximum evaporation
- cold exposure of more than −18 °C in either thermometer or wind chill effect

Whatever season you begin running, per the American College of Sports Science (2009), it may take up to six months to reach the maintenance phase. If you experience any discomfort or pain, inform your instructor and consult your doctor. You may have to modify your program.

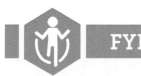

FYI

HOW TO DRESS FOR OUTDOOR RUNNING

The best way to stay warm when running in the winter is to dress in layers for better insulation:

- An inner layer of wool, silk, or synthetic material to keep moisture away from the body.
- A middle layer of wool or synthetic material to provide insulation even when wet.
- An outer wind and rain protection layer that allows some ventilation to prevent overheating.

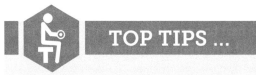

TOP TIPS ...

FOR RELUCTANT RUNNERS

For those people who do not like running, here are a few tips to help you stay on track using a treadmill:

- Go as long as you can keep up the pace without holding on to the treadmill. Get off the treadmill, do your workout, and then return to the treadmill to see how far you can go on the second run.

- Another approach is to run as long as you can and then reduce the treadmill speed to a fast walking pace; catch your breath and then increase the speed until you need to hang on to the treadmill.

- For those who are just starting to run and who prefer resistance training to cardio training: Get on the treadmill for one minute at the highest speed you can, then stop and do three sets (whether it is three sets of one exercise or one set of three exercises). Then, return to the treadmill for another minute. Over the period of an hour, you should be able to do at least 12 minutes of cardio. This approach will get you ready for longer runs on the treadmill.

- Finally, practise the shuttle run outside of class time. Get a group of people together and practise the test in a gym, or set up cones 20 metres apart outdoors and run back and forth to build up your endurance.

> ❝Running is a road to self-awareness and reliance—you can push yourself to extremes and learn the harsh reality of your physical and mental limitations or coast quietly down a solitary path watching the earth spin beneath your feet. ❞
>
> —Doris Brown Heritage, first woman to run a sub 5-minute indoor mile

FINAL THOUGHTS

Ultimately, you should set goals for yourself based on what you want to accomplish this semester. Make sure to incorporate both aerobic and anaerobic activities to meet the criteria for both the health-related components and BFOR requirements set out by your instructor. Use your *Fit for Duty* workbook to keep a record of your progress.

Refer to **assignment 5.3** at www.emond.ca/fitness5e and set up your own cardiorespiratory fitness program.

KEY TERMS

Borg scale
a simple method of rating perceived exertion (RPE) and used as a method for determining the intensity of exercise, used as an alternative to heart rate monitoring

exercising heart rate
your heart rate when your body is in motion during sustained exercise

maximal heart rate (MHR)
your heart rate when your heart beats at maximal effort during a sustained aerobic activity

maximum aerobic capacity (VO$_2$ max or MVO$_2$)
a measure of cardiorespiratory fitness; estimated as the point at which oxygen uptake plateaus and does not increase with further increases in workload

Metabolic Equivalent of a Task (MET)
the physiological measure of the ratio of energy expenditure of a physical activity compared to rest

resting heart rate
your heart rate when you are in a resting state such as sleep

rhabdomyolysis
a rapid breakdown, rupture, and death of muscle tissue due to heat stress and prolonged physical exertion, causing irregular heart rhythms, seizures, and kidney damage

talk test
a method for determining the intensity of exercise, used as an alternative to heart rate monitoring; if a person is breathless and cannot carry on a conversation while exercising, he or she is working too hard

target heart rate (THR) zone
the zone that a person's heart rate must reach during exercise to improve or maintain aerobic fitness

EXERCISES

MULTIPLE CHOICE

1. The formula for determining your target heart rate zone is
   a. MHR × intensity + resting heart rate
   b. (220 − age)
   c. (220 − resting heart rate) × 60–80%
   d. (220 − age) × 60–80%
   e. none of these

2. One positive effect of cardiorespiratory fitness is
   a. your blood pressure increases
   b. it takes less time to return to pre-exercise resting heart rates
   c. your resting heart rate increases
   d. your heart's ability to pump blood decreases
   e. your resting heart rate stays elevated

3. George has a resting heart rate of 62 beats per minute (bpm) at age 25. What is his estimated maximal heart rate (MHR)?
   a. 202 bpm
   b. 205 bpm
   c. 195 bpm
   d. 190 bpm
   e. 200 bpm

4. George has a resting heart rate of 62 beats per minute (bpm) at age 25. What is George's estimated target heart rate?
   a. 100–120 bpm
   b. 120–140 bpm
   c. 117–156 bpm
   d. 127–176 bpm
   e. 150–195 bpm

5. Which of the following is NOT an aerobic exercise?
   a. jogging
   b. bicycling
   c. fitness walking
   d. power lifting
   e. swimming laps

6. The best time to check your heart rate to determine the intensity of your workout is
   a. before beginning your workout
   b. immediately at the end of your warm-up
   c. immediately at the end of your cool-down
   d. immediately at the end of your cardiorespiratory workout
   e. 5 minutes after your cool-down to see whether training effects have occurred

7. Which term describes the greatest amount of oxygen that can be used by your body during intense exercise?
   a. cardiorespiratory endurance
   b. maximum aerobic capacity
   c. cardiorespiratory uptake
   d. maximum endurance
   e. maximum cardiorespiratory uptake

8. Which component of the Physical Readiness Evaluation for Police (PREP) assesses cardiorespiratory capacity?
   a. pursuit and restraint
   b. victim relocation
   c. arm restraint combined with the push–pull machine
   d. shuttle run
   e. running up and down stairs

9. The best example of a situation requiring aerobic fitness in law enforcement is
   a. handcuffing a passive person
   b. chasing down someone who is resisting arrest
   c. following a vehicle in your cruiser
   d. completing your paperwork for your supervisor
   e. bench pressing your body weight

10. HIIT stands for
    a. high-interval intensity training
    b. heavy intense interval testing
    c. high-intensity interval training
    d. high intensity indicator testing
    e. health indicator intensity test

11. You should take your resting heart rate
    a. before you write a test
    b. after you drive to school
    c. after you finish a timed run
    d. just before you go to bed at night
    e. when you first wake up but before you get out of bed in the morning

12. Exercising heart rate can be taken
    a. while you are running
    b. before you go for a run
    c. after completing your cool-down
    d. after completing your warm-up
    e. after completing 30 curl-ups

13. Maximal heart rate refers to
    a. what your heart rate is at before you go out for a run
    b. the rate at which you push your heart rate during a leisure run
    c. the heart rate when you are lying down reading a book
    d. what your heart rate is at maximal effort during a sustained aerobic activity
    e. what your heart rate is at the end of a proper warm-up

14. By resting between HIIT anaerobic sessions, you
    a. enable the oxygen-deprived blood to help clean out the lactic acid from the muscles
    b. enable the oxygen-rich blood to help clean out the lactic acid from your muscles
    c. can catch your breath before the next set
    d. a and c
    e. b and c

15. When preparing for the shuttle run on the treadmill, the starting stage is
    a. 7 kph
    b. 7.5 kph
    c. 8 kph
    d. 8.5 kph
    e. 9 kph

SHORT ANSWER

1. Why is cardiorespiratory fitness important in law enforcement?

2. Identify some of the benefits of cardiorespiratory fitness.

3. Define maximum aerobic capacity (VO_2 max or MVO_2).

4. Explain why it is important to know your target heart rate (THR) zone.

5. Identify some of the conditions in the environment that can affect an exercise program.

6. What are some ways to keep warm when running in the winter?

7. What are three ways in which the body can lose heat?

8. How would you train to pass the shuttle run?

REFERENCES

American College of Sports Medicine (ACSM). (2013). *ACSM's guidelines for exercise testing and prescription*. Philadelphia, PA: Lippincott Williams & Wilkins.

American College of Sports Science. (2009). *Guidelines for graded exercise testing and exercise prescription* (8th ed.). Philadelphia, PA: Lea and Febiger.

Anderson, G.S., Plecas, D., & Segger, T. (2001). Police officer physical ability testing—Re-validating a selection criterion. *Policing: An International Journal of Police Strategies & Management, 24*(1), 8–31.

Armstrong, L.E., Casa, D.J., Millard-Stafford, M., Moran, D.S., Pyne, S.W., & Williams, O. (2007). Exertional heat illness during training and competition. *Medicine & Science in Sports & Exercise, 39*(3), 556–572. Retrieved from http://journals.lww.com/acsm-msse/Fulltext/2007/03000/Exertional_Heat_Illness_during_Training_and.20.aspx

Arnold, C.M., & Faulkner, R.A. (2010, July). The effect of aquatic exercise and education on lowering fall risk in older adults with hip osteoarthritis. *Journal of Aging and Physical Activity, 18*(3), 245–260.

Borg, G. (1998). *Perceived exertion and pain scales*. Champaign, IL: Human Kinetics.

Bouchard, C., Shephard, R.J., Stephens, T., Sutton, J.R., & McPherson, B.D. (Eds.). (1990). *Exercise, fitness, and health: A consensus of current knowledge*. Champaign, IL: Human Kinetics.

Buman, M.P., & King, A.C. (2010, November). Exercise as a treatment to enhance sleep. *American Journal of Lifestyle Medicine, 4*, 500–514.

Bushman, B.A. (2012). How can I use METS to quantify the amount of aerobic exercise? *ACSM's Health & Fitness Journal, 16*(2), 5–7.

Canadian Border Services Agency. (2016). Become a CBSA Officer. Physical abilities standard. Retrieved from http://www.cbsa.gc.ca/job-emploi/bso-asf/phys-eval-apt-phys-eng.html

Canadian Society for Exercise Physiology (CSEP). (2003). *The Canadian physical activity, fitness and lifestyle appraisal: CSEP's guide to healthy living*. Ottawa: Author.

Canadian Society for Exercise Physiology (CSEP). (2011). *Canadian physical activity guideline for adults—18–64 years*. Retrieved from http://www.csep.ca/CMFlles/Guidelines/CSEP_PAGuidelines_adults_en.pdf

Canadian Society for Exercise Physiology (CSEP). (2016). CSEP special supplement—Canadian 24-hour movement guidelines for children and youth: An integration of physical activity, sedentary behaviour, and sleep/Supplément spécial de la SCPE—Directives canadiennes en matière de mouvement sur 24 heures pour les enfants et les jeunes: une approche intégrée regroupant l'activité physique, le comportement sédentaire et le sommei. *Applied Physiology, Nutrition, and Metabolism, 41*, i, 10.1139/apnm-2016-0266. Retrieved from https://indd.adobe.com/view/b82b4a90-6e46-4b1a-b628-d53805688baf

Castellani, J.W., Young, A.J, Ducharme, M.B., Giesbrecht, G.G., Glicman, E., & Sallis, R.E. (2006). ACSM position stand: Prevention of cold injuries during exercise. *Medicine & Science in Sports & Exercise, 38*(11), 2012–2029.

Cooper, K. (1982). *The aerobics program for total well-being*. New York, NY: M. Evans.

Denham, J., Feros, S.A., & O'Brien, B.J. (2015). Four weeks of sprint interval training improves 5-km run performance. *Journal of Strength and Conditioning Research, 29*(8), 2137–2141.

Elley, C.R., & Arroll, B. (2002, April 2). Review: Aerobic exercise reduces systolic and diastolic blood pressure in adults. *Annals of Internal Medicine, 136*(7), 493–503.

Fletcher, G.F, Froelicher V.F., Hartley, L.H., Haskell, W., & Pollock, M. (1990). Exercise standards: A statement for health professionals from the American Heart Association. *Circulation, 82*, 2286–2322.

Galloway, J. (2008). *Galloway's 5k/10k running* (2nd ed.). Aachen, Germany: Meyer & Meyer Sport.

Gibala, M.J., Little, J.P., van Essen, M., Wilkin, G.P., Burgomaster, K.A., Safdar, A., … Tarnopolsky, M.A. (2006). Short-term sprint interval versus traditional endurance training: Similar initial adaptations in human skeletal muscle and exercise performance. *Journal of Applied Physiology, 575*(3), 901–911.

Gibala, M.J., Little, J.P., MacDonald, M.J., & Hawley, J.A. (2012). Physiological adaptations to low-volume, high-intensity interval training in health and disease. *Journal of Physiology, 590*(5), 1077–1084.

Gledhill, N., Jamnik, V., & Shaw, J. (2014) Report on the Revision of the Physical Readiness Evaluation for Policing (PREP) Submitted to the Ministry of Community Safety and Corrections. Draft, Oct. 2014.

Gore, C.J. (Ed.) (2000). *Physiological tests for elite athletes*. Windsor, ON: Human Kinetics.

Government of Canada. (2014). *Air quality; Smog and your health*. Health and the environment. Retrieved from https://www.canada.ca/en/health-canada/services/air-quality/smog-your-health.html?=undefined&wbdisable=false

Gunnarsson, T.P., & Bangsbo, J. (2012). The 10-20-30 training concept improves performance and health profile in moderately training runners. *Journal of Applied Physiology, 113*, 16–24. doi:10.1152/japplphysiol.00334.2012

Hassinen, M., Lakka, T.A., Hakola, L., Savonen, K., Komulainen, P., Litmanen, H., … Rauramää, R. (2010, July). Cardiorespiratory fitness and metabolic syndrome in older men and women. *Diabetes Care, 33*(7), 1655–1657.

Healthy Living Unit. (2008). Public Health Agency of Canada. *The 2008 report on the integrated pan-Canadian healthy living strategy*. Retrieved from http://www.phac-aspc.gc.ca/hp-ps/hl-mvs/ipchls-spimmvs/2008/index-eng.php

Hood, M.S., Little, J.P., Tarnopolsky, M.A., Myslik, F., & Gibala, M.J. (2011). Low-volume interval training improves muscle oxidative capacity in sedentary adults. *Medicine & Science in Sports & Exercise, 43*(10), 1849–1856.

Irwin, M.L., Smith, A.W., McTiernan, A., Ballard-Barbash, R., Cronin, K., Gilliland, F.D., … Bernstein, L. (2008, August 20). Influence of pre- and post-diagnosis physical activity on mortality in breast cancer survivors: The health, eating, activity, and lifestyle study. *Clinical Oncology, 26*(24), 3958–3964.

Jamnik, V.K., Thomas, S.G., Shaw, J.A., & Gledhill, N. (2010). Identification and characterization of the critical physically demanding tasks encountered by correctional officers. *Applied Physiology, Nutrition, and Metabolism, 35*, 45–58.

Larose, J., Sigal, R.J., Khandwala, F., Prud'homme, D., Boulé, N.G., & Kenny, G.P. (2011). Associations between physical fitness and HbA$_{1c}$ in type 2 diabetes mellitus. *Diabetologia, 54*, 93–102.

Léger, L.A., & Lambert, J. (1982). A maximal multistage 20-m shuttle run test to predict VO$_2$ max. *European Journal of Applied Physiology and Occupational Physiology, 49*, 1–12

Léger L.A., Mercier D., Gadoury C., & Lambert J. (1988). The multistage 20 meter shuttle run test for aerobic fitness. *Journal of Sports Sciences, 6*, 93–101.

Léger, L., & Gadoury, C. (1989). Validity of the 20m shuttle run test with 1 min stages to predict VO$_2$ max in adults. *Canadian Journal of Sport Sciences, 14*, 21–26.

Léger, L., Lambert, J., Goulet, A., Rowan, C., & Dinelle, Y. (1984). Aerobic capacity of 6 to 17-year-old Quebecois—20 meter shuttle run with 1 minute stages. *Canadian Journal of Applied Sport Sciences, 9*(2), 64–69.

Mann, S., Beedie, C., & Jimenez, A. (2014). Differential effects of aerobic exercise, resistance training and combined exercise modalities on cholesterol and the lipid profile, synthesis and recommendations. *Sports Medicine, 44*(2), 211–221.

Ministry of Community Safety and Correctional Services (MCSCS). (2015). *PREP. Fit to Serve*. Preparing for the PREP—The Physical Readiness Evaluation for Police. Retrieved from http://www.applicanttesting.com/images/stories/pdf/FittoServe2015Final.pdf

Morris, C.K., Myers, J., Froelicher, V.F., Kawaguchi, T., Ueshima, K., & Hideg, A. (1993). Nomogram based on metabolic equivalents and age for assessing aerobic exercise capacity in men. *Journal of American College Cardiology, 22*, 175–182.

National Institute for Occupational Safety and Health (NIOSH). (2016). NIOSH criteria for a recommended standard: Occupational exposure to heat and hot environments. By Jacklitsch, B., Williams, W.J., Musolin, K., Coca, A., Kim, J-H., & Turner, N. Cincinnati, OH: U.S. Department of Health and Human Services, Centers for Disease Control and Prevention, National Institute for Occupational Safety and Health, DHHS (NIOSH) Publication 2016-106. Retrieved from https://www.cdc.gov/niosh/docs/2016-106/pdfs/2016-106.pdf

Nelson, M.E., Rejeski, W.J., Blair, S.N., Duncan, P.W., Judge, J.O., King, A.C., et al. (2007, August). Physical activity and public health in older adults: Recommendation from the American College of Sports Medicine and the American Heart Association. *Medicine & Science in Sports & Exercise, 8*, 1435–1445.

Nieman, D.C., Henson, D.A., Austin, M.D., & Brown, V.A. (2005). The immune response to a 30-minute walk. *Medicine and Science in Sports and Exercise, 37*, 57–62.

Ontario Ministry of the Solicitor General and Correctional Services. (2015). *Fit to serve: Preparation for the PREP—The Physical Readiness Evaluation for Policing*. Toronto: Author. Retrieved from http://www.applicanttesting.com/images/stories/pdf/FittoServe2015Final.pdf

Papousek, I., & Schulter, G. (2008). Effects of a mood-enhancing intervention on subjective well-being and cardiovascular parameters. *International Journal of Behavioral Medicine, 15*(4), 293–302.

Perceived Exertion (Borg Rating of Perceived Exertion Scale). (2015). Centers for Disease Control and Prevention. Retrieved from https://www.cdc.gov/physicalactivity/basics/measuring/exertion.htm

Ramsbottom, R., Brewer, J., & Williams, C. (1988). A progressive shuttle run test to estimate maximal oxygen uptake. *British Journal of Sports Medicine, 22*(4), 141–144. Retrieved from http://bjsm.bmj.com/content/bjsports/22/4/141.full.pdf

Royal Canadian Mounted Police (RCMP). (2016). 12 week fitness program. Retrieved from http://www.rcmp-grc.gc.ca/en/12-week-fitness-program#pct

RunningWithUs. (n.d.). 5K Training Plans. Cancer Research UK RACE FOR LIFE. https://raceforlife.cancerresearchuk.org/prepare-for-your-event/training-plans/5k

Seguin, R.A. (2015). Factors associated with Success in PARE testing among RCMP officers. *Electronic Thesis and Dissertation Repository.* Paper 2856. Retrieved from http://ir.lib.uwo.ca/etd/2856

Shanely, R.A., Nieman, D.C., Henson, D.A., Jin, F., Knab, A.M., & Sha, W. (2011). Inflammation and oxidative stress are lower in physically fit and active adults. *Scandinavian Journal of Medicine and Science in Sports, 23*, 215–223.

Shephard, R.J. (1997, April). Exercise and relaxation in health promotion. *Sports Medicine, 23*(4), 211–216.

Sigal, R.J., Kenny, G.P., Boulé, N.G., Wells, G.A., Prud'homme, D., Fortier, M., … Jaffey, J. (2007). Effects of aerobic exercise, resistance exercise, or both on glycemic control in type 2 diabetes: A randomized trial. *Annals of Internal Medicine, 147*, 357–369.

Smith, A.J., Phipps, W.R., Thomas, W., Schmitz, K.H., & Kurzer, M.S. (2013). The effects of aerobic exercise on estrogen metabolism in healthy premenopausal women. *Cancer Epidemiology, Biomarkers & Prevention, 22*(5), 756–764. doi: 10.1158/1055-9965

Stubbs, B., Rosenbaum, S., Vancampfort, D., Ward, P.B., & Schuch, F.B. (2016). Exercise improves cardiorespiratory fitness in people with depression: A meta-analysis of randomized control trials. *Journal of Affective Disorders, 190*, 249–253.

Tremblay, M.S., Warburton, D.E.R., Janssen, I., Paterson, D.H., Latimer, A.E., Rhodes, R.E., … Duggan, M. (2011). New Canadian physical activity guidelines. *Applied Physiology, Nutrition, and Metabolism, 36*, 36–46.

Vainio, H., & Bianchini, F. (2002). Weight control and physical activity. *IARC Handbooks of Cancer Prevention*, volume 6. Lyon, France: International Agency for Research on Cancer.

Varady, K.A., & Jones, P.J.H. (2005, August 1). Combination diet and exercise interventions for the treatment of dyslipidemia: An effective preliminary strategy to lower cholesterol levels? *JN: The Journal of Nutrition, 135*(8), 1829–1835.

Veteran Affairs Canada. (2006). Disability benefits: After an illness or injury. 2006 table of disabilities. Chapter 12—Cardiorespiratory impairment. Exercise tolerance and use of METs. Retrieved from http://www.veterans.gc.ca/eng/services/after-injury/disability-benefits/benefits-determined/table-of-disabilities/ch-12-2006 - a05

Warburton, D.E., Gledhill, N., & Quinney, A. (2001a). Musculoskeletal fitness and health. *Canadian Journal of Applied Physiology, 26*, 217–237.

Warburton, D.E., Gledhill, N., & Quinney, A. (2001b). The effects of changes in musculoskeletal fitness on health. *Canadian Journal of Applied Physiology, 26*, 161–216.

Warburton, D.E., McKenzie, D.C., Haykowski, M.J., Taylor, A., Shoemaker, P., Ignaszewski, A.P., & Chan, S.Y. (2005). Effectiveness of high-intensity interval training for the rehabilitation of patients with coronary artery disease. *American Journal of Cardiology, 95*, 1080–1084.

Wells, G.D., Selvanduria, H., & Tien, I. (2009). Bioenergetics provision of energy for muscular activity. *Paediatric Respiratory Reviews, 10*, 83–90. doi:10.1016/j.prrv.2009.04.005

6

RESISTANCE TRAINING

LEARNING OUTCOMES

After completing this chapter, you should be able to:

- Explain the importance of resistance training in law enforcement.

- Explain the benefits of resistance training.

- Understand some of the basic terms and concepts associated with strength, power, endurance, and functional training.

- Understand different training techniques and how to alter and progress on a basic resistance training program.

- Design a resistance training program to meet the job-related demands of law enforcement and improve/maintain an appropriate fitness level.

The health benefits of being physically fit are widely acknowledged. Like cardiorespiratory fitness training, resistance training (strength, endurance, and power training) is important for meeting the occupational requirements of law enforcement. Law enforcement officers are required to go from a sedentary activity to an emergency situation that involves running, detaining, and arresting individuals. They are required to wear a safety vest and a duty belt which can lead to low back issues (Anderson, Zutz, & Plecas, 2011; Brown, Wells, Trottier, Bonneau, & Ferris, 2001). A comprehensive training program helps your performance when you are under physical and mental stress while helping to prevent injury and fix structural imbalances. In this chapter you will learn basic terms and concepts associated with resistance training. This chapter will also enable you to design a training program for yourself that is effective and safe.

THE IMPORTANCE OF RESISTANCE TRAINING

Resistance training is an important part of an overall fitness program. Muscle mass, strength, power, and endurance are essential contributing factors to performing everyday tasks, improving musculoskeletal health, and maintaining mobility (Marcell, 2003). With a regular resistance training program, you can reduce your body fat, increase your lean muscle mass, and burn calories more efficiently. It can be done using your own body weight, or by using equipment like free weights, resistance bands, or machines. Both the American College of Sports Medicine (2009) and the Canadian Society of Exercise Physiology (2011) recommend that you participate in at least two to three sessions of resistance training per week when first starting out.

Resistance training has always been an integral component of training for emergency services. Strength, speed, quickness, and agility are keys to a successful takedown or rescue. Many students learn the basics of resistance training in high school but fail to take them further. Some have no interest in "looking big," many don't have the time to train, and others fail to research and concentrate on proper techniques for developing strength and fitness. Resistance training is not just for meeting the physical demands of the job; it is an important part of remaining fit throughout your career and into retirement.

Many services have emergency response teams (ERTs), tactics and rescue units (TRUs), and provincial emergency response teams (PERTs), all of which require outstanding cardiorespiratory endurance, muscular strength and endurance, and flexibility to meet the demands of the job on a regular basis. In addition to gruelling physical training, officers must learn rappelling, cover and concealment, tracking and searching, dynamic entry, high-risk vehicle assault, and urban and rural stalking (RCMP, 2001).

The physical demands of defensive tactics and arrest and control require a broad-based, general adaptation. This means that officers must be strong, quick to react, fast, accurate, and flexible in order to do their job. While some cases involve aerobic challenges in chasing a suspect, officers are more likely to face situations that involve altercations, which are shorter, more intense, and more threatening in nature, lasting from seconds to a few minutes. So law enforcement training must include workouts that are anaerobic and functional, and that work both the lower and upper extremities as well as training core muscles (see Figure 6.1).

FIGURE 6.1 Physically Meeting the Demands of the Job

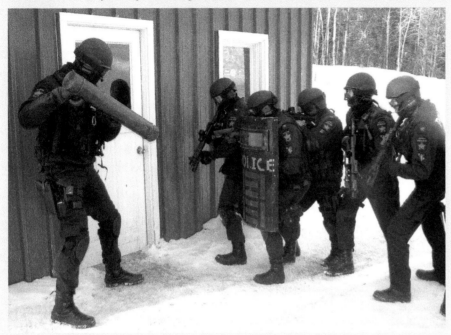

SOURCE: Photo Courtesy of Barrie Police Service, 2017.

As a result, law enforcement agencies have specific BFOR tests for specialized units/teams that assess one's functional abilities. Some of the assessments last up to 30 minutes and include wearing over 23 kg (50 lb.) of equipment; involve walking, running, and crawling; and require enough upper body strength to do single chin-ups and negotiate 1- to 2-m (3.5- to 6-foot) high walls/vault rails, and relocate 85 to 195 lb. mannequins.

Comparing absolute fitness levels between males and females has been an issue for years. A high proportion of female applicants fail entrance fitness tests because of their size, body composition, hemoglobin levels, and muscular strength (Shephard & Bonneau, 2002). BFOR standards have tried to address these issues; however, females, and in some cases smaller males, may still be at a disadvantage if they are not training appropriately. It is important to realize that muscular strength is something that must be continually worked on throughout your career. Statistically, women tend to shy away from strength training (see Women and Strength Training later in this chapter for more information). However, in law enforcement it is very important that all officers have the strength they need to do the job, whether they are physically restraining an individual, applying handcuffs, or pulling themselves over a wall while wearing a uniform, vest, and belt weighing approximately 11 to 23 kg (25 to 50 lb.).

BONA FIDE OCCUPATIONAL REQUIREMENTS (BFORs)

Since the late 1990s, Bona Fide Occupational Requirements (BFORs) (see Chapter 1 for more details) have been the standard for assessing applicants in most of the law enforcement agencies in Canada. BFORs cover elements of the job that require endurance, strength, and stamina. Upper-body strength to restrain and move people is a necessary part of law enforcement (Carlson & Jaenen, 2012; Farenholtz, 1995; Gledhill & Shaw, 1995; Jamnik, Thomas, Burr, & Gledhill, 2010). For this reason, upper-body strength is one of the fitness components tested by law enforcement organizations. Candidates for law enforcement positions are subjected to strength/power tests involving the push/pull machine, the arm-restraint device, body drags, and heavy bag carries.

COMPARISON OF PHYSICAL REQUIREMENTS IN LAW ENFORCEMENT BFORs

Law enforcement agencies require their officers to have a minimal physical fitness level in order to be able to do the specific tasks that are essential to the job. Table 6.1 is a comparison chart of what essential functional tasks are required for the job.

TABLE 6.1 Essential Functional Tasks in Law Enforcement

POLICING	ONTARIO CORRECTIONS	RCMP/CANADIAN BORDER SERVICES	CANADIAN MILITARY
• Pursue a suspect on foot, running a short distance (50–100 m) while negotiating obstacles to apprehend a resisting suspect. • Separate, restrain, and remove a disorderly and/or mentally ill person(s) (push/pull 35.5 kg, arm restraint–grip 14.5 kg, retraction 16 kg). • Conduct a removal of a person (77 kg). • Demonstrate aerobic fitness (stage 7).	• Cell search • Expeditious response • Body control (35.5 kg) • Arm restraint • Inmate relocation • Aerobic assessment (stage 5.5)	• Running • Jumping • Crawling • Balancing • Vaulting • Climbing • Lifting • Carrying (36.3/45.4 kg [80/100 lb.] bag) • Dragging • Pushing/pulling (31.8/36.4 kg [70/80 lb.]) • Fighting	• Escape to cover high–low crawl • Pickets and wire carry • Picking and digging–entrenchment dig • Vehicle extrication casualty evacuation • Sandbag carry

SOURCES: Bonneau & Brown, 1995; Gledhill & Jamnik, 2015; Jamnik, Gumienak, & Gledhill, 2013; Spivock, Reilly, Newton, Blacklock, & Jaenen, 2011.

> **DID YOU KNOW?**
> After the age of 50, sedentary people may begin to lose muscle mass and strength at the rate of approximately 1 to 2 percent per year (Marcell, 2003). This condition is called *sarcopenia*. It contributes to fractures and falls, with the consequent loss of independence, and also decreases metabolic rate and maximum aerobic capacity.

Musculoskeletal endurance influences work capacity when a task requires lifting heavy objects. Lifting and pushing heavy objects requires a metabolic demand which eventually leads to muscular fatigue; this muscular fatigue causes peripheral fatigue (intramuscular energy stores) and central fatigue (glycogen depletion resulting in cognitive impairment) (Sharkey & Davis, 2008) which results in a decrease in performance and work capacity (Astrand, Rodahl, & Dahl, 2003). It is important that you train specifically on these essential tasks in order to demonstrate that you can meet the minimum requirements for a career in law enforcement.

THE BENEFITS OF RESISTANCE TRAINING

In the first two to three weeks of an exercise program, muscles begin to gain strength due to the recruitment of more muscle fibres. Later, after four to six weeks, the muscle fibres increase in size. This is known as hypertrophy. Additional physiological/psychological benefits from resistance training include:

• increased bone mineral density, therefore reducing risk of osteoporosis

- higher resting metabolic rate

- positive body composition changes (increased muscle mass and reduced body fat)

- reduction in the risk of developing metabolic syndrome including cardiovascular disease, hypertension, obesity

- reduction in the risk of developing cancer

- reduction of back pain

- improved glucose utilization, which is important for preventing or controlling diabetes

- improved body image/self-confidence/reduction in depression

- improved athletic performance (in sports and for BFORs)

- reduction in injuries and joint problems (arthritis)

- improved sleep

(Boulé, Haddad, Kenny, Wells, & Sigal, 2001; Calatayud, Borreani, Moya, Colado, & Triplett, 2013; Chang, Lin, & Lai, 2015; Drenowatz, Hand, Sagner, Shook, Burgess, & Blair, 2015; Engelke et al., 2006; Jurca et al., 2004; Kerksick et al., 2010; Paoli, Moro, Marcolin, Neri, Bianco, Palma, & Grimaldi, 2012; Seguin, Eldridge, Lynch, & Paul, 2013; Shiroma, Cook, Manson, Moorthy, Buring, Rimm, & Lee, 2017; Stensvold et al., 2010; Warburton, Nicol, & Bredin, 2006)

THE BASICS OF RESISTANCE TRAINING

Resistance training includes any type of exercise that requires the muscles to move, or attempt to move, against an opposing force. It encompasses weight training but also a much wider range of training activities, including body weight exercises such as push-ups and chin-ups. Most training programs are designed to increase muscular strength or muscular endurance, to alter body composition by increasing muscle size and/or decreasing the percentage of fat in the body.

Athletes train for a variety of reasons. When training for absolute strength, athletes train to lift the heaviest weight possible, regardless of their body weight. When training for relative strength (force generated relative to body weight), athletes consider how strong they are per kilogram of body weight. When an athlete trains for endurance, he or she creates a force such as sustained (isometric) or repeated (isotonic) muscular actions against a submaximal resistance (for example, bicep curls).

Functional strength has become very important both in terms of training and rehabilitation. Functional strength is the amount of strength an individual can use in a sport, doing his/her job, and/or in daily tasks, making them easier, smoother, safer, and more efficient. Functional strength focuses on the strength required for a specific task at hand (for example, relocating a non-compliant individual) (Santana, 2016).

Strength, power, and endurance training focuses on two components of the body: the muscles and the central nervous system (CNS), which causes the muscles to fire and thus to contract. It has been well documented that gains experienced during the first six weeks of training stem primarily from CNS adaptation—the muscles learning to synchronize better with one another. Gains arising from muscular adaptation (improved muscle coordination and movement) occur later (Faulkner & White, 1990; Koutedakis, Stavropoulos-Kalinoglou, & Metsios, 2005).

BASIC PRINCIPLES OF RESISTANCE TRAINING

MUSCULAR STRENGTH

Muscular strength training is defined as *how much* force a muscle can exert. It is measured by the amount of force required for one single maximal effort. The goal of strength training is to stress the muscular and neuromuscular systems through lifting heavy loads for only a few repetitions. Strength training is crucial for all law enforcement officers, as they may be in physical altercations where they need absolute strength for their own safety.

REPETITIONS

A repetition (rep) is one complete movement of an exercise.

SETS

A set is a group of repetitions. For example, "2 sets of 10 reps" means two groups of ten repetitions each, with a rest period between each group.

MUSCULAR ENDURANCE

Muscular endurance is defined as *how long* a muscle can exert a force over time. Athletes who have good endurance levels will have the capacity to maintain force and speed over a longer period of time. This is important for law enforcement officers who may become involved in lengthy foot pursuits and confrontations. It is also important for those officers on tactical units who must respond quickly and maintain speed while wearing approximately 23 kg (50 lb.) of gear and equipment. Figure 6.2 compares strength and endurance training.

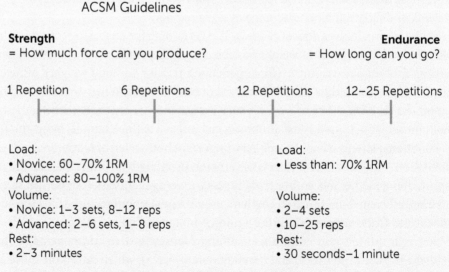

FIGURE 6.2 Comparison of Strength versus Endurance Training Based on ACSM Guidelines

Strength
= How much force can you produce?

Endurance
= How long can you go?

| 1 Repetition | 6 Repetitions | 12 Repetitions | 12–25 Repetitions |

Load:
• Novice: 60–70% 1RM
• Advanced: 80–100% 1RM
Volume:
• Novice: 1–3 sets, 8–12 reps
• Advanced: 2–6 sets, 1–8 reps
Rest:
• 2–3 minutes

Load:
• Less than: 70% 1RM

Volume:
• 2–4 sets
• 10–25 reps
Rest:
• 30 seconds–1 minute

SOURCE: Adapted from ACSM's *Guidelines for Exercise Testing and Prescription*, 2013.

POWER

Muscular power is generating as much force as possible, as quickly as possible. It is the amount of force produced over a period of time. To train for power, an athlete works to build overall body explosiveness and reactive ability. Olympic lifting, such as snatch and clean and jerk, use this power to lift maximum loads as quickly and efficiently as possible. Law enforcement officers need to train for muscular power so that they are prepared to move someone from danger as fast as possible.

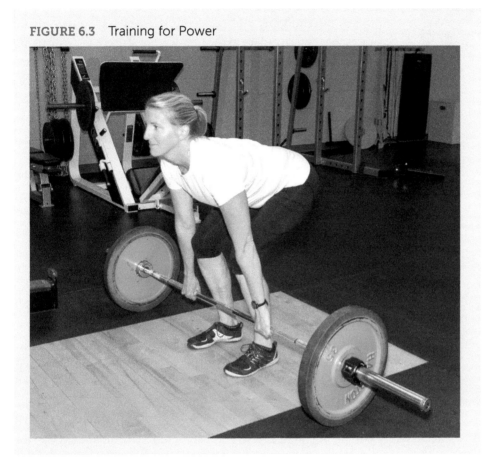

FIGURE 6.3 Training for Power

HYPERTROPHY

Muscular hypertrophy is the increase in size of the skeletal muscle. This is accomplished by lifting heavy loads for approximately 6 to 12 repetitions. The goal is to build muscle mass. When you increase muscle size, the muscle has a greater potential of force. Usually, hypertrophy combined with motor neuron activation—in which the brain recruits more motor units to "fire"—produces greater strength gains.

PLYOMETRICS

Plyometrics, also known as "jump training," involves a lot of fast, bounding type movements. It is based on the principle that the combination of speed and strength is power. It is a method of training that enhances an individual's explosive reaction by means of rapid and powerful muscular contractions through stretch-shortening cycles.

Examples of exercises include 90-degree jumps, lateral skating, one-leg butt kicks, ski tuck jumps, and two-foot side hops. As you become more advanced, you can try activities like decline hops, two-foot hops off a box, bench jumping, rope jumping, and box jumps (see Figure 6.4). Alternating between lunges and sprints on a track also constitutes a form of plyometrics.

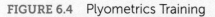

FIGURE 6.4 Plyometrics Training

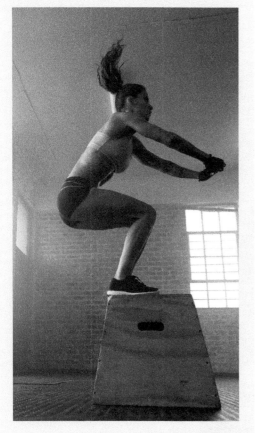

THE PROGRESSIVE OVERLOAD PRINCIPLE

To build muscle mass, a greater than normal load must stress the muscle. This is called the principle of progressive overload. The process of rebuilding and repairing stressed soft muscle tissue causes the tissue to adapt to the new level of stress. Once the tissue has adapted to the new level, additional stress must be placed on it to spur further improvement. Individuals must be cautious in increasing their training load because an abrupt increase in load may go beyond the muscle's ability to adapt, causing injury.

GENERAL ADAPTATION

The general adaptation phase prepares your muscles, joints, tendons, and ligaments for intense training. It is characterized by higher repetitions, lower intensities, and short rest periods, which help the neuromuscular components synchronize so that gains can be seen.

BETWEEN-SET REST

It is important to rest between each set of an exercise. Proper rest periods can affect metabolic, hormonal, and cardiorespiratory responses to strength training. Depending on the exercise, the training program, and your goal, the amount of time you rest between sets can vary. You could be resting anywhere from 30 seconds to 5 minutes. The heavier the load and fewer reps you are completing, the more rest is usually required between sets. You can use this time effectively by completing an exercise that uses a different muscle group (for example, between sets of bench press, you could be doing squats).

ONE REP MAXIMUM (1RM)

One rep maximum (1RM) technique involves determining the maximum load you can lift for a single rep. Because lifting maximum loads can cause injury, this method should be used only under the supervision of your instructor or another certified fitness professional. The purpose of finding your 1RM is to set goals and to determine precise lifting loads.

Refer to **assignment 6.1** (www.emond.ca/fitness5e) to determine your workload for your maximum bench press.

You now can go back to Figure 6.2 and look at the ACSM recommendations for strength and endurance training. This will help you when you create your resistance training program. You can determine your load (how much you might lift) and your volume (how much work you should do) for bench press based on your predicted 1RM.

PROPER BREATHING

Your blood pressure can increase to dangerous levels if you always hold your breath while resistance training. Breathing in and out should occur continuously, and not be trained to a specific exertion effort—this helps to maintain constant abdominal muscle activation and ensure spine stability during all possible situations. (Of course the opposite is true for maximal effort competitive lifting where a valsalva manoeuvre with the breath held is necessary [McGill, 2003].) Just be sure that you are monitoring your breathing and heart rate, and allowing time for them to return to normal between sets.

PERIODIZATION

Periodization is an organized approach to training that involves progressive cycling of various aspects of a training program during a specific period of time to achieve specific goals (such as training for a sport or a law enforcement BFOR). Periodization programs are designed to be very specific to each individual as they plan and progress through different training phases, so as to ensure peak performance at the time of competition or BFOR test.

An example of a periodization training program is shown in Table 6.2. It begins with a "base building/conditioning phase," where the aim is to develop basic hypertrophy and strength, while working on functional sport-specific or job-specific movements. Then training progresses to involve speed and power exercises, along with the strength training in the "pre-competition/pre-BFOR test." During the period of time surrounding the "competition/BFOR test," the intensity of training decreases to a maintenance type of program. The "recovery phase" allows individuals to recover and focus on other aspects of training, such as endurance, mobility, or other goals.

TABLE 6.2 Example of Periodization Training

Base building and conditioning phase
Strength & Coordination—Intensity high/volume high
⇓
Pre-competition/Pre-BFOR phase
Strength, Power, Speed—Intensity high/volume moderate
⇓
Competition/BFOR phase
Maintenance & Recovery—Intensity low/volume moderate
⇓
Recovery phase (off season)
Rehabilitation & Maintenance—Intensity low/volume low

SOURCE: Adapted from B. Martin, 2012.

You may choose to develop your own resistance training program involving periodization. Depending on your goals, a 16-week program would work appropriately with one semester of school and could involve three or four phases. If your program involves a fitness class with a fitness test, you can plan and develop your workouts to prepare accordingly for that fitness test as your "competition phase." Or if you plan on applying to a law enforcement agency while in school, you could use periodization to prepare for that as well. Another option would be to use the summer months as your "base building/conditioning phase," so that you are training hard while you have more time, and then you can use your school months as your "maintenance phase."

FYI

BENEFITS OF PERIODIZATION

There are a number of benefits in utilizing periodization, including:

- reducing the risk of fatigue and overtraining by managing factors such as intensity, load, and recovery,
- the cyclic structure maximizes both general preparation and specific preparation for the sport or job-related testing,
- the ability to optimize performance over a specific period of time, and
- taking into account age, time restraints, and environmental factors.

BASIC GUIDELINES FOR RESISTANCE TRAINING
GETTING STARTED AND SETTING GOALS

Similar to cardiorespiratory training, it is important to begin a resistance training program with what your goals are. What would you like to achieve? Is your goal to be able to pass a specific BFOR to apply for a job? Are you looking to increase your muscle mass? Maybe you would like to increase your endurance training so that you can confidently work 12-hour shifts, with 20 lbs. of gear?

When setting goals, you need to make sure that they follow the SMART principle (see Chapter 2) and that the training will fit into your life. Attending school full-time and working 15 to 20 hours a week does not allow for much training time. Make sure that you set an appropriate goal during school and design a program for yourself that is conducive to your current routine.

Decide on how many days a week you will be able to train. And be realistic. Do not say every day if you cannot make that commitment. Maybe for the first few weeks, it could be every other day. Or even two days during the week and one day on the weekend. If you have a concrete daily routine, then maybe adding in a daily workout fits; but you know yourself best, and need to make sure your training program suits you first. Set yourself up to succeed, not to fail.

For your training to be effective, you must be training regularly, at least two to three times a week. Those who are more advanced, can be training four to five days per week (ACSM, 2009). Remember that is important to allow each muscle group 48 hours to rest after strenuous exercises; otherwise you risk overtraining and will not see the improvements that you wish to see.

Remember that results take time and are sometimes very gradual. Keeping a log may help you monitor your progress. (The *Fit for Duty, Fit for Life* training guide that accompanies this textbook provides a Daily Workout Log that you can use.) Although you will begin to see changes in the first six weeks, it can take at least 16 weeks to see the results you want. If nothing is happening after the first six weeks, you will need to modify your training program (Bickel, Cross, & Bamman, 2011).

DESIGNING A PROGRAM

After deciding on your goals and how many days per week you will train, you need to decide where you will work out and what equipment is available to you. This will allow you to design an appropriate program to suit your goals. Will you have access to a big gym, with every piece of equipment on hand? Or will you be working out in your basement, with a few sets of dumbbells? Many people turn away from strength training simply because they do not have access to a gym and equipment. Do not let that hinder your goals. You can design an incredibly effective program with just a 20 lb. heavy bag and body-based exercises.

WARM-UP AND COOL-DOWN

Your workout must always include a proper warm-up and cool-down. Your warm-up should consist of 5 to 10 minutes of an aerobic activity such as light jogging or bicycling to quicken your heart rate, breathing, and blood flow. Follow with dynamic stretching and movements that mimic the types of exercises you will do in your workout, using light weights to prepare the muscles.

At the end of your workout, take 5 to 10 minutes to cool down and lower your heart rate, breathing, and blood flow. Do some light cardio again, and follow with some stretching, focusing on the muscles that were just exerted.

ARRANGING EXERCISES

When first starting out, choosing what exercises to do can be an overwhelming task for some people. Here are some general rules when it comes to choosing exercises and arranging what order to complete them in:

- For a full body workout, aim for 8 to 12 exercises total. You can complete them in a circuit (which means that you perform each in succession, with minimal rest between exercises) or you can focus on one exercise at a time, resting in between sets. This decision may come down to how much time you have (circuit training is faster) and/or how crowded your training space is (it is hard to circuit train if your gym is busy).

- Ensure that you exercise all the major muscle groups. It is important to achieve a balance between exercising agonists (muscles that move a joint in the desired direction) and antagonists (muscles that simultaneously resist that movement). For example, alternate pushing and pulling exercises (chest presses then rear flys). Similarly, make sure that you are doing upper and lower body exercises, as well as core exercises.

- Exercise the large-muscle groups first so that the small muscles (which are not fatigued) can support the large muscles. Small muscles, such as forearm flexors, recover faster than larger muscles, such as the pectoralis major, and therefore can tolerate more sets without risking soreness or overtraining.

- Do multiple-joint exercises before single-joint exercises, because the former use more muscle groups and better reflect daily activities. Although multiple-joint exercises focus on one particular muscle group, there are many other muscles that act as stabilizers. Examples include squats, deadlifts, bench presses, military presses, rowing, and chin-ups. Single-joint exercises, also known as isolation exercises, engage single-muscle groups. Examples include leg curls, biceps curls, quadriceps extensions, lateral raises, and shoulder shrugs.

- The correct form in resistance training is a steady, controlled execution of the exercise through the full range of motion. It is important to isolate the muscle group you are exercising. For example, if you are doing biceps curls, you need to concentrate on the biceps and not use your back. Control the weight through the concentric and eccentric contraction; it should be your muscle doing the work, not gravity. And resist the urge to lift too fast and bounce the weight.

Choosing the exercises for a program is highly specific to the individual, their goals, and the equipment available to them. Table 6.3 is a list of common exercises for each muscle group. Each muscle group has equipment options: from having no equipment, to simple equipment like dumbbells, bars, and bands, to exercise machines. It is important to recognize that each individual exercise has many different variations available. For example, variations of a basic chest press using a barbell would be doing it on a bench or stability ball, alternating hand locations (narrow grip, shoulder width, or wide grip), changing tempo (down slow, up fast or down fast, up slow) or changing the bench to incline, flat, or decline. You could use dumbbells, cables, bands, kettle bells, heavy bags, or use a chest press machine. Guidelines and examples of exercises will be shown in the *Fit for Duty, Fit for Life* training guide with pictures and descriptions, as well as how they can be incorporated into a resistance training program to prepare for a BFOR.

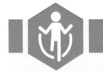 **FYI**

LAW OF DIMINISHING RETURNS

Research has shown that untrained individuals will see greater strength gains initially at a given weight while trained individuals will have to do more repetitions at the same given weight to see changes. This difference is due to neural factors, such as increased recruitment and synchronization and metabolic recovery (Brechue & Mayhew, 2009).

TABLE 6.3 Exercise Options Based on Equipment Available

BODY PART	NO EQUIPMENT	USING FREE WEIGHTS/ BANDS/BALLS	MACHINES
Chest	Push-ups	Chest press Chest flys	Chest press Decline/incline bench press Cable crossover Pec deck fly
Back	Chin-ups Pull-ups Bird-dogs	Rows Stiff leg dead lifts	Lat pull-down Cable row
Shoulders	Handstands Downward dog Push-ups	Shoulder press Upright row Shoulder shrugs Lateral raise Front raise	Seated shoulder press Cable crossovers Cable upright row
Legs	Squats Lunges Jumps Hip bridge Side leg lift Wall sit	Squats Lunges Deadlifts Calf raises	Leg press Leg extension Leg curl Abductor/adductor Calf raises
Arms	Push-ups Chin-ups Dips	Biceps curls Triceps extensions	Biceps curls Cable curls Triceps extensions Cable extensions
Core	Front plank Side bridges Bird-dogs Dead-bugs	Roll-outs Stir-the-pot Suitcase carry Around the world	Wood-chopper

NOTE: Many variations are available for exercises, including variations of grips, machine attachments, hand/foot placement, unilateral versus bilateral, stable versus unstable.

DECIDING ON SETS/REPS

For the first few weeks, most resistance programs should have you aiming to complete 1 to 2 sets of 10 to 15 repetitions until proper exercise form has been developed (Faigenbaum, 2000). After a few weeks, you can gradually increase to 2 to 3 sets and decrease the number of repetitions to 8 to 12. Ultimately, the number of repetitions that one can complete is affected by the subject's age, sex, training status, size of muscle groups, genetics, use of machines or free weights, and movement biomechanics (ACSM, 2009).

Table 6.4 is a very general breakdown on how to decide how many sets, reps, and the amount of rest you may need while training for different goals.

TABLE 6.4 Training Goals

TRAINING GOAL	# OF REPS	# OF SETS	REST BETWEEN SETS
Muscular Endurance	12–25	1–3	30–60 seconds
Hypertrophy	6–12	3–6	30–90 seconds
Strength	1–6	3–6	2–5 minutes
Power	1–5	3–5	2–5 minutes

SOURCES: ACSM, 2009, 2013.

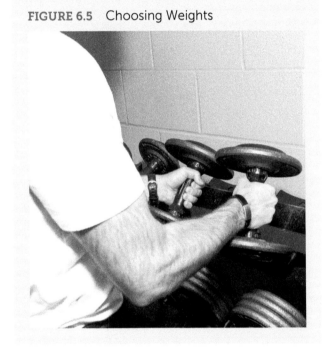

FIGURE 6.5   Choosing Weights

CHOOSING WEIGHTS

It is very common for someone new to resistance training to have no idea what dumbbells to pick up or how many plates to put on the bar. It can be yet another confusing and intimidating process that deters people from starting a resistance training program. Again, it is important to revisit your goals and what you are aiming to achieve at the gym. See Figure 6.5.

For beginners, and for people not interested in lifting maximum or near-maximum loads, here is a simple way to determine your lifting load:

1. Choose a weight that you feel very comfortable that you can lift for 10 repetitions. Do that first set of 10 reps, and consider it your warm-up. How did that weight feel? Was it easy? Or did you struggle to lift the ninth and tenth rep? Don't try to lift more than you are able to even if you didn't reach 10 repetitions. There is less chance of injury lifting a lighter weight to start.

2. Adjust the weight according to what your goals are. (Refer to Table 6.4 for training goals.) Remember that when training for strength, your goal is "how much?" and therefore you want to be choosing a heavier weight and doing anywhere from 3 to 10 reps. When training for endurance, your goal is "how long?" and you are choosing medium to lighter weights and doing 10+ reps.

3. Complete your second set with your adjusted weight and decide if that was a more appropriate load. When it comes to strength, you should always be trying to find a weight that challenges you on your last few repetitions. If you can complete your set without any trouble, you need to be choosing a heavier weight next time.

4. Decide if you want to complete a third set, or if you want to stop at two. On your third set you should have a pretty good idea of the proper load to lift, but remember that your muscles will be fatiguing by that third set, and you may have trouble completing your desired amount of reps. Remember that you don't have to complete all the repetitions—working toward completing the reps can be one of your training goals.

5. At the end of an exercise, record the weight that you used and the sets/ reps. Using a log book like *Fit for Duty, Fit for Life* training guide allows you to record your training and benefits you by saving time and effort trying to remember what you lifted last time. This is vital and one of the greatest internal motivators of resistance training is being able to see your progression.

TABLE 6.5 Example of a Training Log

WORKOUT CARD FOR:										DATE:	
EXERCISE	SET 1		SET 2		SET 3		SET 4		SET 5		
	WEIGHT	REPS	WEIGHT	REPS	WEIGHT	REPS	WEIGHT	REPS	WEIGHT	REPS

For advanced training, there is a more precise method for choosing weights. The widely accepted technique for gauging what weights to lift is based on an athlete's 1RM (one repetition maximum). Once the 1RM is established, the athlete would be training at specific percentages of that 1RM to reach their goals (for example, lifting 4 to 5 reps at 85 percent 1RM [Brechue & Mayhew, 2009]). And then at six- to eight-week intervals, the 1RM would be tested again to determine if changes needed to be made to the training program. It is vital that all of the workouts are recorded in a log book or on your phone, so that you continue to progress and see your accomplishments and gains.

Many trainers are hesitant to subject individuals to 1RM tests because of the high risk of injury. But the benefits of having very specific loads to lift and goals to meet are very encouraging, as long as the 1RM testing is done safely and under the guidance of a certified personal trainer. Your school's instructor or fitness centre can help you find someone qualified.

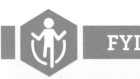

FYI

TOO MUCH, TOO SOON, TOO FAST

One of the most common mistakes people make when beginning a weight training program or returning to a program after a few months off (for example, Christmas break) is that they push too hard on their first trip back to the gym. As tempting as it is to pick up the same weights as your gym-going friend or to challenge yourself to do three sets to failure, it is strongly not advised. This is when injuries occur. Your body will be very sore after a hard workout, and if you have been sedentary prior to this, it may take a while to recover. DOMS (delayed onset muscle soreness) occurs 24 to 48 hours after lifting weights, but has been seen to last 4 to 6 days on untrained individuals who did too much on their first lifting session (Cheung, Hume, & Maxwell, 2003). So be smart. Choose lighter weights and fewer sets/reps until your body gets used to the demands (this could take a couple of weeks). Then progress at a safe pace, so that you don't get injured or become so sore that you get discouraged and never want to return.

TRAINING METHODS

Once you start to feel confident in lifting weights, you can start to modify your training to make your workout more interesting and challenging. A general rule is to modify your workout every six weeks, otherwise, the muscles will adapt and your gains will level off. You can modify your workout (recall the FITT formula in Chapter 5) by altering intensity, the number of sets, the type and speed of muscular action, the type of exercise, the order of exercises, and the length of rest periods between sets and workouts. Changing the type of equipment is one of the easiest modifications you can make as a beginner. For example, if you have been using machines for your first month of training, alter your workout by doing the exact same exercises but with free weights.

Here are several different training techniques you can use to modify your workout. Again, which one you choose depends on your goals and on the amount of time you have to devote to your program.

CIRCUIT TRAINING

Circuit training is structured so that you perform a number of exercises in succession at a submaximal level, with little rest in between. This form of conditioning develops strength, endurance (both aerobic and anaerobic), flexibility, and coordination all in one exercise session. It is a balanced workout that targets all muscle groups while building cardiorespiratory endurance, usually with about 2 to 3 sets of 10 exercises done for 60 seconds each with 15 to 30 seconds of rest in between. Adding a longer cardio component builds in the principles of interval training. By alternating 1 minute of cardio (skipping, steps, sprinting) with ten 1-minute endurance exercises, the athlete pushes the anaerobic system so that the body must adapt to lactic acid fatigue.

LIGHT TO HEAVY TRAINING

With light to heavy training, as you progress through the sets, you increase the weight you are working with. This system carries a low risk of injury. The major drawback is that the muscles may tire during the earlier sets, preventing heavier lifting later.

HEAVY TO LIGHT TRAINING

Heavy to light training has you decrease the amount of weight you are lifting as you progress through your sets. You can also perform a drop set, which means that you decrease the weight you are working with during one set, as you are approaching failure. You could potentially decrease the weight three or four times in a set. The advantage is that you may be able to lift heavier weights. The disadvantage is a high risk of injury if you have not properly warmed up your muscles.

PYRAMID TRAINING

The pyramid training system combines the light to heavy and heavy to light approaches. You begin your workout with the light to heavy approach, followed by the heavy to light approach during the second half. This system is good for developing strength. It can cause injury, however, by tempting people to push too hard to finish their sets.

SUPERSET TRAINING

The superset training system involves performing two exercises in succession, without rest. It is often used to exercise opposing muscle groups. It increases strength and muscle mass of the targeted muscle group. For example, squats followed by leg extensions will increase the size and strength of the quadriceps muscle. Or doing bench press followed by triceps extension targets the triceps muscle. Be careful: if the muscle is pre-fatigued, then you may be pushing it beyond comfortable limits and this is when injuries can occur.

TRISET TRAINING

Trisets are combinations of three exercises done with little rest in between. They can involve working the same muscle group from three different angles, working three different muscle groups, or working different areas of the same muscle from three different angles. Trisets increase training intensity by reducing the average length of rest intervals between sets. Trisets save time and raise the metabolism; however, they are associated with a higher risk of injury. An example of a sequence for the chest and back could be decline dumbbell presses, chin-ups, and incline dumbbell flys.

FUNCTIONAL TRAINING

Functional training adapts or develops exercises which allow individuals to perform daily activities, specific sports, or physically demanding jobs more easily and without injury. It focuses on strengthening a movement, as opposed to a specific body part. The concept behind functional training in law enforcement is to emphasize the movements an officer faces on duty, such as running after a suspect, climbing a wall, running up and down stairs, dealing with a non-compliant individual, and extricating a victim, all while at a high stress level. Examples of exercises that mimic an altercation with an individual that involve pushing would be doing chest presses, push-ups, or pushing a prowler (heavy sled) across a gym.

After an individual has reached their desired fitness level, in regards to strength, size, and power, there comes a time when training needs to have an applicable focus. It may no longer be necessary to be weight lifting just for the sake of it, and if a career in law enforcement is in the individual's future, it makes sense to start concentrating on exercises that will help them to do their job safely. Also, as you age, it is common to see injuries develop due to training too hard, and it is important to limit these injuries by training smart. The focus of training should shift to strength exercises that incorporate stability, coordination, balance, posture, and agility.

A recent study found that law enforcement students wearing a 9 kg weight belt had a significant decrease in acceleration and velocity when doing sprints of the gym versus not wearing a weight belt (Lewinski, Dysterheft, Dicks, & Pettitt, 2015). This means that one focus of an officer's program should be explosive activities through their legs to overcome that decrease in acceleration due to extra gear. Another study that looked at injuries acquired during training in the military resolved that spending more time focusing on exercises that promote balance and ankle control would be helpful in reducing injuries (Bullock, 2010). Officers from specialized teams take functional training one step further by simulating scenarios that allow them to train job-specific movement patterns while under stress. The *Fit for Duty, Fit for Life* training guide shows functional training exercises that allow students to prepare specifically for law enforcement BFORs.

PERSONAL PERSPECTIVE

FUNCTIONAL TRAINING FOR QUALITY OF LIFE

To assist my 87-year-old mother's quality of life after three strokes, we are in the process of functionally training her to do squats in a chair and then behind the chair. This is to assist in improving her balance and muscle strength and decrease her risk of falling. This same approach applies to those who are trying to learn how to use the push–pull or arm restraint machines. It is important to functionally train to mimic the machines in order to use them during the test.

LAW ENFORCEMENT RESISTANCE TRAINING PROGRAMS

In preparation for a career in law enforcement, it is essential that you create a resistance training program. You may want to emphasize endurance, or you may want to include more strength training to meet the demands of the job and BFOR standards to apply for that job.

Provided below are training programs that address the specific areas that will help you complete your specific BFOR requirements. Also, in your *Fit For Duty,*

Fit for Life training guide there are a number of exercises with descriptions and photographs to help you train for tasks such as the push–pull machine and the arm restraint. As you train for your BFOR, you will come to appreciate that technique plays a role and applicants with good strength, coordination, and agility are usually able to get through the protocol without injury. However, it will be up to you to see that you are able to meet the minimum requirements.

These training programs can be found on the specific agency's website in preparation for their BFOR. They can be a great starting point for a beginner, or provide ideas to an intermediate or advanced athlete. These programs can be performed in a circuit training type format or one exercise at a time, and can be used to train for any of the law enforcement BFORs.

PREP TEST/A-PREP

In training for the PREP test, three training programs (beginner, intermediate, and advanced) can be found in the *Fit to Serve Guide* that accompanies the PREP BFOR explanation. They reinforce muscular strength and endurance of the arms, shoulders, core, and legs. Table 6.6 presents the recommended training program for an intermediate level, recommended to be completed three times per week.

TABLE 6.6 Training for the PREP and A-PREP

EXERCISE	SETS	FOR ENDURANCE			FOR STRENGTH		
		REPS	LOAD (% MAX)	REST INTERVAL (SECS)	REPS	LOAD (% MAX)	REST INTERVAL (SECS)
Bench Press	2–3	10–15	60–70	60–120	6–10	80–85	120–180
Leg Press/Lunge	2–3	10–15	60–70	60–120	6–10	80–85	120–180
Shoulder Press	2–3	10–15	60–70	60–120	6–10	80–85	120–180
Front Lats Pull-down	2–3	10–15	60–70	60–120	6–10	80–85	120–180
Triceps Extension	2–3	10–15	60–70	60–120	6–10	80–85	120–180
Abdominal Crunches	2–3	10–15	60–70	60–120	6–10	80–85	120–180
Reverse Chin-ups	2–3	10–15	60–70	60–120	6–10	80–85	120–180
Triceps Bench Dips	2–3	10–15	60–70	60–120	6–10	80–85	120–180

SOURCE: MCSCS, 2015. *PREP: Fit to Serve*: https://www.applicanttesting.com/images/stories/pdf/FittoServe2015Final.pdf

PARE TEST

The resistance training program that prepares you for the PARE BFOR can be found on the RCMP's website. They have two full body workouts: one requiring that you have dumbbells, and one that requires no equipment. They are both recommended to be completed two to four times per week. (See Tables 6.7 and 6.8.)

TABLE 6.7 PARE Total Body Workout #1—Requires Dumbbells

EXERCISE	SETS	REPS	OBJECTIVE
Dumbbell Swing	2–3	10	• Power • Strengthens posterior core chain muscles
One Leg Split Squat (with or without dumbbells)	2–3	10 per side	• Single leg work • Strengthens leg and activates glutes
Chin-ups Medium Grip	2–3	5+	• Upper body vertical pull • Strengthens back
Dumbbell Bench Press	2–3	10	• Upper body horizontal push • Strengthens chest and shoulders
Dumbbell Row	2–3	10 per side	• Upper body horizontal pull • Strengthens back
Dumbbell Biceps Hammer Curl and Shoulder Overhead Press	2–3	10 per side	• Upper body pull and vertical push • Strengthens leg muscles • Strengthens shoulder and back muscles
Stability Ball Roll Out	2–3	10	• Core—bracing • Strengthens front and posterior core chain muscles
Bird-dog	2–3	10 per side	• Core • Strengthens abdominal muscles

SOURCE: RCMP, 2016.

TABLE 6.8 PARE Total Body Workout #2—No Equipment

EXERCISE	SETS	REPS	OBJECTIVE
Jump Squat	2–3	10	• Power • Strengthens leg muscles
Push-up	2–3	10 +	• Horizontal push • Strengthens chest and shoulder
Burpees	2–3	10	• Conditioning/speed • Strengthens full body
One Foot Hip Raise	2–3	10 per side	• Hip dominant • Strengthens core, glutes, and hamstrings
Inverted Row	2–3	10	• Upper body horizontal pull • Strengthens back and stabilizer muscles
Elbow Front Plank	2–3	30–60 secs	• Core • Strengthens core, chest, arms, back, glutes, and legs
Shuffle between 2 cones	2–3	20–30 secs	• Conditioning/agility • Builds leg endurance, agility, and coordination
Walking Lunges	2–3	10 per side	• Single leg work • Strengthens quadriceps, glutes, and hamstrings
Mountain Climber	2–3	10 per side	• Conditioning/core/speed • Strengthens core chain, legs, shoulder, and back
Side Jump over Bench	2–3	10 per side	• Conditioning/power • Strengthens core chain, back, and legs

SOURCE: RCMP, 2016.

FITCO TEST

The resistance training program outlined for the FITCO test is from the Ministry of Safety and Correctional Services' website. It provides seven exercises with three different types of equipment, depending on what you have available, and a six-week program outlining sets/reps/resistance. It recommends completing this workout two to three times per week. (See Table 6.9.)

TABLE 6.9 Training for FITCO

MUSCLE GROUP	BODY WEIGHT	MACHINES/EQUIPMENT	FREE WEIGHTS
Legs	Step-ups/Lunges/Step Lunges	Leg Press	Squats, Lunges
Chest	Push-ups	Bench Press	Dumbbell Chest Press/ Chest Flys
Back	Chin-ups (overhand, underhand)	Seated Row/Front Lats Pull-down	Dumbbell Row
Shoulders	Rubber-band Shoulder Press	Shoulder Press	Dumbbell Shoulder Press
Triceps	Rubber-band Overhead Press	Triceps Press-down	Dumbbell Overhead Triceps Press
Biceps	Rubber-band Arm Curl	Biceps Cable Curl	Dumbbell Biceps Curl
Abdominal/Core	Modified Curl-ups	Stability Ball Crunches	Weighted Abdominal Crunches

	SETS	REPS	RESISTANCE
Week 1	1–2	8	A light weight that can be easily lifted. Proper technique should be emphasized.
Week 2	2	10	Weight increased so 10 reps are completed, where the last rep is difficult to perform.
Week 3	3	10	Weight increased so 10 reps are completed, where the last rep is difficult to perform.
Week 4	3	12	Weight maintained from the previous week.
Week 5	3	15	Weight maintained from the previous week.
Week 6	3	10	Weight increased so 10 reps are completed, where the last rep is difficult to perform.

SOURCE: MCSCS, 2016.

FORCE WORKOUT

In training for the Canadian Armed Forces' FORCE Evaluation, three training programs (beginner, intermediate, and advanced) can be found in the *Bodyweight Training System Manual* (Canadian Forces Morale and Welfare Services, n.d.). They include a 12-week workout plan for body weight training, aerobic training, and core stability training. The body weight training program emphasizes workouts that consist of functional multi-joint movements, such as the squat and lunge, using body weight to develop muscular strength and endurance as opposed to weights or machines. Table 6.10 shows the four body weight training workouts recommended for beginners to be completed at least two times per week. You will find the entire workout including an aerobic and core stability program in the manual.

TABLE 6.10   Beginner FORCE Body Weight Workout

BODYWEIGHT TRAINING #1 CIRCUIT: 2–3 SETS WITH 15–30 SEC REST BETWEEN EXERCISES		BODYWEIGHT TRAINING #2		BODYWEIGHT TRAINING #3 CIRCUIT: 2–3 SETS WITH 15–30 SEC REST BETWEEN EXERCISES		BODYWEIGHT TRAINING #4 TWO CIRCUITS: 2–3 SETS WITH 15–30 SEC REST BETWEEN EXERCISES	
EXERCISE	REPS	EXERCISE	SET/REPS	EXERCISE	REPS	EXERCISE	REPS
Prisoner Squat	8–12	Squat to Walking Lunge	3 sets of 8–12 6–8/leg	Jog quickly on the spot	30 sec	**Circuit 1**	
						Jumping Jacks	20–30
Box or Knee Push-ups	10–12			Y Overhead Sumo Squat	8–12	Prisoner Sumo Squat	8–10
Alternating Lunge	6–8/leg	Good Morning	3 sets/ 12–15	Wide Push-up	Maximum Reps	Push-ups	Maximum Reps
Bent Over Y	5 x 6 sec hold	Butt kicks	5 sets/ 30 sec	Forward Lunge	6–8/leg	Bent Over 3-Position	2 x 4 sec/ position
Jumping Jacks	20–30	Plank to Side Plank	3–6 sets 20 sec hold 10 sec hold	Bird-dog Sweep	8/leg	**Circuit 2**	
Bird-dog	3 x 5–8 sec/side					Linear Jumping Jacks	20
				Plank Downward Dog Exchange	10	Backward Lunge	8/leg
						Lying 3 Position	2 x 3 sec/ position
						Bird-dog Circles	10/side

SOURCE: Canadian Forces Morale and Welfare Services. (n.d.). *Bodyweight Training System CF Fitness Anytime, Anywhere*. https://www.cfmws.com/en/AboutUs/PSP/DFIT/Fitness/BTS Document Library/ENG BTS.pdf

Refer to **assignment 6.2** (www.emond.ca/fitness5e) to start designing your strength, power, and endurance training program.

OTHER CONSIDERATIONS
FUELLING YOUR BODY

Remember the importance of consuming adequate nutrients and fluids before, during, and after exercise. Working out is like driving a car; you wouldn't drive your car without gas, would you? Athletes should be well hydrated and fuelled to help maintain blood glucose concentration during exercise, maximize exercise performance, and improve recovery time. The following are the ACSM (2016) guidelines:

Pre-exercise: Make sure that 1 to 2 hours before working out you drink lots of water and eat some healthy, easily digestible carbohydrates (such as whole grains, fruits, and vegetables).

During exercise: Make sure you stay well hydrated by taking frequent sips of water. Most workouts will not require you to consume any food, and you probably wouldn't want to. However, high intensity exercise lasting longer than 1 hour may require some electrolyte replacement and/or a small high-energy snack.

Post-exercise: Within 1 to 2 hours following a workout it is important to consume some carbohydrates and protein. The carbohydrates will help with your energy and the protein will help repair and grow muscle.

PERFORMANCE-ENHANCING SUBSTANCES

There are three basic types of performance-enhancing substances associated with weight training. *Nutritional aids* include vitamins and minerals, protein and amino acid supplements, carnitine (a substance in your body that helps turn fat into energy), creatine, and caffeine. *Pharmacological aids* include pain-masking drugs, anabolic steroids, prohormones, human growth hormones, and erythropoietin. *Physiological aids* include blood doping and drug masking.

Athletes use amino acids (protein) to assist in the repair and building of muscle tissue and the release of growth hormone. Excessive amounts can lead to a toxic effect due to dehydration. In addition, there is research that shows excessive intake can increase blood pressure, increase risk of cancer (with meat consumption), compromise immune function, and affect renal and liver functions by compromising calcium absorption (Delimaris, 2013). See Chapter 8 for further discussion of amino acids.

Others are using caffeinated products. Original research suggested that caffeine improved endurance by sparing muscle glycogen and increased the use of fats as an energy source. There is new research that caffeine may speed up absorption rates and when combined with energy drinks that contain carbohydrates, it stimulates the utilization of the carbohydrate in the drink as an energy source. For some people, muscle receptors are blocked so they have reduced pain and discomfort. Although it is no longer a banned substance, more caffeine than 3 to 6 mg per kilogram of body weight has been shown to lead to dehydration, jitters, and nausea when consumed in excess (>9 mg per kilogram). The withdrawal symptoms are present when the daily intake is stopped abruptly. The most commonly reported withdrawal symptoms are: headache, fatigue, sleepiness/drowsiness, difficulty concentrating, work difficulty, irritability, depression, anxiety, flu-like symptoms, impairment in psychomotor, vigilance, and cognitive performance (Black, Waddell, & Gonglach, 2015; Goldstein et al., 2010).

Some individuals believe that anabolic androgen steroids, which are synthetic derivatives of the male hormone testosterone, in combination with strength training, may increase muscle fibre numbers and size and improve muscle strength or body composition (lean body mass) (Yu, Bonnerud, Eriksson, Stål, Tegner, & Malm, 2014). However, anabolic androgen steroids have many harmful side effects, including liver damage, increased aggressiveness, acne, stunted growth, gynecomastia (development of breast tissue in males), cardiovascular conditions, stretch marks, and sterility. Tendons can lose elasticity, increasing risk of injury, and bones may stop growing prematurely. In women, anabolic steroids may lead to masculinization including excessive facial hair growth, male pattern baldness, deepening of the voice, and amenorrhea (Canadian Centre for Ethics in Sports, 2017; National Institute on Drug Abuse, 2006). Because the risk factors outweigh the benefits, it is recommended that individuals follow Canada's Food Guide to ensure that they get enough protein rather than take dangerous illegal drugs (see Chapter 8 for more information on nutrition).

WOMEN AND STRENGTH TRAINING

Despite all that we know about the importance and benefits of strength training, the number of women who lift weights is still fairly low compared to their male counterparts (see Figure 6.6). It is much more common to see women doing cardiovascular activities at the gym as opposed to strength training, and of those women that lift weights, most choose to lift light weights as opposed to heavy. Some of the reasons why females are not lifting heavy weights in the gym include:

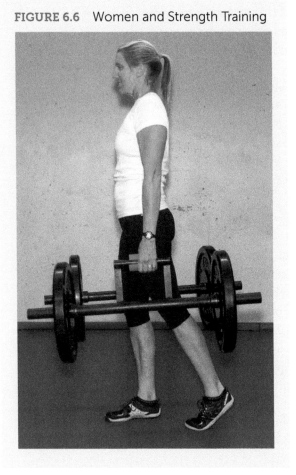

FIGURE 6.6 Women and Strength Training

- They think that they will lose their femininity, as strength training is viewed as a masculine activity.
- They are self-conscious in the gym and think that everyone is watching and judging them.
- They think that they will get big and bulky.
- They think that they are not strong enough to lift weights.
- They are lacking in the knowledge of how to train, what exercises to do, what training methods to use, proper form, etc.

As women watch the way a man's body changes with strength training, some fear that they will develop overly big muscles as well. We know that muscle hypertrophy is induced by testosterone (Cook & Beaven, 2013; Vermeulen, Goemaere, & Kaufman, 1999) and that for the most part, women make ten times less testosterone then men. There should be no fear that women will have the same muscle size response to training as men, yet it is still an ongoing concern for many. We know that the benefits of strength training include reduction in body fat, improved long-term health, and, maybe one of the most important, improved self-esteem, a better attitude, and a reduction in depression. As females who want to pursue a job in law enforcement, it is even more important to be resistance training, to gain strength and endurance for your own safety, and to be able to withstand the demands of the job (Westcott, 2012).

PERSONAL PERSPECTIVE

WEIGHT ROOM CONFIDENCE

I have been lifting weights since I was 16. My goals and motivations were always tied to the sports that I was playing: getting stronger arms for throwing events in track and field, and developing more powerful legs for jumping in basketball and volleyball. In university, I pursued an undergraduate degree in kinesiology, where I took classes in how to design workouts and lift properly, and in my last year I took an extensive course to become a Certified Exercise Physiologist. I have worked for over 15 years in gyms, developing programs and training all sorts of people for all types of goals.

Despite all of this experience and all of this training, I can still be self-conscious lifting weights in a gym. For me, it is twofold: all of the mirrors, and all of the watching that takes place while people are resting between sets. My strategy for this has always been the same. I ALWAYS go into the gym with a plan; I need to know what I am doing, so that when others see me, they know that too. On days where I don't have a plan, I hop on the bike or treadmill and compose what my workout will be before I head into the weights section. I come in focused and intent.

So even though I am fully qualified and have literally lived in gyms, I still can feel the stigma on women and weights. My advice is to plan your workout ahead, keep your head up, and be confident.

FIRST TIME IN THE WEIGHT ROOM

Here are some suggestions on strength training that takes into account the barriers for anyone starting out for the first time:

1. Set a goal. Having a goal will give the training a purpose and will allow you to focus on an outcome that is specific to you. Use something that is measurable like "I want to do 20 push-ups" or "I want to be able to complete the dummy drag of the PREP test." Stay away from goals that you cannot measure like "I want to be toned" or "I want to have strong legs."

2. Develop a program. Based on your goal, decide what you will do for your workout. Don't be afraid to ask for help. This is the perfect time to use a qualified personal trainer to design a workout for you. Write down your program.

3. Be prepared. It is important to have a plan in place when you go to the gym so that you know exactly what exercise you are going to do and how much weight you are going to use. Have your program handy—written down, on your phone, or in a log book. Bring it out into the gym with you. If you don't know the layout of the gym, you can ask a staff member to show you where a certain piece of equipment is.

4. Start small. If you are comfortable in the gym doing cardio or classes, but the thought of going into the weight-lifting section makes you feel uneasy, start small. Pick one upper body exercise and one lower body exercise that requires lifting weights, like bench press and squats with a bar. Do the two exercises back-to-back and then leave. Next time, try to add one more set or one more exercise.

5. Start at home. If you aren't ready or able to use a gym, you can start by working out at home. Get yourself a pair of 5 and 10 lb. dumbbells,

modify your program to use body-based exercises, and use what you have at home.

6. Get some support. Most people, if not everyone, should be doing some sort of resistance training. They may not have the same goals as you, but it is extremely supportive to have a friend, family, or colleague in the gym to talk to while you are lifting weights. Don't be afraid to ask for support. It has been found that people who tell others about their goals are more likely to reach them.

7. Vary the routine. If you feel that you aren't getting anywhere or are frustrated with the program that you have created, don't be afraid to change it up.

8. Reward yourself. It is so important to reward yourself when a goal has been met. Treat yourself for completing what you set out to do and start thinking of what your next goal will be. Remember that as you get more comfortable working out, your confidence (and fitness level) is likely to improve as well.

FINAL THOUGHTS

Resistance training is beneficial for people of all ages and abilities. If you have any health concerns and you are unsure of how to begin, start by speaking with your family doctor. They will be able to provide you with appropriate medical clearance. Then feel free to approach a certified exercise professional who can help you create an appropriate program for your goals and expectations.

KEY TERMS

absolute strength
maximum amount of force exerted, regardless of body size or weight

circuit training
to perform a number of exercises in succession with little to no rest in between

functional strength
focuses on the amount of strength required for a specific job-related task or sport-related skill

functional training
a program that adapts or develops exercises which allows individuals to perform daily activities, specific sports, or physically demanding jobs more easily and without injury

general adaptation
the process of preparing muscles, joints, tendons, and ligaments for intense training by educating the neuromuscular component so that gains can be seen; characterized by higher repetitions, lower intensities, and short rest periods

heavy to light training
decreasing the amount of weight you are lifting as you progress through sets, or even within one set

light to heavy training
increasing the amount of weight you are lifting as you progress through sets

muscular endurance
how long a muscle can repeatedly exert force over time

muscular hypertrophy
the growth and increase of size of a muscle characterized by high training volume with moderate training intensity

muscular power
generating as much force as possible, as quickly as possible

muscular strength
how much force a muscle can produce with a single maximal effort

one rep maximum (1RM)
the maximal amount of weight that can be lifted through the full range of motion, for one repetition, with proper form

periodization
an organized approach to training that involves progressive cycling of various aspects of a training program during a specific period of time

plyometrics
a method of training that enhances an individual's "explosive" reaction through rapid and powerful muscular contractions through stretch-shortening cycles; a concentric action immediately preceded by an eccentric action

principle of progressive overload
refers to training and overloading the muscles that help the body to adapt to more and more stress

pyramid training
a system that combines the light to heavy and heavy to light approaches for weight training

relative strength
maximum amount of force exerted, related to body size or weight

repetition (rep)
one complete movement of an exercise

resistance training
any type of exercise that requires the muscles to move, or attempt to move, against an opposing force

set
a group of repetitions

superset training
a system that involves performing two exercises in succession, without rest; often used to exercise opposing muscle groups, it results in increased strength and muscle mass of the targeted muscle group

trisets
combining three exercises with little rest in between; can involve working the same muscle group from three different angles, working three different muscle groups, or working different areas of the same muscle from three different angles

EXERCISES

MULTIPLE CHOICE

1. Which of the following would not be considered a benefit of resistance training?
   a. better quality of sleep
   b. decreased immune response
   c. decreased risk of cardiovascular disease
   d. positive body composition changes
   e. reduction of back pain

2. Based on BFOR research, what is the most important component needed to restrain and move people?
   a. endurance
   b. power
   c. upper body strength
   d. lower body strength
   e. stamina

3. What is strength, power, and endurance training also known as?
   a. weight training
   b. aerobic training
   c. cardiorespiratory training
   d. resistance training
   e. overload training

4. It is important to rest the muscles for a minimum of how many hours after weight training to avoid overtraining?
   a. 12
   b. 18
   c. 24
   d. 36
   e. 48

5. What is the name of the principle that states that to build muscle mass, the muscle must be subjected to a greater than normal load?
   a. the slow-twitch principle
   b. the isokinetic principle
   c. the recovery principle
   d. the progressive overload principle
   e. the muscle endurance principle

6. What is a group of consecutive repetitions of a resistance exercise called?
   a. a set
   b. a measure
   c. a rep
   d. a sequence
   e. a game

7. Which of the following is poor advice for strength training?
   a. complete a 5- to 10-minute warm-up reflecting the workout you intend to do
   b. try to do as many exercises as you can even when you compromise form
   c. select exercises for all major muscle groups
   d. train initially for endurance if you are a beginner
   e. vary the routine to avoid boredom

8. The maximum amount of force that a muscle can generate at one time is called
   a. power
   b. progression
   c. sticking point
   d. endurance
   e. strength

9. The ability of a muscle to exert a force for a prolonged duration is called
   a. endurance
   b. muscular strength
   c. plyometrics
   d. one repetition maximum
   e. muscle capacity

10. An example of an exercise that trains functional strength would be
    a. perform as many leg press exercises as possible by pressing a heavy weight to exhaustion
    b. do 3 sets of 20 push-ups within 5 minutes
    c. an exercise that simulates a job activity
    d. perform a bench press by lifting the heaviest weight possible
    e. jump repeatedly on and off a box for 1 minute

11. Overload is defined as
    a. overtraining
    b. working the body harder than accustomed
    c. carbohydrate loading for endurance athletes
    d. periodizing exercises in a program
    e. carrying more weight than is necessary for an exercise

12. Plyometrics training involves
    a. a slow progressive repetition of an exercise
    b. a force exerted by a muscle by maintaining a constant level of resistance
    c. an organized approach to training that involves progressive cycling
    d. powerful, explosive movements through jumping and bounding
    e. a process characterized by high training volume with moderate training intensity

13. Based on a study by Shepherd and Bonneau, which component does not put women at a disadvantage with absolute fitness levels?
    a. size
    b. endurance
    c. body composition
    d. hemoglobin levels
    e. strength

14. What is absolute strength?
    a. being able to lift a load once
    b. lifting the greatest load irrespective of your body weight
    c. lifting the greatest load respective to your body weight
    d. lifting the most repetitions irrespective of your body weight
    e. lifting the least repetitions respective to your body weight

MATCH THE TERMS
Match the definition to the term:

Term	Answer	Definition
1. Muscular strength		**A.** one complete movement of an exercise
2. Muscular endurance		**B.** the increase in size of the skeletal muscle
3. Muscular power		**C.** time to rest after each set of exercises
4. Muscular hypertrophy		**D.** a greater than normal load must stress the muscle to build muscle mass
5. Plyometrics		**E.** after training for a period of time you see less gains with your resistance program
6. Progressive overload principal		**F.** a program which adapts or develops exercises which allow individuals to perform daily activities, specific sports, or physically demanding jobs more easily and without injury
7. General adaptation principle		**G.** organized approach to training that involves progressive cycling of various aspects of a training program over a specific time
8. Repetition		**H.** a program which performs a number of exercises in succession at a submaximal level, with little rest in between
9. Sets		**I.** as you progress through the sets, you increase the weight you are working with
10. Between-set-rest		**J.** how long a muscle can exert a force over time
11. One rep maximum		**K.** performing two exercises in succession, without rest
12. Periodization		**L.** a program characterized by higher repetitions, lower intensities, and short rest periods, which helps the neuromuscular components synchronize so that gains can be seen
13. Law of diminishing returns		**M.** a program which combines the light to heavy and heavy to light approaches to training
14. Circuit training		**N.** how much force a muscle can exert
15. Light to heavy training		**O.** a program with combinations of three exercises done with little rest in between
16. Heavy to light training		**P.** known as "jump training," involves a lot of fast, bounding type movements
17. Pyramid training		**Q.** the maximum load that you can lift for a single rep
18. Superset training		**R.** also known as drop set training, decreasing the weight you are working with as you are approaching failure
19. Triset training		**S.** generating as much force as possible, as quickly as possible
20. Functional training		**T.** a group of repetitions

SHORT ANSWER

1. Define "progressive overload principle."

2. How should you warm up before a workout?

3. What is the difference between muscular endurance and muscular strength and how do you develop a program (including number of sets, reps, and rest) for each?

4. What are some of the advantages of circuit training?

5. What are some benefits of resistance training?

6. What are some basic guidelines for resistance training?

7. What are the benefits of periodization training?

8. What is functional strength and does it apply to training for a BFOR test?

REFERENCES

American College of Sports Medicine (ACSM). (2009). Progression models in resistance training for healthy adults. *Medicine and Science in Sports and Exercise, 41*(3), 687–708.

American College of Sports Medicine (ACSM). (2013). *ACSM's Guidelines for exercise testing and prescription* (9th ed.). Philadelphia, PA: Lippincott Williams & Wilkins.

American College of Sports Medicine (ACSM). (2016). Nutrition and athletic performance. Joint position statement. *Medicine & Science in Sports & Exercise, 48*(3), 543–568. doi: 10.1249/MSS.0000000000000852

Anderson, G., Zutz, A., & Plecas, D. (2011). Police officer back health. *The Journal of Criminal Justice Research, 2*(1), 1–17.

Astrand, P., Rodahl, K., & Dahl, H.A. (2003). *Textbook of work physiology* (4th ed., pp. 521, 529–535). Champaign, IL: Human Kinetics.

Bickel, C.S., Cross, J.M., & Bamman, M.M. (2011, July). Exercise dosing to retain resistance training adaptations in young and older adults. *Medicine and Science in Sports and Exercise, 43*(7), 1177–1187.

Black, C.D., Waddell, D.E., & Gonglach, A.R. (2015). Caffeine's ergogenic effects on cycling: Neuromuscular and perceptual factors. *Medicine & Science in Sports & Exercise, 47*(6), 1145–1158.

Bonneau, J., & Brown, J. (1995). Physical ability, fitness and police work. *Journal of Clincial Forensic Medicine, 2*(3), 157–164.

Boulé, N., Haddad, E., Kenny, G., Wells, G.A., & Sigal, R.J. (2001, September). Effects of exercise on HbA1C and body mass in type 2 diabetes mellitus: A metaanalysis of controlled clinical trials. *Journal of the American Medical Association, 286*(10), 1218–1227.

Brechue, W.F., & Mayhew, J.L. (2009). Upper-body work capacity and 1RM prediction are unaltered by increasing muscular strength in college football players. *Journal of Strength and Conditioning Research, 23*(9), 2477–2486.

Brown, J., Wells, G., Trottier, A., Bonneau, J., & Ferris, B. (2001). Back pain in a large Canadian police force. *Health Services Research, 23*(7), 821–827.

Bullock, S. (2010). Prevention of physical training-related injuries recommendations for the military and other active populations based on expedited systematic reviews. *American Journal of Preventive Medicine, 38*(1 Suppl), S156–S181.

Canadian Centre for Ethics in Sport. (2017) Steroids: Toxic effects. Retrieved from http://cces.ca/steroids

Canadian Forces Morale and Welfare Services. (n.d.). *Bodyweight training system CF fitness anytime, anywhere.* Retrieved from https://www.cfmws.com/en/AboutUs/PSP/DFIT/Fitness/BTS Document Library/ENG BTS.pdf

Canadian Society of Exercise Physiology (CSEP). (2011). *Canadian physical activity guidelines for adults 18–64 years.* Retrieved from http://www.csep.ca/english/view.asp?x=804

Calatayud, J., Borreani, S., Moya, D., Colado, J.C., & Triplett, N.T. (2013). Exercise to improve bone mineral density. *Strength and Conditioning Journal, 35*(5), 70–74.

Carlson, M.J., & Jaenen, S.P. (2012). The development of a preselection physical fitness training program for Canadian special operations regiment applicants. *Journal of Strength & Conditioning Research, 26*, S2–S14.

Chang, W.-D., Lin, H.-Y., & Lai, P.-T. (2015). Core strength training for patients with chronic low back pain. *Journal of Physical Therapy Science, 27*(3), 619–622. http://doi.org/10.1589/jpts.27.619

Cheung, K., Hume, P.A., & Maxwell, L. (2003). Delayed onset muscle soreness treatment strategies and performance factors. *Sports Medicine, 33*(2), 145–164.

Cook, C.J., & Beaven, C.M. (2013). Salivary testosterone is related to self-selected training load in elite female athletes. *Physiology & Behavior, 116–117,* 8. doi:10.1016/j.physbeh.2013.03.013

Delimaris, I. (2013). Adverse effects associated with protein intake above the recommended dietary allowance for adults. *ISRN Nutrition, 2013.* doi:10.5402/2013/126929

Drenowatz, C., Hand, G.A., Sagner, M., Shook, R.P., Burgess, S., & Blair, S.N. (2015). The prospective association between different types of exercise and body composition. *Medicine & Science in Sports & Exercise, 47*(12), 2535–2541. doi: 10.1249/MSS.0000000000000701

Engelke, K., et al. (2006). Exercise maintains bone density at spine and hip EFOPS: A 3-year longitudinal study in early postmenopausal women. *Osteoporosis International, 17,* 133–142.

Faigenbaum, A.D. (2000). Strength training for children and adolescents. *Clinics in Sports Medicine, 19,* 593–619.

Farenholtz, D. (1995). *Correctional Officer's Physical Abilities Test (COPAT): Physical training, conditioning, and maintenance program.* Ottawa: National Headquarters, Correctional Service of Canada.

Faulkner, J.A., & White, T.P. (1990). Adaptations of skeletal muscle to physical activity. *Proceedings of the international conference on exercise, fitness, and health* (pp. 265–275). Champaign, IL: Human Kinetics.

Gledhill, N., & Shaw, C. (1995, October). Constable Selection Project. Final report: Medical, physical, skills and abilities project. Race Relations and Policing Unit. Toronto: Ministry of the Solicitor General and Correctional Services.

Gledhill, N., & Jamnik, R. (2015) Technical Guide: Physical Readiness Evaluation for Police Constable Applicants (PREP). Ontario Association of Chiefs of Police Constable Selection System. Toronto: Ontario Ministry of Community Safety and Correctional Services.

Goldstein, E.R., Ziegenfuss, T., Kalman, D., Kreider, R., Campbell, B., Wilborn, C., … Antonio, J. (2010). International society of sports nutrition position stand: Caffeine and performance. *Journal of the International Society of Sports Nutrition, 7*(5). DOI: 10.1186/1550-2783-7-5.

Jamnik, V., Gumienak, R., & Gledhill, N. (2013). Developing legally defensible physiological employment standards for prominent physically demanding public safety occupations: A Canadian perspective. *European Journal of Applied Physiology, 113*(10), 2447–2457.

Jamnik, V.K., Thomas, S.G., Burr, J.F., & Gledhill, N. (2010). Construction, validation, and derivation of performance standards for a fitness test for correctional officer applicants. *Applied Physiology, Nutrition, and Metabolism, 35,* 59–70.

Jurca, R., et al. (2004). Associations with muscle strength and aerobic fitness with metabolic syndrome in men. *Medicine and Science in Sports and Exercise, 36,* 1301–1307.

Kerksick, C.M., et al. (2010). Changes in weight loss, body composition and cardiovascular disease risk after altering macronutrient distributions during a regular exercise program in obese women. *Nutrition Journal, 9,* 59–78.

Koutedakis, Y., Stavropoulos-Kalinoglou, A., & Metsios, G. (2005). The significance of muscular strength in dance. *Journal of Dance Medicine and Science, 9*(1), 29–34.

Lewinski, W.J., Dysterheft, J.L., Dicks, N.D., & Pettitt, R.W. (2014). The influence of officer equipment and protection on short sprinting performance. *Applied Ergonomics, 47,* 65–71.

Marcell, T.J. (2003). Sarcopenia: Causes, consequences and preventions. *Journal of Gerontology, 58A*(10), 911–916.

Martin, B. (2012). Strength training for running: Planning and strategy. Running technique tips. Retrived from http://www.runningtechniquetips.com/2012/07/strength-training-for-running-planning-and-strategy

Mayhew, J.L., Ball, T.E., Arnold, M.D., & Bowen, J.C. (1992). Prediction of 1RM bench press from relative endurance performance in college males and females. *Journal of Applied Sports Science Research, 6,* 200–206.

McGill, S. (2003). Enhancing low-back health through stabilization exercise. Retrieved from http://www.ahs.uwaterloo.ca/~mcgill/fitnessleadersguide.pdf

Ministry of Community Safety and Correctional Services. (2015). PREP: Fit to serve. Retrieved from https://www.applicanttesting.com/images/stories/pdf/FittoServe2015Final.pdf

Ministry of Community Safety and Correctional Services. (2016). Becoming a correctional service officer: FITCO—Fitness test for correctional officer. Retrieved from https://www.mcscs.jus.gov.on.ca/english/corr_serv/careers_in_corr/become_corr_off/FITCO/cs_FITCO.html#muscular

National Institute on Drug Abuse. (2006, August). Anabolic steroid abuse. Research Report Series. Retrieved from http://www.drugabuse.gov/PDF/RRSteroids.pdf

Paoli, A., Moro, T., Marcolin, G., Neri, M., Bianco, A., Palma, A., & Grimaldi, K. (2012). High-Intensity Interval Resistance Training (HIRT) influences resting energy expenditure and respiratory ratio in non-dieting individuals. *Journal of Translational Medicine, 10*, 237. http://doi.org/10.1186/1479-5876-10-237

Royal Canadian Mounted Police (RCMP). (2001). Emergency response team: Selection criteria. Retrieved from http://www.rcmp-grc.gc.ca/ert-gti/prog-eng.htm

Royal Canadian Mounted Police (RCMP). (2016). 12 week fitness program. Retrieved from http://www.rcmp-grc.gc.ca/en/12-week-fitness-program

Santana, J.C. (2016). Functional training: Exercises and programming for training & performance. Champaign, IL.: Human Kinetics.

Seguin, R.A., Eldridge, G., Lynch, W., & Paul, L.C. (2013). Strength training improves body image and physical activity behaviors among midlife and older rural women. *Journal of Extension, 51*(4), 4FEA2.

Sharkey, B.J., & Davis, P.O. (2008). Hard work: Defining physical work performance requirements. Windsor, ON: Human Kinetics.

Shephard, R., & Bonneau, J. (2002). Assuring gender equity in recruitment standards for police officers. *Applied Physiology, Nutrition and Metabolism, 27*(3),263–295.

Shiroma, E.J., Cook, N.R., Manson, J.E., Moorthy, M.V., Buring, J.E., Rimm, E.B., & Lee, I-M. (2017). Strength training and the risk of type 2 diabetes and cardiovascular disease. *Medicine & Science in Sports & Exercise, 49*(1), 40–46.

Spivock, M., Reilly, T., Newton, P., Blacklock, R., & Jaenen, S. (2011). Project FORCE. Phase I Report: Identification of common essential, physically demanding tasks in the CF. Retrieved from https://www.cfmws.com/en/AboutUs/PSP/DFIT/PSP_Resources/Documents/Project FORCE Phase I Report with signature sheet.pdf

Stensvold, D., et al. (2010). Strength training versus aerobic interval training to modify risk factors of metabolic syndrome. *Journal of Applied Physiology, 108*, 804–810.

Vermeulen, A., Goemaere, S., & Kaufman, J.M. (1999). Testosterone, body composition and aging. *Journal of Endocrinological Investigation, 22*(5 Suppl), 110–116.

Warburton, D.E.R., Nicol, C.W., & Bredin, S.S.D. (2006). Health benefits of physical activity: The evidence. *CMAJ: Canadian Medical Association Journal, 174*(6), 801–809. http://doi.org/10.1503/cmaj.051351

Westcott, W.L. (2012) Resistance training is medicine: Effects of strength training on health. American College of Sports Medicine. *Current Sports Medicine Reports, 11*(4), 209–216. Retrieved from http://journals.lww.com/acsm-csmr/toc/2012/07000

Yu, J.-G., Bonnerud, P., Eriksson, A., Stål, P.S., Tegner, Y., & Malm, C. (2014). Effects of long term supplementation of anabolic androgen steroids on human skeletal muscle. *PLoS ONE, 9*(9), e105330. http://doi.org/10.1371/journal.pone.0105330

PART 3

BODY COMPOSITION AND NUTRITION

CHAPTER 7 Body Composition

CHAPTER 8 Nutrition

BODY COMPOSITION

LEARNING OUTCOMES

After completing this chapter, you should be able to:

- Understand the issues surrounding overweight and obesity in Canada.

- Distinguish between the concepts of overfat and overweight.

- Describe the three somatotypes (body types).

- Explain how basal metabolism affects body composition.

- Explain eating disorders, including anorexia nervosa, bulimia nervosa, binge eating disorder (BED), and the female athlete triad.

- Describe several methods for measuring body composition.

Canadians have been battling the bulge for decades, but despite better food labelling, healthier food options in schools, reduced amounts of trans fats in processed foods, and tax incentives to promote physical activity, the costs of obesity to the Canadian health-care system have risen. Three factors contribute to this burden: the increase in numbers of individuals who are obese; rising costs of treatments specific to obesity-related illnesses; and a demographic shift, with a general trend for older individuals (our fastest-growing population demographic) to be obese. Understanding the underlying causes of chronic diseases associated with tackling the circumstances leading to obesity may help people to be proactive to make healthier choices and seek help when needed to live a healthier life.

UNDERSTANDING CHRONIC DISEASE

Chronic diseases, such as cardiovascular disease, diabetes, cancer, etc., represent a major fiscal and productivity risk for a country's economy. It affects health spending and family income, and lowers labour productivity due to illness. We need to focus on prevention of these diseases rather than providing sufficient medical care. Treatment of chronic diseases consumes 67 percent of all direct health-care costs in Canada, or $190 billion annually, of which $68 billion was attributed to treatment while the remainder was in lost productivity (Elmslie, 2012).

Figure 7.1 gives a better understanding of the pathways to chronic diseases and the underlying drivers that lead to behaviours that affect our health.

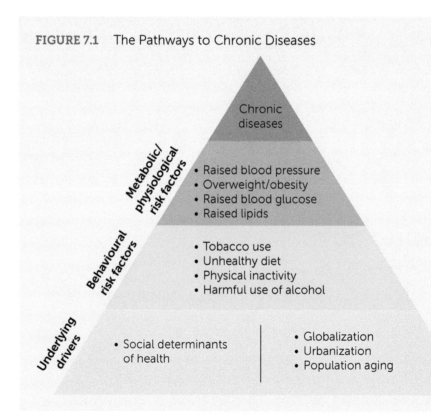

FIGURE 7.1   The Pathways to Chronic Diseases

The prevalence of obesity in Canadian adults has steadily increased. Obese people are at risk of hypertension, type 2 diabetes, sleep apnea, cancer, and premature death (Bray, 2004; Guh et al., 2009; Katzmarzyk & Ardern, 2004; Luo et al., 2007).

There is clear evidence that we can reduce the four common modifiable risk factors that lead to overweight and obesity issues (tobacco use, unhealthy diet, physical inactivity, and harmful use of alcohol) through low-cost solutions and help fight heart disease, strokes, cancers, diabetes, and chronic lung diseases. In fact, 80 percent of heart disease, diabetes, and respiratory diseases and 40 percent of cancers are preventable by eliminating these four common risk factors (WHO, 2010).

FYI

CHRONIC DISEASES AND COMMON RISK FACTORS

		COMMON RISK FACTORS			
		TOBACCO USE	UNHEALTHY DIET	PHYSICAL INACTIVITY	HARMFUL USE OF ALCOHOL
CHRONIC DISEASES	CARDIOVASCULAR DISEASE	✓	✓	✓	✓
	DIABETES	✓	✓	✓	✓
	CANCER	✓	✓	✓	✓
	RESPIRATORY DISEASES	✓			

SOURCE: WHO. (2010). Raising the priority of non-communicable diseases in development work at global and national levels. http://www.who.int/ncdnet/events/booklet_20100224.pdf

Ultimately, it will be up to each of us, in all facets of life, to change our behaviour and reduce the negative impact of the growing burden of disease in Canada by modifying the determinants (like transportation, education, urban planning, workplace, etc.) that affect health over a lifetime (Elmslie, 2012). It is important to play an active role in your life to stay healthy, fit, and well.

This chapter examines obesity, eating disorders, and other weight-related issues more closely by delving into the question of what constitutes a healthy body composition.

MISGUIDED VIEWS OF THE BODY

Weight is an issue that we all think about, and potentially struggle with, in different ways. While many Canadians are justly concerned about being overweight, many others who are within a healthy weight range are obsessed with weight loss. The media equates beauty with thinness in women and muscularity in men, ideals that fuel the obsession with weight (CSEP, 1996). Many people compare their bodies to models and celebrities, who always seem to have flat tummies and perfect figures. The stress and anxiety caused by unrealistic weight-loss goals can lead to serious eating disorders, such as anorexia, bulimia, and yo-yo dieting. Weight teasing is associated with higher rates of disordered binge eating behaviours among adolescent boys and girls (Neumark-Sztainer, 2002). Weight stigmatization often leads to increased food consumption as coping strategies among individuals (Puhl, 2012).

Recent research suggests that we have nurtured an obesity epidemic (Sharma & Kushner, 2009). With our sedentary work habits and lifestyles, a constant time crunch, and our fast-food culture, we have turned obesity into a chronic disease. People struggle to maintain a healthy body weight. If eating healthy and exercising worked for everyone, there would not be so many fad diets on the market. The simplistic lifestyle advice to "eat less—move more" (ELMM) is not very effective—a fact well known to most people who have tried this approach. The reality is that many factors can hinder your ability to lose weight, including mental illness, chronic pain, family or social barriers, and environmental conditions. It is not always easy to make healthy choices. Like smoking cessation, effective obesity prevention may require a multifaceted, long-term approach involving interventions that operate on multiple levels and in complementary ways (PHAC, 2011).

There has been a significant increase in the combined overweight/obesity rate among youth in Canada over the past 30 years, increasing from 14 percent to 29 percent. In addition, young people of Indigenous origin (off-reserve) have a significantly high combined overweight/obesity rate of 41 percent. In 2014, 20.2 percent of Canadians adults, roughly 5.3 million adults, reported height and weight that classified them as obese while 40.0 percent of men and 27.5 percent of women were classified as overweight (Statistics Canada, 2015).

The health consequences of excess weight include increased risk for type 2 diabetes, cardiovascular disease, high blood pressure, some cancers, and gallbladder disease. Obesity is also associated with increased risk of chronic back pain, sleep apnea, and osteoarthritis. The emotional and mental effects of obesity are also significant and lead to low self-esteem, depression, anxiety, and isolation (Kalra, De Sousa, Sonavane, & Shah, 2012; Okifuji & Hare, 2015; PHAC, 2011).

FACTS TO THINK ABOUT

BODY WEIGHT

Body weight is affected by our genetic makeup, our eating choices, our level of physical activity, and our social, cultural, physical, and economic environments. Where we live, learn, play, and work are all factors that affect our body weight. Consider the following data:

- Statistics Canada has determined that those with less than a secondary education eat less fruit and vegetables and have higher rates of obesity.
- In terms of socio-economic status, obesity rates are higher among Canadian women in middle- and upper-middle-income households compared with highest-income households, while men in lower-middle-income households are less obese than those in highest-income households.
- Physical activity levels are higher among Canadians who have a positive social support network and are in more frequent contact with their friends and family.
- People who work in physically active jobs have a lower likelihood of being obese.
- Neighbourhoods that have better street lighting, sidewalks, recreational facilities, and playgrounds have more physically fit individuals living in them.
- Indigenous people experience higher rates of diseases such as heart disease, diabetes, cancer, and asthma, and obesity rates are expected to grow at more than twice the rate of the general population.
- Mental health problems are associated with eating disorders such as anorexia, bulimia, and binge eating. Girls and women are affected more than boys and men.
- The mean total hospital stay for an eating disorder was 37.9 days.
- If nothing new and effective is done to mitigate obesity among adults, objectively measured obesity will rise over the next two decades to more than one in three Canadian adults by 2031.

SOURCES: Addy et al., 2004; CIHI, 2006; Health Canada, 2002; King et al., 2001; Pan et al., 2009; PHAC, 2011; PHAC, 2015; Roberts, Shields, deGroh, Aziz, & Gilbert, 2012; Shields, 2005; Shields et al., 2010; Tjepkema, 2006; Toulany et al., 2015.

Although body image is often assumed to be a women's problem, research has revealed that men are increasingly dissatisfied, preoccupied, and impaired by concerns over their appearance. One study found that the percentage of men who are dissatisfied with their overall appearance (43 percent) had nearly tripled over 25 years (Pope, Phillips, & Olivardia, 2000). There is also a growing form of male *body dysmorphic disorder* (excessive concern about a perceived defect in one's physical features) called *muscle dysmorphia*, which is a preoccupation that one's body is too small and inadequately muscular (Phillips & Castle, 2001). Muscle dysmorphia may lead to potentially dangerous abuse of anabolic steroids, and studies indicate that 6 to 7 percent of high school boys have used these drugs (Kanayama & Pope, 2012). While the cause of body dysmorphic disorder is unknown and is probably multifactorial, involving genetic, neurobiological, evolutionary, and psychological factors, social pressures for boys and men to be large and muscular almost certainly contribute to the development of muscle dysmorphia (Kanayama & Pope, 2012; Phillips & Castle, 2001). This disorder may be accompanied by an eating disorder.

> **DID YOU KNOW?**
> - Forty-two million children (under the age of 18) worldwide are overweight or obese.
> - Obese children are likely to become obese adults.
> - Being overweight during childhood is associated with increased risk of coronary artery disease in adulthood.
>
> SOURCE: Langford, 2010.

BODY COMPOSITION

Body composition refers to the proportion of lean tissue to fat in the body. Determining this proportion can provide an indicator of overall health and fitness in relation to weight and age. Many factors, including sex, age, heredity, activity, overall nutrition, and eating patterns, affect body composition.

Your body needs fat for fuel and other purposes, but if you consume too much fat and neglect physical activity, you end up with non-essential fat stored in various areas of your body. Adults over 30 tend to carry more fat on their frames than younger people do. Generally, women accumulate more fat than men do, and it tends to be distributed more evenly over the entire body (among men, the fat tends to accumulate more on the trunk and less on the extremities). Abdominal obesity is one of the six components of metabolic syndrome—a cluster of risk factors that increase an individual's likelihood of developing cardiovascular diseases, diabetes, and several other conditions (Grundy, Brewer, Cleeman, Smith, & Lenfant, 2004).

But being overweight is not the same as being obese, because many physically fit people are overweight from muscle gain (muscle is heavier than fat). Of course, people can be overweight because they carry excess fat, but it is important to distinguish between the concepts of overfat and overweight.

All fat in your body is classified as either essential or non-essential fat. Essential fat is required for normal functioning of your body. Deposits of this fat can be found in your muscles, heart, brain, spinal cord, nerves, lungs, and liver. Fat serves as an energy reserve, a regulator of body functions, an insulator against heat loss, and a protector against physical shock.

Non-essential or storage fat is stored below the surface of the skin and around major organs. Although some fat is vital for insulation and organ protection, too much can put you at risk for disease.

Recent research has suggested that obese individuals who are otherwise healthy—free of all obesity-related comorbidities such as pre-diabetes, pre-hypertension, occasional difficulty breathing, and mental illness—could live just as long as their lean counterparts (Kuk et al., 2011). Kuk and colleagues (2011) found that it is better to engage in a healthy lifestyle that includes physical activity rather than repeatedly trying to lose weight, because most people regain the weight they lose. It is believed that the cycle of weight loss and gain may be more detrimental than maintaining an elevated body weight and exercising if the person has no other health issues.

SOMATOTYPES

Your body composition is affected by your somatotype (body type). Most people have a genetic predisposition toward a specific somatotype, although it is often mixed with some traits of a second somatotype. Although your somatotype is inherited and cannot be changed, diet and exercise can reduce the percentage of fat in your body. There are three somatotypes: endomorphic, mesomorphic, and ectomorphic (see Figure 7.2).

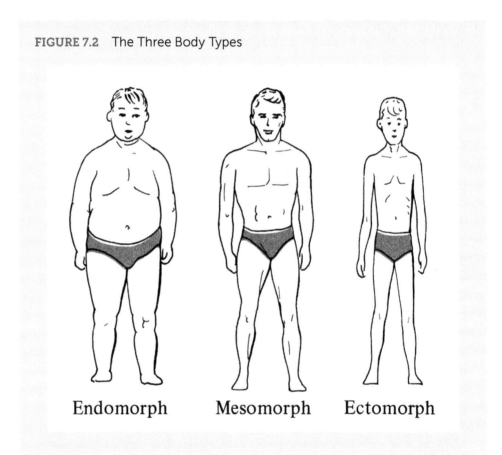

FIGURE 7.2   The Three Body Types

Endomorph   Mesomorph   Ectomorph

TABLE 7.1 Comparing Somatotypes

	ENDOMORPH	**MESOMORPH**	**ECTOMORPH**
FAT PERCENTAGE	High	Low to medium	Low
MUSCLE PERCENTAGE	Low	High	Low
BONE SIZE	Large	Medium to large	Small
METABOLIC RATE	Low	Medium to high	High

- With a light build and slight muscular development, *ectomorphs* usually have a harder time gaining weight, and spend more time on strength training and less on cardiorespiratory training.

- Many *mesomorphs* have a large chest and long torso, and can build muscle easily.

- *Endomorphs* tend to have a stocky build, wide hips, and a tendency to gain weight. Because this weight gain accumulates around the middle, endomorphs have difficulty losing weight. They need to pay close attention to their diet, and focus on cardiorespiratory training over strength training.

METABOLISM

Metabolism describes the chemical processes that occur within a living cell or organism that are necessary for maintaining life. Some substances are broken down to yield energy for vital processes (for example, carbohydrates are broken down into glucose), while other substances are synthesized (such as muscle tissue and cells).

BASAL METABOLISM

Body composition is also affected by basal metabolism, the amount of energy a body at rest needs to maintain essential functions. The basal metabolic rate (BMR) is the speed at which energy is used by the body. Factors affecting the BMR include age, sex, and level of physical activity.

Your basal metabolic rate represents roughly 60 percent of your daily energy expenditure. The more you weigh, the higher your metabolism rate. These are calories burned at rest, just to breathe, think, and live. For example:

- a 150-lb. (68-kg) man might have a BMR of 1600 kcal/day
- a 200-lb. (90-kg) man might have a BMR of 1900 kcal/day

What's important to know is that BMR can differ up to 15 percent from person to person. This means the 200-lb. person may have a friend of equal weight whose BMR is 300 kcal/day more or less than them, depending on their metabolism.

Your metabolism affects your ability to lose or gain weight. A high metabolic rate makes it easier to burn fat and lose weight. If your metabolism is slow or inefficient, you will find it more difficult to keep your weight stable or to lose weight.

Cutting calories lowers your metabolic rate. Your body senses the reduction in energy intake and slows down the burning of fat to protect the fat it has. After about three months your metabolic rate levels off and you no longer lose weight. If you return to your old eating habits, your body will store more fat than it used to because the metabolic rate remains depressed. Eventually you may gain back all the weight, and even put on more.

When you fast, the body protects its fat reserves by starting to break down protein instead of fat for energy. Because protein is an important constituent of muscle and other tissues, fasting harms key parts of the body. (This is true to an even greater extent in the extreme cases of anorexia and bulimia.)

The key to maintaining a healthy weight is to combine proper eating (as described in Chapter 8) with a good exercise program. A program of cardiorespiratory exercise 30 minutes every day, will improve your cardiovascular system, increase your metabolic rate, and burn fat. Weight and strength training for 20–30 minutes a day, three to five days a week, will increase your muscular strength and endurance, make you leaner, and have a beneficial effect on bone density.

MEASURING BODY COMPOSITION

In the 1960s and 1970s, insurance companies based their life and health premiums on height–weight tables. The more you weighed within a certain height class, the more you paid. The insurance companies did not take bone size into account, nor did they look at fat as a percentage of body weight. They simply assumed that higher weight equalled higher risk. But research in the 1990s led health experts to the idea that there are many kinds of healthy body shapes and sizes, and to the notion that each person has an "acceptable weight range." We no longer look simply at weight, but now consider the percentages of fat, bone, and muscle in our bodies. Further, being overweight for your height does not necessarily mean that you are unfit.

BODY MASS INDEX (BMI)

Health Canada (2003) developed a weight classification system to identify weight-related health risks in populations and individuals over 18 years old. This system categorizes individuals' risks based on body weight and height, and is measured by body mass index (BMI) and the level of abdominal fat as determined by waist circumference (WC).

BMI is calculated by dividing your body weight in kilograms by the square of your height in metres (Health Canada, 2000). For example, someone who is 1.8 metres tall and weighs 71 kilograms would have a BMI of 21.9 (that is, $71/1.8^2 = 21.9$).

Refer to **assignment 7.1** at www.emond.ca/fitness5e and determine your BMI.

BMI is a popular method among health-care professionals for determining whether, and to what extent, a person is overweight or obese, but disregards frame size and muscle mass. Excluding pregnant women and those under age 18, whose rate of growth varies, the BMI puts individuals into four categories: underweight, normal weight, overweight, and obese. The obese category is divided further into three classes. See Table 7.2 for an overview of body weight classifications.

TABLE 7.2 Canadian Guidelines for Body Weight Classification in Adults

CLASSIFICATION	BMI CATEGORY (KG/M²)	RISK OF DEVELOPING HEALTH PROBLEMS
Underweight	< 18.5	Increased
Normal weight	18.5–24.9	Least
Overweight	25.0–29.9	Increased
Obese Class I	30.0–34.9	High
Obese Class II	35.0–39.9	Very high
Obese Class III	≥ 40.0	Extremely high

SOURCES: Health Canada, 2000; adapted from WHO, 2000.

Under the current Canadian guidelines for body weight classification, the term *underweight* refers to an adult with a BMI of less than 18.5. Being underweight increases the risk of undernutrition, osteoporosis, infertility, and impaired immunocompetence (Health Canada, 2003). A very low BMI also alerts health-care professionals to the possibility of anorexia or similar problems.

The term *overweight* refers to anyone with a BMI of 25.0 to 29.9. The term *obese* refers to someone with a BMI of 30 or more (Health Canada, 2000). Canadians rank in the middle of the G8 countries in terms of the proportion of the population that is obese.

It is important to note that a high BMI is not necessarily a problem for competitive athletes and bodybuilders (whose BMI may be high because their muscle mass is greater than average), pregnant or lactating women, children, and sedentary elderly people. Other tools are needed to assess the body composition of these groups. We do know that overweight status indicates some risks to health. Research suggests that regular physical activity can decrease the risk of several health problems. Equally, a nutritious diet has been shown to decrease some of the risks associated with being overweight.

EDMONTON OBESITY STAGING SYSTEM

Recent research has shifted the health focus from how big people are to how sick they are. Sharma and Kushner (2009) developed a more holistic understanding of the potential impact of weight on an individual's health and functioning. The Edmonton Obesity Staging System (EOSS) categorizes obesity-related comorbidities in five stages (0 to 4) to complement anthropometric indices (measurements of the percentage of fat a person has) and determine the best course of treatment for a specific individual. Known as the 4Ms, treatment is based on the amount the following issues are affecting you:

1. metabolic complications (dyslipidemia, metabolic syndrome, nonalcoholic fatty liver disease, hypertension, and polycystic ovary syndrome),

2. mechanical complications (sleep apnea, sleep disordered breathing, gastroesophageal reflux disease, and musculoskeletal pain and dysfunction),

3. mental health issues (social isolation, bullying, depression, anxiety, dysregulated eating behaviours, body dissatisfaction), and

4. social milieu (school difficulties, family factors including poor family functioning, lack of emotional support, parental physical and mental health) (Hadjiyannakis et. al., 2016; Padwal, Padewski, Allison, & Sharma, 2011).

WAIST CIRCUMFERENCE

Waist circumference (WC) is an indicator of health risks associated with excess abdominal fat. A waist circumference of 102 centimetres (40 inches) or more in men, or 88 centimetres (35 inches) or more in women, is associated with health problems such as type 2 diabetes, heart disease, and high blood pressure. WC measurement can be used for individuals with a BMI in the 18.5 to 34.9 range. For BMIs equal to or exceeding 35.0, WC measurements do not provide additional information regarding the level of risk.

DID YOU KNOW?

Each five-unit increment in BMI above 25 kg/m² is associated with increases of 29 percent risk for overall mortality, 39 percent for liver cancer, 41 percent for vascular mortality, 210 percent for diabetes-related mortality, and increased risk of cardiovascular disease. In Canada, between the ages of 18 and 55, 61.8 percent of men (8.2 million) and 46.2 percent (6.1 million) of women are classified as overweight or obese.

SOURCES: Canoy et al., 2013; Wang, Wang, Shen, Fan, & Cao, 2012; Yusuf et al., 2005.

DID YOU KNOW?

Since 1985, the prevalence of obesity has increased by 200 percent in Canada, with the highest increases occurring in the excessive weight categories. By 2019, it is predicted that about 21 percent of the Canadian adult population will be obese. This does not include the overweight category.

SOURCES: Twells, Gregrory, Reddigan, & Midodzi, 2014.

See Figure 7.3 and refer to **assignment 7.2** at www.emond.ca/fitness5e to determine your waist circumference (WC).

FIGURE 7.3 Measuring Waist Circumference

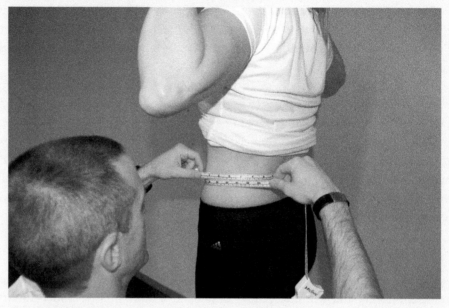

TABLE 7.3 Waist Circumference Cut-offs Based on Nationality and Country

POPULATION AND COUNTRY SPECIFIC GROUPS	MEN (CM)	WOMEN (CM)
Canada, United States	≥102 (40 inches)	≥88 (35 inches)
European, Middle Eastern, sub-Saharan African, Mediterranean	≥94 (37 inches)	≥80 (31.5 inches)
Asian, Japanese, South and Central American	≥90 (35.4 inches)	≥80 (31.5 inches)

SOURCE: Canadian Diabetes Association Clinical Practice Guidelines Expert Committee, 2013.

WAIST-TO-HIP RATIO MEASUREMENT

Waist-to-hip ratio (WHR) measurement is based on the relationship between the girth of the waist and the girth of the hips. Most people store excess fat either around the middle (making the body apple-shaped) or on the hips (making the body pear-shaped). It is generally accepted that people who carry their extra weight around the abdomen face a greater health risk than those who carry it on the hips. Nevertheless, obese people are at greater risk than non-obese people, no matter where the excess fat is stored.

See Figure 7.3 and refer to **assignment 7.3** at www.emond.ca/fitness5e and determine your waist-to-hip ratio (WHR).

For men, a WHR greater than 0.9 indicates that excess fat is being carried around the middle, increasing the health risks associated with hypokinetic diseases

(diseases related to lack of physical activity). For women, the crucial number is 0.85 or greater (WHO, 2011).

HEALTH RISK CLASSIFICATION

Excess fat around the waist and upper body (also described as an apple-shaped body) is associated with greater health risks than excess fat in the hip and thigh area (a pear-shaped body). A WC at or above guidelines (see Table 7.3), set by Diabetes Canada (Canadian Diabetes Association Clinical Practice Guidelines Expert Committee, 2013) based on population and ethnic specific cut-offs, is associated with an increased risk of developing health problems such as type 2 diabetes, heart disease, and high blood pressure.

Individuals who are overweight but not obese and who have a WC under the cut-off are in a low-risk category. In other words, their muscle weighs more, and they are at less risk if they keep abdominal fat off. However, even if a person's BMI falls within the normal weight range, a high WC indicates some health risk. A marked weight change—either a gain or loss—may place someone at risk even if he or she remains within the same BMI category. Unhealthy weight-loss practices, such as restrictive eating habits, can also increase a person's risk of health problems, even for those of normal weight (Health Canada, 2003).

SKINFOLD MEASUREMENT

The Canadian Society for Exercise Physiology (1996) recommends skinfold measurement for determining whether people whose BMI is greater than 25 are considered overweight or overfat. Unlike BMI measurement, skinfold measurement takes body type into account. The procedure involves using calipers to measure skinfolds at five points on the body (see Figure 7.4). Fitness club staff or your college fitness instructor may be available to assess your body composition this way.

FIGURE 7.4 Measuring Skinfolds

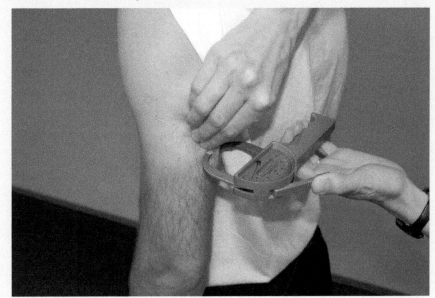

BIOELECTRIC IMPEDANCE

Bioelectric impedance is a commonly used method for measuring body composition, specifically body fat (see Figure 7.5). By determining the resistance to an electric current, they can predict how much fat-free and fat mass you have. Fat-free mass contains mostly water (less resistance), while fat contains very little water (more resistance).

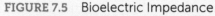

FIGURE 7.5 Bioelectric Impedance

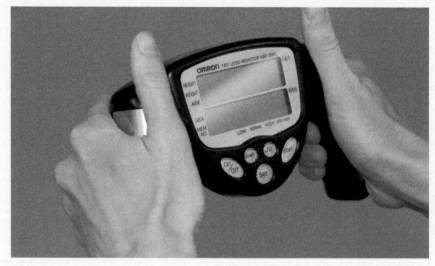

BODPOD

The bodpod is an apparatus that the individual sits in and computerized sensors determine the amount of air displaced by the person's body (similar to underwater weighing, see below) to determine body fat (see Figure 7.6).

FIGURE 7.6 Bodpod

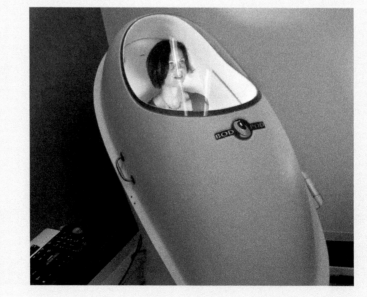

HYDROSTATIC WEIGHING

Hydrostatic weighing or underwater weighing is used to calculate percentage of body fat by measuring the density of the body. This is accomplished by weighing the person underwater while expelling all their air compared to their dry weight (see Figure 7.7).

FIGURE 7.7   Hydrostatic Weighing

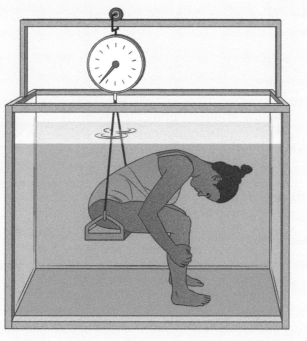

EATING DISORDERS

Being overweight or obese is not the only kind of body image problem that occurs in our society. Western society's obsession with thinness as the ideal—as seen in magazines, movies, and advertisements—causes many people, both male and female, constant anxiety about their weight and body shape. Many assume that being thin equates with being attractive, successful, in control, and popular, while being overweight signifies being weak-willed, lazy, and out of control. (Of course, this assumption is untrue, as many thin people feel unhappy, unhealthy, and unpopular!) Poor self-image and underlying emotional problems may cause an individual to develop an eating disorder.

Eating disorders carry with them a high risk of other mental and physical illnesses that can even lead to death. It is not only about food and weight or a means to seek attention. Eating smaller or larger portions of food than usual is common, but for some people, portion size turns into a compulsion and their eating behaviours become extreme. If they succeed in losing weight, they gain a temporary sense of achievement. But because caloric deprivation lowers basal metabolic rate and increases the likelihood of binge eating, such people tend to regain the weight, causing them greater dissatisfaction and lower self-esteem. Losing and regaining weight then becomes a vicious cycle.

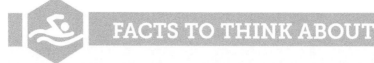

FACTS TO THINK ABOUT

DIETING AND WEIGHT LOSS

- At any given time, 70 percent of women and 35 percent of men are dieting.
- One out of five women in Ontario between the ages of 20 and 34 is underweight.
- 40 percent of nine-year-old girls have dieted, despite being within healthy weight ranges.
- 80 percent of 18-year-old women have dieted.
- Approximately 3 percent of women will be affected by an eating disorder during their lifetime.
- Surveys have shown that 7.7 percent of men have a strong fear of being overweight, compared to 18.5 percent of women.
- The biggest risks to an individual's health were a weight change of more than ten pounds in the previous six months and skipping meals almost every day, reported by 22 percent of men and 13 percent of women, respectively.
- Subclinical disordered eating behaviours (including binge eating, purging, laxative abuse, and fasting for weight loss) are nearly as common among males as they are among females.
- Men with eating disorders often suffer from comorbid conditions such as depression, excessive exercise, substance disorders, and anxiety.
- Body dissatisfaction and weight change behaviours have been shown to predict later physical and mental health difficulties, including weight gain and obesity on the one hand and the development of eating disorders on the other.

SOURCES: Bushnik, 2016; Gadalla & Piran, 2007; Health Canada, 2002; Mond, Mitchison, & Hay, 2014; NEDIC, 2014; Weltzin et al., 2014.

Extreme and repetitive dieting can exact a physical toll, including anemia (low iron in the blood), delayed or absent menstruation, dehydration, high cholesterol, hair loss, nail destruction, and change of liver function. Muscle and lean tissue are lost first, because the body protects its fat, which is required for hormonal functions. Fluctuation in body weight is associated with higher mortality and a higher rate of cardiovascular events independent of traditional cardiovascular risk factors (Bangalore et al., 2017; NEDIC, 2014).

Psychologically, dieting can cause depression, mood swings, reduced sexual interest, and impaired concentration and judgment. Some people develop alcohol dependency and anxiety disorders, particularly if bullying is a factor in their compulsion to lose weight. In extreme cases, bullying has led to suicide and even murder—all because of how people looked and felt.

Law enforcement officers may come to recognize several eating disorders as they deal with individuals in their community. These include anorexia nervosa, bulimia nervosa, binge eating disorder, body dysmorphic disorder, and female athlete triad disorder. Treatment of eating disorders usually involves hospitalization and behavioural therapy to help the person regain control over his or her perception of body image, eating habits, and self-esteem in relation to friends and family (NEDIC, 2014).

FYI

WARNING SIGNS OF EATING DISORDERS

The following behaviours may indicate that someone you care about has an eating disorder:

1. a marked decrease or increase in weight that is not related to a medical condition
2. a preoccupation with food
3. unusual eating habits, such as cutting up food into tiny pieces, playing with food, or hiding/disguising uneaten food
4. hiding or hoarding of large amounts of food in unusual places (for example, bedroom, closet)
5. a preoccupation with weight
6. constant dissatisfaction with weight and body size/image despite weight loss, clothing size, etc.
7. negative and self-critical comments about body shape, size, and physical appearance
8. behavioural changes including isolation, depression, irritability, or loss of trust in friends
9. frequent trips to the washroom, especially after meals
10. smell of vomit in the washroom or on the breath
11. abuse of laxatives, diet pills, or diuretics
12. excessive exercising or multiple, daily trips to the gym
13. wearing of baggy clothes to mask weight gain or loss

HELP IS AVAILABLE

Help for eating disorders is available, for you and the person you care about. Contact:

- EatRightOntario: http://www.eatrightontario.ca/en/default.aspx
- What's Eating You?: http://www.whatseatingyou.com
- National Eating Disorder Information Centre: http://www.nedic.ca
- Dieticians of Canada: http://www.dietitians.ca
- Nutrition—Centers for Disease Control: http://www.cdc.gov/nutrition
- Kids Help Phone: http://www.kidshelpphone.ca
- Eating Disorders Foundation of Canada: http://www.edfofcanada.com
- Bulimia Anorexia Nervosa Association (BANA): http://www.bana.ca
- Eating Disorders of York Region (EDOYR): http://www.edoyr.com
- Body Sense: http://www.bodysense.ca
- The National Association for Males with Eating Disorders: http://www.namedinc.org

ANOREXIA NERVOSA

Anorexia nervosa is a serious medical and psychiatric disorder. People who suffer from it do not get enough calories to maintain a healthy body weight. They usually begin at a normal or slightly above-average weight, and then starve themselves and exercise excessively to burn calories. These individuals refuse to maintain a normal body weight and have a distorted perception of the shape or size of their bodies (American Psychiatric Association, 1994). Anorexia often begins during adolescence, characterized by maladaptive eating behaviours as well as psychological disturbances involving mood, obsessionality, and body image due to fear of weight gain. Many resort to cosmetic surgery to help them change the way they look.

BULIMIA NERVOSA

People who suffer from bulimia nervosa may be able to maintain a normal weight but have an intense fear of being overweight and overfat. They have a distorted body image. Bulimia is characterized by two types of compensation: the most prevalent is a purging type in which the individual partakes in uncontrollable binge eating followed by self-induced vomiting or misuse of laxatives, diuretics, or enemas; while the second is a non-purging type where compensation is through fasting or excessive exercise. Many bulimics rely on laxatives and diuretics to prevent food from being absorbed by their bodies. The majority of bulimics are women in their late teens or early 20s. Cultural ideals and social attitudes toward body appearance are likely to contribute, as well as self-evaluation based on body weight and shape (Statistics Canada, 2012). Bulimics have difficulty handling emotions like depression, loneliness, and anger. They can have low self-esteem and may come from families with high expectations. They may have also suffered from a critical incident (traumatic event faced by an individual that causes unusually strong emotional reactions. See Chapter 12 for more information). The eating disorder may be an attempt to gain control over one part of their life.

Besides bingeing and purging, symptoms of bulimia include fluctuations in weight, dental decay, salivary gland enlargement, bowel problems or digestive complaints, and feelings of guilt and depression (American Psychiatric Association, 1994; Jacobi, Hayward, de Zwaan, Kraemer, & Agras, 2004; Stice, 2002).

BODY DYSMORPHIC DISORDER

Body dysmorphic disorder (BDD) is a relatively common disorder where individuals obsess about some aspect of their appearance that they deem to be severely flawed and take exceptional measures to hide or fix it. Many seek reassurance from others, take photos of themselves, and review in their minds how people look at them. They engage in compulsive behaviours of excessive grooming, cosmetic surgery, excessive shopping for flattering clothing, excessive exercise, and potential use of steroids. Males are more likely to describe involvement in sports as being catalysts for their disorder (Arnow et al., 2017). Poor quality of life (mental health and emotional well-being) and social isolation can lead to risky behaviours of suicide, substance abuse, and violence (Bjornsson, Didie, & Phillips, 2010; Conroy, Menart, Fleming-Ives, Modha, Cerullo, & Phillips, 2008; Phillips, Menard, Fay, & Pagano, 2005).

BINGE EATING DISORDER

Binge eating disorder (BED) is diagnosed if the binge eating is not followed by compensatory behaviours such as vomiting, excessive exercise, or laxative abuse. This disorder is associated with obesity. BED usually starts during adolescence or young adulthood. Men are more likely to be affected by BED than by other eating disorders. Individuals with BED who are obese must contend with negative societal attitudes toward obesity. As a result, many become isolated and lose self-esteem. They are hungry because they have been dieting or restricting their eating in response to that hunger. Many overeat to comfort themselves, to avoid uncomfortable situations, or to numb their feelings. Embarrassed, they eat alone and when they are unable to stop eating become depressed and feel ashamed.

DID YOU KNOW?

Muscle dysmorphia (also known as bigorexia), a subtype of body dysmorphic disorder, is an emerging condition that primarily affects male bodybuilders. Such individuals obsess about being muscular. Compulsions include spending many hours in the gym, squandering excessive amounts of money on supplements, abnormal eating patterns, or use of steroids.

SOURCE: Cafri, Blevins, & Thompson, 2006.

FEMALE ATHLETE TRIAD

The female athlete triad was first described in the early 1990s. This condition is defined by three signs: disordered eating, amenorrhea, and osteoporosis. Although researchers are still debating the prevalence of female athlete triad, many women who suffer from it may not be diagnosed (Yeager, Agostini, Nattiv, & Drinkwater, 1993). The concern is not only for the performance of these athletes but also for their future health.

DISORDERED EATING

The first sign in the female athlete triad is the precipitating event for the triad (Yeager et al., 1993). "Disordered eating" refers to a broad spectrum of abnormal eating behaviours (Sanborn, Horea, Siemers, & Dieringer, 2000). At the severe end of the spectrum are athletes who meet the diagnostic criteria for anorexia or bulimia. At the other end of the spectrum are athletes who consume fewer calories than their body requires. They may appear to be eating a healthy diet, but they are not consuming enough calories. Whichever end of the spectrum applies to a woman, this mismatch of energy needed versus what she is consuming creates an energy drain on the endocrine system, which in turn leads to the second and third signs of the triad.

AMENORRHEA

Amenorrhea is the cessation of menstrual periods for three or more consecutive cycles. It is the result of insufficient estrogen production by the ovaries. Missing periods is a warning sign that something is not right in the female body. Confirmation by medical diagnosis is important and should not be ignored. Women who do not menstruate for more than three or four months can lose bone strength.

Amenorrhea is associated with a condition known as *anorexia athletica*, in which people exercise excessively because they believe this will help them master their bodies and give them a sense of power, control, and self-respect. These excessive behaviours may lead to amenorrhea. Some of the symptoms include over-exercise, being fanatical about weight and diet, taking time away from school, work, and relationships to exercise, a focus on the outcome of exercising rather than the fun of participating, a belief that self-worth is dependent on physical results, disappointment with training outcomes, and making statements such as, "It's okay to exercise this much because I'm an athlete" (NEDIC, 2015).

OSTEOPOROSIS

Osteoporosis is another consequence of inadequate estrogen. Yeager and colleagues (1993) describe osteoporosis in the female athlete triad as "premature bone loss or inadequate bone formation." They point out that the failure to build bone at a normal rate or losing bone density at a young age leads to short- and long-term problems, including stress fractures and early bone mineral density loss. At least one in three women and one in five men will suffer from an osteoporotic fracture during their lifetime. Peak bone mass is achieved at an early age, ages 16 to 20 in girls and ages 20 to 25 in young men. After your mid-30s, you can expect to lose an average of 0.5 percent of bone density per year, a rate that accelerates to 2 percent for women after menopause (Osteoporosis Canada, 2017). Without estrogen, these young athletes may never be able to maximize bone mineral density.

TREATMENT

Treatment for eating disorders takes multiple approaches. In addition to medical diagnosis and supervision, the athlete requires nutritional education and some form of counselling to deal with the disorder and the underlying causes.

It is important for athletes not to skip meals and snacks; they need to maintain enough energy for competition. Snacking on foods such as bagels, cheese, unsalted nuts and seeds, raw vegetables, fruit, and granola bars will aid in acquiring the required amount of iron, calcium, and protein. It is also important for female athletes to keep track of their menstrual periods and to discuss any irregularities with a physician.

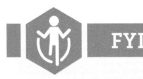

FYI

Relative Energy Deficiency Syndrome (RED-S) (of which the Female Athlete Triad is part) refers to impaired physiological functioning caused by relative energy deficiency and includes but is not limited to impairments of metabolic rate, menstrual function, bone health, immunity, protein synthesis, and cardiovascular health in both females and males. Overtraining, negative influence of sport performance, and disorder eating or an eating disorder are attributed to the cause.

The American College of Sport Medicine and the IOC emphasize that energy availability is the cornerstone for optimum health and fitness. Without correction, the impact of this syndrome is significant. Increasing dietary intakes and reducing training volumes are key to treatment.

SOURCES: Barrack, Ackerman, & Gibbs, 2013; M. Mountjoy, 2015; Weiss Kelly & Hecht, 2016.

FINAL THOUGHTS

If you recognize the symptoms of any eating disorder in yourself or a friend, do not hesitate to do something about it. There are excellent counselling services available that can help individuals get back on track and get proper medical attention. As a law enforcement officer, while you are not qualified to make diagnoses, you can watch for signs that should not be ignored. These may include physical or sexual abuse, emotional abuse (teasing, harassment, or bullying), perfectionism, behavioural rigidity, and substance abuse in elite-performance and competitive sports, in which body shape and size are factors.

KEY TERMS

amenorrhea
the cessation of menstrual periods for three or more consecutive cycles

anorexia nervosa
an eating disorder in which individuals do not eat enough to maintain a healthy body weight

basal metabolic rate (BMR)
the speed at which energy is used by the body

basal metabolism
the amount of energy a body at rest needs to maintain essential functions

binge eating disorder (BED)
an eating disorder associated with obesity, where the person alternately eats obsessively and then diets and restricts eating; the disorder is diagnosed if the person does not follow the binge eating with compensatory behaviours such as vomiting, excessive exercise, or laxative abuse

body composition
the proportion of lean tissue to fat in the body

body dysmorphic disorder (BDD)
a relatively common disorder where individuals obsess about some aspect of their appearance that they deem to be severely flawed and take exceptional measures to hide or fix it

body mass index (BMI)
a method for assessing body composition, based on weight and height

bulimia nervosa
an eating disorder in which individuals have an intense fear of being overweight and overfat that causes binge eating followed by self-induced vomiting or the non-purging type where compensation is through fasting or excessive exercise

disordered eating
a broad spectrum of abnormal eating behaviours

female athlete triad
an eating disorder among female athletes that is defined by three conditions: disordered eating, amenorrhea, and osteoporosis

metabolic syndrome
a cluster of risk factors that increase an individual's likelihood of developing cardiovascular diseases, diabetes, and several other conditions

metabolism
describes the chemical processes that occur within a living cell or organism that are necessary for maintaining life

skinfold measurement
measurement of fat just below the skin surface at five points on the body to determine the percentage of body fat

somatotype
there are three somatotypes (body types): ectomorphic, mesomorphic, and endomorphic

waist circumference (WC)
an indicator of health risk associated with abdominal fat around the waist

waist-to-hip ratio (WHR) measurement
a method for assessing body composition, based on the relationship between the girth of the waist and the girth of the hips

EXERCISES

MULTIPLE CHOICE

1. The following signs all indicate an eating disorder except
   a. unusual eating behaviours such as cutting up food into very small pieces, playing with food, or hiding or disguising food that is uneaten
   b. disordered eating, amenorrhea, and osteoporosis
   c. an intense fear of being overweight and overfat
   d. satisfaction with body weight and body shape or size
   e. uncontrollable binge eating followed by self-induced vomiting

2. What is one health risk associated with obesity?
   a. type 2 diabetes
   b. glaucoma
   c. nerve disorder
   d. indigestion
   e. hernia

3. Which of the following is true about overweight?
   a. It is defined as "excessive abdominal fat."
   b. It is possible to be obese and not overweight.
   c. Overweight and obesity mean the same thing.
   d. It is possible to be overweight but not obese.
   e. Overweight is the same as being underweight.

4. Which of the following is a characteristic of anorexia nervosa?
   a. intense fear of fat
   b. denial of appetite
   c. avoidance of food
   d. excessive exercising
   e. all of the above

5. The female athlete triad is characterized by
   a. disordered eating, amenorrhea, and osteoporosis
   b. disordered eating, dysmenorrhea, and weight gain
   c. weight gain, amenorrhea, and excessive exercise
   d. weight gain, amenorrhea, and osteoporosis
   e. none of the above

6. Basal metabolic rate (BMR) is
   a. the sum of all the processes by which food energy is used by the body
   b. the body's total daily energy expenditure
   c. the energy required to digest a meal
   d. the speed at which energy is used by the body
   e. the energy required to start your day

7. The body mass index (BMI) is determined by
   a. skinfolds
   b. body weight
   c. body height
   d. body weight and body height
   e. body weight and skinfolds

8. The three somatotype bodies are
   a. ectomorphic, endomorphic, and mesomorphic
   b. ectomorphic, endomorphic, and mendomorphic
   c. ectomorphic, mesomorphic, and cytomorphic
   d. endomorphic, mesomorphic, and octomorphic
   e. endomorphic, mesomorphic, and mendomorphic

9. A high BMI may indicate
   a. a low immune system
   b. overweight
   c. anorexia
   d. a healthy body
   e. none of the above

10. The waist-to-hip ratio (WHR) provides an estimate of
    a. fatness
    b. location of regional fat deposition
    c. cholesterol
    d. athletic potential
    e. the percentage of fat in your body

11. Bulimia nervosa is associated with all the following except
    a. fear of becoming obese
    b. restricted eating patterns
    c. periods of bingeing and purging
    d. high levels of physical activity
    e. suffering from a critical incident

12. The body mass index measures
    a. the relationship between height and weight
    b. bioelectrical impedance
    c. girth (or circumference) at various body sites
    d. anorexia nervosa
    e. percentage of body fat

13. An eating disorder characterized by excessive preoccupation with food, self-starvation, and/or extreme exercising to achieve weight loss is known as
    a. bulimia nervosa
    b. anorexia nervosa
    c. binge eating disorder
    d. social physique anxiety
    e. satiety

14. Jadie is 1.65 metres tall and weighs 60 kilograms. Her BMI is approximately
    a. 20
    b. 21
    c. 22
    d. 23
    e. 24

15. Those who suffer from female athletic triad see the effects of osteoporosis
    a. when they are young
    b. both when they are young and when they reach menopause
    c. when they reach menopause
    d. after they are 80 years old
    e. only if they don't stop poor eating habits

SHORT ANSWER

1. What issues surround overweight and obesity in Canada?

2. Describe the three somatotypes.

3. Explain the terms *body mass index* and *waist-to-hip ratio*.

4. Determine the BMI for an adult female who is 1.70 metres tall and weighs 55.0 kilograms. Comment on the result.

5. What is the waist circumference a measure for? What is a healthy circumference for men? For women? Why?

6. Why is fasting a poor way to lose weight? What is a more appropriate way to modify body weight?

7. How are eating disorders not just physical problems? How might this affect your job as a law enforcement officer?

8. What methods are available to assess your body composition?

REFERENCES

Addy, C.L., Wilson, D.K., Kirtland, K.A., Ainsworth, B.E., Sharpe, P., et al. (2004). Associations of perceived social and physical environmental supports with physical activity and walking behavior. *American Journal of Public Health, 94*(3), 440–443.

American Psychiatric Association. (1994). *Diagnostic and statistical manual of mental disorders* (4th ed.). Washington, DC: Author.

Arnow, K.D., et al. (2017). A qualitative analysis of male eating disorder symptoms. *The Journal of Treatment & Prevention, Apr 10*, 1–13.

Bangalore, S., Fayyad, R., Laskey, R., DeMicco, D.A., Messerli, F.H, & Waters, D.D. (2017). Body-weight fluctuations and outcomes in coronary disease. *New England Journal Medicine, 376*, 1332–1340.

Barrack, M.T., Ackerman, K.E., & Gibbs, J.C. (2013). Update on the female athlete triad. *Current Reviews in Musculoskeletal Medicine, 6*(2), 195–204.

Bjornsson, A.S., Didie, E.R., & Phillips, K.A. (2010). Body dysmorphic disorder. *Dialogues in Clinical Neuroscience, 12*(2), 221–232.

Bray, G.A. (2004). Medical consequences of obesity. *Journal of Clinical Endocrinology & Metabolism, 89*, 2538–2539.

Bushnik, T. (2016). Women in Canada: A Gender-based Statistical Report. The health of girls and women. Statistics Canada. Cat. No. 89-503-X. Retrieved from http://www.statcan.gc.ca/pub/89-503-x/2015001/article/14324-eng.pdf

Cafri, G., Blevins, N., & Thompson, J.K. (2006). The drive for muscle leanness: A complex case with features of muscle dysmorphia and eating disorder not otherwise specified. *Eating and Weight Disorders, 11*(4), 117–118.

Canadian Diabetes Association Clinical Practice Guidelines Expert Committee. Canadian Diabetes Association 2013 Clinical Practice Guidelines for the Prevention and Management of Diabetes in Canada. *Canandian Journal of Diabetes, 37*(suppl 1), S1–S212.

Canadian Institute for Health Information (CIHI). (2006). *Hospital morbidity database*. Ottawa: Author.

Canadian Society for Exercise Physiology (CSEP). (1996). *Canadian standardized test of fitness interpretation and counselling manual*. Ottawa: Author.

Canoy, D., Cairns, B.J., Balkwill, A., Wright, F.L., Green, J., Reeves, G., et al. (2013). Body mass index and incident coronary heart disease in women: A population-based prospective study. BMC Med*icine, 11*, 87.

Conroy, M., Menard, W., Fleming-Ives, K., Modha, P., Cerullo, H., & Phillips, K.A. (2008). Prevalence and clinical characteristics of body dysmorphic disorder in an adult inpatient setting. *General Hospital Psychiatry, 30*, 67–72.

Elmslie, K. (2012). *Against the growing burden of disease*. Ottawa: Public Health Agency of Canada, Centre for Chronic Disease Prevention.

Gadalla, T., & Piran, N. (2007). Co-occurrence of eating disorders and alcohol use disorders in women: A meta analysis. *Archives of Women's Mental Health, 10*(4), 133–140.

Grundy, S.M., Brewer, H.B. Jr., Cleeman, J.I., Smith, S.C. Jr., & Lenfant, C. (2004). Definition of metabolic syndrome: Report of the National Heart, Lung, and Blood Institute/American Heart Association Conference on Scientific Issues Related to Definition. *Circulation, 109*(3), 433–438.

Guh, D.P., Zhang, W., Bansback, N., et al. (2009). The incidence of co-morbidities related to obesity and overweight. A systematic review and meta-analysis. *BMC Public Health, 9*, 88.

Hadjiyannakis, S., Buchholz, A., Chanoin, J.-P., Jetha, M.M., Gaboury, L., Hamilton, J., et al. (2016). The Edmonton Obesity Staging System for Pediatrics: A proposed clinical staging system for paediatric obesity. *Paediatrics & Child Health*, 21(1), 21–26.

Health Canada. (2000). *Canadian guidelines for weight classification in adults*. Ottawa: Author.

Health Canada. (2002). *A report on mental illnesses in Canada*. Catalogue no. 0-662-32817-5. Ottawa: Author.

Health Canada. (2003). *Canadian guidelines for body weight classification in adults*. Ottawa: Author.

Jacobi, C., Hayward, C., de Zwaan, M., Kraemer, H., & Agras, W.S. (2004). Coming to terms with risk factors for eating disorders: Application of risk terminology and suggestions for a general taxonomy. *Psychological Bulletin*, 130(1), 19–65.

Kalra, G., De Sousa, A., Sonavane, S., & Shah, N. (2012). Psychological issues in pediatric obesity. *Industrial Psychiatry Journal, 21*(1), 11–17. Retrieved from http://doi.org/10.4103/0972-6748.110941

Kanayama, G., & Pope, H.G. Jr. (2012). Illicit use of androgens and other hormones: Recent advances. *Current Opinion in Endocrinology, Diabetes and Obesity, 19*(3), 211–219.

Katzmarzyk, P.T., & Ardern, C.I. (2004). Overweight and obesity mortality trends in Canada 1985–2000. *Canadian Journal of Public Health, 95*, 16–20.

King, G.A, Fitzhugh, E.C., Bassett, D.R., McLaughlin, J.E., Strath, S.J., et al. (2001). Relationship of leisure-time physical activity and occupational activity to the prevalence of obesity. *International Journal of Obesity and Related Metabolic Disorders, 25*, 606–612.

Kuk, J.L., Ardern, C.I., Church, T.S., Sharma, A.M., Padwal, R., et al. (2011). Edmonton Obesity Staging System: Association with weight history and mortality risk. *Applied Physiology, Nutrition and Metabolism, 36*, 570–576.

Langford, E. (2010). *Did you know…About Obese Children and Atherosclerosis*. Cardiac Health Foundation of Canada. Retrieved from http://cardiachealth.ca/templates/content/pages/didyouknow5.html

Luo, W., Morrison, H., de Groh, M., et al. (2007). The burden of adult obesity in Canada. *Chronic Diseases in Canada, 27*, 135–144.

Mond, J.M., Mitchison, D., & Hay, P. (2014). Prevalence and implications of eating disordered behavior in men. In L. Cohn & R. Lemberg, *Current findings on males with eating disorders*. Philadelphia, PA: Routledge.

Mountjoy, M., Sudgot-Borgen, J., Burke, L., Carter, S., Constantini, N., Lebrun, C., Meyer, N., Sherman, R., Steffen, K., Budgett, R., Ljungqvist, A., & Ackerman, K. (2015). The IOC relative energy deficiency in sport clinical assessment tool. *British Journal of Sports Medicine*; 49: 417-420.

National Eating Disorder Information Centre (NEDIC). (2014). Statistics: Understanding Statistics on Eating Disorders. Retrieved from http://nedic.ca/know-facts/statistics

National Eating Disorder Information Centre (NEDIC). (2015). Compulsive Exercising. Informal Definitions. http://nedic.ca/informal-definitions

Neumark-Sztainer, D. (2002). Weight-teasing among adolescents: Correlations with weight status and disordered eating behaviours. *International Journal of Obesity and Related Metabolic Disorders, 26*(1), 123.

Okifuji, A., & Hare, B.D. (2015). The association between chronic pain and obesity. *Journal of Pain Research, 8*, 399–408.

Osteoporosis Canada (2017). Osteoporosis Facts & Statistics. Retrieved from http://www.osteoporosis.ca/osteoporosis-and-you/osteoporosis-facts-and-statisticsh

Padwal, R.S., Padewski, N.M., Allison, D.B., & Sharma, A.M. (2011). Using the Edmonton Obesity Staging System to predict mortality in a population-representative cohort of people with overweight and obesity. *Canadian Medical Association Journal, 183*(4), 1059–1066. doi:10.1503/cmaj.110387

Pan, S.Y., Cameron, C., DesMeules, M., Morrison, H., Craig, C.L., et al. (2009). Individual, social, environmental and physical environmental correlates with physical activity among Canadians: A cross-sectional study. *BMC Public Health, 9*, 21. doi:10.1186/1471-2458-9-21

Phillips, K.A., & Castle, D.J. (2001). Body dysmorphic disorder in men. *British Medical Journal, 323*, 1015–1016.

Phillips, K.A., Menard, W., Fay, C., & Pagano, M.E. (2005). Psychosocial functioning and quality of life in body dysmorphic disorder. *Comprehensive Psychiatry, 46*, 254–260.

Pope, H.G., Phillips, K.A., & Olivardia, R. (2000). *The Adonis complex: The secret crisis of male body obsession*. New York, NY: Free Press.

Public Health Agency of Canada (PHAC). (2011). *Obesity in Canada. A joint report from the Public Health Agency of Canada and the Canadian Institute for Health Information.* Catalogue no. hps-107/2011 E-PDF. Ottawa: Authors.

Public Health Agency of Canada (PHAC). (2015). Evidence brief: Trends and projections of obesity among Canadians. *Health Promotion and Chronic Disease Prevention in Canada: Research, Policy and Practice, 35*(7).

Puhl, R.M. (2012). Weight-based victimization among adolescents in the school setting: Emotional reactions and coping behaviours. *Journal of Youth and Adolescence, 41*(1), 27.

Roberts, K.C., Shields, M., deGroh, M., Aziz, A., & Gilbert, J. (2012). Overweight and obesity in children and adolescents: Results from the 2009 to 2011 Canadian Health Measures Survey. *Statistics Canada; Health Reports, 23*(3). Catalogue no. 82-003-X.

Sanborn, C.F., Horea, M., Siemers, B.J., & Dieringer, K.I. (2000). Disordered eating and the female athlete triad. *Clinics in Sports Medicine, 19*(2), 199–213.

Sharma, A.M., & Kushner, R.F. (2009). A proposed clinical staging system for obesity. *International Journal of Obesity, 33*(3), 289–295.

Shields, M. (2005). Overweight Canadian children and adolescents. *Nutrition: Findings from the Canadian Community Health Survey.* Catalogue no. 82-620-MWE2005001. Ottawa: Statistics Canada.

Shields, M., Tremblay, M.S., Laviolett, M., Craig, C.L., Janssen, I., & Gorber, S.C. (2010). Fitness of Canadian adults: Results from the 2007–2009 Canadian Health Measures Survey. *Health Reports, 21*(1), 1–15. Catalogue no. 82-003-X

Statistics Canada. (2012). *Health State Descriptions for Canadians: Mental Illness–Section D: Eating Disorders.* Catalogue no. 82-619-M. Ottawa: Authors. Retrieved from http://www.statcan.gc.ca/pub/82-619-m/2012004/sections/sectiond-eng.htm - a1

Statistics Canada. (2015). *Overweight and Obese Adults (self-reported) 2014.* Catalogue no. 82-625-X2015001. Ottawa: Authors. Retrieved from http://www5.statcan.gc.ca/olc-cel/olc.action?objId=82-625-X&objType=2&lang=en&limit=0

Stice, E. (2002). Risk and maintenance factors for eating pathology: A meta-analytic review. *Psychological Bulletin, 128*(5), 825–848.

Tjepkema, M. (2005). Measured obesity: Adult obesity in Canada. *Nutrition: Findings from the Canadian Community Health Survey.* Catalogue no. 82-620-MWE2005001. Ottawa: Statistics Canada.

Tjepkema, M. (2006). Adult obesity. *Health Reports, 17*(3), 9–25.

Toulany, A., Wong, M., Katzman, D.K., Akseer, N., Steinegger, C., Hancock-Howard, R., & Coyte, P.C. (2015). *Canadian Medical Association Journal Open, 3*(2): E192–E198. doi: 10.9778/cmajo.20140086

Twells, L.K., Gregory, D.M., Reddigan, J., & Midodzi, W.K. (2014). Current and predicted prevalence of obesity in Canada: A trend analysis. *Canadian Medical Association Journal, 2*(1), E18–E26. doi.10.9778/xmJO.20130016

Wang, Y., Wang, B., Shen, F., Fan, J., & Cao, H. (2012). Body mass index and risk of primary liver cancer: A meta-analysis of prospective studies. *The Oncologist, 17*(11), 1461–1468.

Weiss Kelly, A.K., Hecht, S., & Council on Sports Medicine and Fitness. (2016). The female triad. *Pediatrics, 138*(2).

Weltzin, T., Carlson, T., et al. (2014). Treatment issues and outcomes for males with eating disorders. In L. Cohn & R. Lemberg, *Current findings on males with eating disorders.* Philadelphia, PA: Routledge.

World Health Organization (WHO). (2000). *Obesity: Preventing and managing the global epidemic: Report of a WHO consultation on obesity.* Geneva: Author.

World Health Organization (WHO). (2010) Raising the priority of non-communicable diseases in development work at global and national levels. Retrieved from http://www.who.int/ncdnet/events/booklet_20100224.pdf

World Health Organization (WHO). (2011). *Waist circumference and waist-hip ratio. Report of a WHO expert consultation.* Geneva: Author.

Yeager, K.K., Agostini, R., Nattiv, A., & Drinkwater, B. (1993). The female athlete triad: Disordered eating, amenorrhoea, osteoporosis. *Medicine and Science in Sports and Exercise, 25*(7), 775–777.

Yusuf, S., et al. (2005). Obesity and the risk of myocardial infarction in 27,000 participants from 52 countries: A case-control study. *Lancet, 366*(9497), 1640–1649.

NUTRITION

LEARNING OUTCOMES

After completing this chapter, you should be able to:

- Describe nutritional trends in Canada.
- Understand the importance of maintaining a healthy weight, and the role of portion sizes and food labelling.
- Describe the role of the six basic nutrients: water, carbohydrates, protein, fats, vitamins, and minerals.
- Understand glycemic index and glycemic load.
- Explore the role of sodium within the body and effects of having too little or too much
- Describe the role of fibre in a healthy diet.
- Make better food choices using *Eating Well with Canada's Food Guide*.
- Explain the importance of proper nutrition while working shifts.
- Determine which nutrition information, including websites, is valid and reliable.
- Understand serving sizes and how to read nutrient labels when grocery shopping.
- Identify nutritional consideration regarding appropriate snacking and caffeine consumption.

Over the past 30 years, law enforcement officers—like other Canadians—have become better informed about nutrition. Yet, most Canadians' dietary and exercise habits remain substandard. Based on the Canadian Community Health Survey (CCHS), the diet quality of Canadians is "poor." The majority of Canadians still have low intakes of vegetables and fruit, milk and alternatives, and whole grains. Research found that 30 percent of total calories are consumed from food and beverages not recommended in the *Eating Well with Canada's Food Guide*, such as those high in fat, sugar, or salt, and up to 25 percent of the daily energy intake was snacks (Health Canada, 2015). A 2011 survey reported that 78 percent of Canadians believe they eat nutritiously, yet "the preponderance of skipped meals, rushed meals, and meals without fresh fruits or vegetables; the expansive consumption of soft drinks; the excessive intake of caffeine, and the lack of portion control seen … suggest otherwise" (Canadian Council of Food and Nutrition, 2011). Today, we are still struggling.

Shift work has traditionally created barriers to accessing healthy foods. In large urban areas there are 24-hour grocery stores; however, in small communities, individuals must plan better to ensure that they eat well. Given the demands of shift work and the unforeseen lack of breaks and requests for overtime, there is a tendency for officers to consume fast-food meals, which are high in fat, sugar, and sodium, between stressful calls. Compounded with the lack of regular exercise and high stress, these habits put them at risk for high cholesterol, elevated triglycerides, increased insulin sensitivity, and overall body fat, potentially leading to diabetes and cardiovascular disease (see Chapters 9 and 10). Planning and eating balanced meals and snacks at appropriate times and choosing healthy foods, such as fruits, vegetables, and whole grains, help to keep your energy levels stable during your working hours and may promote more restful sleep.

This chapter addresses the topic of nutrition with the view that good dietary choices are made over the course of a lifetime and are especially important to keep on track during your career.

MAINTAINING A HEALTHY WEIGHT

A person's weight is the result of many factors, including height, genes, metabolism, behaviour, and environment. It is important that you learn how to balance the energy that you take in (calories) with the energy that you expend (exercise). For most people, maintaining this balance means consuming fewer calories and exercising more. In addition to making healthy food choices that are lower in fats, cholesterol, added sugars, and salt, Canadians need to pay attention to portion sizes. These topics will be covered later in this chapter.

Poor lifestyles and diets have led to a condition known as metabolic syndrome. Metabolic syndrome (MetS) is a cluster of medical conditions that increase the risk of many chronic illnesses including diabetes, hypertension, cardiovascular diseases, chronic kidney disease, and dyslipidemia. Nearly one in five Canadians meet the criteria of MetS (Metabolic Syndrome Canada, 2017; PHAC, 2014). MetS is diagnosed when a patient has three of the following five conditions:

- High blood pressure (≥130/85 mm Hg, or receiving medication)
- High blood glucose levels (A1C levels ≥5.6 mmol/L, or receiving medication)
- High triglycerides (≥1.7 mmol/L, or receiving medication)

- Low HDL-cholesterol (≥1.0 mmol/L in men, ≥1.3 mmol/L in women)
- Large waist circumference (≥102 cm in men, ≥88 cm in women; range varies according to ethnicity)

If you are overweight or obese, losing as little as 10 percent of your current weight can lower your risks for these chronic diseases. It is reasonable and safe to lose one-half to one kilogram per week. Losing more per week puts you at risk for gaining the weight back. Along with making healthier eating choices, you need to make a commitment to increase your level of physical activity (see Chapter 2 on goal setting and behavioural changes). Although weight-loss medication and weight-loss surgery may be an option for a small percentage of the population, for most people, changing eating habits and becoming more active are the key to sustained weight loss. There are, however, metabolic issues that are not affected by increased exercise and eating less. Some of those include insulin resistance, low serotonin, high estrogen, low testosterone, high cortisol brought on by chronic stress, and hypothyroidism. If your goal is to lose weight, whatever your circumstances, you should check with your doctor or a nutritionist.

FACTS TO THINK ABOUT

NUTRITION IN CANADA

- According to recent data, overweight and obese adult Canadians—61.8 percent of men and 42 percent of women—are at increased health risk because of excess weight. The prevalence of overweight and obesity combined is greater in Indigenous men (71 percent) and Indigenous women (64 percent) living off-reserve in Ontario and western provinces.
- In children, body weight and self-esteem are inversely related. For each BMI unit increase, self-esteem scores decrease by 4.8 percent. Children who have more screen time are particularly susceptible to weight gain. Those who take medications for mental health issues may experience increased appetite, making healthy dietary changes difficult to accomplish.
- Canadian families spend approximately 10.4 percent of their yearly income on food expenditures. Millennials are spending approximately 44 percent of their food dollars on eating out.
- Sixty percent of Canadians eat out once or more a week, spending a national average of $8.80 each time. Forty-five percent of Canadians buy at least one item from a fast-food restaurant every day. After tax, eating out three times a week could add up to about $2000 a year.
- The highest consumers of fast food are men aged 19 to 30. The most popular items include pizza, hamburgers, hot dogs, chicken wings, french fries, coffee, and soft drinks.
- Women are more likely than men to consume fruit and vegetables. In 2010, 49.9 percent of females consumed fruit and vegetables five or more times daily, compared to 36.4 percent of males. Canada's Food Guide recommends greater consumption of dark green and orange vegetables, yet the most common ones chosen by Canadians are potatoes, salad, and corn. Fruit choices tend to be seasonal and consumed as a snack or dessert.
- In choosing protein foods, Canadians are more likely to select high-fat, high-sodium processed meats (sausages, ham, bacon) rather than fish or legumes (lentils and beans).
- When people eat alone, they tend to eat things that are convenient yet less nutritious—more packaged and processed foods, including fewer basic food groups (grains, protein, fruits and vegetables, dairy products).

SOURCES: Dietitians of Canada, 2010; Garriguet, 2007, 2012; Panagiotopoulos, Ronsley, Elbe, Davidson, & Smith, 2010; Pérez, 2002; PHAC, 2010a, 2010b; Statistics Canada, 2016, 2017; United States Department of Agriculture, 2016; Visa Canada Corporation, 2012; Wang, Wild, Kipp, Kuhle, & Veugelers, 2009.

IMPACT OF DIET, NUTRITION, AND PHYSICAL ACTIVITY ON CANCER

Figure 8.1 provides a summary of strong evidence from the World Cancer Research Fund International on the impact of lifestyle choices on the risk and prevention of cancer.

FIGURE 8.1 Impact of Diet, Nutrition, and Physical Activity on the Prevention of Cancer

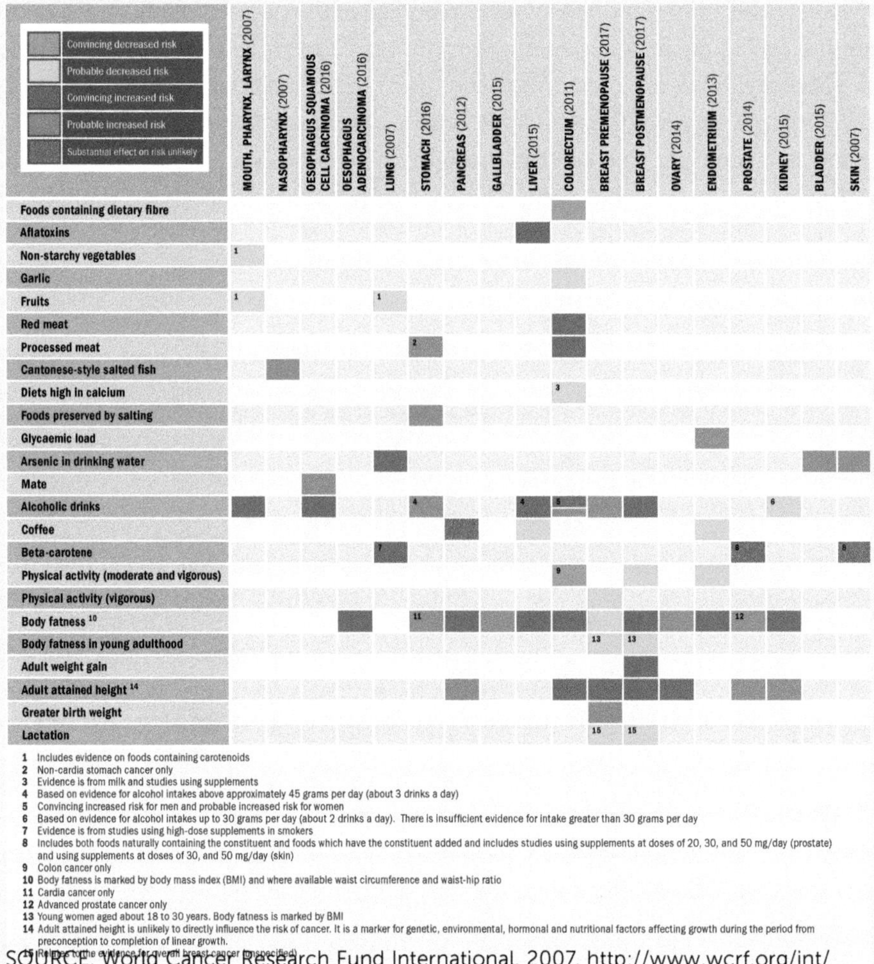

1 Includes evidence on foods containing carotenoids
2 Non-cardia stomach cancer only
3 Evidence is from milk and studies using supplements
4 Based on evidence for alcohol intakes above approximately 45 grams per day (about 3 drinks a day)
5 Convincing increased risk for men and probable increased risk for women
6 Based on evidence for alcohol intakes up to 30 grams per day (about 2 drinks a day). There is insufficient evidence for intake greater than 30 grams per day
7 Evidence is from studies using high-dose supplements in smokers
8 Includes both foods naturally containing the constituent and foods which have the constituent added and includes studies using supplements at doses of 20, 30, and 50 mg/day (prostate) and using supplements at doses of 30, and 50 mg/day (skin)
9 Colon cancer only
10 Body fatness is marked by body mass index (BMI) and where available waist circumference and waist-hip ratio
11 Cardia cancer only
12 Advanced prostate cancer only
13 Young women aged about 18 to 30 years. Body fatness is marked by BMI
14 Adult attained height is unlikely to directly influence the risk of cancer. It is a marker for genetic, environmental, hormonal and nutritional factors affecting growth during the period from preconception to completion of linear growth.
15 Breast cancer (however lower cancer types specified)

SOURCE: World Cancer Research Fund International, 2007. http://www.wcrf.org/int/research-we-fund/continuous-update-project-findings-reports/continuous-update-project-cup-matrix

For more information on diet and lifestyle impact on cancer go to:

- World Cancer Research Fund International http://www.wcrf.org
- Canadian Cancer Society http://www.cancer.ca

FUNCTION OF FOOD

Most Canadians have abundant choices with respect to food: grocery stores, cafeterias and restaurants, even vending machines. College and university students face obstacles in ensuring a nutritious diet (time constraints, lack of cooking facilities, money pressures), but education, motivation, and determination can make a difference. See Figure 8.2.

FIGURE 8.2   Deciding What Is Good Nutrition

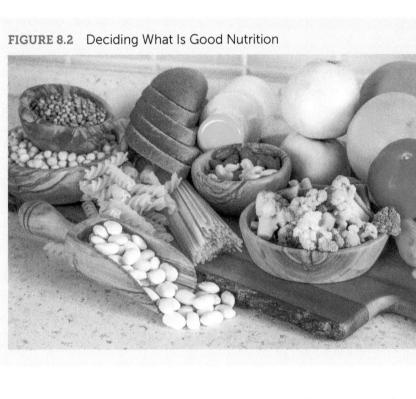

Food provides nutrients that have physiological and biochemical functions in the body. There are six basic nutrients: water, carbohydrates, protein, fats, vitamins, and minerals. Their functions are:

- *To promote growth and development of muscle, soft tissues, and organs.* Protein does most of the work for growth and repair, with the assistance of calcium and phosphorus in the skeletal building blocks.
- *To provide energy to the body.* Carbohydrates and fats contribute predominantly, although protein assists as a fuel source if needed.
- *To regulate metabolism.* Your body's enzymes are proteins that work with vitamins and minerals to regulate your metabolism.

Maintaining your energy balance and a nutrient-dense diet, a prudent training regime, proper timing of nutrient intake, and adequate rest and recovery are cornerstones to enhancing performance and seeing gains in your physique. It is important that you understand the basics of nutrition if you want to succeed in becoming and staying fit throughout your career.

BASIC NUTRIENTS

Our bodies require six basic nutrients to function efficiently: water (the most important), carbohydrates, protein, fats, vitamins, and minerals. In total, these substances provide 45 essential nutrients, which our bodies assimilate through digestion. Failing to consume the right nutrients in appropriate quantities inevitably leads to ill health.

WATER

Water is the transportation medium in the body. Our bodies are about 60 percent water (the brain is composed of approximately 70 percent water, while our bones have about 22 percent water). Children have a higher percentage of water than

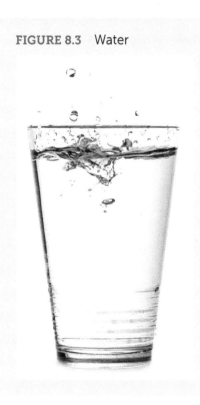

FIGURE 8.3 Water

adults. Women have less water than men, and people who have more fatty tissue have less water than those with less fatty tissue. Water cools and purifies the body's tissues, carries carbohydrates and protein through the bloodstream, participates in biochemical reactions, aids in digestion and absorption, and helps regulate body temperature. Water helps in getting rid of waste through urine, and drinking a lot of water correlates with a lower risk of developing kidney stones and colon and bladder cancer. Water also acts like a lubricant and a cushion for the joints. It protects sensitive tissue like the spine and is the fluid in the eye.

Law enforcement officers are often required to stand outdoors in hot weather for hours at a time. Dehydration (lack of body fluids) can quickly set in, so always carrying a source of water is important. Even a loss of 2 percent of your body weight through perspiration results in a decline in performance; a loss of 5 percent can result in fatigue, weakness, lethargy, dizziness, headache, and elevated heart rate. These symptoms can progress to cramps, confusion, inability to swallow or move, and failing kidney function. If you are thirsty, you are already dehydrated.

In general, men should be drinking 3 L (12 cups) of water per day, and women 2.2 L (9 cups) (Dietitians of Canada, 2014). Those who are exercising, on a weight-loss program, or ill need more water. It is advisable to drink at least 500 millilitres of water before any physical activity that lasts an hour or more, and to consume more fluids afterward, including those that restore electrolyte balance, such as sports drinks and juices. The most common electrolytes are sodium, potassium, magnesium, chloride, and calcium. Electrolytes assist in heart and nerve functions, muscle control, coordination, and the body's ability to absorb fluid.

Deficiency of sodium is called hyponatremia; other electrolyte imbalances can happen with low calcium (hypocalcemia) and potassium (hypokalemia). Electrolyte imbalance rarely occurs through physical activity, but may result from other conditions such as severe burns, prolonged diarrhea or vomiting, or liver or kidney disease. Adequate consumption of properly formulated electrolyte-containing beverages as part of a fluid replacement regime may help prevent or reduce the risk of hyponatremia (Tipton, 2006).

Hydrating for an athletic event or when you are doing specialized job-related tasks such as a canine search or crowd control for long hours, is slightly different from general hydration. It is recommended to avoid dehydration during exercise/ activities by continually consuming fluids, and a more practical approach is to consume about 500 millilitres of water two hours before going to bed the night before an exercise or event, and another 500 millilitres of fluid (juice, milk, or water) first thing the next morning. Then, one should drink (a) just enough water to maintain optimal hydration, (b) 300 to 500 millilitres of a diluted sports drink (3–4 percent) one hour before, and then (c) an additional 300 to 500 millilitres (1–2.5 percent) 25 minutes before the event.

DID YOU KNOW?

Besides dehydration, electrolyte imbalance can also be caused by hyperhydration, or water intoxication. This is related to extreme endurance events where individuals are not getting enough electrolytes. Consuming too much water can result in a potentially fatal disturbance in brain function when electrolytes, specifically sodium, are diluted beyond safe limits. As your water level rises, the cells begin to swell, and the brain cannot handle the swelling. Symptoms of water intoxication include headache, nausea, vomiting, fatigue, restlessness, muscle weakness, spasms or cramps, and decreased consciousness or coma.

CARBOHYDRATES

Carbohydrates are the sugars, starches, and fibres found in fruits, grains, vegetables, and milk products. They are called *carbohydrates* because, at the cellular level, they contain carbon, hydrogen, and oxygen. Carbohydrates are needed primarily in the diet to provide energy to the body. The brain and central nervous system (CNS) use only carbohydrates for fuel. During high-intensity exercises, muscular energy requires carbohydrates for immediate energy.

There are two types of carbohydrates: simple and complex. Simple carbohydrates are small and consist of either one or two molecules of sugar. They digest easily and give quick energy. Simple carbohydrates are found naturally in fruit and milk, but have also been added to soft drinks, candy, and many other processed foods to increase sweetness.

Complex carbohydrates consist of chains of sugar molecules, called starches and fibre. They are also broken down into sugar molecules, but take longer to digest because of their large chain structure. Starches are found naturally in grains, vegetables, and legumes. Fibre is found in fruits, vegetables, and grains (and will be discussed later in the chapter).

The digestive system handles all carbohydrates in a similar fashion. It breaks them down into single sugar molecules for absorption. The pancreas releases

TOP TIPS ...

WAYS TO REDUCE SUGAR IN YOUR DIET

- Remove sugar (white and brown), high fructose corn syrup, honey, agave, maple sugar, molasses, and anything ending with an "ose" from your diet.
- Cut back on the amount of sugar added to things you eat or drink like cereal, pancakes, muffins, coffee, and tea.
- Enhance foods with spices instead of sugar; try cinnamon, nutmeg, allspice, or ginger.
- Try substituting zero-calorie naturally occurring Stevia, as a replacement for sugar.
- When baking, cut the sugars called for in the recipe by one-third to one-half.
- Do your own baking. Store-bought treats have so much more sugar in them then you would add.
- Use unsweetened applesauce for sugar in recipes (use equal amounts).
- Choose fresh fruit or fruit canned in water or natural fruit juice over those canned in syrup, especially heavy syrup.
- Replace pop and juice with unsweetened teas or water infused with fresh fruit (a 20-oz bottle of Coca-Cola contains 65 g of sugar; see Table 8.1).

insulin to allow cells to take up sugar and use it for fuel for physical activity and proper organ function. The liver and muscles also take up glucose and store it as glycogen to be used later. When sugar is consumed in excess, the body stores it as fat.

Complex carbohydrates can also be further divided into natural whole grains or refined (processed) whole grains. Refinement strips away essential parts of the grain, losing important vitamins, minerals, and fibre. Natural whole-grain options include whole wheat, brown rice, 100 percent rye bread, spelt, buckwheat, and quinoa. Unrefined grains take longer to digest and therefore keep you feeling fuller longer, lessening the chance of overeating. Consuming whole-grain products every day reduces the risk of heart disease, diabetes, high blood pressure, and cancer (Aune et al., 2011; Rautiainen, Larsson, Virtamo, & Wolk, 2012).

TABLE 8.1 Sugar Content in Common Drinks

	TEASPOONS OF SUGAR	GMS OF CHO	CALORIES FROM SUGAR (KCAL)	*TOTAL CALORIES (KCAL)
1% Milk (250 mL)	4	12	104	110
1% Chocolate Milk (250 mL)	8.5	26	128	170
Apple Juice (360 mL)	10	40	160	160
Orange Juice (360 mL)	12	42	160	160
Pop (600 mL—Medium)	15	59	238	238
Fruitopia (600 mL)	24	64	230	230
Powerade (591 mL)	8.2	32	131	131
Gatorade (591 mL)	9	36	140	140
Ice Tea (609 mL)	10	40	260	260
McDonald's® Caramel Cappuccino (354 mL)	8.75	35	140	230
McDonald's® Coffee Iced Frappé (376 mL)	13.5	54	216	370
Tim Hortons® Latte (354 mL)	5	15	60	99
Tim Hortons® Iced Capp® (Cream) (380 mL)	8.25	33	132	250
Starbucks® Iced Chai Latte (354 mL)	8.25	33	132	190
Starbucks® Ice Coffee & Milk (325 mL)	6	24	96	110
Starbucks® Caffè Mocha (354 mL)	8.5	34	136	290
Starbucks Midnight Mint Mocha Frappuccino® Blended Coffee (354 mL)	9.5	38	152	310
*TOTAL calories (calories from carbohydrates, proteins, and fats).				

SOURCES: Coca-Cola, 2017; McDonalds, 2017; PepsiCo, 2017; Starbucks, 2015; Tim Hortons, 2013.

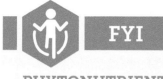

FYI

PHYTONUTRIENTS

Phytonutrients are compounds, found in vegetables and fruits, that are not used for normal functions of the body but have a beneficial effect on health or disease. An example is flavonoids, which are found in berries, herbs, and vegetables, and are associated with a decreased risk for cancer owing to their antioxidant and anti-inflammatory effects.

UNDERSTANDING THE GLYCEMIC INDEX

The glycemic index (GI) relates to how the body digests food—that is, how much the carbohydrate-rich foods raise blood glucose levels in the first two hours of digestion (Jenkins et al., 1981). Your body's response depends on several factors, including age, activity level, insulin levels, time of day, amount of fibre and fat in the food, how processed the food is, and what you have ingested with the food (see Figure 8.4).

> **DID YOU KNOW?**
> Your brain uses only glucose as a source of energy; without it, your ability to think is compromised. This is why many school boards have adopted breakfast programs. It also explains why diets that cut out carbohydrates leave you feeling angry, emotional, and upset.

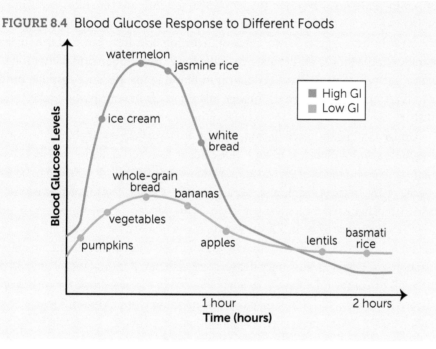

FIGURE 8.4 Blood Glucose Response to Different Foods

Foods that rank high on the glycemic index cause the blood sugar to increase rapidly (foods on the blue line), which often leads to a rush of energy and a steep increase in insulin levels—and is consequently followed by a crash in energy. This is especially dangerous for diabetics, who are susceptible to spikes in blood sugar and insulin levels, meaning that people who suffer from diabetes must be very careful about where their foods rank on the glycemic index. Foods on the green line have a lower glycemic index, which keep blood sugar levels more even.

The following factors affect the glycemic index:

1. *Processing*   Grains that are milled and refined (had the bran and germ removed) will have a higher glycemic index than whole grains.

2. *Type of starch*   Some starches are easier to break down than others. For example, mashed potatoes (GI=85) are digested and absorbed faster than sweet potato (GI=51).

3. *Fibre content*   The higher the fibre content, the less digestible the carbohydrate. Hence, less sugar is delivered.

4. *Ripeness*   The riper the fruit or vegetable, the higher the glycemic index. For example, an underripe banana has a GI of 30, whereas an overripe banana has a GI of 48.

5. *Fat and acid content*   The more fat or acid a food or meal has, the slower the carbohydrates are converted to sugar and absorbed.

6. *Physical form*   Finely ground grain is more rapidly digested than a more coarsely ground grain, making it more glycemic.

The glycemic index ranges from 0 to 100, with glucose being 100. High-glycemic foods—those that are starchy or sugary, such as simple carbohydrates—will increase the body's sugar levels rapidly. Within 30 minutes of ingestion, your body senses that energy levels are declining, which leaves you hungry again and running to the fridge (or fast-food outlet), even if you've just eaten loads of calories. Low-glycemic foods slowly increase sugar levels in the blood. These foods are generally lower in fat and higher in fibre, and are a rich source of vitamins, minerals, and antioxidants. A lower glycemic index suggests slower rates of digestion and absorption of the sugars and starches in the foods. This translates into a lower insulin demand, better long-term blood glucose control, and a reduction in blood lipids. Because insulin's other job is to tell your body to store fat, higher insulin levels in your blood make you more likely to convert your food to body fat rather than usable energy.

Understanding the glycemic index (Table 8.2) will help you if you are trying to lose weight or control diabetes. If your blood sugar rises too quickly, your brain signals your pancreas to release more insulin, which opens the cells to glucose to be used as energy by the muscles, while any excess gets stored as fat. The more glucose your cells take in, the higher your blood sugar. Then, as the pancreas slows the release of insulin, your blood glucose dips. This is the reason that when you eat a chocolate bar, you first feel an energy rush, then feel lethargic and hungry. Excess secretion of insulin leads to fatigue, weight gain, and potentially, type 2 diabetes. Besides overweight and diabetes, high-glycemic index foods have been linked to increased risk for coronary heart disease (Beulens et al., 2007), macular degeneration (Chiu, Milton, Klein, Gensler, & Taylor, 2009), colorectal cancer (Higginbotham et al. 2004), and ovulatory infertility (Chavarro, Rich-Edwards, Rosner, & Willett, 2007).

The glycemic index only tells part of the story. To understand a food's complete effect on blood sugar, you need to know both how quickly the food makes glucose enter the bloodstream (glucose index), and how much glucose is delivered (glucose load). The glycemic load (GL) is a measure of how quickly a food is converted into sugar in relation to how much sugar the food contains. The glycemic load is determined by multiplying the grams of a carbohydrate in a serving by the glycemic index, then dividing by 100. A glycemic load of 10 or below is considered low; 20 or above is considered high. Watermelon, for example, has a high glycemic index (80). But a serving of watermelon has so little carbohydrate (6 grams) that its glycemic load is only 5.

Eating carbohydrates often and in large quantities is known to increase the risk of diabetes and coronary heart disease. As a result, high-protein diets, such as

Atkins and South Beach, have led people to believe that all carbohydrates are bad for you, but this is an oversimplification. Easily digested carbohydrates—such as white bread, white rice, pastries, sugared sodas, and other highly processed foods—may indeed contribute to weight gain and interfere with weight loss. But whole grains, beans, fruits, vegetables, and other intact carbohydrates do just the opposite: they promote good health.

TABLE 8.2 Examples of Low-, Medium-, and High-Glycemic Index Foods

FOOD GROUP	LOW-GLYCEMIC INDEX FOODS (<60*)	MEDIUM-GLYCEMIC INDEX FOODS (60–85*)	HIGH-GLYCEMIC INDEX FOODS (>85*)
Sugars	• Fructose	• Sucrose	• Glucose
Breads and cereals	• Pumpernickel bread • All-Bran cereal • Barley • Oatmeal and oat bran	• Bagel • Bran muffins • Shredded Mini Wheats • Instant oatmeal (porridge) • Long-grain white rice (boiled 15–25 minutes)	• White bread • French baguette • Corn Flakes • Rice Krispies • Instant white rice
Dairy products	• Milk (skim and full-fat) • Yogurt	• Low-fat ice cream	
Fruits, vegetables, and legumes	• Unripe banana • Apple, berries, apple juice • Peach (fresh), pear • Yams • Black beans • Chickpeas (garbanzo beans) • Lentils (dhal), peas • Soybeans • Peanuts	• Overripe banana • Mango • Orange juice • Papaya • Peaches in heavy syrup • New potatoes (white or red)	• Carrots • Parsnips • Baked potato (russets) • Instant potatoes • Watermelon
Processed foods	• White spaghetti noodles • Vermicelli • Tomato soup	• Popcorn • Soft drinks • Most cookies	• Jelly beans • Rice cakes

* Glycemic index scores are based on a score out of 100.

SOURCES: Adapted from Foster-Powell, Holt, & Brand-Miller, 2002; University of Sydney, 2017.

TOP TIPS ...

MAKING GOOD CHOICES

- Start the day with whole grains such as steel-cut oats, whole wheat bread, or whole oats. Also use whole-grain breads for lunches and snacks.
- Try quinoa for breakfast or after a workout. It offers complete protein and low-glycemic carbohydrates.
- Try whole barley in place of refined white rice. In addition to being a low-glycemic food, barley has cholesterol-lowering fibre.
- Limit potatoes to only a few days a week. Instead, try brown rice, bulgur, wheat berries, millet, and hulled barley.

- Try whole wheat pasta. If it is too chewy, mix it with white pasta.
- Add more beans, peas, and lentils to your diet. They are a good source of slowly digestible carbohydrates and contain protein and minerals as well.
- Nuts such as almonds, walnuts, and pistachios help lower cholesterol and reduce heart disease risk.
- A low-carbohydrate diet can and should include daily portions of low-glycemic foods such as fruits, vegetables, and whole grains for essential vitamins, minerals, and phytonutrients.

DIETARY FIBRE

Dietary fibre is the term for food components that cannot be digested. All fibre-containing foods contain a combination of insoluble and soluble fibre. Dietary fibre is a carbohydrate and is found exclusively in plants. When we consume refined grains, the fibre has been removed and what is left lacks a number of nutrients (including zinc, vitamin E, and magnesium). One indicator that you are consuming too many refined products is that as the day goes on, you experience abdominal bloating.

Insoluble fibre helps promote regularity and a healthy digestive system. It is fibre that will not dissolve in water and is not broken down in the digestive tract. It is found in wheat bran and wheat bran cereals, brown rice, whole-grain foods, fruits (such as raspberries and blackberries), and vegetables (such as broccoli and green peas). Insoluble fibre helps push food through the intestinal tract, promoting regularity and preventing constipation. This is important in chronic conditions such as irritable bowel syndrome, colitis, and diverticulitis.

Soluble fibre helps lower blood cholesterol and control blood sugar. When mixed with water, soluble fibre forms a gel. It binds to fatty substances in the intestine and carries them out as waste. It is found in oat bran, oatmeal, legumes (dried beans, peas, and lentils), pectin-rich fruit (apples, strawberries, and citrus fruits), and psyllium (a popular ingredient in breakfast cereals). Soluble fibre is important in lowering low-density lipoproteins (LDL, or "bad" cholesterol) in the prevention of cardiovascular disease. As well, it helps regulate the body's use of sugars, keeping hunger and blood sugar in check. This helps prevent and treat diabetes. A high fibre diet may also help prevent colon cancer. See Table 8.3.

TABLE 8.3 Best High Fibre Foods

FOOD	PER CUP (OR AS SHOWN)	PER 100G	FOOD	PER CUP (OR AS SHOWN)	PER 100G
Millet	17 g	8.5 g	Edamame	8 g	5 g
Oats	16.5 g	10.6 g	Coconuts	7 g	5.4 g
Split peas	16.3 g	8.3 g	Whole wheat pasta	6.3 g	10.6 g
Lentils	15.6 g	7.9 g	Pears	5.5 g/pear	3.1 g
Black beans	15 g	8.9 g	Broccoli	5.1 g	2.6 g
Lima beans	13 g	7 g	Apples	4.4 g/apple	2.4 g
Chickpeas	12.5 g	7.6 g	Sweet potatoes	3.8 g/med size	2.5 g
Kidney beans	11.3 g	6.4 g	Brown rice	3.5 g	1.8 g
Almonds	11 g	12.5 g	Dark chocolate	3.1 g/oz.	10.9 g
Avocados	10 g	6.7 g	Bananas	3.1 g/banana	2.6 g

SOURCES: Diabetes Canada, 2017; Dietitians of Canada, 2016.

One way to tell if you are consuming enough fibre is your regularity. For proper bowel function you should be going one to three times daily. Less than that indicates constipation, which means sugars and fat have more time to sit in your intestine to be absorbed. Moving one's bowels more often than that, on the other hand, may indicate that the nutrients from food are not being absorbed. It is important to keep the fibre moving through your system by consuming enough water.

Recommended daily intake of fibre will vary with age and health status (such as pregnancy). So far, there is no upper limit for fibre so a high intake of fibre-rich foods is not a problem for healthy people. It helps you feel full for a longer time, which helps with appetite and weight control. See Table 8.4.

Here are some ways to improve your fibre intake:

- Check food labels for fibre-filled whole grains like whole oats or whole wheat. Make sure that whole grains are the first ingredient listed and contain at least 3 grams of fibre per serving.

- To reach your daily fibre goal, you'll need to include fibre-rich foods at every meal. An average side salad of iceberg lettuce, tomatoes, cucumber, and onion yields only 2.6 grams of fibre for each 2-cup serving.

- Choose whole fruit instead of juice. Not only do fruits have more fibre, they have fewer calories than their liquid counterparts. Pressing fruit to obtain juice leaves much of the fibre behind. Five prunes contain 3 grams of fibre, while a half-cup of canned prune juice has only 1 gram.

- While whole wheat bread has three times the fibre of white bread, one slice of whole wheat bread still has only 1.6 grams of fibre.

- Fluids are important and water is the ideal choice, but you can also supply some of your fluid requirements with milk, juice, soup, and even tea. Drinking more fluids is especially important when increasing fibre intake.

- Try to eat more beans. They are a cheap source of fibre, complex carbohydrates, protein, and other important nutrients.

- Introduce flax seeds slowly into your diet. Flax is a soluble fibre that results in constipation in the beginning if you eat too much and don't consume enough water.

TABLE 8.4 How Much Fibre Do I Need?

AGE GROUP	RECOMMENDED DAILY INTAKE (GRAMS)
Teenage boys (14–18 years old)	38
Teenage girls (14–18 years old)	26
Men (19–50 years old)	38
Women (19–50 years old)	25

SOURCE: Eatrightontario.ca, 2016.

A word of caution: Consuming too much fibre can lead to certain risks in those with digestive disorders (e.g., Crohn's), including dehydration (if the fibre absorbs too much water), reduced bodily absorption of important minerals, and nutritional and energy deficiencies if the fibre replaces other foods. So when starting a high-fibre diet it is important to go at it slowly and drink plenty of water. One of the side effects is increased gas and bloating until your body adjusts to the increased intake.

TABLE 8.5 Top Meatless Protein Sources

FOOD	SERVING/MEASUREMENT
Nut butters	8 g/per 30 mL (2 tbsp)
Oatmeal	6 g/per 237 mL (1 cup)
Greek yogurt	10 g/per 100 g
Beans	15 g/per 180 g serving (3/4 cup)
Eggs	6 g/per egg
Nuts	6 g/per handful
Cauliflower	5 g/per 180 g serving (3/4 cup)
Broccoli	5 g/per 180 g serving (3/4 cup)
Seeds	6 g/per handful
Spinach	5 g/per 180 g serving (3/4 cup)
Soy beans	14 g/per 64 g serving (1/2 cup)

SOURCES: Dietitians of Canada, 2017; EatrightOntario, 2017.

PROTEIN

Protein is found throughout your body in muscles, bones, skin, and hair. It makes up enzymes that power many biochemical reactions and builds hemoglobin, which carries oxygen in your blood. Protein is made up of 22 building blocks called amino acids that provide the raw material to build over 10,000 proteins in your body.

Unlike carbohydrates or fats, which are stored in your body, you do not store protein and therefore require a daily supply. Children and infants need protein for growth, and adults need it to maintain health. Under certain extreme circumstances, such as starvation, the body may use amino acids as fuel.

Proteins that contain all the amino acids needed to build new proteins are called complete proteins and are found in animal sources—meat and fish, milk and cheese products. Incomplete protein sources lack one or more of the essential amino acids and are found in fruits, vegetables, grains, and nuts (see Table 8.5). This means that you have to combine protein sources from cereals and grains with legumes to obtain all essential amino acids from plant sources. One exception is the soybean, which is a complete protein, and is also high in folate, omega-3 fatty acids, and minerals.

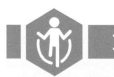

FYI

VEGETARIANISM

People choose to be vegetarians for a number of reasons. Some do it to reduce the risks of obesity, heart disease, hypertension, type 2 diabetes, and certain cancers (particularly colorectal cancer). Others do not want to eat animals that have been slaughtered, while others find handling raw meat or chewing meat difficult.

A well-planned vegetarian diet carries some nutritional benefits, such as a lower level of saturated fats, cholesterol, and animal protein, as well as higher levels of carbohydrates, fibre, magnesium, potassium, folate (a water-soluble B vitamin), antioxidants such as vitamins C and E, and phytochemicals (American Dietetic Association and Dietitians of Canada, 2003). There are a number of variations of vegetarianism, including pesco-vegetarianism (which allows some fish in the diet), lacto-ovo vegetarianism (includes dairy products and eggs), and veganism (eating only plant-based foods).

Vegetarians run the risk of deficiencies in some areas: protein, iron, calcium, zinc, and B vitamins. If you are contemplating a vegetarian diet, be sure to investigate alternative sources of these nutrients (such as soy products for protein and iron from spinach and other vegetables; see Table 8.5 for alternate protein sources).

HOW MUCH PROTEIN DO WE NEED?

Our bodies need to consume approximately 0.8–1 gram of protein per kilogram of body weight over the course of the day. For example, an adult who weighs 70 kg would need to consume about 56 to 70 grams of protein per day. Consuming less than this amount may result in the body going into starvation mode and breaking down muscle instead of fat stores as a fuel source. If not enough protein is consumed, growth failure, loss of muscle mass, decreased immunity, and weakening of the heart and respiratory systems can result, which can lead to death. Protein

malnutrition can also lead to a condition known as kwashiorkor (a childhood malnutrition disease).

Too much protein in your diet may lead to high cholesterol, heart disease, and
other diseases such as gout. A high-protein diet may put additional strain on the
kidneys when extra waste matter (the end product of protein metabolism) is excreted in urine. This is why high-protein diets and over-consumption of protein
supplements may not be healthy.

When choosing protein-rich foods, pay attention to what comes along with the
protein. Meatless sources of protein like beans, nuts, and whole grains also offer
fibre, vitamins, and minerals. The best animal protein choices are fish and poultry
(see Figure 8.5). Lean cuts of red meat, in moderate-sized portions, may be eaten
occasionally. A 200-gram (6-ounce) steak has about 40 grams of protein but also
about 38 grams of fat, 14 of them being saturated (which equates to about 60 percent
of your recommended daily fat intake). The same amount of salmon has 34 grams
of protein and 18 grams of fat, 4 of them saturated. Of concern is that moderate
consumption of red meats is linked to colon cancer (World Cancer Research Fund
International, 2007), heart disease, and diabetes (Aune, Ursin, & Veierod, 2009).

It is important to get protein from a variety of sources. Vegetarians must be sure to
consume the proper combination of plant proteins (dry beans, lentils, nuts, soy foods,
sprouted seeds, grains, spirulina, and chlorella or blue-green algae) to achieve this
balance. While most people who follow Canada's Food Guide will get enough protein
in their diet, protein supplements may be useful for some individuals. The most efficient protein supplement is protein powder, which is more concentrated than pills.

FIGURE 8.5 Lean Protein Sources

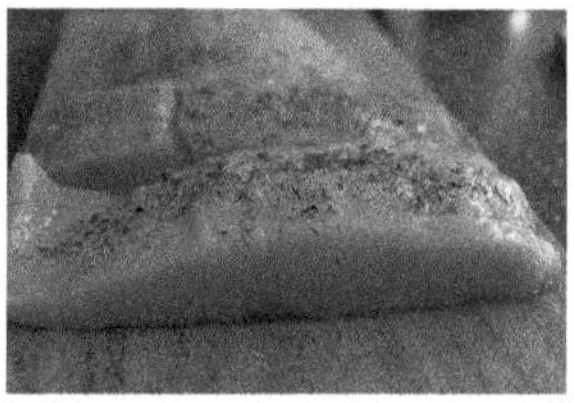

34 grams of protein

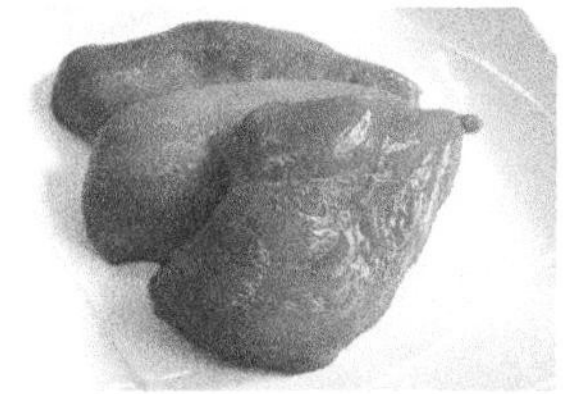

27 grams of protein

11 grams of protein

Fish
Skinless Chicken Breast
Turkey
Egg Whites
Cottage Cheese
Greek Yogurt
Beans and Lentils

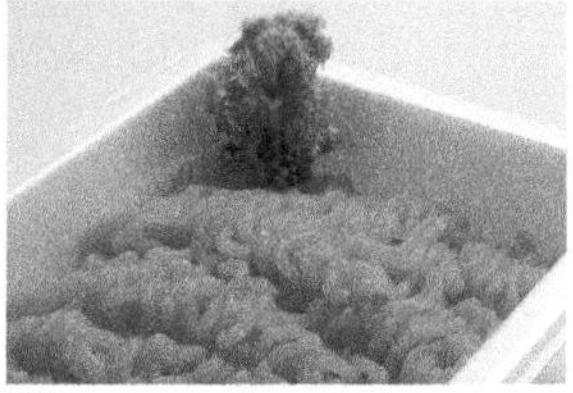

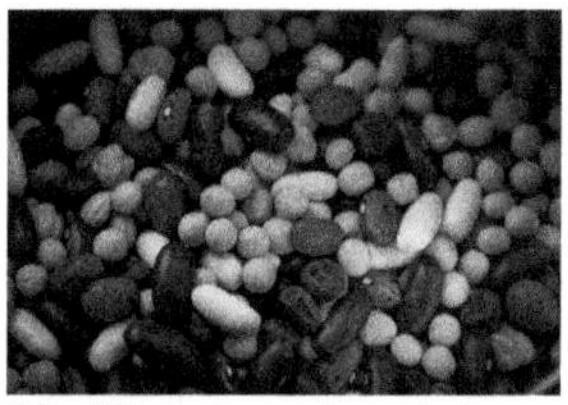

Remember that although protein
builds, maintains, and restores
muscles, you need to consume
these foods with carbohydrates to
provide the body with energy. If
you don't, your body will tap the
protein for energy.

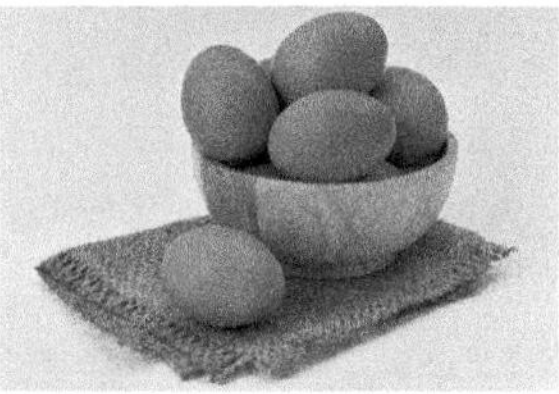

31 grams of protein

12–15 grams of protein

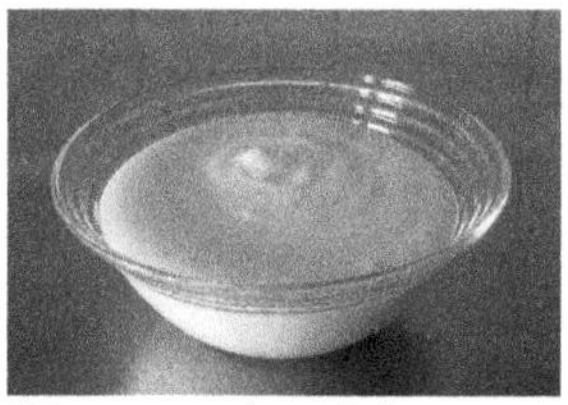

10 grams of protein

NOTE: The gram measurements are for 1 serving size according to Canada's Food Guide. It only takes 75 g (2.5 oz.) of meat,
fish, poultry; 175 mL (0.75 cup) cooked beans; 2 eggs; or 245 g (8 fl. oz.) of yogurt to make up one Food Guide serving.

FYI

HIGH-PROTEIN, "LOW-CARB" DIETS FOR WEIGHT LOSS

High-protein, low-carbohydrate diets have become popular in recent years. They permit foods rich in fat as well as protein, but prohibit consumption of starchy foods, legumes, fruits, and sugar.

These diets may result in rapid and substantial weight loss, but the weight is likely to be regained quickly. A loss of 2 to 4 kilograms in the first week is common (mainly due to water loss), but weight loss is slow after that. Fatigue, constipation, and high blood cholesterol levels are some of the side effects.

Concerns about high-protein diets include the fact that they are high in saturated fats, very low in calcium (increasing the risk of osteoporosis), and low in fibre; fibre intake is usually less than 10 grams per day.

When deprived of carbohydrates, your body responds in a fashion similar to fasting. The breakdown of protein and fats produces ketone bodies, which can lead to kidney damage. Thus, it is important to consume more water than the diet may recommend. Finally, high-protein diets lack many essential vitamins and minerals due to a lack of vegetables, fruits, and grains.

In choosing a protein supplement, make sure it uses high-quality protein isolated from whey (extracted at low temperatures to prevent the breakdown of the amino acids themselves), if you do not have a dairy allergy. Protein supplements consist of whole protein (such as egg, milk, rice, hemp, or soy protein), individual amino acids, or combinations of individual amino acids. These do not have an advantage over food sources of protein, but they may offer convenience.

PROTEIN SUPPLEMENTATION TO BUILD MUSCLE TISSUE

The timing of protein intake is important. Protein needs to be consumed throughout the day, not just in one dose/meal, but in every meal. Research shows that protein consumed with carbohydrates within an hour after exercise stimulates the release of insulin and growth hormone, and therefore, the growth of muscle mass (Poole, Wilborn, Taylor, & Kerksick, 2010).

Athletes training at high intensities can consume between 1.4 and 2.0 grams per kilogram of body weight (Kleiner, 2000). Research does not support protein intake in excess of 2.0 grams per kilogram of body weight. Excess protein intake is associated with dehydration and may be related to excessive urinary calcium losses and inadequate carbohydrate intake.

FATS

Fats play an essential role in your body, including hormone production, cell growth and maintenance, and transportation and storage of fat-soluble vitamins (A, D, E, and K). Fats break down into fatty acids (chains of carbon molecules with hydrogen atoms attached) and are stored in your body to be used as a vital source of energy. Without physical activity, high-fat diets lead to weight gain and sometimes obesity, which can result in increased risk for heart disease and diabetes.

Knowing how much of which fats to include in your diet has become increasingly difficult. It's not just the amount that matters but the type that makes the difference—some fats are good at lowering the risk of certain diseases. Since Canadian legislation regulates the labelling of all prepackaged foods, manufacturers are now required to indicate unhealthy trans fatty acids on labels—in the past, we consumed them without knowing. Each gram of fat contains nine calories, no matter which fat it is. Some fats make food taste good, while other fats make us feel full (it takes longer for them to leave the stomach).

UNDERSTANDING THE DIFFERENCES AMONG FATS

Fat is an important part of a healthy diet, providing energy (calories) as well as fatty acids. The body uses one fat—cholesterol—as a starting point to make estrogen, testosterone, vitamin D, and other vital compounds. Fat influences how our muscles will respond to insulin's signal to open up cells and allow sugar in. Over one-quarter of Canadians aged 31 to 50 get more than 35 percent of their total calories from fat, the threshold beyond which health risks increase (Garriguet, 2007).

There are four main types of fatty acids: saturated fatty acids, monounsaturated fatty acids, polyunsaturated fatty acids, and trans fatty acids. Most fats and oils contain a mixture of all four types, but such mixtures usually have a higher proportion of one particular type of fatty acid (see Figure 8.6).

FIGURE 8.6 Do You Know Your Fats?

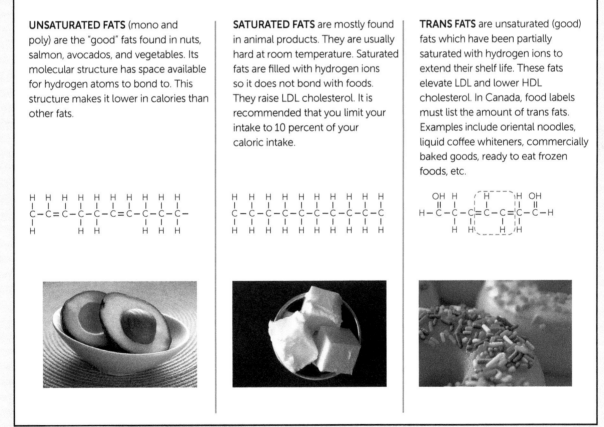

Essential fatty acids are those needed by the human body and only obtained through foods. Some are helpful to our body while others are harmful.

UNSATURATED FATS (mono and poly) are the "good" fats found in nuts, salmon, avocados, and vegetables. Its molecular structure has space available for hydrogen atoms to bond to. This structure makes it lower in calories than other fats.

SATURATED FATS are mostly found in animal products. They are usually hard at room temperature. Saturated fats are filled with hydrogen ions so it does not bond with foods. They raise LDL cholesterol. It is recommended that you limit your intake to 10 percent of your caloric intake.

TRANS FATS are unsaturated (good) fats which have been partially saturated with hydrogen ions to extend their shelf life. These fats elevate LDL and lower HDL cholesterol. In Canada, food labels must list the amount of trans fats. Examples include oriental noodles, liquid coffee whiteners, commercially baked goods, ready to eat frozen foods, etc.

SOURCE: Fats. Adopted from Eat Right Ontario https://www.eatrightontario.ca/en/Articles/Fat.aspx

SATURATED FATS

Saturated fats are a chain of carbon atoms, each having two hydrogens and no double bonds. This type of chain structure means that saturated fats are solid at room temperature. They raise the level of low-density lipoproteins (LDL, or "bad" cholesterol) and increase a person's risk for heart disease. LDLs carry cholesterol from the liver to the rest of the body. When there are too many in the bloodstream, they begin to deposit on the artery walls. Foods that have saturated fats include animal products (for example, poultry, steak, eggs, and full-fat dairy), as well as tropical oils such as coconut, palm, and palm kernel oils. If you consume 1,800 calories a day, you should be getting a maximum of 60 grams total of fat per day and only 20 grams of saturated fats (180 kcal). Food guides are advocating for less than 10 percent of your diet to come from saturated fats (US Department of Health and Human Services; US Department of Agriculture, 2015). Humans have consumed animal products and tropical oils as long as they have been on this earth. The trouble now is the excess amount that we eat and the amount of processing that occurs. The healthy choice for saturated fats would be unrefined tropical oils and pasture raised meat and dairy.

UNSATURATED FATS

Unsaturated fats have one or more double bonds in their chains and therefore have a kink in their chain. They are liquid at room temperature and are subcategorized as either monounsaturated or polyunsaturated. In general terms, monounsaturated and polyunsaturated fatty acids tend to lower the risk of heart disease.

Monounsaturated fats protect against heart disease and cancer by lowering LDL levels. Olive oil, avocados, and nuts such as peanuts, almonds, and hazelnuts are excellent sources of these fats (see Figure 8.7).

Polyunsaturated fats (PUFAs) are subdivided into three categories: omega-3 fatty acids, omega-6 fatty acids, and omega-9 fatty acids. Because the body can't make these, we need to consume them in our diet.

FIGURE 8.7 Unsaturated Fats

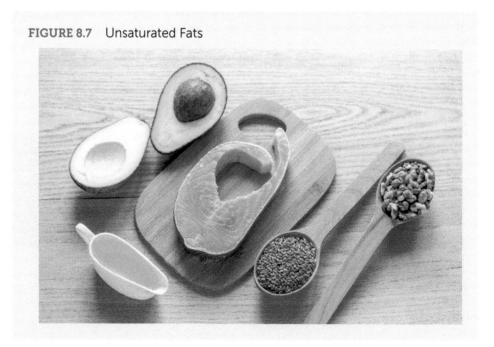

Omega-3 fatty acids are three fatty acids—eicosapentaenoic acid (EPA), docosahexaenoic acid (DHA), and alpha-linolenic acid (ALA). These fatty acids help prevent heart disease by lowering harmful triglycerides and blood pressure, reducing heart rhythm abnormalities, and preventing blood clots (thus reducing the risk of strokes and embolisms). They also have anti-inflammatory properties, thus reducing inflammation in rheumatoid arthritis and colitis. They are believed to help fight wrinkles and depression. Food sources include oily, cold-water fish such as salmon, mackerel, herring, and sardines for EPA and DHA. You can find ALA in flax seeds and flaxseed oils, canola oil, soybeans and soybean oil, and walnuts, and in smaller amounts in dark green, leafy vegetables.

Omega-6 fatty acids are a family of pro-inflammatory and anti-inflammatory polyunsaturated fatty acids like linoleic acid. They help lower LDL cholesterol but need to be eaten in moderation, as in large quantities they can lower HDL ("good") cholesterol. They are important for reduction of inflammation in the body and are used to treat diabetic neuropathy, rheumatoid arthritis, allergies, eczema, and breast cancer. Sources include safflower, sunflower, corn, soybean, and sesame oils, as well as almonds, pecans, Brazil nuts, sunflower seeds, and sesame seeds. It is also found in evening primrose, borage, and blackcurrant seed oils.

There is concern that we are consuming too much omega-6, so there is now a push to consume more omega-3s. The recommended ratio of omega-6 to omega-3 fatty acids in a healthy diet is 4:1. The conservative estimate is that Canadians are getting 10:1, and those who consume a fast-food diet may be consuming between 14:1 and 25:1 (Dyerberg, & Passwater, 2012). This higher concentration is found in refined sources, especially soybean oil, and not from whole foods. For a good source of essential fatty acids, the ideal serving size of nuts is 60 millilitres, or one-quarter cup (Health Canada, 2012c). Look at your diet to see if you need to up your omega-3 consumption.

Unlike omega-3 and omega-6, omega-9 fatty acids are a family of unsaturated fatty acids that are classified as non-essential. They are found in olive oil (oleic acid) and canola and refined sunflower oils (erucic acid), the latter two of which were developed for cooking at high temperatures.

UNDERSTANDING CHOLESTEROL

Cholesterol is a waxy, fat-like substance that is important for normal body function. It aids cellular function and hormone production. Cholesterol travels through the blood packaged with other fats and proteins. When blood cholesterol is too high, it settles on the inside walls of blood vessels, clogging them (atherosclerosis; see Chapter 10). The recommended intake for cholesterol consumption is less than 300 milligrams per day (Canadian Food Inspection Agency, 2016a). Twenty-five percent of our cholesterol is dietary cholesterol (from exogenous, or outside, sources), while seventy-five percent is blood cholesterol, manufactured by the body (endogenous source). Familial hypercholesterolemia (genetic high blood cholesterol) is believed to be due to a mutant gene, which releases cholesterol in the body and increases the risk of heart attacks. Most people make more cholesterol in their bodies than they consume in their diet. These cholesterols travel as lipoproteins (Durstine, 2005). There are two key kinds of lipoproteins:

- Low-density lipoprotein (LDL) cholesterol, often referred to as "bad" cholesterol, is linked to heart disease and stroke. Although approximately one-half of LDL is removed by the liver within two to six hours after its formation, the rest can travel for approximately two days with the chance of binding to arteries and veins. This form of cholesterol is decreased through diet by decreasing fat intake, increasing dietary fibre, and maintaining good body composition through aerobic activity.

- **High-density lipoprotein (HDL) cholesterol** is known as the "good" form of cholesterol. These particles scavenge cholesterol from the bloodstream and the arterial walls and take it back to the liver for disposal. It is increased through exercise, cessation of smoking, and weight reduction.

Total blood cholesterol levels should not exceed 6.2 mmol/L. LDL cholesterol should not be above 4.14 mmol/L, and HDL cholesterol should be greater than 0.9 mmol/L. Many people have their cholesterol levels checked by their doctor, but many are also not aware of what levels are acceptable. RCMP officers are required to have their levels checked for their annual physical. You can ask your doctor what your levels are, and if they are high, what you can do about them. It is your right to know and make educated decisions about this aspect of your health and reduce your risk of cancer and cardiovascular diseases.

TRANS FATTY ACIDS

Trans fatty acids, often called trans fats, are created when a vegetable oil undergoes hydrogenation, a chemical process in which hydrogen is added at high temperature to make the oil solid. The process is commonly used in food processing to prolong the shelf life of packaged products and keep them more solid and resistant to chemical change. Fried foods and fast foods tend to be higher in trans fats. Trans fats are commonly found in baked goods, hard margarine, coffee whitener, garlic spreads, and snack foods, including donuts.

Trans fatty acids consumption is associated with an increased risk in all-cause mortality, cardiac heart disease (CHD) mortality, coronary artery disease, type 2 diabetes, and cancer (Adams & Standridge, 2006; de Souza, et al., 2015; Healthy Canadians, 2016).

In 2007, Health Canada made it mandatory for Canadian food companies to place the amount of trans fatty acids on their Nutrition Facts labels. Prior to 2007, it appeared as "hydrogenated" or "partially hydrogenated fats" or "vegetable shortening" on labels. Canada was the first country to introduce mandatory labelling of trans fat. The intent was to help Canadians make healthier choices and force food companies to reduce or eliminate trans fats from their products (Health Canada, 2016). Canada has reduced the consumption of trans fats from approximately 3.7 percent of daily energy intake in the mid-1990s to 1.42 percent in 2012; however, we still have not achieved the 1 percent target set by the World Health Organization (Krenosky, L'Abbé, Lee, Underhill, Vigneault, Godefroy, & Ratnayake, 2012) or the recommended 0 grams of trans fats per day.

WAYS TO MINIMIZE YOUR RISKS AND REDUCE FAT

Many people who have made an effort to lower their fat intake have still become obese. The so-called "Western diet" is low in fruits, vegetables, and whole grains, and high in red meat, processed meats, refined grains, potatoes, and sugary drinks—the opposite of the Mediterranean diet, which is high in unsaturated fats, vegetables, fruit, legumes, nuts, whole grains, olives/olive oil, yogurt, and some cheese. Western dietary habits increase the risk for metabolic syndrome, which can lead to heart disease and type 2 diabetes (Kastorini et al., 2011).

Here are some tips to ensure that your diet has no more than 10 percent saturated fats and a maximum of 35 percent total dietary fat:

- Avoid full-fat dairy foods, fried foods, and high-fat bakery products.

- Choose lower-fat dairy products, less red meat, leaner meats, and foods prepared with little or no fat.

- Eat one or more good sources of omega-3 fats every day—such as fish, walnuts, canola oil, ground flax seeds, or flaxseed oil—to help prevent heart disease.

- Read the labels on packages before you buy. This practice is important for products such as cookies and crackers that advertise themselves as "low-fat." Many have replaced fat with added sugars, refined flour, salt, and trans fats. Avoid foods with labels that list "hydrogenated" or "partially hydrogenated" oils.

- If you are going to buy soft margarines, make sure that they are labelled as being free of trans fatty acids or made with non-hydrogenated fat. In cooking and at the table, use liquid vegetable oils rich in polyunsaturated and monounsaturated fats, such as olive, canola, sunflower, safflower, corn, and peanut oils.

- Fry foods less often. Try baking, broiling, and poaching instead.

- Do not replace high-fat foods with highly processed or refined carbohydrate foods like white bread, white rice, or potatoes. Just eat smaller portion sizes of products like skim milk and low-fat cheeses and low-fat meats.

- When you eat out, ask about the fat content of foods on the menu. Fast-food restaurants must now make their caloric content available for customers to read.

VITAMINS AND MINERALS

VITAMINS

A vitamin is an essential, non-caloric, organic nutrient needed in small amounts in the diet. Vitamins act as facilitators for other nutrients, helping digestion, absorption, metabolism, and the building of structures in the body. Vitamins fall into two categories, based on how they are absorbed, transported, and stored in the body—fat soluble and water soluble. Fat-soluble vitamins (A, D, E, and K) are found in the fats and oils of food and are generally absorbed into the lymph system with the help of bile. They travel in the blood in association with protein carriers. Fat-soluble vitamins are stored in the liver or fatty tissue and can build up to toxic concentrations. Water-soluble vitamins are absorbed directly into the bloodstream and, instead of being stored to any great extent, are excreted in the urine. Water-soluble vitamins

(B vitamins and vitamin C) can be easily leached out of food by cooking and washing with water. Although foods do not supply toxic levels of water-soluble vitamins, supplements may result in toxic levels.

Vitamins are important in many different ways and are found mostly in food. B vitamins, found in legumes, oats, and leafy green vegetables, help convert food to energy and promote healthy skin, hair, muscles, and brain function. However, vitamin B12 is found only in animal sources (such as meat, fish, milk, and eggs) or fortified products, so a strict vegan needs to be aware of possible deficiencies in B12, which are linked to heart disease and stroke (Humphrey, Fu, Rogers, Freeman, & Helfand, 2008). Vitamin C, found in foods such as citrus fruits, tomatoes, leafy green vegetables, and sweet peppers, helps the body form collagen, a protein that is the primary component of the body's white fibrous connective tissue. Vitamin C also contributes to the formation of teeth, bones, cartilage, skin, and capillaries (the smallest blood vessels), and strengthens the immune system. Vitamin D is made in the body when it is exposed to sunlight. But living in Canada, we do not get enough sunlight to meet our daily requirement of vitamin D; therefore, it is important to obtain it in fortified food (such as eggs, juice, or milk) or from a vitamin D supplement.

Table 8.6 summarizes key information about vitamins.

MINERALS

Minerals, which are found in all body tissues and fluids, play a role in nerve function, muscle contraction, and metabolism. They are responsible for fluid and electrolyte balance (increased sodium concentration in response to water loss) and acid–base balance or pH (the kidneys control pH balance by excreting more or less acid). Minerals are the main components of bones and teeth. The major minerals include calcium, chloride, magnesium, phosphorus, potassium, sodium, and sulphur. Trace minerals include iodine, iron, zinc, selenium, fluoride, chromium, copper, manganese, and molybdenum. We require very small amounts of minerals—an excess of any mineral can create imbalances with other minerals and become toxic.

Table 8.7 summarizes key facts about minerals.

UNDERSTANDING THE ROLE OF SODIUM

Sodium is a mineral necessary for transmission of nerve impulses, muscle contraction, maintaining pH balance and, at the cellular level, pumping nutrients (like potassium) and fluid in and out. Yet, over-consumption of sodium can lead to high blood pressure—a major risk factor for stroke, heart disease, and kidney disease. According to the 2013 Global Burden of Disease Study (Campbell et al., 2016), hypertension and dietary sodium are the third leading risk factor for death and disability in Canada. High sodium intake is also associated with vascular and cardiac damage independent of high blood pressure, detrimental effects on calcium and bone metabolism, increased risk of stomach cancer, and increased severity of asthma (Health Canada, 2012b; Strazzullo, D'Elia, Kandala, & Cappuccio, 2009).

TABLE 8.6 Major Vitamins

	VITAMIN	MAJOR FUNCTIONS	FOOD SOURCES	DEFICIENCY SIGNS AND SYMPTOMS	TOXICITY SIGNS AND SYMPTOMS
FAT-SOLUBLE	A	Vision, antioxidant, growth, reproduction, immune system	Fortified dairy products, liver, eggs, dark green leafy vegetables, yellow vegetables	Poor vision in dim light, blindness, anemia, diarrhea, poor growth, frequent infections	Blurred vision, growth retardation, abdominal cramping, pain in calves
	D	Bone and tooth development and growth	Fortified milk, eggs, liver, exposure to sun	Rickets (deformed bones)	Mental and physical retardation, excessive thirst, kidney stones
	E	Antioxidant, protects cell membranes	Vegetable oils, whole grains, green and leafy vegetables	Anemia, leg cramps, muscle degeneration	Discomfort, mimics the effects of anti-clotting medication
	K	Synthesis of blood-clotting proteins, assists in regulating blood calcium	Leafy green vegetables, liver, milk, cabbage-type vegetables	Hemorrhage	Jaundice, interference with anti-clotting medication
WATER-SOLUBLE	**Thiamine (B1)**	Energy metabolism, normal appetite function	Pork, liver, nuts, dried beans and peas, whole-grain cereals	Beriberi (paralysis), edema, chronic constipation, heart failure, confusion, depression	Sweating, nausea, restlessness, tightness of the throat
	Riboflavin (B2)	Energy metabolism, supports normal vision and healthy skin	Milk, yogurt, leafy green vegetables, meats, whole-grain and enriched breads and cereals	Enlarged purple tongue, hypersensitivity to light, skin rash	Bloodshot eyes, abnormal sensitivity to light, lesions of the skin
	Niacin (B3)	Increases levels of HDL in the blood and modestly decreases the risk of cardiovascular events	Dairy products, eggs, enriched breads and cereals, fish, lean meats, legumes, nuts, and poultry	Pellagra characterized by diarrhea, dermatitis, and dementia; mild deficiency slows metabolism, decreases tolerance to cold, and causes irritability, poor concentration, anxiety, apathy	Skin flushing, itching, dry skin and skin rashes including eczema; persistent toxicity may lead to dyspepsia (indigestion), nausea, and liver toxicity
	B6	Coenzyme for fat and protein metabolism, helps make red blood cells	Protein-rich foods, green and leafy vegetables, whole grains	Anemia, skin rash, irritability, muscle twitching	Depression, fatigue, nerve damage, headaches
	Folate (B9)	DNA production, anti-stress vitamin; prevents neural tube defects and assists in a healthy nervous system	Green leafy vegetables, oranges, nuts, liver	Anemia, depression, spina bifida in developing embryo	Itching, rashes, mental changes, shortness of breath, sleep disturbances
	B12	Coenzyme in new cell synthesis, maintains nerve cells	Animal products (meat, milk, cheese, eggs)	Anemia, fatigue, nerve degeneration	Diarrhea, blood clots, signs of allergic reactions
	C	Antioxidant, scar tissue formation, bone growth, strengthens immune system, aids in iron absorption	Citrus fruit, dark green vegetables, cabbage-type vegetables, strawberries, cantaloupe, tomatoes	Anemia, frequent infections, bleeding gums, failure of wounds to heal	Nausea, abdominal cramps, diarrhea, gout symptoms; deficiency symptoms may appear at first with withdrawal of high doses

SOURCES: Adapted from Dietitians of Canada, 2012; National Institutes of Health, Office of Dietary Supplements, n.d.; Sizer & Whitney, 2013.

TABLE 8.7 Major Minerals

MINERALS	MAJOR FUNCTIONS	FOOD SOURCES	DEFICIENCY SIGNS AND SYMPTOMS	TOXICITY SIGNS AND SYMPTOMS
Calcium	Builds and maintains bones and teeth, needed for muscle and nerve activity, regulates blood pressure and blood clotting	Milk products, fortified tofu and soy milk, salmon, broccoli, dried beans	Weak bone growth, rickets, stunted growth, muscle spasms, osteoporosis	Kidney stones, decreased zinc absorption
Sodium	Maintains acid–base balance in body fluids, needed for muscle and nerve activity	Salt, cured foods, bread, milk, cheese	Muscle cramps, headaches, weakness, swelling	Hypertension, kidney disease, heart problems
Potassium	Necessary for nerve function, maintains fluid balance	Whole grains, fruits (bananas), vegetables	Muscular weakness, confusion	Heart failure, death
Magnesium	Regulates enzyme activity, necessary for nerve function	Green leafy vegetables, whole grains, nuts	Muscular weakness, convulsions, confusion	Risk increases with kidney failure; nausea, diarrhea, appetite loss, muscle weakness, extremely low blood pressure and irregular heartbeat
Zinc	Component of several enzymes and the hormone insulin, maintains immune function, necessary for sexual maturation and reproduction	Meat, fish, poultry, whole grains, vegetables	Improper healing of wounds, poor growth, failure to mature sexually	Gastrointestinal problems, anemia, cardiovascular vessel diseases
Selenium	Component of an enzyme that functions as an antioxidant	Seafood, liver, vegetables and grains grown in selenium-rich soil	Gastrointestinal problems, hair loss, diarrhea, cirrhosis, and fatigue	Nerve damage
Iron	Component of hemoglobin, involved in the release of energy	Liver, red meats, and enriched breads and cereals	Anemia	Hemochromatosis (a rare iron metabolism disease)

SOURCES: Adapted from Dietitians of Canada, 2012; National Institutes of Health, Office of Dietary Supplements, n.d.; Sizer & Whitney, 2013.

Sodium is mainly consumed in the salts added to food. While the recommended maximum daily intake is 1,500 milligrams per day, the average Canadian consumes about 3,400 milligrams of sodium (Health Canada, 2017b). Over 75 percent of the sodium we consume is found in processed foods, such as deli meats, pizza, sauces, and soups. It is found in condiments and dressings, and occurs naturally in milk, fresh meats, fruits, and vegetables (see Figure 8.8).

Health Canada (2017c) started an initiative to encourage the food industry to reduce sodium content in prepackaged foods including cereals, breads, vegetable juices, soups, and infant and toddler's food. Although there has been progress, foods like french fries, hash browns, and deli meats are having difficulty meeting the 35 percent reduction target (Health Canada, 2017a). It is important to learn to read labels to know how much you are consuming (see Figure 8.9).

FIGURE 8.8   Six Foods High in Sodium

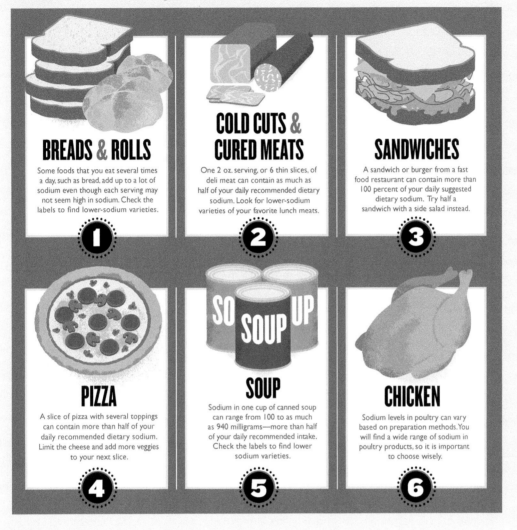

BREADS & ROLLS

Some foods that you eat several times a day, such as bread, add up to a lot of sodium even though each serving may not seem high in sodium. Check the labels to find lower-sodium varieties.

1

COLD CUTS & CURED MEATS

One 2 oz. serving, or 6 thin slices, of deli meat can contain as much as half of your daily recommended dietary sodium. Look for lower-sodium varieties of your favorite lunch meats.

2

SANDWICHES

A sandwich or burger from a fast food restaurant can contain more than 100 percent of your daily suggested dietary sodium. Try half a sandwich with a side salad instead.

3

PIZZA

A slice of pizza with several toppings can contain more than half of your daily recommended dietary sodium. Limit the cheese and add more veggies to your next slice.

4

SOUP

Sodium in one cup of canned soup can range from 100 to as much as 940 milligrams—more than half of your daily recommended intake. Check the labels to find lower sodium varieties.

5

CHICKEN

Sodium levels in poultry can vary based on preparation methods. You will find a wide range of sodium in poultry products, so it is important to choose wisely.

6

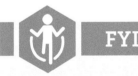 **FYI**

THE DASH DIET

The **Dietary Approaches to Stop Hypertension (DASH) diet** is a flexible and balanced eating plan that was developed to lower high blood pressure through reduction of sodium consumption. An excellent plan for weight loss, it emphasizes healthy foods and is heavy on fruits and vegetables, while balanced with the right amount of protein. Improved blood pressure results were obtained by cutting back on the "empty carbs" and adding in more protein and/or heart healthy fats (National Institutes of Health, 2006, 2015). It focuses on low-fat or non-fat dairy with whole grains, while emphasizing a high-fibre and low- to moderate-fat diet that is rich is potassium, calcium, and magnesium. The Heart and Stroke Foundation of Canada and Diabetes Canada endorse the DASH diet (Canadian Diabetes Association, 2017; Heart and Stroke Foundation of Ontario, 2012), which reflects the principles of Canada's Food Guide. To see the publication *Your Guide to Lowering Your Blood Pressure with DASH,* go to the link listed under DASH Eating Plan in the appendix at the end of this chapter.

Refer to **assignment 8.1** (at www.emond.ca/fitness5e) to gain a greater awareness of your sodium intake.

TOP TIPS ...

FOR LOWERING SODIUM INTAKE

- Buy unsalted and low-sodium foods whenever possible. Look for words such as "sodium free," "low sodium," or "no added salt" on the package.
- Compare food labels. Buy products with the lowest amounts of sodium. Look for foods that contain less than 360 milligrams of sodium per serving.
- You can also use the "% Daily Value" (% DV) on the label to compare products to see whether the food has a little or a lot of sodium. Here is a good guide: 5 percent DV or less is a little and 15 percent DV or more is a lot, so look for products with a sodium content of less than 15 percent DV.
- Check food labels often, because product ingredients may change.
- Buy fresh or frozen vegetables over canned ones (choose low-sodium if you have to buy canned products) and look for low-sodium content if you buy canned or bottled vegetable juices.
- Enjoy grains such as barley, quinoa, and rice, which are naturally sodium free.
- Buy unseasoned meats, poultry, fish, seafood, and tofu. Choose unsalted nuts. Pick fresh and frozen poultry that is not injected with sodium solution. Check the fine print for terms like "broth," "saline," or "sodium solution."
- Choose condiments carefully. For example, soya sauce, bottled salad dressings, dips, ketchup, jarred salsas, mustard, pickles, olives, and relish can be high in sodium. Either use reduced versions or flavour your food with lemon or pepper.
- At restaurants, ask for gravy, sauces, salad dressing, and other condiments on the side. Ask for food to be cooked without salt or monosodium glutamate (MSG), a seasoning very high in sodium. Taste your food before adding salt.
- Check the restaurant's nutritional information for menu items with a low sodium content. Watch out for words like pickled, brined, barbequed, cured, smoked, broth, au jus, soya sauce, miso, or teriyaki sauce. Choose foods that are steamed, baked, grilled, poached, or roasted.
- When cooking, use onions, garlic, herbs, spices, citric juices, and vinegars in place of some or all of the salt to add flavour to foods.
- Drain and rinse canned beans (like chickpeas, kidney beans, etc.) and vegetables before cooking with them as it can cut the sodium content by 40 percent.

SOURCES: American Heart Association, 2017; Arcand, Au, Schermel, & L'Abbe, 2014; Health Canada, 2017a, 2017b; Healthy Canadians, 2011a, 2011b.

For more information about sodium and ways to reduce it in your diet, go to the Healthy Canadians website at www.healthycanadians.gc.ca/init/sodium/index-eng.php or visit Hypertension Canada's website at http://www.hypertension.ca

CALORIES

Also known as a kilocalorie (kcal), a calorie is a measure of the amount of energy in food. An individual's energy needs are the number of calories he or she must consume to maintain health based on age, sex, weight, height, and activity level (Institute of Medicine, 2005). Just as gasoline powers your car, proper energy is required for your body. In terms of nutritional labelling (discussed below), nutritional energy is recorded in kilocalories and kilojoules (kJ).

Carbohydrates, fats, and proteins are the nutrients that contain calories and thus are the main energy sources for your body. In terms of energy density, food components have estimated energy values, while other substances found in food (water, non-digestible fibre, minerals, and vitamins) do not contribute to calculated energy density (Health Canada, 2007).

UNDERSTANDING THE CALORIC VALUE OF NUTRIENTS

Nutrients have different caloric value per gram. Caloric estimates are as follows:

- Fat has 9 kcal/g.
- Alcohol has 7 kcal/g.
- Protein has 4 kcal/g.
- Carbohydrate has 4 kcal/g.
- Polyols (sugar-free sweeteners) have 2.4 kcal/g.

The calories you eat are either converted to physical energy or stored within your body as fat after your limited carbohydrates are restored. Unless you lose those stored calories either by reducing caloric intake or by increasing physical activity so that you burn more calories, this fat remains in your body. Reducing the amount of sugar and fat in your diet is one way to limit your overall caloric intake. However, it is also important to reduce your overall food intake to reduce calories. Just because a product is fat free doesn't mean that it is calorie free.

NUTRITION FACTS AND LABELLING

In 2007, Canada made nutritional labelling on prepackaged foods mandatory. Each label had a nutrition facts table and the list of ingredients by weight, with an optional nutritional claims section.

In 2017, the nutritional facts table changed to include (see Figure 8.9):

- making the serving size more consistent so it's easier to compare similar foods and more realistic to what we actually are eating (e.g., Did you know that there were four servings in a Kraft® Dinner box?)
- making information on serving size and calories easier to find (larger font) and bolded under calories
- revising the % daily values based on updated science
- adding a new % daily value for total sugars
- updating by removing vitamins A and C, as most Canadians get enough of these nutrients
- adding the amount in milligrams (mg) for potassium, calcium, and iron; potassium is linked to maintaining healthy blood pressure
- adding a footnote at the bottom of the table about % daily value around consumption of other nutrients (like sodium) and how much sugar is in the product (5 percent or less is a little and 15 percent or more is a lot)

In the past, it was difficult to compare foods. For example, one label would indicate four crackers while another would indicate two crackers. The intent of this new label is to standardize a serving size. This means you are comparing by weight (grams) rather than the number of crackers. (See Figure 8.10.)

FYI

HOW TO READ A NEW NUTRITION LABEL

FIGURE 8.9 Nutrition Facts

ORIGINAL

Nutrition Facts
Valeur nutritive
Per 250 mL / par 250 mL

Amount Teneur	% Daily Value % valeur quotidienne
Calories / Calories 110	
Fat / Lipides 0 g	**0 %**
Saturated / saturés 0 g + Trans / trans 0 g	**0 %**
Cholesterol / Cholestérol 0 mg	
Sodium / Sodium 0 mg	**0 %**
Carbohydrate / Glucides 26 g	**9 %**
Fibre / Fibres 0 g	**0 %**
Sugars / Sucres 22 g	
Protein / Protéines 2 g	
Vitamin A / Vitamine A	**0 %**
Vitamin C / Vitamine C	**120 %**
Calcium / Calcium	**2 %**
Iron / Fer	**0 %**

NEW

Nutrition Facts
Valeur nutritive
Per 1 cup (250 mL)
pour 1 tasse (250 mL)

Calories 110	% Daily Value* % valeur quotidienne*
Fat / Lipides 0 g	**0 %**
Saturated / saturés 0 g + Trans / trans 0 g	**0 %**
Carbohydrate / Glucides 26 g	
Fibre / Fibres 0 g	**0 %**
Sugars / Sucres 22 g	**22 %**
Protein / Protéines 2 g	
Cholesterol / Cholestérol 0 mg	
Sodium 0 mg	**0 %**
Potassium 450 mg	**10 %**
Calcium 30 mg	**2 %**
Iron / Fer 0 mg	**0 %**

*5% or less is **a little**, 15% or more is **a lot**
*5% ou moins c'est **peu**, 15% ou plus c'est **beaucoup**

Calories is larger and stands out more with bold line below

mg amounts are shown

New % Daily Value footnote

Serving size stands out more and is more similar on similar foods

Daily Values updated

New % Daily Value for total sugars

Updated list of minerals of public health concern

SOURCE: Government of Canada, 2016.

FIGURE 8.10 Comparing Different Products

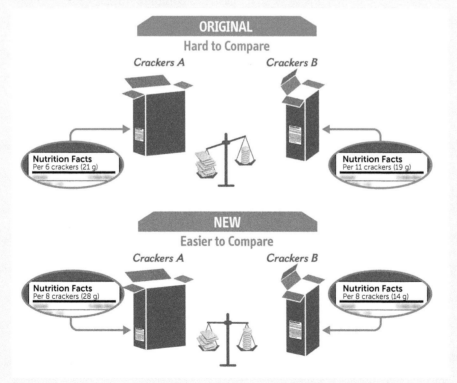

Health Canada also felt it was important that Canadians are aware of the sugar content of their foods. Labels are now required to list all sugars together so individuals have a better understanding of how much sugar really is in a product. (See Figure 8.11.)

FIGURE 8.11   List of Ingredients

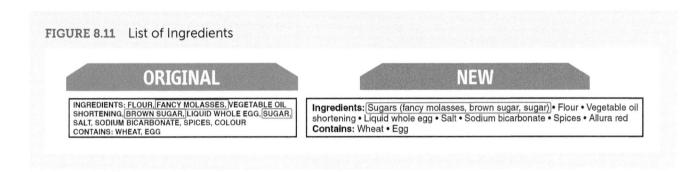

NUTRIENT CONTENT CLAIMS

Nutritional claims on labels and packaging, such as "free," "low," or "reduced," can signal that a food has less of a certain component, such as calories, fat, saturated fat, or sodium. Such labels can help consumers moderate their intake of these components. Some labels also provide information on better options regarding fibre, vitamins, and minerals. Labelling can help people with diabetes choose foods lower in calories and sugar.

Table 8.8 includes key words found on labels and what criteria they have for being labelled that way.

Refer to **assignment 8.2** (at www.emond.ca/fitness5e) to learn more about how to assess your foods.

TABLE 8.8 Nutritional Terms for Food

KEY WORDS	WHAT IT MEANS	NUTRIENT CRITERIA
Free No 0 Zero Without	The food provides an amount of a nutrient that is so small it likely won't have any effect on your body.	• Less than 5 calories • Less than 5 mg • Less than 0.5 g fat • Less than 0.2 g saturated fatty acids and less than 0.2 g of trans fatty acids • Less than 2 mg of cholesterol and less than 2 g of saturated and trans fatty acids combined • Less than 0.5 g of sugar and less than 5 calories
Low Little Few	The food provides a very small amount of the nutrient.	• 40 calories or less • 3 g or less of fat • 2 g or less AND 15% or less energy from the sum of saturated fatty acids and trans fatty acids combined • 20 mg or less of cholesterol • 140 mg or less of sodium • No more than 1 g protein per 100 g of the food

KEY WORDS	WHAT IT MEANS	NUTRIENT CRITERIA

Reduced
Less
Lower
Lower in
Fewer
	The food is processed/modified so that it contains at least 25% less of the nutrient.	• At least 25% less calories than the food to which it is compared
		• At least 25% less
		  • fat
		  • trans fatty acids
		  • cholesterol
		  • sodium
		  • sugars

Lightly	The food provides at least 50% less of the added nutrient.	• At least 50% less added sodium than the food to which it is compared
Source contains	The food provides a significant amount of the nutrient.	• At least 100 calories • 20+ g protein • 0.3+ g omega-3 • 2+ g omega-6 • 2 + g fibre source • 5+% recommended daily intake of vitamin/mineral
More Higher Higher in	At least 25% more of a nutrient compared with a similar product.	• 25+% more calories totalling at least 100 calories than the food to which it is compared • 25+% more fibre totalling at least 1 g more • At least 2 g fibre if no fibre source is identified • Protein rating of 20 or more and contains at least 25% more protein, totalling at least 7 g more than the food to which it is compared
Good source	At least 15% of the recommended daily intake.	• At least 15% of the recommended daily intake except at least 30% of the recommended daily intake for vitamin C
High in High source of	The food contains at least 4 g of fibre.	• At least 4 g of fibre if no fibre or fibre source is identified in the statement or claim OR • At least 4 g of each identified fibre or fibre from an identified source
Excellent source Very high Very high in Very high source Rich Rich in	The food provides a very large amount of the nutrient.	• Protein rating of 40 or more • At least 6 g of each identified fibre or fibre from an identified source • At least 25% of the recommended daily intake except at least 50% of the recommended daily intake for vitamin C
Light	The food is processed/modified so that it contains at least 25% less of the nutrient.	• At least 25% less calories than the food to which it is compared • At least 25% less fat than the food to which it is compared
Lean	Contains 10% or less fat.	• The food is meat or poultry that has not been ground, a marine or fresh water animal, or a product of any of these
Extra lean	Contains 7.5% or less fat.	• The food is meat or poultry that has not been ground, a marine or fresh water animal, or a product of any of these

SOURCE: Government of Canada, 2012.

Tables for different nutrients, vitamins, and minerals within the Nutrition Facts Table can be found with the Nutrition Labelling of the Food Labelling and Advertising at http://www.inspection.gc.ca/food/labelling/food-labelling-for-industry/nutrition-labelling/elements-within-the-nutrition-facts-table/eng/13892 06763218/1389206811747.

EATING WELL FOR LIFE

Good nutrition, like regular physical activity, is something you practise over the course of a lifetime. The beneficial habits that will help carry you through your career and into retirement can be formed now, during your student years.

CANADA'S FOOD GUIDE

Canada's Food Guide first appeared during the Second World War, when food was rationed, as a way to ensure that Canadians did not become nutritionally deficient. Canada's Food Guide offers practical advice for healthy eating patterns. It also emphasizes physical activity to reduce the risk of obesity, type 2 diabetes, heart disease, certain cancers, and osteoporosis.

Based on scientific evidence to ensure that people are meeting their nutritional needs, Canada's Food Guide recommends the number of servings people should eat from each of the four food groups (vegetables and fruit, grain products, milk and alternatives, and meat and alternatives), plus a small amount of added oils and fats. Recommended servings differ for different ages, and there is a difference between males and females. People who are very active can choose extra servings from the four food groups, but must still ensure that their intake is low in fat, sugar, and salt.

SERVING SIZES AND RECOMMENDED SERVINGS

The reality of the 2007 version of Canada's Food Guide is that it was not effective in providing nutritional guidance. Even though it provided guidelines, Canadians are not eating enough vegetables, fruit, whole grains, or milk and alternatives, and certain nutrients such as calcium and fibre are being under-consumed. Roughly 30 percent of calories come from foods that are high in sugar, fat, and sodium. With a push to lower sodium intake, eliminate trans fats, and increase potassium intake, during 2017-2018, Health Canada worked to develop healthy eating recommendations and a more updated dietary guideline. Go to the Government of Canada website (http://www.canada.ca/) and search for Canada's Food Guide to see the new guidelines for recommended servings.

It is very important to understand what a serving size entails. Table 8.9 gives suggested serving sizes and Figure 8.12 provides an easy way to gauge what amounts of food look like.

Canada's Food Guide provides acceptable ranges for macronutrients (carbohydrate, protein, and fat) in the diet, based on age group. This approach offers flexibility for those who choose different diets to meet their physical needs. For example, the higher end of the range for protein may address athletes' needs. 25 percent of male and 23 percent of female adults have fat intakes above the acceptable ranges, while 32 percent of male and 21 percent of female adults have carbohydrate intakes below the acceptable range (Health Canada, 2012c).

FIGURE 8.12   Easy Ways to Measure Portions: Hand Guide For Portion Control

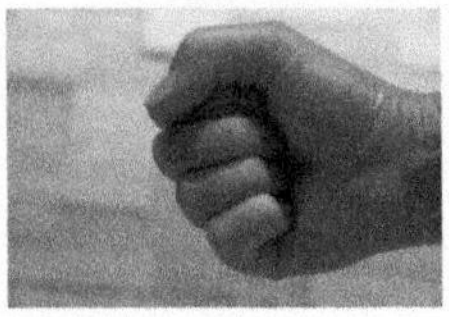	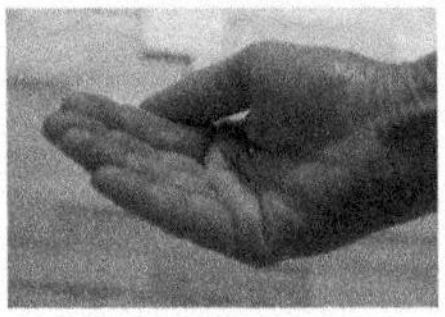	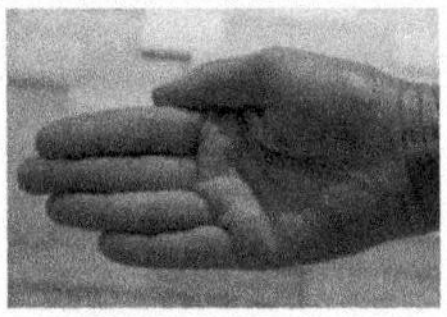	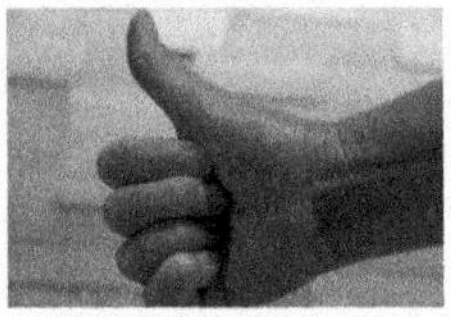	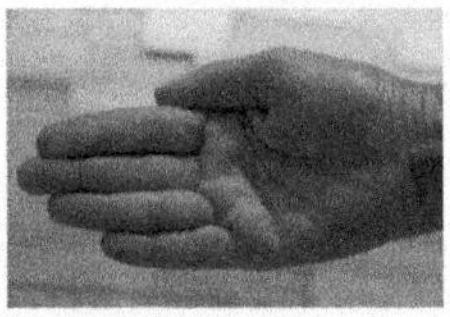
Serving Size: 236.5 ml 1 cup	Serving Size: 118 ml 1/2 cup	Serving Size: 85 gms 3 ounces	Serving Size: 14.5 ml 1 tablespoon	Serving Size: 15.4 cm 6 inches
Visual aid: Fist	Visual aid: Cupped hand	Visual aid: Palm	Visual aid: Thumb	Visual aid: Hand
• Rice • Cooked vegetables • Tea/coffee • Soups • Fresh fruit • Salads • Popcorn	• Pasta • Quinoa • Couscous • Potatoes • Pudding • Ice cream • Walnuts • Almonds • Yogurt	• Beef • Chicken • Fish • Pork • Poultry	• Salad dressing • Peanut butter • Cheese • Cream • Mayonnaise	• Bread • Pita bread • Pizza • Sandwich • Burger • Flatbreads like roti & paratha

Differentiating between Portion and Serving Size

• Portion is how much food you choose to eat at one time, whether in a restaurant, from a package or in your own kitchen. A portion is 100 percent under our control. Many foods that come as a single portion actually contain multiple servings.

• Serving Size is the amount of food listed on a product's Nutrition Facts label. So all of the nutritional values you see on the label are for the serving size the manufacturer suggests on the package.

GROCERY SHOPPING 101

Supermarkets can be overwhelming and intimidating. Here are a few tips when you are shopping and trying to follow the Canada Food Guide:

- For the best nutritional content and taste, look for fresh produce. However, many factors affect nutritional content, including crop variety, growing conditions, ripeness, how food is stored, and how it is processed and transported. For example, some vegetables—such as broccoli, green beans, kale, tomatoes, and soft fruits like peaches—lose nutrients more quickly when they travel long distances. So try to buy locally first if you can. Look for firm and blemish free vegetables. Hardier foods—like apples, oranges, grapefruit, and carrots—can travel long distances and still keep their nutrients.

- When you visit the grocery store, shop around the outside of the store and avoid the middle aisles. You will be able to get your whole, real foods that way: fresh fruits and vegetables, meat, seafood, and dairy.

TABLE 8.9 Making Wise Choices

FOOD GROUP	GUIDELINES	EXAMPLES OF ONE SERVING
Vegetables and fruit	• Eat dark green and orange vegetables daily. • Choose vegetables and fruit prepared with little or no added fat, sugar, or salt. • Have vegetables and fruit more often than juice.	• 125 mL (0.5 cup) fresh, frozen, or canned vegetable or fruit or 100% juice • 250 mL (1 cup) leafy raw vegetables or salad • 1 piece of fruit
Grain products	• Make at least half your grain products whole grain each day. • Choose grain products that are low in fat, sugar, and salt.	• 1 slice (35 g) bread or half a bagel (45 g) • half a pita (35 g) or half a tortilla (35 g) • 125 mL (0.5 cup) cooked rice, pasta, or couscous • 30 g cold cereal or 175 mL (0.75 cup) hot cereal
Milk and alternatives	• Drink skim, 1%, or 2% milk at least twice daily. • Choose low-fat alternatives to milk, including cheeses and yogurt.	• 250 mL (1 cup) milk or fortified soy beverage • 175 g (0.75 cup) yogurt • 50 g (1.5 oz.) cheese
Meat and alternatives	• Try meat alternatives such as beans, lentils, and tofu. • Eat at least two food servings of fish each week (check Guide for mercury warnings) such as Arctic char, herring, mackerel, salmon, sardines, and trout. • Select lean meats and alternatives prepared with little or no added fat or salt.	• 75 g (2.5 oz.)/125 mL (0.5 cup) cooked fish, shellfish, poultry, or lean meat • 175 mL (0.75 cup) cooked beans • 2 eggs • 30 mL (2 tbsp.) peanut butter

SOURCE: Health Canada, 2012c.

- Real, whole foods should have an expiry date. Foods that can last months or even years on your shelf or in your fridge have been processed to accommodate that shelf life. Make sure that you are buying foods that have not expired.

- During the months of April to November most cities and towns have farmers' markets. These are great places to buy locally grown food.

- It is hard as a student to buy healthy groceries when you are on a limited budget. Watch flyers, get a coupon app on your phone, buy in bulk and freeze. Go shopping with a friend who is willing to split the cost of foods that are sold in bulk (e.g., a bag of oranges). Remember that your body is still growing and needs proper nutrients now more than ever.

- If a store has a nutritionist/dietitian on staff, take advantage of the programs they have to offer like one-on-one nutrition counselling, food demonstrations, and educational grocery store tours.

- Learn to read labels. Know what you are buying and decide if the convenience of food in a box is nutritionally worth the purchase.

- Buy what you are going to eat in the next three or four days. Twenty to thirty percent of produce that we buy never gets consumed. From the flyer, make a list based on what is on sale that you need, so you don't impulse buy because you're hungry or see something while waiting in the checkout line.

THE BENEFITS OF OTHER NUTRIENTS IN YOUR DIET

A career in law enforcement is stressful and shift work can add to the stress load. Particular nutrients and foods that may help you manage the stresses of work/school include the following (before considering supplementing, you should consult your physician/dietitian):

- *Antioxidants* help repair, prevent, or limit oxidative damage—loss of electrons from atoms and molecules caused by free radicals (unstable molecules that may damage cells and lead to heart disease and cancer). Some of the best-known antioxidants include vitamins C and E, selenium (a trace mineral that helps reduce LDL cholesterol levels), and carotenoids (natural red, yellow, and orange pigments found in fruits and vegetables that help protect vitamin A and cells). The best sources of antioxidants include blueberries, cranberries, blackberries, raspberries, artichokes, raisins, and prunes.

- *B vitamins* promote wakefulness throughout the day or shift and encourage restful sleep. Vitamin B–rich foods include breads and beans, as well as various fruits, vegetables, and grains (see Table 8.6). If you take B vitamin supplements, it is important that you not consume them with coffee and take them with food during the day, not just before going to sleep.

- *Calcium*, besides building strong, healthy bones and teeth, is involved in muscle contraction and relaxation, blood clotting, and blood pressure. As you get older, calcium supplements only help you keep what bone you have left; they can no longer add to it. This is a concern with the physical demands of all fields of law enforcement. You can add calcium in your diet by choosing calcium-rich snacks like cheese and yogurt, desserts such as puddings and custards, and by using skim milk powder or evaporated milk in baking, sauces, and shakes (see Table 8.7). Of special note: caffeinated drinks increase the excretion of calcium that is stored in the body, specifically the bones.

- *Iron* deficiency can lead to decreased immune function, loss of energy, and reduced capacity to learn. Iron-deficiency anemia is more prevalent in females and is characterized by a pale complexion, listlessness, irritability, and mental and physical fatigue. Iron can be found in meat, fish, and poultry, all of which contain heme iron, which is more easily absorbed by the body. It is also found in vegetables and grains (see Table 8.7).

- *Magnesium* is one of the most abundant minerals in the body. If you lack magnesium you may feel anxious, fatigued, and moody, and experience muscle and joint pain and restless legs syndrome. Foods rich in magnesium include Brazil nuts, soybeans, wheat bran, millet, seafood, legumes, and dark green vegetables like kale or Swiss chard (see Table 8.7). If you take a magnesium supplement, be sure to take it with calcium, and later in the day rather than earlier, as it will make you drowsy.

- *Tyrosine* is one of the amino acids used to synthesize proteins. It is important for lucid and swift thinking. It releases dopamine, a neurotransmitter that increases heart rate and blood pressure, and stimulates metabolism and many of the body's energy reserves. Dopamine releases chemicals (for example, endorphins) that allow us to feel pleasure. A massive disturbance of dopamine regulation in the brain can result in the inability to respond emotionally or express feelings appropriately. Lack of dopamine is associated with conditions such as Parkinson's disease, schizophrenia, autism, and attention disorders. Tyrosine is found in eggs, soy products, fish, turkey, almonds, and avocados.

- *Tryptophan* is an amino acid that aids in releasing serotonin, a hormone that helps produce a stable mood and healthy sleep. It also helps in making niacin (vitamin B3), which facilitates the function of the digestive system, skin, and nerves. It helps with mental alertness and in converting food to energy. Serotonin triggers the release of melatonin, a natural chemical that helps you sleep. Tryptophan-rich foods include turkey, cheese, sesame and pumpkin seeds, yogurt, peanuts, and warm milk. If you take melatonin supplements, you should take them only for short periods when your shifts are changing, 30 minutes to one hour prior to going to sleep.

SNACKING

For people who work shifts, snacking is a double-edged sword. Eating small amounts of healthy food at appropriate intervals can keep your energy levels stable during working hours. But snacking too much, or snacking on the wrong foods, can lead to consumption of empty and extra calories that result in weight gain.

Without a healthy snack, our bodies experience a drop in blood sugar that decreases your energy and concentration levels. Reach this level of hunger, and you're apt to gobble up the first edible thing within reach. Here are some points to consider when reaching for a snack (Dietitians of Canada, 2010):

- Eat no more than three snacks per day, and keep each under 200 calories. Include foods from at least two of the four food groups.

- Eating empty calories from sweet, sugary foods will leave you unsatisfied. Boost your satisfaction and your satiety by choosing delicious and nutritionally dense snacks. Nuts, full of healthy unsaturated fats and protein, will fill you up. So will whole-grain breads or cereals and fruits and veggies, since they're packed with fibre that your body digests slowly.

- Think of snacks as mini-meals. Rather than pumping a bunch of empty extra calories into your daily tally, think of snacks as fuel to fill you up and to serve a nutritional purpose.

- Drink water often. Water has no calories. It quenches your thirst and helps you feel full. Being dehydrated often masks itself as hunger or headaches.

- Make snacks as convenient to eat as possible. Put snacks into baggies at the beginning of the week. Select finger foods, like freshly popped popcorn with minimal salt; nuts and seeds; low-fat cheese sticks; and whole-grain crackers, pita, or English muffins. Or, pack a travel-sized spoon for scooping from a yogurt cup.

- Before the start of your workweek, cut up vegetables so that they are ready to go whenever you are, whether to take to work or for eating right out of the fridge.

- Give your body a break between snacks. Eat a small serving, and then stow any remaining food out of sight. We tend to eat more when food is right in front of us.
- Skip individually prepackaged foods. For example, buy a large box of low-fat, low-sodium whole-grain crackers and place them in small baggies. Include a jar of natural peanut butter to stash at work.

CAFFEINATED DRINKS

Caffeine, although not a nutritional food or supplement, is ubiquitous in our culture. Not only do we consume it in coffee and tea, but it is also added to some carbonated drinks and certain drug products, such as cold and headache remedies. Caffeine is found naturally in the leaves, seeds, and fruit of a number of plants, including cocoa, kola, guarana, and yerba mate (the last two being herbs that are not always listed as caffeinated ingredients).

Caffeine is adrenaline (or stress) in a mug. It stimulates us and, theoretically at least, makes us more alert and wakeful with clearer thinking and better general body coordination. In some people, it can improve speed, endurance, and reaction time. Caffeine relieves pain. However, too much caffeine can result in restlessness, headaches, and dizziness, as well as insomnia, loss of fine motor control, and rapid breathing. Not only do caffeinated drinks dehydrate us, they also raise our cortisol (stress hormone) levels and decrease our metabolic rate. Caffeine can have a laxative effect on the digestive system, making it "lazy" and preventing the absorption of important nutrients. It can also interfere with the absorption of medication and iron. It fits the definition of an addictive substance because habituated individuals experience withdrawal symptoms, an increased tolerance over time, and physical cravings. As a result, three 8-oz cups of coffee should be an adult's daily limit—that is, 400 milligrams of caffeine per day. Recent recommendations for children and adolescents suggest a daily intake of no more than 2.5 milligrams per kilogram of body weight (Health Canada, 2012a).

One major concern today is the popularity of "energy drinks." They not only contain caffeine, which must by law be labelled, they often also include caffeine-containing herbs that do not have to be listed among the ingredients. This means that some drinks can have two or three times the caffeine content that is listed on the container. Some people ingest these as sports drinks to enhance their performance, mistakenly thinking that they provide energy and replenish electrolytes. Worse, some consume them when they are out drinking alcohol with friends in an attempt to delay alcohol's depressant effect and stay alert and awake.

In reality, these drinks cause irregular heartbeat, high blood pressure, and jitteriness. They can interfere with insulin sensitivity and cause headaches and fatigue. In extreme circumstances, energy drinks have caused death (Seifert, Schaechter, Hershorin, & Lipshultz, 2011). Given the physical demands and training required of law enforcement officers, and the concern about the negative effects of consuming these drinks prior to participation in physical activity or testing for a Bona Fide Occupational Requirement, waivers now include a clause stipulating that the participant must not have consumed an energy drink for at least two hours prior to participation in fitness class, testing, or competition.

Staying awake on night shifts and then trying to sleep during the day is a challenge for officers who work shifts. Here are some caffeine-related tips that can apply to your career as a student, as well:

- Don't consume caffeinated products within six hours of going to sleep. If you want to have a caffeinated beverage, stick to decaffeinated coffee or tea, as it has a slight amount of caffeine compared to the regular options.

- For every cup of caffeinated drink consumed, drink two cups of water.

- Manage your diet to gain more energy. Eat smaller meals, eat healthier, and drink more water. Rather than have a cup of coffee, eat fruit on an empty stomach to boost your glucose levels and raise your energy.

- When you feel drowsy, take a short exercise break. This means getting out of the cruiser every hour or so to walk around.

- Whether or not they are caffeinated, stay away from soft drinks (carbonated or non-carbonated). They provide empty calories and tons of sugar, and have been linked to fatty liver disease (Nseir, Nassar, & Assy, 2010).

FYI

FINDING THE MOST TRUSTWORTHY HEALTH INFORMATION ON THE INTERNET

Finding trustworthy health information on the Internet can be overwhelming. Here are some guidelines to help you determine the reliability and quality of the information you are reading.

1. Is the resource credible?
   - Are the author's name and professional credentials clearly stated? Is there contact information for the author or organization? Is the organization reputable? Is medical information provided by a medical professional? Is evidence (scientific studies, research) provided to support the information? Who sponsors the website (government agency, education institution, professional organization)?

2. Does the site reflect a broad view of health?
   - Does the cited research recognize that health has many different facets, is dynamic and changing, is unique to different demographics, and is determined by many diverse factors? Does it present facts and not opinions?

3. Is the resource timely?
   - Is the information continually reviewed and updated? Is the date of the last revision clearly marked?

4. Is there clear and adequate disclosure?
   - Is the mandate of the information clearly stated? For example, is it a non-profit organization trying to promote nutrition, exercise, and active living, or is it a product company trying to sell you its goods? Are there commercial links or sponsorships tied to the site, or links you must access before entering the intended site? If a site is collecting or requesting information about you, does it tell you exactly why it wants the information? Are the site's privacy guidelines stated? If you have to register to use the site, is the reason clear and is your privacy ensured? Is the information for consumer or health-related professionals?
   - Is the article biased or based on a conflict of interest? Are both sides of the issue presented? (For example, promotion of a vegetarian diet should indicate that there are other dietary options or clearly state that the viewpoint is just one side of a multifaceted issue.)

5. Are there clear caution statements?
   - Does the site state that health information should not be a substitute for visiting a health professional? If there are fees associated with use of the resources on the site, are they clearly explained?

6. Is the site user-friendly?
   - Is information presented in a clear manner? Can you contact the author/organization for additional information?

SOURCE: Adapted from Medical Library Association, 2017.

WELLNESS INITIATIVES

Many private sector companies are beginning to encourage their employees to make healthy food choices and engage in physical activity. Some companies provide flexible time schedules so that employees can participate in physical fitness programs throughout the day; nutritional counselling as a benefit option; and on-site fitness centres, weight-loss programs, and cafeteria facilities with healthy food selections. Some services in Ontario have fitness and lifestyle consultants as well as nutritionists/dietitians who work with employees to improve their health. Refer to the appendix below for a list of Canadian resources available to you.

FINAL THOUGHTS

The bottom line comes down to making educated and healthy choices for yourself. Shift work can affect the availability of health-promoting foods; however, if you plan appropriately and prepare meals and snacks ahead of time, you can avoid the pitfalls of poor nutrition. If you want to stay healthy, follow the guidelines set out by Canada's Food Guide and ensure that you exercise. Make sure you read widely about nutrition and ask questions. If you need assistance to get on track with better eating habits, contact your doctor or a dietitian for advice.

APPENDIX: FURTHER INFORMATION ON NUTRITION

Here are some Canadian websites that can provide you with more health and nutrition information.

5 to 10 a Day

http://www.5to10aday.com

A campaign aimed at helping Canadians of all ages eat more fruits and vegetables as part of a healthy diet and active lifestyle.

Active Healthy Kids Canada

http://www.activehealthykids.ca

"Powering the movement to get kids moving." The 2012 Active Healthy Kids Canada Report Card looks at how physical activity affects such outcomes as mental health and body weight, which in turn affect levels of physical activity.

Canadian Cancer Society

http://www.cancer.ca

Provides cancer patients, their friends and family, and the general public with up-to-date information about cancer and cancer prevention.

Canadian Centre for Ethics in Sport; Sport Nutrition

http://cces.ca/sport-nutrition

Clear and consistent guidance on fuelling the body for athletic performance.

Canadian Diabetes Association

http://www.diabetes.ca

Information on nutrition and physical activity for the prevention and management of diabetes.

Canadian Diabetes Association; Diet and Nutrition

http://www.diabetes.ca/diabetes-and-you/healthy-living -resources/diet-nutrition

Created to help diabetics eat tasty and healthy meals for good health and diabetes management. The manual contains information on a wide variety of topics, from eating out to recipe makeovers and physical activity.

Canadian Food Inspection Agency

http://www.inspection.gc.ca

Dedicated to safeguarding food, animals, and plants to enhance the health and well-being of Canada's people, environment, and economy.

Canadian Foundation for Dietetic Research

http://www.cfdr.ca/sharing/CCFNLibrary.aspx

Information and advocacy on policy matters and critical food and nutrition issues in Canada.

DASH Eating Plan

http://www.nhlbi.nih.gov/health/public/heart/hbp/dash/new_dash.pdf

A guide to lowering blood pressure and reducing the amount of sodium you consume.

Dietitians of Canada

http://www.dietitians.ca

Interactive tools, tips, and fact sheets for healthy eating. Check out the Eating & Activity Tracker (eaTracker; see below) to get personalized advice about your current food choices. The website can also help you find a nutrition professional in your area.

eaTracker

http://www.eatracker.ca

An initiative of Dietitians of Canada to help Canadians track their daily food and activity choices, and track their progress. The eaTracker tool provides personalized feedback on calories, essential nutrients, activity levels, and body mass index (BMI).

Eat Right Ontario

http://www.eatrightontario.ca

Information on popular nutrition and healthy eating. Its monthly email newsletter provides timely updates. The site offers access to a dietitian via email or phone for specific information.

Facts About Fats

http://www.hc-sc.gc.ca/fn-an/nutrition/gras-trans-fats/index-eng.php

Health Canada's information on trans fats, including frequently asked questions and information on the trans fat task force.

Food Allergy Canada

http://foodallergycanada.ca

Dedicated to helping people with severe allergies.

Food and Consumer Products of Canada

http://www.fcpc.ca

Works with government agencies and industry to provide support to the government's commitment to nutrition, healthy lifestyles, and workplace wellness.

Health Canada

http://www.hc-sc.gc.ca

Federal department responsible for helping Canadians maintain and improve their health while respecting individual choices and circumstances. Provides high-quality research on long-term health care and disease prevention, and encourages physical activity and healthy eating.

Healthy Buddies

http://www.healthybuddies.ca

Empowers elementary school children to live healthier lives by informing them about the three components of health: physical activity, nutrition, and mental health.

Heart & Stroke Health Check

http://www.heartandstroke.ca

A not-for-profit food information program that provides information on choosing foods in grocery stores and restaurants that can be part of a healthy diet. On the home page, scroll down under "Manage Your Health" and click on "Health Information" and choose "Health Check."

Leslie Beck

http://www.lesliebeck.com

Leslie Beck, a Canadian registered dietitian and nutritionist, provides information about nutrition and exercise.

Nutritional Labelling

http://www.canada.ca/en/health-canada/services/food -nutrition/food-labelling/nutrition-labelling.html

Information regarding the regulation of and compliance with nutritional labelling for most prepackaged foods.

Nutrition Resource Centre (NRC)

http://opha.on.ca/Nutrition-Resource-Centre/Home.aspx

An initiative of the Ontario Public Health Association, funded by the Ontario Ministry of Health and Long-Term Care, NRC was established to increase the level of coordinated provincial support of nutritional promotion programming, resource development, dissemination, and support services for nutrition professionals.

Osteoporosis Canada

http://www.osteoporosis.ca

Information on nutrition and physical activity for the prevention of osteoporosis.

Sodium 101

http://www.sodium101.ca

Information for consumers on sodium, including label reading, health effects, and tips for reducing sodium intake.

Sodium Reduction Strategy for Canada

http://www.canada.ca/en/health-canada/services/food -nutrition/healthy-eating/sodium/related-information/ reduction-strategy.html

Based on research, this Sodium Reduction Strategy for Canada is a multi-staged approach to reduce sodium in the Canadian diet.

KEY TERMS

amino acids
the fundamental constituents of proteins; amino acids can be divided into two types—complete (essential) and incomplete

blood cholesterol
the cholesterol produced by the liver

cholesterol
a waxy, fat-like substance important for normal body function that travels through the blood and is linked to atherosclerosis

DASH diet
a diet that follows Canada's Food Guide in order to reduce sodium, cholesterol, and fat in Canadians' diet

dietary cholesterol
the cholesterol in food

dietary fibre
food components that cannot be digested, found exclusively in plants; the two types of dietary fibre are insoluble and soluble

fatty acids
the fundamental constituents of fats; fatty acids can be divided into two types—saturated and unsaturated

glycemic index (GI)
the amount of blood glucose (sugar) levels of certain foods within two hours of digestion

glycemic load (GL)
a measure of how quickly a food is converted into sugar in relation to how much sugar it contains

high-density lipoprotein (HDL) cholesterol
"good" cholesterol; it helps clean out undesirable LDL deposits

hyperhydration
water "intoxication," characterized by an abnormal increase in the body's water content

kilocalorie (kcal)
a measure of the amount of energy in food; also referred to as a calorie

low-density lipoprotein (LDL) cholesterol
"bad" cholesterol; it can build up in the arteries and cause health problems

metabolic syndrome
is a cluster of medical conditions that increase the risk of many chronic illnesses including diabetes, hypertension, cardiovascular diseases, chronic kidney disease, and dyslipidemia

six basic nutrients
the basic nutrients that the body requires to function efficiently: water, carbohydrates, protein, fats, vitamins, and minerals

trans fats
unsaturated fatty acids that have been hydrogenated to give them a longer shelf life; diets high in trans fats increase the risk of atherosclerosis and coronary heart disease

EXERCISES

MULTIPLE CHOICE

1. According to Canada's Food Guide, over half of your daily calories may come from
   a. vitamins
   b. minerals
   c. fats
   d. carbohydrates
   e. proteins

2. What is the best advice for someone participating in a regular fitness program?
   a. eat as much as you can
   b. eat more protein
   c. eat a balanced diet
   d. eat fewer carbohydrates
   e. reduce all fats

3. The guidelines in Canada's Food Guide do not include
   a. enjoying a variety of foods from each of the four food groups daily
   b. choosing higher-fat foods more often
   c. emphasizing grain products, vegetables, and fruit
   d. consuming a small amount of oils and fats
   e. limiting salt, alcohol, and caffeine

4. Carbohydrates are stored in the liver and muscles in the form of
   a. fatty acids
   b. amino acids
   c. glycogen
   d. LDL
   e. HDL

5. A good source of protein is _____.
   a. oranges
   b. lettuce
   c. meat

   d. strawberries
   e. squash

6. The body cannot survive without which nutrient for a prolonged period of time?
   a. carbohydrates
   b. proteins
   c. fats
   d. water
   e. minerals

7. According to Canada's Food Guide, one serving of grain products would consist of
   a. one large hamburger bun
   b. one cup of hot cereal
   c. three saltine crackers
   d. one-half cup of cooked rice
   e. one toasted bagel

8. Which is least likely to be true of complex carbohydrates?
   a. they are high in fibre
   b. they are low in calories
   c. they are low in nutrients
   d. they are low in saturated fats
   e. they are low in amino acids

9. Which of the following is good advice for weight control?
   a. eat as fast as you can so you don't think about food
   b. space meals out equally throughout the day
   c. skip lunch or breakfast if you don't feel hungry
   d. eat a large dinner and a small lunch and breakfast
   e. read a book while eating to take your mind off of food

10. "Empty calories" refers to
    a. food that does not make you fat
    b. calories with a low caloric content
    c. regurgitation of food to prevent weight gain
    d. food that is low in nutrients and high in calories
    e. the apparent inability of thin people to gain weight

11. Which of the following is true of dietary fat?
    a. it is an essential part of the diet
    b. it should never be consumed by an athlete
    c. it should make up 40 percent of your total caloric intake
    d. it should be primarily saturated
    e. it has fewer calories per gram than carbohydrates

12. How many calories are found in a 4-gram serving of fat?
    a. 12 kcal
    b. 15 kcal
    c. 27 kcal
    d. 36 kcal
    e. 40 kcal

13. Complete proteins, containing all the essential amino acids, are found in
    a. legumes
    b. nuts
    c. animal products
    d. wild rice
    e. leafy green vegetables

14. Most experts agree that there is a link between excessive sodium intake and
    a. cancer
    b. hypotension
    c. blood clotting
    d. diabetes
    e. hypertension

15. Which is worst for you?
    a. butter
    b. tub margarine
    c. stick margarine
    d. low-sodium whipped butter
    e. light tub margarine

16. Four of these strategies have been clearly shown to keep blood pressure from rising. Which hasn't?
    a. cutting salt
    b. losing excess weight
    c. eating potassium-rich foods
    d. getting adequate calcium
    e. exercising regularly

17. _____ are high in saturated fats.
    a. Corn oil and soybean oil
    b. Broccoli and cauliflower
    c. Whole milk and cheeses
    d. Bread and potatoes
    e. White and whole-grain rice

18. Which of the following is the best source for omega-3 fatty acids?
    a. wheat products
    b. berries
    c. corn oil
    d. pork
    e. sardines

SHORT ANSWERS

1. What are the six basic nutrients?

2. What constitutes a balanced and healthy diet?

3. What factors affect the glycemic index?

4. Why is fibre important to your diet?

5. What is the distinction between blood cholesterol and dietary cholesterol?

6. What are some ways to reduce fat in your diet?

7. What are vitamins and minerals, and why are they important in your diet?

8. What are the benefits and risks of consuming caffeine?

9. What is the basis of the DASH diet?

10. What are five ways to improve your nutritional value when you go shopping?

REFERENCES

Adams, S.M., & Standridge, J.B. (2006). What should we eat? Evidence from observational studies. *Southern Medical Journal*, 99(7), 744–748.

American Dietetic Association and Dietitians of Canada. (2003). Position of the American Dietetic Association and Dietitians of Canada: Vegetarian diets. Public policy statement. *Canadian Journal of Dietetic Practice and Research, 64*(2).

American Heart Association (2017). How to reduce sodium. Retrieved from https://sodiumbreakup .heart.org/how_to_reduce_sodium

Arcand, J., Au, J.T.C., Schermel, A., & L'Abbe, M.R. (2014). A comprehensive analysis of sodium levels in the Canadian packaged food supply. *American Journal of Preventive Medicine, 46*(6), 633–642. Retrieved from http://doi.org/10.1016/j.amepre.2014.01.012

Aune, D., et al. (2011). Dietary fibre, whole grains, and risk of colorectal cancer: Systematic review and dose-response meta-analysis of prospective studies. *British Medical Journal, 343,* d6617. Retrieved from http://www.ncbi.nlm.nih.gov/pubmed/22074852

Aune, D., Ursin, G., & Veierod, M.B. (2009). Meat consumption and the risk of type 2 diabetes: A systematic review and meta-analysis of cohort studies. *Diabetologia, 52,* 2277–2287.

Beulens, J.W., et al. (2007). High dietary glycemic load and glycemic index increase risk of cardiovascular disease among middle-aged women: A population-based follow-up study. *Journal of the American College of Cardiology, 50,*14–21.

Campbell, N.R., Khalsa, T., Lackland, D.T., Miebylski, M.L., Nilsson, P.M., Redburn, K.A., ... Weber, M.A. (2016). High blood pressure 2016: Why prevention and control are urgent and important. The World Hypertension League, International Society of Hypertension, World Stroke Organization, International Diabetes Foundation, International Council of Cardiovascular Prevention, *The Journal of Clinical Hypertension, 18*(8), 714.

Canadian Council of Food and Nutrition. (2011). Home plate. What consumers are eating behind closed doors. An initiative of the Canadian Council of Food and Nutrition. Retrieved from http://www.cfdr.ca/downloads/ccfn-docs/home-plate-jan-28-final.aspx

Canadian Diabetes Association. (2017). Dash diet. Retrieved from http://www.diabetes.ca/diabetes -and-you/healthy-living-resources/diet-nutrition/dash-diet

Canadian Food Inspection Agency. (2016a). Daily intake; information within the nutrition facts table. Retrieved from http://www.inspection.gc.ca/food/labelling/food-labelling-for-industry/nutrition -labelling/information-within-the-nutrition-facts -table/eng/1389198568400/1389198597278?chap=6

Canadian Food Inspection Agency (2016b). Specific nutrient content claim requirements: Fat claims. food labelling and advertising. Retrieved from http://www.inspection.gc.ca/food/labelling/food-labelling-for-industry/nutrient-content/specific-claim-requirements/eng/1389907770176/1389907817577?chap=4

Chavarro, J.E., Rich-Edwards, J.W., Rosner, B.A., & Willett, W.C. (2007). Diet and lifestyle in the prevention of ovulatory disorder infertility. *Obstetrics and Gynecology, 110,* 1050–1058.

Chiu, C.J., Milton, R.C., Klein, R., Gensler, G., & Taylor, A. (2009). Dietary compound score and risk of age-related macular degeneration in the Age-Related Eye Disease Study. *Ophthalmology, 116*(5), 939–946.

Coca-Cola. (2017). Product facts. Powerade. Retrieved from http://www.coca-colaproductfacts.com/en/coca-cola-products/powerade/

de Souza R.J., et al. (2015). Intake of saturated and trans unsaturated fatty acids and risk of all cause mortality, cardiovascular disease, and type 2 diabetes: Systematic review and meta-analysis of observational studies. *British Medical Journal, 351,* h3978. Retrieved from http://www.bmj.com/content/351/bmj.h3978.long

Diabetes Canada. (2017). Fibre. Retrieved from http://diabetes.ca/diabetes-and-you/healthy-living -resources/diet-nutrition/fibre

Dietitians of Canada. (2010). Healthy snacks for adults. Retrieved from http://www.dietitians.ca/downloads/Factsheets/Healthy-Snacks-for-Adults.aspx

Dietitians of Canada. (2012). Functions and food sources of some common vitamins. Retrieved from http://www.dietitians.ca/downloads/Factsheets/Functions-Sources-Common-Vitamins.aspx

Dietitians of Canada. (2014). Guidelines for drinking fluids to stay hydrated. Retrieved from https://www.dietitians.ca/Your-Health/Nutrition-A-Z/Water/Why-is-water-so-important-for-my-body--Know-when-.aspx

Dietitians of Canada. (2016). Food sources of fibre. Retrieved from https://www.dietitians.ca/Your-Health/Nutrition-A-Z/Fibre/Food-Sources-of-Fibre.aspx

Dietitians of Canada. (2017). Vegetarian diets. Retrieved from https://www.dietitians.ca/Your-Health/Nutrition-A-Z/Vegetarian-Diets.aspx

Durstine, L. (2005). Understanding blood cholesterol. In *Action plan for high cholesterol* (pp. 1–12). American College of Sports Medicine. Champaign, IL: Human Kinetics.

Dyerberg, J., & Passwater, R. (2012). *The Missing Wellness Factors: EPA and DHA: The most important nutrients since vitamins*. Laguana Beach, CA: Basic Health Publications.

EatrightOntario. (2016). Focus of fibre. Retrieved from http://www.eatrightontario.ca/en/Articles/Fibre/Focus-on-Fibre.aspx

EatrightOntario. (2017). Introduction to protein and high protein foods. Retrieved from http://www.eatrightontario.ca/en/Articles/Protein/Introduction-To-Protein-And-High-Protein-Foods.aspx

Foster-Powell, K., Holt, S.H., & Brand-Miller, J.C. (2002). International table of glycemic index and glycemic load values: 2002. *American Journal of Clinical Nutrition, 76,* 5–56.

Garriguet, D. (2007). Overview of Canadians' eating habits. In *Nutrition: Findings from the Canadian Community Healthy Survey.* Ottawa: Statistics Canada Cat. no. 82-003-x/2006004. Retrieved from http://www.statcan.gc.ca/pub/82-003-x/2006004/article/habit/9609-eng.pdf

Garriguet, D. (2012). Eating habits and nutrient intake of Aboriginal adults aged 19–50, living off-reserve in Ontario and the western provinces. In *Health and Nutrition Surveys* from Canadian Community Health Survey. Ottawa; Statistics Canada. Catalogue no: H164-122/2012E-PDF. Retrieved from http://www.hc-sc.gc.ca/fn-an/alt_formats/pdf/surveill/nutrition/commun/aboriginal-aborigene-eng.pdf.

Government of Canada. (2012). Nutrition content claims: What they mean. Retrieved from https://www.canada.ca/en/health-canada/services/understanding-food-labels/nutrient-content-claims-what-they-mean.html

Government of Canada. (2016). Food labelling changes. Retrieved from http://www.healthycanadians.gc.ca/eating-nutrition/label-etiquetage/changes-modifications-eng.php?_ga=1.50892841.1671999758.1485374439

Health Canada. (2007). Guide to developing accurate nutrient values. Retrieved from http://www.canada.ca/en/health-canada/services/food-nutrition/food-labelling/nutrition-labelling/regulations-compliance/guide-developing-accurate-nutrient-values.html

Health Canada. (2012a). Caffeine in foods. Retrieved from http://www.canada.ca/en/health-canada/services/food-nutrition/food-safety/food-additives/caffeine-foods.html

Health Canada. (2012b). Do Canadian adults meet their nutrient requirements through food intake alone? Cat. No.: H164-112/3-2012E-PDF. Retrieved from https://www.canada.ca/en/health-canada/services/food-nutrition/food-nutrition-surveillance/health-nutrition-surveys/canadian-community-health-survey-cchs/canadian-adults-meet-their-nutrient-requirements-through-food-intake-alone-health-canada-2012.html

Health Canada. (2012c). *Eating well with Canada's Food Guide.* Retrieved from http://www.hc-sc.gc.ca/fn-an/alt_formats/hpfb-dgpsa/pdf/food-guide-aliment/view_eatwell_vue_bienmang-eng.pdf

Health Canada. (2015). Evidence review for dietary guidance: Summary of results and implications for Canada's Food Guide. Cat.: H164-193/2016E-PDF. Retrieved from https://www.canada.ca/content/dam/canada/health-canada/migration/publications/eating-nutrition/dietary-guidance-summary-resume-recommandations-alimentaires/alt/pub-eng.pdf

Health Canada. (2016). Canadian nutrient file. Retrieved from http://www.canada.ca/en/health-canada/services/food-nutrition/healthy-eating/nutrient-data/canadian-nutrient-file-2015-download-files.html

Health Canada. (2017a). Sodium. Retrieved from https://www.canada.ca/en/health-canada/services/nutrients/sodium.html

Health Canada. (2017b). Sodium in Canada. Retrieved from http://www.canada.ca/en/health-canada/services/food-nutrition/healthy-eating/sodium.html

Health Canada. (2017c). Symposium on Sodium Reduction in Foods Meeting Report (2016). Cat.: H164-204/2017E-PDF. Retrieved from https://www.canada.ca/content/dam/themes/health/campaigns/sodium/symposium-sodium-eng.pdf

Healthy Canadians. (2011a). Choosing foods with less sodium: At the grocery store. Retrieved from https://www.canada.ca/en/health-canada/services/nutrients/sodium.html

Healthy Canadians. (2011b). Choosing foods with less sodium: When eating out. Retrieved from https://www.canada.ca/en/health-canada/services/nutrients/sodium.html

Healthy Canadians. (2016). FATS. Retrieved from http://healthycanadians.gc.ca/eating-nutrition/healthy-eating-saine-alimentation/nutrients-nutriments/fats-lipides-eng.php?_ga=2.127081933.1753045385.1499873221-1568368488.1439990706

Heart and Stroke Foundation of Ontario. (2012). The DASH diet to lower high blood pressure. Retrieved from http://www.heartandstroke.ca/get-healthy/healthy-eating/dash-diet

Higginbotham, S., et al. (2004). Dietary glycemic load and risk of colorectal cancer in the Women's Health Study. *Journal of the National Cancer Institute, 96*(3), 229–233.

Humphrey, L.L., Fu, R., Rogers, K., Freeman, M., & Helfand, M. (2008). Homocysteine level and coronary heart disease incidence: A systematic review and meta-analysis. *Mayo Clinical Proceedings, 83*(11), 1203–1212.

Institute of Medicine. (2005). *Dietary reference intakes for energy, carbohydrate, fiber, fat, fatty acids, cholesterol, protein and amino acids.* Washington, DC: National Academies Press.

Jenkins, D.A., et al. (1981). Glycemic index of foods: A physiological basis for carbohydrate exchange. *American Journal of Clinical Nutrition, 34*, 362–366.

Kastorini, C.M., et al. (2011). The effect of Mediterranean diet on metabolic syndrome and its components: A meta-analysis of 50 studies and 534,906 individuals. *Journal of the American College of Cardiology, 57*,1299–1313.

Kleiner, S. (2000). Bodybuilding. In Rosenbloom, C. (Ed.), *Sports nutrition: A guide for the professional working with active people* (3rd ed.). Chicago: American Dietetic Association.

Krenosky, S., L'Abbé, M., Lee, N., Underhill, L., Vigneault, M., Godefroy, S.B., & Ratnayake, N. (2012). Risk assessment of exposure to trans fat in Canada. *International Food Risk Analysis Journal, 19*, 10. DOI: 10.5772/56127

McDonalds. (2017). Nutrition centre. Retrieved from http://www.mcdonalds.ca/ca/en/food/nutrition_centre.html

Medical Library Association. (2017). For health consumers and patients: Find good health Information. Retrieved from http://www.mlanet.org/resources/userguide.html

Metabolic Syndrome Canada. (2017). Pathophysiology of metabolic syndrome. Retrieved from https://www.metabolicsyndromecanada.ca/professionals

National Institutes of Health. (2006). DASH eating plan: Your guide to lowering your blood pressure with DASH. US Department of Health and Human Services. NIH Publications no. 06-4082. Retrieved from http://www.nhlbi.nih.gov/files/docs/public/heart/new_dash.pdf

National Institutes of Health. (2015). Explore DASH eating plan. National Heart, Lung and Blood Institute. Retrieved from https://www.nhlbi.nih.gov/health/health-topics/topics/dash

National Institutes of Health, Office of Dietary Supplements. (n.d.). Nutrient recommendations: Dietary reference intakes (DRI). Retrieved from http://ods.od.nih.gov/Health_Information/Dietary_Reference_Intakes.aspx

Nseir, W., Nassar, F., & Assy, N. (2010). Soft drinks consumption and non-alcoholic fatty liver disease. *World Journal of Gastroenterology, 16*(21), 2579–2588.

Panagiotopoulos, C., Ronsley, R., Elbe, D., Davidson, J., & Smith, D.H. (2010). First do no harm: Promoting an evidence-based approach to atypical antipsychotic use in children and adolescents. *Journal of the Canadian Academy of Child and Adolescent Psychiatry, 19*, 124–137.

PepsiCo. (2017). The facts about your favourite beverages. Retrieved from http://www.pepsicobeveragefacts.com/home/find

Pérez, C.E. (2002). Fruit and vegetable consumption. *Health Reports, 13*(3). Statistics Canada Cat. no. 82-003 (pp. 23–31). Retrieved from http://www.statcan.gc.ca/pub/82-003-x/2001003/article/6103-eng.pdf

Poole, C., Wilborn, C., Taylor, L., & Kerksick, C. (2010). The role of post-exercise nutrient administration of protein and glycogen synthesis. *Journal of Sports Science and Medicine, 9*, 354–363. Retrieved from http://www.jssm.org/vol9/n3/1/v9n3-1pdf.pdf

Public Health Agency of Canada (PHAC). (2010a). Fruit and vegetable consumption. Canadian Community Health Survey, 2010 Health Fact sheets. Cat. no. 82-625-X. Retrieved from http://www.statcan.gc.ca/pub/82-625-x/2011001/article/11461-eng.htm

Public Health Agency of Canada (PHAC). (2010b). Overweight and obese adults (self-reported). Canadian Community Health Survey, 2010 Health Fact sheets. Cat no. 82-625-X. Retrieved from http://www.statcan.gc.ca/pub/82-625-x/2011001/article/11461-eng.htm

Public Health Agency of Canada (PHAC). (2014). Metabolic syndrome and chronic disease. *Chronic Diseases and Injuries, 34*(1). Retrieved from http://www.phac-aspc.gc.ca/publicat/hpcdp-pspmc/34-1/ar-06-eng.php

Rautiainen, S., Larsson, S., Virtamo, J., & Wolk, A. (2012). Total antioxidant capacity of diet and risk of stroke: A population-based prospective cohort of women. *Stroke, 43*(2), 335–340. Retrieved from http://www.ncbi.nlm.nih.gov/pubmed/22135074

Seifert, S.M., Schaechter, J.L., Hershorin, E.R., & Lipshultz, S.E. (2011). Health effects of energy drinks on children, adolescents and young adults. *Pediatrics, 127*(3), 511–528. doi:10.1542/peds.2009-3592.

Sizer, F., & Whitney, E. (2013). *Nutrition: Concepts and controversies* (13th ed.). Belmont, CA: Wadsworth.

Starbucks. (2015). Explore our menu. Retrieved from https://www.starbucks.com/menu/catalog/nutrition?drink=all

Statistics Canada. (2016). Overweight and obese adults (self-reported), 2014. Health Fact Sheet. Catalogue No. 82-625-X. Retrieved from http://www5.statcan.gc.ca/olc-cel/olc.action?objId=82-625-X&objType=2&lang=en&limit=0

Statistics Canada. (2017). Average household expenditure 2015 (Canada). CANSIM, table 203-0021 and Catalogue no. 62F0026M. Retrieved from http://www.statcan.gc.ca/tables-tableaux/sum-som/l01/cst01/famil130a-eng.htm

Strazzullo, P., D'Elia, L., Kandala, N.-B., & Cappuccio, F. P. (2009). Salt intake, stroke, and cardiovascular disease: Meta-analysis of prospective studies. *The British Medical Journal, 339*, b4567. Retrieved from http://doi.org/10.1136/bmj.b4567

Tim Hortons. (2013). Tim Hortons nutrition guide. Retrieved from https://www.timhortons.com/ca/en/pdf/TH_Nutrition_Guide_CE_2013_-_FINAL.pdf

Tipton, C.M. (Ed.). (2006). Physiological systems and their responses to conditions of heat and cold. In *ACSM's Advanced Exercise Physiology* (pp. 550–551). Baltimore, MD: Lippincott, Williams & Williams.

University of Sydney. (2017). International GI database. Retrieved from http://www.glycemicindex.com

US Department of Health and Human Services; US Department of Agriculture. (2015). *2015-2020 Dietary guidelines for Americans*. 8th ed. Washington, DC: US Dept of Health and Human Services. Retrieved from http://www.health.gov/DietaryGuidelines

United States Department of Agriculture. (2016). Food expenditures. Retrieved from https://www.ers.usda.gov/data-products/food-expenditures.aspx

Visa Canada Corporation. (2012). Canadians who buy lunch spend $8.80 on average, according to Visa Canada—An expense that adds up. Retrieved from http://www.newswire.ca/news-releases/canadians-who-buy-lunch-spend-880-on-average---an-expense-that-adds-up-510456691.html

Wang, F., Wild, T.C., Kipp, W., Kuhle, S., & Veugelers, P.J. (2009). The influence of childhood obesity on the development of self-esteem. Statistics Canada Cat. no. 82-003-XPE. *Health Reports, 20*(2). Retrieved from http://www.statcan.gc.ca/pub/82-003-x/2009002/article/10871-eng.pdf

World Cancer Research Fund International. American Institute for Cancer Research. (2007). *Food, nutrition, physical activity, and the prevention of cancer: A global perspective*. Washington, DC: Author. Retrieved from http://www.dietandcancerreport.org

PART 4

UNDERSTANDING AND MANAGING POTENTIAL HEALTH PROBLEMS

CHAPTER 9   Diabetes

CHAPTER 10   Cardiovascular Disease

CHAPTER 11   Back Health

CHAPTER 12   Stress

CHAPTER 13   Shift Work and Sleep

CHAPTER 14   Common Injuries

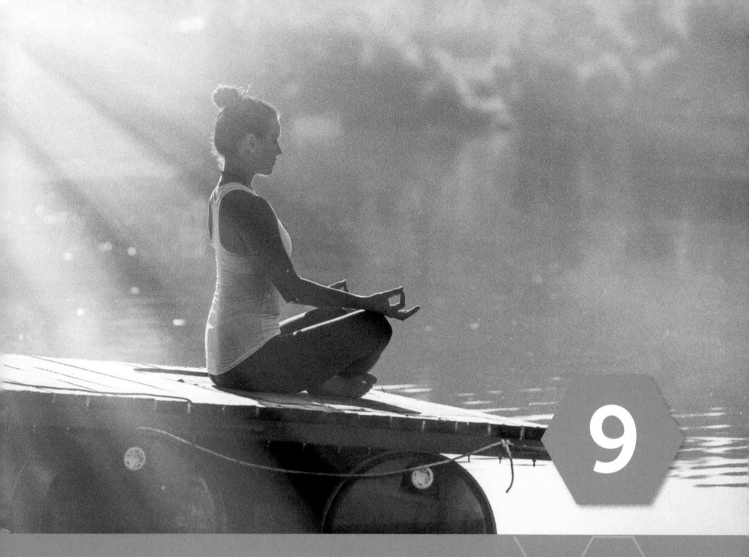

DIABETES

LEARNING OUTCOMES

After completing this chapter, you should be able to:

- Understand the facts about diabetes as a disease.

- Describe the four types of diabetes.

- Describe signs and symptoms associated with diabetes.

- Explain the risk factors associated with diabetes.

- Describe the complications associated with diabetes.

- Describe lifestyle modifications that officers who have diabetes must make in order to perform shift work.

Diabetes is a chronic disease in which the body cannot properly use glucose for energy. Glucose, a component of carbohydrates and the main source of energy for the brain, comes from foods such as breads, cereals, pasta, rice, potatoes, fruits, and some vegetables. To use glucose for energy, your body needs insulin, a hormone produced in the pancreas. When your body has little or no insulin, the glucose builds up in your blood instead of being used for energy. This causes high blood glucose levels, also known as hyperglycemia.

Normal glucose levels are between 4.0 and 7.0 mmol/L when fasting and between 5.0 and 10.0 mmol/L two hours after eating (Diabetes Canada, 2011b). When blood glucose levels are consistently above 10 mmol/L, a person is hyperglycemic, which can lead to serious medical conditions (discussed below). These can have an impact on a law enforcement career—for example, the ability to drive a vehicle or deal with an emergency. Illnesses such as a cold, flu, or infection can raise your blood glucose as a stress response. Emotional stress (excitement, anger, worry) can also increase blood glucose.

Low blood sugar—hypoglycemia—is also associated with diabetes. When blood glucose levels are between 2.5 and 4.0 mmol/L, a person is hypoglycemic (discussed below in more detail). Individuals who skip meals, eat poorly (not enough carbohydrates), are more active than usual, or take more diabetes medication than normal will experience a drop in blood glucose. People whose blood glucose is this low should not drive or operate machinery, as their responses are impaired. Below 2.5 mmol/L, individuals are severely hypoglycemic and may experience loss of consciousness or seizures. (See Figure 9.1.)

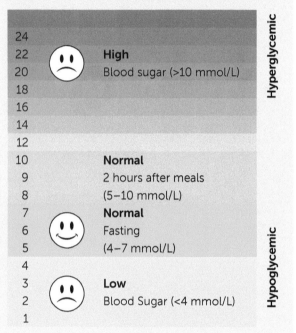

FIGURE 9.1 Blood Glucose Levels

TYPES OF DIABETES

There are four types of diabetes (Diabetes Canada, 2011b): type 1 diabetes, type 2 diabetes, gestational diabetes, and prediabetes (the newest type identified).

Type 1 diabetes (T1D) is an autoimmune disease in which a person's pancreas stops producing insulin, a hormone that enables people to get energy from food. The body's immune system attacks and destroys the insulin-producing cells in the pancreas, called beta cells. About 10 percent of people with diabetes have this type. Type 1 diabetes usually begins in the first two decades of life. A combination of genetic factors and environmental stressors such as viruses are believed to trigger this form of diabetes. Its onset has nothing to do with diet or lifestyle. Treatment requires a strict diet, planned physical activity, home blood glucose testing several times a day (Figure 9.2), and multiple daily insulin injections. Type 1 diabetes has huge implications for an individual's health. The pain and discomfort of blood glucose monitoring and needle injections often lead to anxiety and fear. In fact, between 30 percent and 50 percent of insulin users avoid injections because of anxiety (Kruger, LaRue, & Estepa, 2015). Type 1 diabetes can result in a drastic reduction in one's quality of life, and shortens the average lifespan by 15 years (PHAC, 2009, 2011). Researchers continue to work hard to find out what causes type 1 diabetes. It is known that having a family member (parent, sibling) with type 1 diabetes slightly increases the risk; however, definite risk factors are currently not known.

Although type 1 diabetes can develop in children only a few months old, it is somewhat rare for children under five years to develop this disease. The incidence increases with age through childhood and adolescence, and then decreases during adulthood. Usually, people are diagnosed with type 1 diabetes before the age of 30, most often during childhood or their teens.

FIGURE 9.2   Blood Glucose Monitor

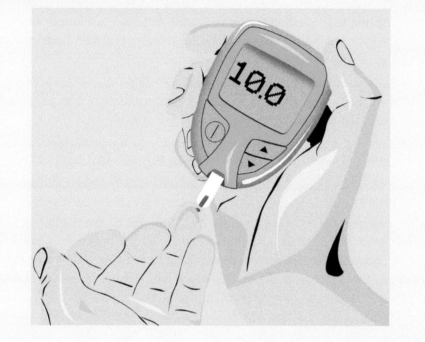

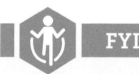 **FYI**

BRITTLE DIABETES MELLITUS (OR LABILE DIABETES)

Brittle diabetes is a subtype of type 1 diabetes that is particularly hard to control due to insulin absorption issues, malfunctioning hormones, delayed stomach emptying, and drug interactions, resulting in frequent, extreme swings in blood sugar levels, causing hyperglycemia or hypoglycemia. This type of diabetes can preclude you from being hired in many law enforcement agencies.

SOURCE: Diabetes.co.uk, 2017.

Type 2 diabetes (T2D, formerly known as adult-onset diabetes mellitus) occurs when the pancreas cannot produce enough insulin or the body is unable to use the insulin effectively. About 90 percent of diabetics have this type. This form of diabetes is now widely considered to be one of the components of a group of disorders called *metabolic syndrome*, which includes central obesity (extra weight around the middle of the body), insulin resistance, high cholesterol, lipid disorders, high blood pressure, a high risk of blood clotting, and disturbed blood flow to many organs (Health Canada, 2000). Obesity, physical inactivity, poor diet, aging, hormonal changes, and stress significantly increase the risk of type 2 diabetes. The disease can be controlled by diet, exercise, and oral medication. In addition, some people may require insulin injections. Weight loss can also help to bring blood sugar into the normal range, as approximately 80 to 85 percent of people who develop type 2 diabetes are overweight (Diabetes Canada, 2011a). Life expectancy is also reduced in people with type 2 diabetes.

The mechanisms of type 2 diabetes are not fully understood. However, some experts believe it happens in three stages (American Diabetes Association, 2007):

- The first stage is called *insulin resistance*. Although insulin can attach to the liver and muscle receptors, this stage prevents insulin from moving glucose from the blood into the cells.

- The second stage is called *postprandial hyperglycemia*, which occurs when the pancreas cannot produce enough insulin and there is an abnormal rise in blood sugar after a meal.

- The third stage is termed *fasting hyperglycemia*, a state of elevated glucose levels most of the time. Elevated glucose impairs and possibly destroys beta cells, thereby stopping insulin production and causing full-blown diabetes.

Gestational diabetes is a temporary condition that occurs during pregnancy (generally after the 24th week) and resolves after delivery. Hormonal changes associated with pregnancy and the growth demands of the fetus increase insulin needs to two to three times the normal level. Gestational diabetes occurs in 2 to 10 percent of all pregnancies (Centers for Disease Control and Prevention, 2011). If gestational diabetes is diagnosed in a pregnant woman but not addressed, her baby is likely to be larger than normal (over 4 kilograms or 9 pounds), born with low glucose levels, and born prematurely. It increases the risk to both mother and child of developing type 2 diabetes. Women who gain over 14 kilograms (30 pounds) during pregnancy have an increased risk. Gestational diabetes may result in respiratory distress syndrome, low blood calcium, neonatal hypoglycemia (low blood sugar in the newborn infant), and pre-eclampsia (toxemia of pregnancy, a life-threatening condition). Many babies born with diabetes die within their first year of life despite receiving medical care (Billionnet et al., 2017; Diabetes Canada, 2017f).

Prediabetes is a term for impaired fasting glucose or impaired glucose tolerance. It refers to blood glucose levels that are consistently higher than normal, but not at diabetic levels yet. Although not everyone with higher glucose levels will develop type 2 diabetes, many will, especially when combined with other metabolic syndrome risk factors such as high blood pressure, high levels of low-density lipoprotein cholesterol (LDL, or "bad" cholesterol) and triglycerides, low levels of high-density lipoproteins (HDL, or "good" cholesterol), and a tendency toward abdominal obesity. Usually, those who have prediabetes have no symptoms but if glucose levels are not lowered, they are at increased risk for developing diabetes within ten years. There is good news, though: you can reduce the risk of getting diabetes, and even return to normal blood glucose levels, with modest weight loss and moderate physical activity.

DID YOU KNOW?

Studies have shown that through lifestyle changes, including moderate weight loss and regular exercise (a combination of aerobic and resistance training), the onset of type 2 diabetes can be delayed by up to 58 percent.

SOURCE: Hamman et al., 2006.

DID YOU KNOW?

Diabetics who cannot control their blood glucose levels may have their driver's licence revoked. For more information, contact Diabetes Canada.

SOURCE: Diabetes Canada, 2012.

SYMPTOMS OF DIABETES

Some of the symptoms of diabetes that individuals experience include the following (Diabetes Canada, 2017g):

- unusual thirst
- frequent urination
- unusual weight loss or weight gain
- extreme fatigue or lack of energy
- blurred vision
- fruity odour on the breath (a sign of diabetic ketoacidosis)
- heavy or laboured breathing
- frequent or recurring infections
- cuts and bruises that are slow to heal
- tingling or numbness in hands or feet
- stupor or unconsciousness

Note: many people who have type 2 diabetes display no symptoms.

WHAT HAPPENS WHEN YOU ARE HYPOGLYCEMIC OR HYPERGLYCEMIC?

Insulin shock is another term used for the condition of hypoglycemia or low blood sugar. Symptoms include shakes, sweating, trembling, dizziness, irritability, confusion, blurred vision, and hunger. In severe cases, low blood sugar may cause you to pass out. It is common in diabetics who take too much insulin, skip meals, drink too much alcohol, and exercise too vigorously. Treatment includes providing the individual with something to ingest that contains a high amount of glucose; this will increase blood sugar levels adequately in order to improve mental status. Such treatment can include tablets made of glucose or dextrose (these can be obtained at health food stores), fruit juices such as orange juice or apple juice, milk, 100 millilitres of regular pop, or table sugar (10–15 grams or 2–3 teaspoons) with water. Bystanders should not try to administer fluids by mouth to someone who is unconscious, because this may cause the person to aspirate (inhale the fluid into the lungs, which can cause serious complications).

One of the most significant issues is unrecognized hypoglycemia, which may be disruptive to children's performance and participation in physical activity (Pacaud, 2002). This may lead to metabolic control problems. Education, regular monitoring, and lifestyle choices can help regulate metabolism.

Hyperglycemia is a condition caused by greater than normal glucose in the blood. This condition comes on slowly and can be brought on by circumstances such as taking too little insulin, eating too much food, or during stressful times or illness. Symptoms include increased thirst, frequent urination, dry mouth, nausea, vomiting, shortness of breath, and fatigue. Prolonged high levels can lead to ketoacidosis, which results when fat is used as the energy source rather than glucose, resulting in ketones (a chemical byproduct of the breakdown of fat) in the urine.

This is more common in type 1 diabetes, and can lead to serious dehydration and coma. In addition to the signs listed above, someone that is suffering from ketoacidosis will have a slightly sweet breath odour (which smells like nail-polish remover) (Diabetes Canada, 2007).

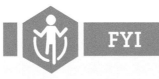

FYI

LOW BLOOD SUGAR

Someone with low blood sugar looks a lot like someone who is drunk or mentally incapacitated. They are not getting any sugar to their brain, and therefore cannot think or speak clearly. If you ever come across someone who is having trouble communicating, it might be a good idea to ask if they are diabetic and if you can, get them some sugar.

RISK FACTORS ASSOCIATED WITH DIABETES

Some of the risk factors for developing diabetes include the following (Diabetes Canada, 2017e):

- *Family history* The genetic link for type 2 diabetes is stronger than for type 1. Having a parent or sibling with the disease particularly increases the risk (Scott et al., 2013).

- *Age* Incidence increases with age—throughout childhood and adolescence for type 1, and after 40 years of age in adults for type 2.

- *Being overweight* A BMI greater than 27 indicates a risk for developing type 2 diabetes and other health problems, including cardiovascular disease and premature death. In Canada, 62 percent of adults and 31 percent of children and youth are overweight or obese (Diabetes Canada, 2016b).

- *Metabolic syndrome* Metabolic syndrome is a common condition characterized by a cluster of risk factors occurring together, including high fasting blood sugar, obesity around the waist, high triglycerides, low HDL-C (high density lipoprotein cholesterol), and high blood pressure. Individuals who carry most of their weight in the trunk of their bodies (apple-shaped bodies) tend to have a higher risk of diabetes than those of similar weight with pear-shaped bodies (excess fat carried mainly in the hips and thighs). A waist measurement of more than 102 centimetres (40 inches) in men, and 88 centimetres (35 inches) in women suggests an increased risk (Alberti et al., 2009).

- *Having a sedentary lifestyle* Lack of exercise and sitting for long periods of time can lead to being overweight, which increases the risk of diabetes and impedes glucose uptake. In Canada, only 22 percent of adults and

9 percent of children and youth are achieving the recommended level of physical activity (Diabetes Canada, 2015b).

- *Belonging to a high-risk group* Some populations are at higher risk of type 2 diabetes, such as those of South Asian, Asian, African, Hispanic, or Indigenous descent, those who are overweight, older, or have low income. Diabetes rates are three to five times higher in Indigenous peoples than in the general population, a situation compounded by barriers to care for Indigenous peoples (Canadian Diabetes Clinical Practice Guidelines Expert Committee, 2013). On Canadian Indigenous reserves, 74 percent of adults and 43 percent of children and youth are overweight or obese (Diabetes Canada, 2015b).

  Factors that pose a risk to Indigenous populations are lifestyle and heredity. The relatively recent shift from traditional diets high in animal protein to "modern urban diets" high in carbohydrates, combined with decreased physical activity and higher smoking rates has resulted in high levels of obesity that compound pre-existing risks for diabetes.

- *History of diabetes during pregnancy* Every year, between 3 percent and 20 percent of pregnant women across Canada develop gestational diabetes. After having gestational diabetes, and/or delivering a baby that weighs more than 4 kilograms (9 pounds), as many as 30 percent of women will develop type 2 diabetes within 15 years. (Diabetes Canada, 2017f).

- *Dyslipidemia (high cholesterol) or other fats in the blood* More than 40 percent of people with diabetes have abnormal levels of cholesterol and similar fatty substances that circulate in the blood. These abnormalities appear to be associated with an increased risk for cardiovascular disease.

- *Impaired glucose tolerance* If blood sugar control and reaction to sugar loads are abnormal, there is a higher risk of developing type 2 diabetes within five years and developing cardiovascular disease (Centers for Disease Control and Prevention, 2003).

- *High blood pressure* Up to 60 percent of people with undiagnosed diabetes have high blood pressure (Centers for Disease Control and Prevention, 2003).

- *Prediabetes* In this condition, blood sugar levels are higher than normal but not high enough to be classified as type 2 diabetes. Left untreated, prediabetes often progresses to type 2 diabetes.

- *Tobacco use* Tobacco use is an independent risk factor for type 2 diabetes. Smoking also accelerates the development of complications in people with diabetes. Higher rates of tobacco use occur in Atlantic Canada and among men, young adults, Indigenous groups, and lower-income earners (Diabetes Canada, 2015b). People who smoke 25 or more cigarettes daily have double the risk of type 2 diabetes over non-smokers, regardless of whether they have other risk factors (Zhang et al., 2011).

Refer to **assignment 9.1** at www.emond.ca/fitness5e and assess your risk for diabetes.

THE CHANGING FACE OF DIABETES IN CANADA
WHAT DOES THE FUTURE HOLD?

While the prevalence of diabetes in Ontario increased so much between 1995 and 2005 that it exceeded the predicted global rate set for 2030, the mortality rate fell by 25 percent in the same period (Lipscombe & Hux, 2007). This means that more people are living with the disease longer. Currently, one in four Canadians live with diabetes or prediabetes. If nothing is done to stem the tsunami, by 2020, it will be one in three (Diabetes Canada, 2009; see Diabetes, 2011a). With a further 7 million people developing diabetes each year, the rate is now expected to reach 438 million by 2030 (Diabetes Canada, 2015a).

The financial burden of diabetes and its complications is enormous. Diabetics have two to three times higher medical costs over their lifetime. The cost of medication and supplies can reach $15,000 a year. Of greater concern is the cost to the Canadian health-care system, predicted to reach $16.9 billion a year by 2020 for diabetic care and related complications (Diabetes Canada, 2015a). See Table 9.1.

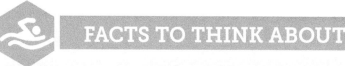

FACTS TO THINK ABOUT

DIABETES

- Diabetes is the sixth leading cause of death in Canada (Statistics Canada, 2015).

- Canada has the third-highest rate of mortality among 20 peer countries (behind Austria and the United States). Diabetes is a contributing factor in the deaths of approximately 41,500 Canadians each year. The gap between the death rates of diabetics and non-diabetics is greater in younger age groups.

- Mortality rates for adults aged 45–79 are two to three times higher for individuals with diabetes. Diabetic children ages 1 to 19 have about a ten-year reduction in life expectancy.

- Approximately 80 percent of people with diabetes will die as a result of heart disease or stroke.

- As age increases, so does prevalence of the disease, with more men being affected than women.

- In 2010, 185,430 Canadians were newly diagnosed with diabetes, translating into an incidence rate of 6.3 per 1,000 people–an equivalent of 1 person diagnosed every 3 minutes (PHAC, 2014).

- Notably, one in three people with diabetes don't know they have it. On average, people have diabetes for seven years before diagnosis.

- More than 9 million Canadians live with diabetes or prediabetes. With more than 20 people being newly diagnosed with the disease every hour of every day, chances are that diabetes affects you or someone you know.

SOURCES: Diabetes Canada, 2009; Health Canada, 2003; PHAC, 2009.

TABLE 9.1 Prevalence of Diabetes in Canada

KEY STATISTICS	2000	2006	2016	2026 ESTIMATED
Diabetes and pre-diabetic prevalent cases (rate)	1.2 million	9 million (21%)	11 million (29%)	13.9 million (33%)
Cost of diabetes to health-care system			$3.4 billion	$5 billion
2006 to 2016 estimated increase in diabetes prevalence		72%		
2016 to 2026: estimated increase in diabetes prevalence			41%	

SOURCES: Diabetes Canada, 2011a, 2015a, 2016b.

COMPLICATIONS ASSOCIATED WITH DIABETES

Long-term complications of diabetes develop gradually. The longer you have diabetes—and the less control you have over your blood sugars—the higher the risk of complications. Many aspects of quality of life may be affected by diabetes. Possible complications include (Diabetes Canada, 2016a, 2017b):

- *Depression* This condition is twice as common in people with diabetes as in the general population. About 25 percent of patients with diabetes have symptoms of depression, and major depression is present in at least 15 percent of those afflicted.

- *Heart disease and stroke* Compared to the general population, diabetics have cardiovascular problems at a younger age and die from these events at rates much higher than people without diabetes (three times higher for men and five times higher for women). In general, a 40-year-old diabetic has the same level of risk as a 50- to 55-year-old non-diabetic (Diabetes Canada, 2011a; Stone, Fitchett, Grover, Leawnchzuk, & Lin, 2013).

- *Digestive problems* These are relatively common among people with diabetes. Constipation affects 60 percent of diabetics. Diabetes is also linked to diarrhea, and is one of the most common causes of gastroparesis (delayed emptying of the stomach), which affects up to 75 percent of people with diabetes. Gastroparesis can cause bloating, loss of appetite, vomiting, dehydration, heartburn, nausea, an early feeling of fullness when eating, weight loss, erratic blood glucose levels, reflux, and spasms of the stomach wall.

- *Dental problems* Diabetes can contribute to dry mouth and a burning sensation on the tongue, which can lead to irritation of the lining of the mouth. If blood glucose levels are poorly managed, toothaches, bleeding of the gums, infection of the gum and bone tissues, and delayed healing responses may result.

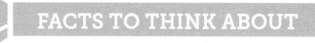

DIABETES COMPLICATIONS

Hospitalization data indicates that adults diagnosed with diabetes were also diagnosed with the following:

- 3 times the rate of hypertension
- 3 times the rate of ischemic heart disease
- 3 times the rate of stroke
- 4 times the rate of heart attacks/failure
- 6 times the rate of chronic kidney disease
- 20 times the rate of lower-limb amputation
- 12 times the rate of hospitalization for end-stage kidney disease
- 25 times more likely to become blind

SOURCES: Canadian Diabetes Clinical Practice Guidelines Expert Committee, 2013; Institute for Clinical Evaluative Sciences, 2003; PHAC, 2009, 2011; Thommann, Marks, & Adamczyk, 2001.

- *Compromised men's sexual health* Diabetes causes damage to the walls of the blood vessels, which affects circulation and blood flow. Fifty percent of men will experience erectile dysfunction (ED) within ten years of a diagnosis of diabetes. In fact, in up to 12 percent of men with diabetes, ED is the first sign that leads to the diagnosis of diabetes.

- *Thyroid disorders* Approximately one-third of people with type 1 diabetes have thyroid disease. The thyroid is a butterfly-shaped gland in the lower neck (just beneath the skin in the front of the windpipe) that regulates the body's metabolism. An overactive thyroid (hyperthyroidism) may increase insulin requirements, while an underactive thyroid (hypothyroidism) may decrease insulin requirements.

- *Diabetic retinopathy and other eye conditions* Diabetic retinopathy is the most common cause of blindness in people under age 65. About one in four people with diabetes experience this problem. Those who develop diabetes are also more likely to develop cataracts at a younger age and are twice as likely to develop glaucoma (increased intra-ocular pressure causing irreversible optic nerve damage). Nearly all people with type 1 diabetes and 60 percent of those with type 2 develop some form of diabetic retinopathy during the first 20 years they have the disease (Diabetes Canada, 2017b; PHAC, 2011). It is the leading cause of vision loss in Canadians under 50 (PHAC, 2011) and of adult blindness in Canada (Diabetes Canada, 2017b). Diabetes causes the arteries in the retina to weaken and begin to leak, forming dot-like hemorrhages. Vision may begin to blur, floaters (caused by blood leaking into the retina) may drift in front of the visual field, and eyesight may decrease. With abnormal vessel growth and scar tissue, some people develop retinal detachment (separation of the sensory and pigment layers) and glaucoma.

- *Neuropathy* Damage to sensory nerves of the extremities can affect the transmission of nerve impulses and lead to loss of sensation, making people more prone to injury. Numbness and tingling in the feet is often the first sign, though symptoms vary depending on the nerve(s) and the part of the body affected. Because of poor circulation, wounds heal slowly or ineffectively. Some people suffer from pressure sores. Gangrene and amputation are more common in people with this complication.

- *Skin infections* These include bacterial infections (styes, boils, folliculitis, carbuncles, and nail infections) caused by *Staphylococcus*, as well as yeast-like fungal infections between the fingers and toes, corners of the mouth, armpits, groin, and so on.

- *Diabetic foot* This complication manifests as infection in the skin, muscles, or bones of the foot, resulting in poor circulation and neuropathy. The diabetic's compromised immune system can lead to the loss of sensation in the foot, reduced blood circulation, poor wound healing, death of the tissue, severe infection, gangrene, and potential amputation. Approximately 15 percent of individuals with diabetes will develop foot ulceration at some point in their life (American Podiatric Medical Association, 2017), and a third of all leg amputations occur in people with diabetes (Canadian Institute for Health Information, 2013).

- *Diabetic nephropathy* This is the most common cause of chronic kidney failure, which accounted for 35 percent of all new kidney failure cases (PHAC, 2011). The kidneys lose the ability to filter out waste products, leading to a buildup of waste in the blood and, ultimately, end-stage kidney disease. Early intervention can prevent or delay the advance of diabetic kidney disease.

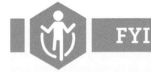

FYI

DIABETIC DERMOPATHY

Diabetic dermopathy, also known as shin spots or pigmented pretibial patches, is a skin condition usually found on the lower legs of people with diabetes. It is thought to result from changes in the small blood vessels that supply the skin and from minor leakage of blood products from these vessels into the skin. Many diabetics have problems with their feet, must keep them clean and dry, and must keep their toenails in good condition.

LIVING WITH DIABETES AND SHIFT WORK

The province of Ontario designates certain medical conditions as possible grounds for disqualification to be hired as a police constable, for example, dialysis dependence or insulin dependence. In the latter case, the applicant will be referred to a specialist to determine whether he or she meets the medical standards for driving (in accordance with the driving fitness guidelines of the CMA and Diabetes Canada). Those candidates who are non-insulin-treated diabetics and do not understand how to control insulin levels through diet, medication, and exercise may be considered ineligible as well. (To learn more about medical requirements for constables and special constables, refer to Ontario Association of Chiefs of Police, 2016, in the References.) Many of the other law enforcement agencies (Corrections, Canadian Border Services, Transport Canada Transportation Security, Fishery Officers, RCMP) must pass an Occupational Health Evaluation with the Treasury Board of Canada. Refer to each service's website for particulars.

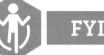

FYI

ONTARIO CORRECTIONAL OFFICER MEDICAL REQUIREMENTS

The following conditions would be considered as not meeting the bona fide occupational requirements for the position of a correctional officer (as of 2017):

Hearing: less than 15dB (500–4000Hz), corrected

Eye Sight:

- Distance Acuity (best, corrected): visual acuity at least 20/25 (6/7.5) with both eyes open and not less than 20/30 (6/9) with the better-seeing eye alone
- Near Acuity, 40 cm (best, corrected): visual acuity at least 20/25 (6/7.5) with both eyes open and not less than 20/25 (6/7.5) with each eye alone

Epilepsy: seizure in the last two years

Diabetes: brittle diabetics

For more information contact the Correctional Services Recruitment Unit. For Ontario Police medical requirements go to http://www.mcscs.jus.gov.on.ca/english/police_serv/const_select_sys/Self-Assess-MedicalRequirementsforCandidates/Self_Assess.html.

SOURCES: Streppel, Anthony, Manager Occupational Fitness, Crisis Response Training Ontario Correctional Services College (OCSC), Correctional Services Recruitment Unit (CSRU), Ministry of Community Safety and Correctional Services (personal communication, July 12, 2017).

Shift work can be hard on everyone, but it can be especially challenging for those with diabetes. Shift work can cause changes in appetite, weight loss or weight gain, and digestive problems like constipation, diarrhea, indigestion, and heartburn. When you eat and sleep at different times it affects how well your body can keep blood glucose levels at a healthy level. Mental and physical stress that sometimes comes with shift work might also affect your blood glucose levels. Shift work will increase your risk of a hypoglycemic incident. This pattern of work influences the body's circadian (daily) rhythms, which regulate processes such as hunger and fatigue, thus disrupting your body's internal clock and affecting blood glucose control from physical and mental stress.

It is the responsibility of the individual to be in control of their blood sugar and able to manage their diabetes sensibly. Putting a plan in place will help you deal effectively with diabetes and shift work (Diabetes Canada, 2017a; Diabetes UK, 2006; Eat Right Ontario, 2016):

- Prepare a written plan that you can share with your supervisor, including a medical plan and personal health identification.

- Wear personal health identification (such as a medical alert bracelet).

- Carry quick, easy-to-eat food and drinks that you can consume following a check of your blood glucose level.

- Have regularly planned meals. Snacking and strict adherence to certain mealtimes may not be as critical for people on regular, intermediate-acting, or premixed insulins; however, this approach is very important for somebody taking oral medications in place of injections. Avoid eating large meals during the night as this can lead to heartburn and constipation.

- Don't rely on vending machines, cafeterias, and fast food restaurants that don't offer healthy alternatives (and sell food and drinks high in fats and sugars). For example, a 355-mL soft drink contains approximately 40 grams (about 10 teaspoons) of sugar.

- Carry your blood glucose meter, and juice boxes or glucose tablets with you. When you are driving for work or operating machinery (such as on a bike, snowmobile, or water patrol), it is best that you check your levels every couple of hours to know how much insulin you need rather than risk a hypoglycemic reaction.

- Make sure everyone on your shift (specifically your partner) understands your condition and knows how to help you if needed. Show them where you keep your blood glucometer and sugar. Make sure they know the signs of low blood sugar and how to assist.

- Take regular active-rest breaks.

- Engage in regular physical activity. This is very important, especially if you are working the night shift.

- Manage your stress. Stress can increase your body's production of hormones that block the effects of insulin, causing your blood sugar to rise. As well, prolonged stress may lead to illness and depression.

If you are diabetic, Table 9.2 lists some simple guidelines that you can follow to control your blood sugar and reduce your risk of diabetes-related health complications.

TABLE 9.2 Managing your ABCDEs

ABCDEs	REDUCE YOUR RISK OF DIABETES-RELATED HEALTH PROBLEMS
A – A1C	Glucose control target is usually seven or less (A1C is a blood test that is an index of your average blood glucose level over the preceding 120 days).
B – Blood Pressure (BP)	Control your blood pressure (less than 130/80* mmHg). Limit intake of salt and alcohol.
C – Cholesterol	LDL (bad) cholesterol target is 2.0* mmol/L or less.
D – Drugs (prescribed heart medication)	Blood pressure pills (ACE inhibitors or ARBs), cholesterol-lowering pills (statins), Aspirin (prevents blood clots), Clopidogrel (blood thinner). Speak with your health-care team about medications to protect against heart attack or stroke.
E – Exercise	Regular physical activity, healthy diet, achievement and maintenance of a healthy body weight.* Exercise uses blood sugar for energy.
S – Smoking and Stress	Stop smoking and manage stress effectively.

*Discuss your target values with your health-care team.
Note that A1C targets for pregnant women, older adults, and children (under 12) are different.

SOURCES: Diabetes Canada, 2017c; NIDDK, n.d.; Type2Diabetes.com, 2017.

A couple of great resources for more information on managing your weight, alcohol intake, blood pressure, cholesterol, and nutritional concerns such as eating out, glycemic index, and basic carbohydrates, are Diabetes Canada at www.diabetes.ca and Eat Right Ontario at www.eatrightontario.ca.

Despite all the latest advancements in the treatment of diabetes, there are still complications that may preclude you from your career. Those who have foot problems may find it difficult to wear steel-toed boots on cold concrete for 12-hour shifts. Retinopathy may impair your vision, making it difficult to drive. Finally, shift rotation can be stressful. It is best to have shifts that rotate every two to three days and move "forward" (from morning to afternoon to night). The stress of shift work can be further compounded by adding court days to regular shifts.

Remember that *you* must take care of you. Research suggests that lifestyle and type 2 diabetes are closely linked. This means that you can help prevent or delay the onset of the disease. A healthy diet, weight control, exercise, and stress management are important preventive steps.

FINAL THOUGHTS

With early diagnosis, you can manage diabetes well. It is important that you learn as much about the disease as you can in order to make healthier life choices, and be sure to get tested every three years after you reach age 40.

You need to know what, when, and how much to eat to manage your blood sugar levels. You may need to add pills, insulin, or both to your lifestyle changes to achieve your blood glucose targets. You must also maintain a healthy weight, especially if you have type 2 diabetes. Exercise is known to lower blood sugar and enhance overall fitness. This will also help to keep your blood pressure at or below 130/80 and your cholesterol levels down.

Here are some additional suggestions to help prevent, delay, or manage diabetes:

- If you smoke, make a serious effort to quit.
- See an eye specialist on a regular basis to check for signs of eye disease.
- Exercise proper foot care, have your feet checked regularly by your physician, and keep your vaccinations up to date.
- Be nutritionally conscious when you are at work and home. You can find diabetes-friendly recipes on the website of Diabetes Canada (2017), or research the DASH (Dietary Approaches to Stop Hypertension) diet at the National Heart, Lung, and Blood Institute (n.d.) (see References).
- Speak to a specialist if you are feeling overwhelmed or depressed about how diabetes is negatively affecting you.
- If your extremities feel numb or if you experience "pins and needles," advise your physician.
- Have your urine tested regularly for early signs of kidney disease.
- Have your teeth cleaned twice a year.

Stay healthy by asking your doctor the right questions. Be a proactive patient who is informed.

KEY TERMS

diabetes
a chronic disease in which the body cannot properly use glucose for energy

gestational diabetes
a temporary condition in which hormonal changes associated with pregnancy and the growth demands of the fetus increase insulin needs to two to three times the normal level; generally occurs after the 24th week of pregnancy and resolves after delivery

glucose
a simple form of sugar that acts as fuel for the body

hyperglycemia
high blood sugar (glucose) levels

hypoglycemia
low blood sugar (glucose) levels

prediabetes
impaired fasting glucose or impaired glucose tolerance; refers to blood glucose levels that are consistently higher than normal but not over 7.0 mmol/L

type 1 diabetes
diabetes that occurs when the pancreas no longer produces insulin or produces very little

type 2 diabetes
diabetes that occurs when the pancreas cannot produce enough insulin or the body is unable to use the insulin effectively

EXERCISES

TRUE OR FALSE?

1. You can help prevent or delay type 2 diabetes.

2. By far the most common form of diabetes is type 2 diabetes mellitus.

3. Risk factors for type 1 diabetes mellitus include family history, obesity, inactivity, and being a member of a high-risk population.

4. Type 1 diabetes mellitus is caused by an autoimmune reaction that destroys the beta cells of the pancreas.

5. Type 2 diabetes mellitus was previously called juvenile-onset or insulin-dependent diabetes.

6. When a pregnant woman develops diabetes mellitus it is called gestational diabetes.

7. Babies born to mothers with gestational diabetes often exhibit excessive birth weight.

8. In type 2 diabetes mellitus the body tissues become less sensitive to the effects of insulin.

9. Blurred vision is a symptom of low blood sugar.

10. Type 1 diabetes can be prevented or delayed through weight loss and exercise.

MULTIPLE CHOICE

1. What symptom(s) may indicate that you should get checked for diabetes?
   a. your feet swell up
   b. you feel more energized than usual
   c. you may be extra thirsty and lose weight quickly
   d. you gain weight and are hungry
   e. you experience heart palpitations

2. How often should you test your blood glucose?
   a. it depends on the individual
   b. every 24 hours
   c. every couple of hours
   d. before you eat
   e. when you first get up and when you go to bed

3. What does diabetes have to do with your nerves?
   a. it makes them more aware of your surroundings
   b. it affects the transmission of nerve impulses
   c. it interferes with blood flow to the tissues
   d. it has nothing to do with your nerves
   e. it sends feedback to the brain

4. What is the greatest risk factor for diabetes?
   a. poor lifestyle choices
   b. ethnic background and genetic susceptibility
   c. eating too much sugar
   d. smoking and drinking
   e. exercising too much

5. What does diabetes have to do with erectile dysfunction?
   a. it is not involved in sexual dysfunction
   b. no one really understands the link
   c. nerve damage affects the blood flow to the penis
   d. it prevents the dysfunction
   e. blood flow to the groin is decreased

6. What does diabetes have to do with dental care?
   a. diabetes is unrelated to dental care
   b. diabetes can cause gum disease and teeth problems
   c. dentists want to be involved in your health care
   d. diabetes affects the alignment of your teeth
   e. diabetes medication promotes good dental health

7. What is diabetic ketoacidosis?
   a. the name of a diabetic research project
   b. a life-saving condition
   c. a form of indigestion caused by too much acid
   d. the breakdown of protein to use as an energy source in place of glucose
   e. the breakdown of fat to use as an energy source in place of glucose

8. What do diabetes pills do?
   a. they treat pancreas problems
   b. they help keep blood glucose in the target range
   c. they help to keep you regular
   d. they reduce pain
   e. they help digestive enzymes

9. How does diabetes affect your eyes?
   a. lack of insulin interferes with brain signals to the eyes
   b. lack of insulin reduces energy levels to the brain
   c. high blood glucose levels can damage blood vessels in the retina
   d. low blood glucose levels can cause cornea damage
   e. low blood glucose causes headaches behind the eyes

10. Who should check your blood glucose levels?
   a. only your doctor
   b. your doctor and a diabetic educator
   c. you
   d. you, your doctor, and a diabetic educator
   e. you don't have to check your levels outside of a medical checkup

11. How does diabetes affect your feet?
   a. it causes athlete's foot
   b. it causes feet to become very sweaty
   c. it causes blisters on the feet
   d. it affects the arch in your foot
   e. it causes nerve damage to the feet

12. Can children and young people develop type 2 diabetes?
   a. yes, but mostly adults develop type 2 diabetes
   b. yes, but they grow out of it
   c. no, only adults get type 2 diabetes
   d. no, because they exercise too much
   e. yes; children first develop type 1, which then becomes type 2

13. How does diabetes affect your kidneys?
   a. it affects the liver rather than the kidneys
   b. high blood glucose levels can affect the kidneys' filter system
   c. insulin gets blocked in the kidneys
   d. fat cells get blocked by the kidneys
   e. protein cells get blocked by the kidneys

14. Why is it important to check blood glucose levels with diabetes?
   a. regular checks don't change the condition of the disease
   b. regular checks ensure that blood glucose remains at a normal level
   c. regular checks ensure that you don't need to take insulin
   d. regular checks take your blood glucose levels down
   e. regular checks ensure you have enough fluids in your body

15. How is type 2 diabetes controlled?
   a. through insulin injections
   b. you don't need to do anything
   c. exercise and diet alone
   d. insulin, exercise, diet, and healthy lifestyle choices
   e. through a high carbohydrate diet

16. Which statement regarding prediabetes is incorrect?
    a. Prediabetes is a term for impaired fasting glucose or impaired glucose tolerance.
    b. More than 9 million Canadians live with diabetes or prediabetes.
    c. Symptoms show up quickly for those who develop prediabetes.
    d. Abdominal fat increases your risk of becoming prediabetic.
    e. Blood sugar levels are higher than normal but not high enough to be classified as type 2 diabetes.

17. If you have diabetes in your family, are you at risk?
    a. you definitely will get diabetes
    b. you aren't at any risk for diabetes
    c. if one person has diabetes, everyone will have diabetes
    d. you are at low risk for developing the disease
    e. you are at higher risk for developing the disease

18. What is neuropathy?
    a. sensory nerve damage
    b. the study of the brain
    c. nervous system surgery
    d. the study of kidney nerves
    e. the pathway of nerve transmissions

19. What signs might you see if someone is experiencing low blood glucose?
    a. the person is out of breath after a 1.5-mile run
    b. the person becomes emotional
    c. the person gets confused and may lose consciousness
    d. the person is not hungry
    e. the person can't do more than ten curl-ups

20. How do you know if you have type 2 diabetes?
    a. you are more thirsty than normal and have blurry vision
    b. you feel energetic but not very hungry
    c. a friend tells you that you have diabetes
    d. you are energetic and able to work out vigorously
    e. you are not thirsty after working out

SHORT ANSWER

1. What is the prevalence of diabetes in Canada?

2. Describe the difference between type 1 and type 2 diabetes.

3. Explain what prediabetes is and the impact it could have on your career.

4. What are five risk factors associated with type 2 diabetes?

5. What are five of the signs or symptoms of diabetes?

6. How does shift work affect diabetes?

7. Describe five ways to regulate your blood sugar levels.

8. What are three severe complications of diabetes?

9. How can you moderate diabetes risks?

REFERENCES

Alberti, K., Eckel, R.H., Grundy, S.M., et al. (2009). Harmonizing the metabolic syndrome. A joint interim statement of the International Diabetes Federation Task Force on Epidemiology and Prevention; National Heart, Lung and Blood Institute; American Heart Association; World Heart Association; International Atherosclerosis Society; and International Association for the Study of Obesity. *Circulation, 120*(16), 1640–1645. Retrieved from http://circ.ahajournals.org/content/120/16/1640.long

American Diabetes Association. (2007). Diagnosis and classification of diabetes mellitus. *Diabetes Care, 30,* 42–47.

American Podiatric Medical Association. (2017). Facts on diabetes and the foot. Retrieved from http://www.apma.org/Learn/FootHealth.cfm?ItemNumber=980

Billionnet, C., Mitanchez, D., Weill, A., Nizard, J., Alla, F., Hartemann, A., & Jacqueminet, S. (2017). Gestational diabetes and adverse perinatal outcomes from 716,152 births in France in 2012. *Diabetologia, 60,* 636. doi:10.1007/s00125-017-4206-6

Canadian Diabetes Association Clinical Practice Guidelines Expert Committee. (2013). Canadian Diabetes Association 2013 clinical practice guidelines for the prevention and management of diabetes in Canada. *Canadian Journal of Diabetes, 37*(suppl 1).

Canadian Institute for Health Information. (2013). *Compromised wounds in Canada.* Ottawa, ON: Author. Retrieved from https://secure.cihi.ca/free_products/AiB_Compromised_Wounds_EN.pdf

Centers for Disease Control and Prevention. (2003). National diabetes fact sheet: National estimates and general information on diabetes and prediabetes in the United States, 2003. Atlanta, GA: US Department of Health and Human Services.

Centers for Disease Control and Prevention. (2011). National diabetes fact sheet: National estimates and general information on diabetes and prediabetes in the United States, 2011. Atlanta, GA: US Department of Health and Human Services. Retrieved from http://diabetes.niddk.nih.gov/dm/pubs/statistics

Diabetes Canada. (2007). About diabetic ketoacidosis. Retrieved from http://www.diabetes.ca

Diabetes Canada. (2009). Economic tsunami: The cost of diabetes. Research report 2009, 7. Retrieved from http://www.diabetes.ca/publications-newsletters/advocacy-reports/economic-tsunami-the-cost-of-diabetes-in-canada

Diabetes Canada. (2011a). Diabetes: Canada at the tipping point—Charting a new path. Retrieved from https://www.diabetes.ca/CDA/media/documents/publications-and-newsletters/advocacy-reports/canada-at-the-tipping-point-english.pdf

Diabetes Canada. (2011b). Diabetes and you. What is diabetes? Retrieved from http://www.diabetes.ca/diabetes-and-you

Diabetes Canada. (2012). Driving & your rights. Retrieved from http://www.diabetes.ca/diabetes-and-you/know-your-rights/driving-your-rights

Diabetes Canada. (2015a). Diabetes statistics in Canada. Retrieved from http://www.diabetes.ca/how-you-can-help/advocate/why-federal-leadership-is-essential/diabetes-statistics-in-canada

Diabetes Canada. (2015b). *Report on Diabetes: Driving change.* Toronto, ON: CDA. Retrieved from https://www.diabetes.ca/getmedia/5a7070f0-77ad-41ad-9e95-ec1bc56ebf85/2015-report-on-diabetes-driving-change-english.pdf.aspx

Diabetes Canada. (2016a). *2016 Report on diabetes in Ontario.* Toronto, ON: CDA. Retrieved from http://www.diabetes.ca/getmedia/a45fe16a-3967-416c-bef5-d810f00ddb65/Diabetes-in-Ontario_FINAL.pdf.aspx

Diabetes Canada. (2016b). Diabetes in Canada. Retrieved from https://www.diabetes.ca/getmedia/513a0f6c-b1c9-4e56-a77c-6a492bf7350f/diabetes-charter-backgrounder-national-english.pdf.aspx

Diabetes Canada. (2017a). Diabetes & shift work. Retrieved from http://www.diabetes.ca/diabetes-and-you/healthy-living-resources/general-tips/diabetes-shift-work

Diabetes Canada. (2017b). Diabetes and you: Complications. Eye damage (diabetic retinopathy). Retrieved from http://www.diabetes.ca/diabetes-and-you/complications/eye-damage-diabetic-retinopathy

Diabetes Canada. (2017c). Heart disease and stroke. Retrieved from http://www.diabetes.ca/diabetes-and-you/complications/heart-disease-stroke

Diabetes Canada (2017d). Recipes. Retrieved from http://www.diabetes.ca/diabetes-and-you/recipes

Diabetes Canada. (2017e). Risk factors. Are you at risk? Retrieved from http://www.diabetes.ca/about-diabetes/risk-factors/are-you-at-risk

Diabetes Canada. (2017f). Risk factors. Mothers at risk. Retrieved from https://www.diabetes.ca/about-diabetes/risk-factors/mothers-at-risk

Diabetes Canada. (2017g). Signs and symptoms. Retrieved from http://www.diabetes.ca/about-diabetes/signs-and-symptoms

Diabetes.co.uk. (2017). Brittle diabetes (labile diabetes). Retrieved from http://www.diabetes.co.uk/brittle-diabetes.html

Diabetes UK. (2006). *Diabetes and the police officer: Guidance for the recruitment and employment of police officers with diabetes.* Retrieved from http://www.diabetes.org.uk/Documents/Reports/police_Guidance_FINAL.pdf

Eat Right Ontario. (2016). Retrieved from https://www.eatrightontario.ca/en/Diabetes.aspx

Hamman, R.F., Wing, R.R., Edelstein, S.L., et al. (2006). Effect of weight loss with lifestyle intervention on risk of diabetes. *Diabetes Care, 29*(9), 2102–2107.

Health Canada. (2000). *Diabetes among Aboriginal (First Nations, Inuit and Métis) people in Canada: The evidence.* Ottawa, ON: Author.

Health Canada. (2003). *Responding to the challenge of diabetes in Canada.* Catalogue no. H39-4/21-2003E. Ottawa, ON: Author.

Institute for Clinical Evaluative Sciences. (June 2003). Diabetes in Ontario: An ICES practice atlas. Retrieved from http://www.ices.on.ca/Publications/Atlases -and-Reports/2003/Diabetes-in-Ontario.aspx

Kruger, D.F., LaRue, S., & Estepa, P. (2015). Recognition of and steps to mitigate anxiety and fear of pain in injectable diabetes treatment. *Diabetes, Metabolic Syndrome and Obesity: Targets and Therapy, 8*, 49–56. http://doi.org/10.2147/DMSO.S71923

Lipscombe, L., & Hux, J. (2007). Trends in diabetes prevalence, incidence and mortality in Ontario, Canada 1995–2005: A population-based study. *Lancet, 369*(9563), 750–756.

National Heart, Lung, and Blood Institute. (n.d.). Healthy eating. [The DASH diet.] Retrieved from https://www .nhlbi.nih.gov/files/docs/public/heart/hbp_low.pdf

National Institute of Diabetes and Digestive and Kidney Disease (NIDDK). (n.d.) 4 Steps to manage your diabetes for life. Retrieved from https://www.niddk .nih.gov/health-information/diabetes/overview/ managing-diabetes/4-steps

Ontario Association of Chiefs of Police (OACP). (2016, December). Constable selection system: Self assess! Medical requirements for candidates. Retrieved from http://www.mcscs.jus.gov.on.ca/sites/default/files/ content/mcscs/docs/ec075034.pdf

Pacaud, D. (2002). Hypoglycemia: The Achilles heel of the treatment of children with type 1 diabetes. *Canadian Journal of Diabetes, 26*(3), 215–222.

Public Health Agency of Canada (PHAC). (2009). *Report from the National Diabetes Surveillance System: Diabetes in Canada, 2009.* Catalogue no. HP32-2/1-2009E-PDF. Ottawa, ON: Centre for Chronic Disease Prevention and Control.

Public Health Agency of Canada (PHAC). (2011). *Diabetes in Canada: Facts and figures from a public health perspective, 2011.* Catalogue no. HP35-25/2011E-PDF. Ottawa, ON: Author.

Public Health Agency of Canada (PHAC). (2014). Canadian Chronic Disease Surveillance System 1999/2000–2010/2011; open data [Internet]. Ottawa, ON: Author. Retrieved from http://open.canada.ca/ data/en/dataset/9525c8c0-554a-461b-a763 -f1657acb9c9d?_ga=2.173365987.155000125.14966 73554-1207302661.1493655802

Scott, R., Langenberg, C., Sharp, S., Franks, P., Rolandsson, O., Drogan, D., … Wareham, N. (2013). The link between family history and risk of type 2 diabetes is not explained by anthropometric, lifestyle or genetic risk factors: The EPIC-InterAct Study. *Diabetologia, 56*(1), 60–69. http://doi.org/10.1007/s00125-012-2715-x

Statistics Canada. (2015). Table 012-0561. Vital statistics—Death database. Ranking, number and percentage of death for the 10 leading causes of death in Canada, 2000, 2011 and 2012. Retrieved from http://www.statcan.gc.ca/pub/82-625-x/ 2015001/article/14296-eng.htm

Stone, J.A., Fitchett, D., Grover, S., Leawnchzuk, R., & Lin, P. (2013). Canadian Diabetes Association 2013 Clinical Practice Guidelines for the Prevention and Management of Diabetes in Canada: Vascular protection in people with diabetes. *Canadian Journal of Diabetes, 37*(suppl 1), S100–S104.

Thomann, K.H., Marks, E.S., & Adamczyk, D.T. (2001). Primary eye care in systemic disease. New York, NY: McGraw-Hill. Retrieved from http://www.cdc.gov/ diabetes/ndep/pdfs/ppod-guide-eye-care -professionals.pdf

Type2Diabetes.com. (2017). Learning the ABCDEs of diabetes. Retrieved from https://type2diabetes.com/ what-is-t2d/abcdes/

Zhang, L., Curhan, G.C., Hu, F.B., et al. (2011). Association between passive and active smoking and incident type 2 diabetes in women. *Diabetes Care, 34*, 892–897.

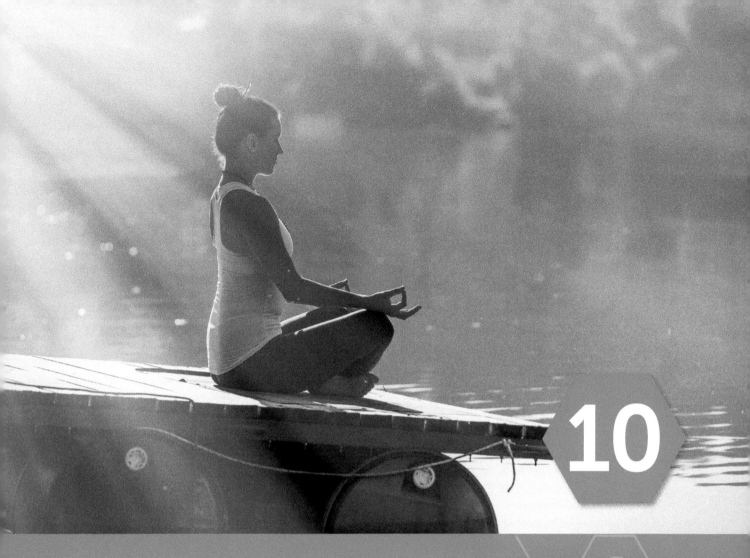

CARDIOVASCULAR DISEASE

LEARNING OUTCOMES

After completing this chapter, you should be able to:

- Comment on the impact of cardiovascular disease on Canadian society.

- Understand the basic anatomy of the heart and the etiology of various cardiovascular diseases.

- Describe four common cardiovascular diseases: arteriosclerosis, coronary heart disease, stroke, and hypertension.

- Describe the controllable and uncontrollable risk factors associated with cardiovascular diseases.

- List some of the signs and symptoms of heart attacks, strokes, and hypertension.

- Make appropriate health decisions regarding your heart.

The term *cardiovascular disease* (CVD) applies to any condition or disease of the circulatory system. Although much research—and media attention—has focused on diseases such as cancer, HIV/AIDS, and hepatitis B and C, cardiovascular disease was the leading cause of death in Canada until 2005 (Statistics Canada, 2011, p. 6) when it took second place to cancer. The four most common types of CVD are ischemic heart disease, myocardial infarction or heart attack, congestive heart failure, and cerebrovascular disease (Public Health Agency of Canada, 2016).

While mortality rates have declined in recent years, as of 2012, 25 percent of all deaths in Canada were due to cardiovascular disease and strokes combined (Statistics Canada, 2015a). Figure 10.1 shows the proportion of deaths attributable to the ten leading causes of death in Canada (Statistics Canada, 2015d). Mortality rates have dropped from 584 per 100,000 population in 1960 to 131 in 2009. The decline in mortality rates is attributed to medical advances, new pharmaceuticals, and reduction in major risk factors, such as a decline in tobacco use (Elmslie, 2012).

FIGURE 10.1   Top Ten Leading Causes of Death in Canada in 2011

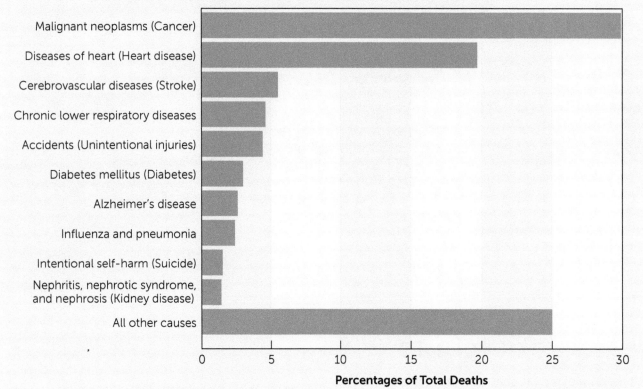

THE IMPACT ON OUR HEALTH-CARE SYSTEM

Here are some facts regarding health-care costs for cardiovascular diseases and strokes:

- Cardiovascular disease and strokes remain the number one causes of hospitalization in the country (CIHI, 2011).
- Three out of five Canadians adults have a chronic disease and heart and stroke diseases are in greater numbers in our older population.

- Treatment of chronic disease consumes 67 percent of all direct health-care costs, and costs the Canadian economy $190 billion annually—$68 billion is attributed to treatment and the remainder to lost productivity (Elmslie, 2012).

- High blood pressure or hypertension is the number one risk factor for stroke and a major risk factor in heart disease (risk factors are discussed later in the chapter). The prevalence of high blood pressure is trending upwards in Canada.

- In 2013, one in seven Canadians suffered from high blood pressure (Elmslie, 2012).

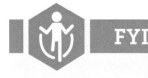

FYI

ON THE JOB

In the spring of 2002, the RCMP's "O" Division had its officers' blood cholesterol levels tested. Almost 50 percent of those tested had high LDL cholesterol readings. This finding had serious implications: combined with any other risk factors, high LDL cholesterol can be life threatening. The stresses of shift work, the lack of available nutritious foods on night shifts, and, for some officers, limited involvement in exercise programs—especially for those who live and work in isolated locations—can be a deadly combination. Nutrition and exercise was the focus in the 2000s while now the focus is more on wellness and resiliency (R. Seguin, RCMP "O" Division Fitness and Lifestyle Coordinator, personal communication, 2017). As an officer, you need to be aware of the risks associated with the career that you have chosen and make healthier choices to reduce your risks.

THE DEMOGRAPHICS OF THOSE WITH CARDIOVASCULAR DISEASE

Canadians run a high risk of developing cardiovascular diseases. We know that nine out of ten Canadians have at least one risk factor associated with cardiovascular disease (smoking, alcohol, physical inactivity, overweight or obesity, high blood pressure, high blood cholesterol, less than recommended daily consumption of vegetables and fruit, diabetes, stress). We've gone from one in ten Canadians having three or more risk factors in 2003, to two in five Canadians by 2009 (Government of Canada, 2017; HSFC, 2003; PHAC, 2009).

Cardiovascular disease is not restricted to elderly people. It is the number two killer for ages 25 to 64 years, the number five killer for ages 15 to 24 years, and the number six killer for ages 0 to 14 years (Statistics Canada, 2012).

Young people carry a high level of risk factors. Only 9 percent of Canadian youth aged 5 to 17 get the 60 minutes of heart-pumping activity they need each day. For those over 18 years old, 61.8 percent of men and 46.4 percent of women are either overweight or obese (Statistics Canada, 2015b). In 2014, 18.1 percent of Canadians aged 12 and older (21.4 percent of males and 14.8 percent of females) smoked cigarettes daily (Statistics Canada, 2015c).

Excessive weight gain during adolescence and young adulthood may be one of the most important determinants of future development of heart disease and stroke (Committee on Physical Activity and Physical Education in the School Environment; Food and Nutrition Board; Institute of Medicine, 2013). Dr. Douglas Lee and colleagues (2009), of the Institute for Clinical Evaluative Sciences, say projections suggest that the rising prevalence of obesity in the current generation of adolescents will increase the prevalence of coronary heart disease by 5 to 16 percent by 2035. Many cardiac rehabilitative exercise therapists are seeing increasing numbers of patients who are between 25 and 50 years of age (J. Pepe, CSEP Certified Exercise Physiologist, personal communication, 2017).

Income and education also affect the prevalence of cardiovascular diseases. Those with higher levels of education tend to have increased knowledge and skills to undertake healthier behaviours. Individuals who live in poverty, however, must cope with meeting basic needs, and their lack of income may limit their ability to purchase healthy foods, engage in physical activity, and acquire medications that can improve health problems such as high blood pressure and diabetes.

The gap between men and women in the prevalence and number of deaths from heart disease and stroke has reversed:

- More women than men are dying within a year after a cardiovascular event such as a heart attack or stroke: 38 percent of women compared to 25 percent of men (HSFC, 2016c; Statistics Canada, 2012; Women's Heart Foundation, 2007).

- If a woman becomes hypertensive, it increases the risk of cardiovascular disease by 2.5 times over that of a woman with normal blood pressure (PHAC, 2010).

- Women and men with high blood pressure at age 50 develop heart disease seven years earlier and die on average five years earlier than people with normal blood pressure at this age (Maas & Appelman, 2010).

- Combine hypertension, dyslipidemia, and obesity with diabetes, and the risk of developing cardiovascular disease becomes two to four times greater than that for women without diabetes (Centers for Disease Control and Prevention, 2011).

- Older women face the greatest danger because the risk of cardiovascular disease quadruples after menopause (Terry et al., 2005). At menopause, the ovaries gradually stop producing the heart-protective hormone estrogen. There may be an increase in LDL or "bad" cholesterol and triglyceride levels, and a decrease in HDL or "good" cholesterol. Blood pressure also starts creeping up. Reduced estrogen may lead to an increase in body fat above the waist, which affects the way blood clots and the way the body handles sugars (prediabetes).

- Although smoking is at its lowest level in more than four decades of monitoring smoking rates (Canadian Cancer Society, 2010; US Department of Health and Human Services, 2014), when combined with oral contraceptives there is an increased risk of blood clots and strokes in women (Stampfer, Hu, Manson, Rimm, & Willett, 2003; McGinley, Morales-Vidal, Biller, & Levine, 2015).

PERSONAL PERSPECTIVE

STROKES AND SMOKING

A few years ago, a female graduate at our college suffered a mild stroke. She was 21 years old. The doctors determined that smoking, social drinking, and taking birth control pills contributed to her stroke. With a strong will, she has struggled with regaining her speech and the use of her arm and foot.

We all need to understand that what we consume can directly affect our bodies. Statistics indicate that women smokers who use birth control pills are 10 to 20 times more likely to have heart attacks or strokes than non-smoking women (HSFC, 2006d).

Here are some self-help resources to assist you if you are a smoker and are interested in quitting:

- One Step at a Time: Canadian Cancer Society http://www.cancer.ca/en/support-and-services/resources/publications
- How to Quit Smoking: Ontario Lung Association http://www.lung.ca
- Tobacco: Public Health Agency of Canada http://www.phac-aspc.gc.ca/chn-rcs/tobacco-tabagisme-eng.php
- Physicians for a Smoke-Free Canada http://www.smoke-free.ca
- Government of Canada. You can quit smoking. We can help https://www.canada.ca/en/health-canada/services/smoking-tobacco/quit-smoking/tips-help-someone-quit-smoking/you-can-quit-smoking-we-can-help.html
- Quit Smoking Support http://www.quitsmokingsupport.com
- Quit 4 Life: Health Canada https://www.canada.ca/en/health-canada/services/health-concerns/tobacco/youth-zone/quit4life.html
- Stopsmoking http://www.ontario.ca/page/support-quit-smoking
- Women's Health Matters http://www.womenshealthmatters.ca

ANATOMY OF THE HEART

Located between your lungs, slightly to the left and behind your sternum, is your heart. It weighs between 200 and 425 grams and is about the size of your fist.

Your heart is designed to circulate blood. It pumps oxygen-rich blood to the rest of your body through a complex network of arteries, arterioles, and capillaries; deoxygenated (oxygen-poor) blood is carried back to the heart through the veins to send to the lungs to pick up oxygen and remove carbon dioxide.

HOW THE HEART FUNCTIONS

Your heart is a pump with four chambers. The two upper chambers are referred to as the left and right atria, and the lower ones are the left and right ventricles. Separating the left and right sides of the heart is a wall of muscle called the septum. There are four valves that separate each chamber and prevent the blood from coming back when the heart is at rest (see Figure 10.2).

In order to supply oxygen and nutrients to the rest of the body, oxygen-poor blood returns from the body through the superior and inferior vena cava to the right side of the heart through the right atrium to the right ventricle. From there the blood goes to the lungs through the pulmonary arteries to get rid of carbon dioxide and pick up oxygen. The oxygen-rich blood returns through the pulmonary veins to the left atrium and then the left ventricle pumps the blood to the rest of the body through the aorta.

DID YOU KNOW?

The average heart beats approximately 100,000 times a day, distributing about 7,200 litres (1,900 gallons) of blood. In your lifetime, it will beat approximately 2.5 billion times.

FIGURE 10.2 Diagram of the Heart

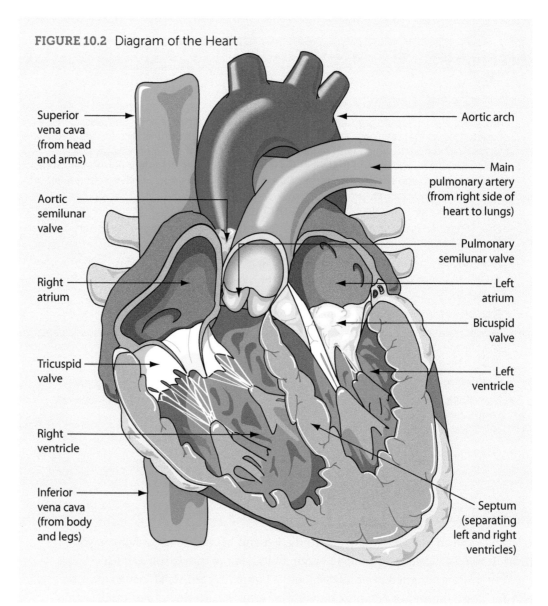

An electrical impulse starts each heartbeat and causes the atria to contract. The impulse begins in a group of cells called the sinoatrial node (SA node). This node is the pacemaker of the heart. The electrical impulse spreads across into the lower part of the heart, stimulating the atrioventricular node (AV node), which causes the ventricles to contract and send blood pumping out with great force.

The heart has its own blood vessels, called coronary arteries, which run along the outside of the heart muscle. The coronary arteries supply blood to the heart.

TYPES OF CARDIOVASCULAR DISEASE

Cardiovascular disease refers to diseases of the heart and blood vessels throughout the body. The remainder of this chapter examines four of them: arteriosclerosis/atherosclerosis, coronary heart disease, stroke, and hypertension. Ischemic heart disease is the condition in which blood flow and oxygen are restricted or reduced by narrowing of the coronary (heart) arteries (that specifically feed the heart).

ARTERIOSCLEROSIS/ATHEROSCLEROSIS

Arteriosclerosis is not a single disease but a group of ischemic cardiovascular diseases characterized by a narrowing or hardening of the arteries. In these diseases, blood flow to vital organs is restricted by a progressive blockage of the arteries.

Atherosclerosis is a common type of arteriosclerosis, a slow, progressive disease that may start in childhood, in which arterial blockage results from fatty deposits collecting in the arteries. The deposits are typically composed of cholesterol, cellular debris, fibrin (a clotting material in the blood), and calcium. Atherosclerosis is not restricted to one area of the body, although some areas may experience a greater degree of blockage than others. This buildup of deposits in the arteries is called plaque (see Figure 10.3). There are two types of plaque. Hard plaque causes the artery walls to thicken and harden. Soft plaque is more likely to break apart from the walls and enter the bloodstream, which can cause a blood clot that can partially or totally block the flow of blood in an artery. If this happens, the tissue past the blockage is deprived of blood and oxygen, and it may either die or suffer severe damage.

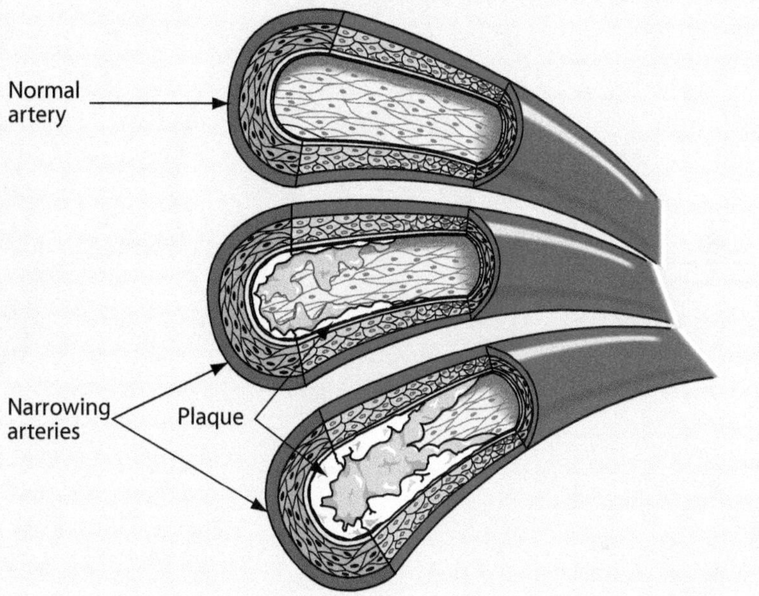

The causes of atherosclerosis are complicated. It is believed that the inner lining of the arteries becomes damaged and the body reacts by laying down the fatty deposits. Over time, the blood vessels become progressively thicker. High blood pressure, cholesterol, triglycerides in the blood, and smoking can contribute to the development of plaque.

FIGURE 10.3 Atherosclerosis: Cross-Sectional View of an Artery

Symptoms may not be apparent until the disease is far enough advanced to block a large part of the vessel. In the arteries of the heart (coronary arteries) it may cause angina (chest pain), and the blockage can lead to coronary heart disease. In the brain or carotid arteries (the two large arteries on either side of the head that carry blood to the brain), it can cause a stroke. Narrowed or blocked arteries may also cause problems in your intestines, kidneys, and legs.

CORONARY HEART DISEASE

Coronary heart disease, a type of ischemic cardiovascular disease, occurs when fatty deposits block one or more coronary arteries (arteries supplying the heart). When the blockage becomes severe enough to restrict the blood flow, insufficient oxygen reaches the heart and the person may experience angina, which may be infrequent or constant, depending on the severity of the restriction.

In the most extreme cases, no oxygen can get past the blockage. When this happens, a heart attack (myocardial infarction) occurs (see Figure 10.4). The cells past the blockage become damaged or die. The number of damaged and dead cells determines the seriousness of the attack—the greater the damage, the smaller the chance of recovery. Damage to the ventricles may cause the heart to quiver rapidly (ventricular fibrillation), preventing the heart from delivering oxygenated blood to other organs and tissues, especially the brain. Permanent brain damage can occur within five minutes if the heart does not resume pumping blood to the brain. Myocardial infarction may lead to cardiac arrest (the heart stops pumping).

FIGURE 10.4 Diagram of Myocardial Infarction (Heart Attack)

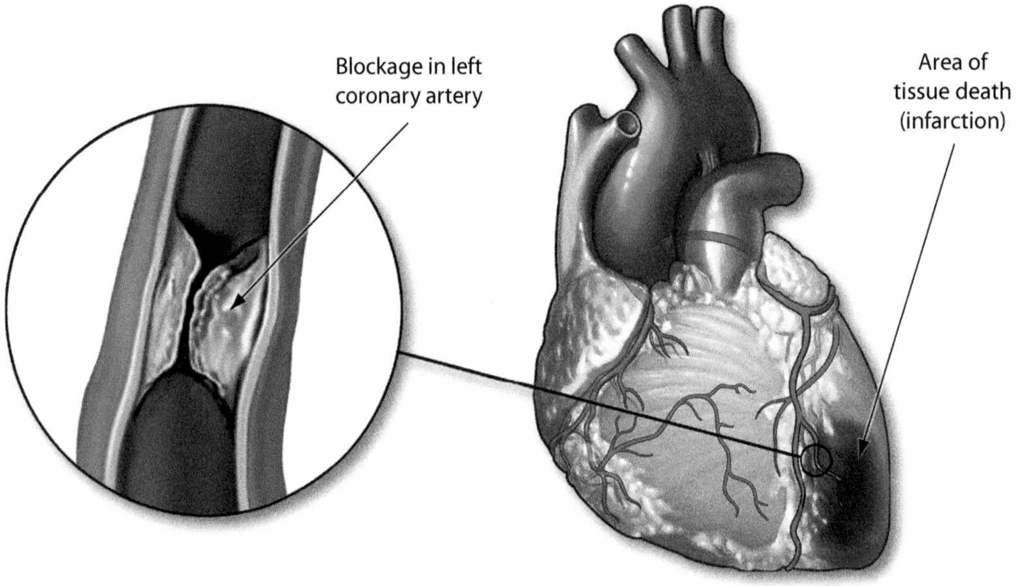

Blockage in left coronary artery

Area of tissue death (infarction)

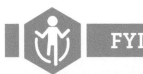

THE FRAMINGHAM HEART STUDY

The objective of the Framingham Heart Study, which began in 1948, was to identify the common factors or characteristics that contribute to cardiovascular disease by following its development over a long period of time in a large group of participants who had not yet developed overt symptoms of cardiovascular disease or suffered a heart attack or stroke. Researchers recruited men and women between the ages of 30 and 62 from the town of Framingham, Massachusetts, and began the first round of extensive physical examinations and lifestyle interviews, which they would later analyze for common patterns related to the development of cardiovascular disease.

Since the study's inception, the subjects have continued to return to Framingham every two years for a detailed medical history, physical examination, and laboratory tests. In fact, the third generation of these families is now being recruited and examined to understand how genetic factors relate to cardiovascular disease. This study, which has gone on for over six decades, is viewed throughout the world as pioneering research. It has led to identification of major CVD risk factors, as well as valuable information on blood pressure, blood cholesterol and triglyceride levels, age, gender, and psychosocial issues.

For more information about the study, go to http://www.framinghamheartstudy.org.

RECOGNIZING THE SIGNS OF A HEART ATTACK

Thousands of Canadians die from heart attacks each year because people do not recognize the signs and symptoms. These are not always sudden or severe. Quick recognition of the symptoms may reduce the severity of damage and prevent death. For some, a heart attack starts as muscular soreness or flu-like symptoms, but can progress to include those listed in Figure 10.5.

FIGURE 10.5 Recognizing the Signs and Symptoms of a Heart Attack

MEN...	WOMEN...
• Uncomfortable pressure, squeezing, fullness, or pain in the centre of the chest • Pain that spreads to the shoulders, neck, arms, teeth, or jaw • Lightheadedness, possible fainting • Pain that feels like heartburn • Sweating • Nausea or vomiting • Shortness of breath • A feeling of extreme anxiety and fear, or denial that anything is wrong	• Shortness of breath or difficulty breathing • Nausea, vomiting • Dizziness • Back or jaw pain • Unexplained anxiety • Palpitations, cold sweats, or paleness • Mild, flu-like symptoms • Inability to sleep • Unusual weakness, or fatigue
Trigger: Men most often report physical exertion prior to heart attacks	**Trigger:** Women most often report emotional stress prior to heart attacks

The majority of women (78 percent) experience at least one symptom for more than one month prior to their heart attack. Only 30 to 35 percent report the classical symptoms listed in the men's column (McSweeney et al., 2003; Roger et al., 2012). As well, some heart attack tests and treatments may not work as well for women as for men.

If emergency medical personnel reach a heart attack victim in time, they can administer medication to limit the damage and open up the coronary artery. If treatment occurs early enough, damage to the heart muscle is minimized, and the pumping ability of the undamaged tissue is not as greatly impaired, which means that the heart attack survivor is able to enjoy a higher quality of life. If left untreated, the dead or damaged areas of the heart muscle are replaced by scar tissue, which weakens the pumping action of the heart and can lead to heart failure and other complications. The heart may develop an arrhythmia (irregular heartbeat or rhythm), causing ventricular fibrillation. Survival rates are highest for those victims able to receive clot-busting medication within an hour of a heart attack.

For women, education (including the role of the mass media) about risks and symptoms, poverty, geography, women's roles and control over their lives, and equality of access to services needs to be addressed.

SURGICAL PROCEDURES FOR CARDIOVASCULAR DISEASES

Cardiac research really got a jump-start in the 1970s in Canada. In addition to life-style changes and medications, there are medical procedures that may be used to treat heart disease including:

- Coronary (balloon) angioplasty is a procedure in which a balloon-tipped catheter is insert into the artery and moved to the site of the blockage. It is expanded to open the clogged artery and improve blood flow. A stent (small metallic tube) is inserted to help keep the artery open. See Figure 10.6.

FIGURE 10.6 Balloon Angioplasty

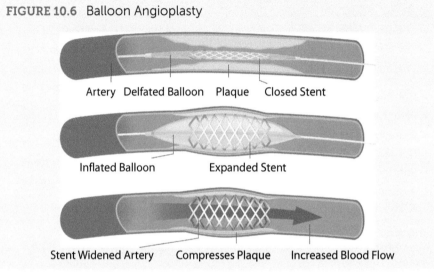

Artery   Delfated Balloon   Plaque   Closed Stent

Inflated Balloon   Expanded Stent

Stent Widened Artery   Compresses Plaque   Increased Blood Flow

- Coronary bypass surgery or coronary artery bypass graft (CABG) is the procedure used to replace the arteries that feed your heart. It involves taking arteries or veins from elsewhere in the body to create a detour or bypass around the blocked portion of the coronary artery. Bypass surgery doesn't cure the underlying heart disease but with lifestyle change and medication, it may reduce atherosclerosis and blood clot formation to help prevent another blockage and buy you some time. See Figure 10.7.

FIGURE 10.7 Coronary Artery Bypass Graft (CABG)

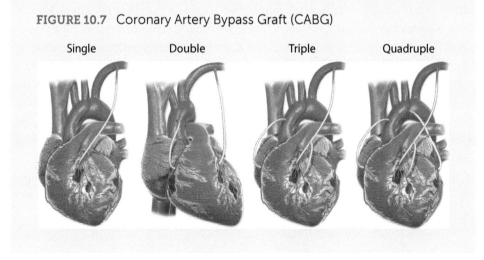

Single   Double   Triple   Quadruple

- A pacemaker is a small device that is placed in the chest or abdomen to help control abnormal heart rhythms (treat arrhythmias). This device uses low-energy electrical pulses to get the heart to beat at a normal rate. See Figure 10.8.

FIGURE 10.8 Pacemaker/ICD

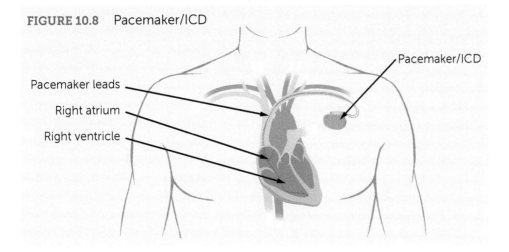

- In cases where a person suffers from abnormal arrhythmias, an implantable cardioverter defibrillator (ICD) may have to be implanted in the chest or abdomen. It uses electrical pulses or shocks to help control life-threatening arrhythmias, especially those that cause cardiac arrest. The size and implanted location is very similar to a pacemaker. See Figure 10.8 for location of a pacemaker and an ICD.

CARDIAC ARREST

Sudden cardiac arrest is a major cause of death in Canada. Each year, more than 45,000 Canadians suffer from a sudden cardiac arrest (Heart and Stroke Foundation of Manitoba, 2011). During cardiac arrest, the heart is not beating effectively and so death occurs within minutes after the heart stops due to lack of oxygen to the tissues, especially the brain. Arrhythmias, such as ventricular fibrillation, cause most sudden cardiac arrests. Ventricular fibrillation is a heart rhythm problem that occurs when the heart beats with rapid, erratic electrical impulses. This causes the pumping chambers in your heart (the ventricles) to quiver uselessly, instead of pumping blood through the heart.

The time between the onset of cardiac arrest and the performance of defibrillation is the major determinant for success in any resuscitation attempt. While cardiopulmonary resuscitation (CPR) is an emergency procedure that supports circulation and ventilation through chest compressions and artificial ventilation for a short period of time, it is unlikely to convert ventricular fibrillation to a normal heart rhythm. Early defibrillation is the intervention that is most likely to save lives. If the heart is not restarted within a few minutes, brain damage and death will occur. Of those who suffer a sudden cardiac arrest that happens out of the hospital (85 percent of cardiac arrests occur in public places or at home), fewer than one in ten people survive the trip to hospital because of delays in recognizing the cardiac emergency and gaining access to the appropriate care (Heart and Stroke Foundation of Canada, 2016a, 2016e).

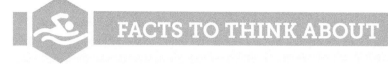

FACTS TO THINK ABOUT

CAUSES OF CARDIAC ARREST

Cardiac arrest is triggered by an electrical malfunction in the heart that causes an irregular heartbeat (arrhythmia). With the pumping action of the heart disrupted, the heart cannot pump blood to the brain, lungs, and other organs.

- Ventricular fibrillation—due to erratic impulses, the heart quivers uselessly, instead of pumping blood
- Coronary heart disease
- Myocardial infarction (heart attack)
- Congestive heart failure—a weakness of the heart that leads to a buildup of fluid in the lungs and surrounding body tissue
- Aortic stenosis (narrowing of the aortic valve in the heart)
- Cardiomyopathy (diseases of the heart)
- Myocarditis (inflammation of the heart)
- Respiratory arrest
- Choking
- Trauma
- Electrocution
- Drowning

An **automated external defibrillator (AED)** is a portable device the size of a laptop computer that checks the heart rhythm and can send an electric shock to the heart to try to restore a normal rhythm, aiding in rescuing people having sudden cardiac arrest. Once the machine's adhesive pads are attached to a victim, the AED analyzes the heart rhythm, advises the rescuer of the need for defibrillation, and prompts the rescuer to press a button to deliver a controlled shock, or series of shocks, as required, or tells the rescuer to keep administering CPR (Figure 10.9). Restoration of the rhythm requires defibrillation to be administered within a few minutes of the cardiac arrest. The use of external defibrillators with CPR within the first three minutes of cardiac arrest can increase the chance of survival by up to 75 percent (Weisfeldt et al., 2010). On average, early use of an AED defibrillation before emergency medical services arrives seems to nearly double a victim's odds of survival. Every minute that passes reduces the chances of survival by 7 to 10 percent and after more than 12 minutes of ventricular fibrillation (irregular, rapid, and chaotic firing of the ventricles), the survival rate is less than 5 percent (Hazinski, Markenson, & Neish, 2004).

Administering CPR before emergency personnel arrive, even in the absence of an AED, until advanced life support measures can be taken, increases the victim's likelihood of survival, and for this reason everyone should know CPR. The flow of oxygen to the brain can be sustained and the amount of permanent damage can be reduced.

FIGURE 10.9 AED Shocking Heart to Go from Ventricular Fibrillation to Sinus (Regular) Rhythm

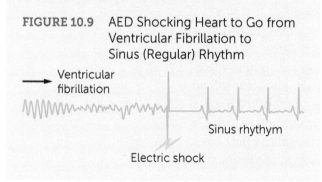

RISK FACTORS ASSOCIATED WITH CORONARY HEART DISEASE

Coronary heart disease risk factors are conditions or habits that raise your risk of coronary heart disease and heart attack. There are some risks that you cannot control, while others you can. On their own, one risk factor will not mean that you will have a disease, but in combination with others these risk factors will increase the chance of you suffering a cardiovascular event/disease.

UNCONTROLLABLE RISK FACTORS FOR CORONARY HEART DISEASE

The major uncontrollable risk factors for heart disease are the following:

- *Family history of coronary heart disease* Having a family history of cardiovascular disease appears to increase your risk significantly. If your father or brother had a heart attack before age 55, or if your mother or sister had one before age 65, you are more likely to get heart disease yourself.

- *Ethnicity* South Asians, Indigenous peoples (First Nations, Inuit, and Métis), and South Africans are at greater risk for hypertension and thus are at higher risk for cardiovascular disease. These groups may develop high blood pressure, diabetes, or heart disease earlier in life, and have a worse chance of surviving heart attacks (HSFC, 2016a).

- *Gender* Men have a greater risk of suffering cardiovascular disease in their younger years. Women catch up to men quickly after reaching menopause because the protection of female hormones is removed. Some women increase their risk before menopause if they smoke and take oral contraceptives.

- *Age* Your risk increases as you get older. The risk of coronary artery disease rises in men after the age of 45 and in women after the age of 55 (HSFC, 2017a).

FYI

LAW ENFORCEMENT EDUCATIONAL PROGRAMS

Many law enforcement agencies now offer educational programs to help officers assess their risk of developing coronary heart disease and to modify risky behaviours. Smoking-cessation programs, cholesterol assessments, blood pressure clinics, and the fitness pin award offered by the Police Fitness Personnel of Ontario are some of the initiatives that have been undertaken.

CONTROLLABLE RISK FACTORS FOR CORONARY HEART DISEASE

Here are some of the risk factors for coronary heart disease that you *can* control:

- *Smoking* Smoking poses the greatest risk for heart disease. Smokers increase their risk for cardiovascular disease by 70 percent. Exposure to second-hand smoke may increase the risk of cardiovascular disease by 25 to 30 percent (US Department of Health and Human Services, 2014).

There are two possible explanations: first is that carbon monoxide in cigarette smoke may cause a deficiency of oxygen in the body, causing the heart to work harder, and secondly nicotine and tar released in cigarette smoke cause damage to the blood vessel walls and allow cholesterol and plaque to build up.

- *Physical inactivity* Individuals who do not participate in moderate to vigorous physical activity increase their risk for cardiovascular disease. Exercise increases levels of "good" (HDL) cholesterol, improves serum lipids and blood pressure, helps people manage stress, and improves the efficiency of the heart, lungs, and muscles. Exercise also reduces body weight and risk of diabetes. Individuals who are having difficulty becoming physically active should seek professional assistance (such as a certified personal trainer), and those who have been diagnosed with heart disease or who have identified risk factors should seek professionally trained personnel who are familiar with these issues (such as a certified exercise physiologist).

- *High blood pressure* Defined as blood pressure greater than 140/90, high blood pressure is a major risk factor for stroke, coronary heart disease, peripheral vascular disease (including kidney disease), and congestive heart failure. We know that those who are overweight, are physically inactive, drink heavily, and consume excessive salt have a higher risk of developing high blood pressure. There is also a higher risk of metabolic cardiovascular risk factors, which include insulin resistance, obesity, hyperuricemia (an excess of uric acid in the blood, often producing gout), and dyslipidemia (an abnormal concentration of lipids or lipoproteins in the blood) (Kaur, 2014). A startling statistic is that one in three people with high blood pressure don't even know that they have it (Mozaffarian et al., 2015).

- *Diabetes* People with diabetes tend to have elevated blood fat levels and increased atherosclerosis. Because overweight individuals have an increased risk for diabetes, it becomes more difficult to differentiate the effects on cardiovascular disease. Cardiovascular disease is in fact the leading cause of death in diabetics. Diabetes increases the risk of high blood pressure, strokes, and heart and vascular diseases. There are also added risks of peripheral vascular disease, eye problems, and kidney disease. After the age of 50, the percentage of men with diabetes is higher than the percentage of women (HSFC, 2003).

- *Obesity* Being overweight puts additional strain on your entire body. If you are more than 13.5 kilograms (30 pounds) overweight, you are at higher risk for heart disease and stroke (HSFC, 2001). Your heart must work harder to push blood through extra capillaries that feed the excess fat and you are at higher risk for developing high blood pressure, high blood lipids, and diabetes, all of which put you at a high risk for cardiovascular or heart disease. Among individuals aged 18 to 64, being overweight (having a body mass index [BMI] of 25.0–29.9) or obese (BMI ≥ 30.0) is one of the most common factors that influences the development of high blood pressure and diabetes (Hall et al., 2014).

- *Stress* Depression, anxiety, and uncontrolled stress are growing risk factors (Cohen, Edmondson, & Kronish, 2015). As discussed in Chapter 12, people who have especially high stress levels are considered time bombs for a heart attack. When under stress, the body produces stress chemicals, which in turn increase blood pressure. Chronic hostility and aggression are two key personality factors related to the greatest risk.

- *Inadequate consumption of fruits and vegetables* As discussed in Chapter 8, *Canada's Food Guide* (Health Canada, 2012) recommends that everyone eat one dark green and one orange vegetable each day; choose vegetables and fruit prepared with little or no added fat, sugar, or salt; prepare vegetables by steaming, baking, or stir-frying, rather than deep-frying; and consume vegetables and fruit more often than juice. Fruits and vegetables are associated with reduced risk of cardiovascular diseases. They are important for intake of natural vitamins, antioxidants, and fibre. Potassium, which is present in many fruits and vegetables (for example, white beans, spinach, dried apricots, avocados, bananas, tomatoes, and sweet potatoes), has been shown to be protective, particularly against strokes, and might reduce risk of CVD (D'Elia, Barba, Cappuccio, & Strazzullo, 2011).

- *Sleep deprivation* Sleep deprivation (less than 5 hours) is now associated with a higher risk of hypertension in middle-aged adults (Cappuccio et al., 2007). Studies have shown that if you sleep less than 6 hours per night and have disturbed sleep, you stand a 48 percent greater chance of developing or dying from heart disease and a 15 percent greater chance of developing or dying from a stroke, because of the hormonal and chemical changes that take place in the body in the absence of sleep (Miller & Cappuccio, 2007).

- *High blood cholesterol* Abnormally elevated low-density lipoproteins (LDL) and triglycerides, and low levels of high-density lipoproteins (HDL) were linked to increased risk factors for developing vascular diseases, particularly coronary heart disease. However, there isn't clear supportive evidence for current cardiovascular guidelines to encourage high consumption of polyunsaturated fatty acids and low consumption of saturated fats (Chowdhury et al., 2014; Samis, 2016). Canada has never set an upper-limit guideline as there is no evidence-based research to show that saturated fats increase the risk for CVD. In 2015, the Heart and Stroke Foundation of Canada put out a position paper which supported the use of saturated fats through whole foods rather than processed foods which may contain high sugar content (Heart and Stroke Foundation, 2016d). There is proof regarding reducing trans fats as this fat raises LDL (bad) cholesterol and lowers HDL (good) cholesterol. One way to do this is by eating unprocessed foods (Samis, 2016).

STROKE

A **stroke** occurs when blood flow to an area in the brain is cut off. When this happens, brain cells begin to die from lack of oxygen and the parts of the body they control stop functioning. It is one of the leading causes of death in Canada. Over

50,000 people suffer a stroke in Canada each year, and 15 of every hundred die (HSFC, 2012). Of the survivors, only a third make a full recovery. Not only elderly people die from a stroke; in 2007, 10.3 percent of all stroke deaths occurred in people under age 65. For every 100,000 Canadian children under the age of 19, there are 6.7 childhood strokes (Statistics Canada, 2011).

TYPES OF STROKES

There are two main categories of strokes: ischemic and hemorrhagic (Table 10.1 and Figure 10.10). When you have a stroke, the brain cells and tissue past that point begin to die within minutes due to lack of oxygen and nutrients. The area where the tissue has died is called an *infarct*.

A transient ischemic attack (TIA), also known as a mini-stroke, occurs when the blood supply to the brain is temporarily interfered with. About 15,000 Canadians each year suffer a TIA. These attacks can last for seconds or hours and can happen for a variety of reasons. The clot may dissolve on its own or get dislodged so that it stops causing the symptoms. They usually do not cause permanent neurological damage and should be considered a warning sign of an impending stroke. People who have had a TIA are five times more likely than the general population to have a full-blown stroke within two years (HSFC, 2006c).

TABLE 10.1   Categories, Types, and Causes of Strokes

CATEGORY OF STROKE	TYPE OF STROKE	CAUSES
Ischemic stroke (about 87 percent of all strokes) • occurs when a blood vessel that supplies the brain becomes blocked or clogged, impairing the blood flow.	**Thrombotic stroke** (about 80 percent of all strokes)	• caused by a blood clot that develops in the blood vessels of the brain. • these are seen in older people with high cholesterol and atherosclerosis or diabetes.
	Embolic stroke	• caused by a blood clot or plaque debris that develops elsewhere in the body and travels through the bloodstream until it becomes stuck in the small blood vessels in the brain. • embolic strokes often result from heart disease or heart surgery.
Hemorrhagic stroke • occurs when a blood vessel in the brain ruptures and bleeds. • the tissues are deprived of oxygen and pressure builds up from the swelling, which can lead to further brain injuries.	**Intracerebral hemorrhage**	• result of bleeding from the blood vessels within the brain. • usually caused by hypertension (high blood pressure) and occur suddenly and rapidly.
	Subacrachnoid hemorrhage	• result of bleeding within the subarachnoid space (space between the brain and the membranes that cover them). • often caused by an **aneurysm** (excessive localized enlargement of an artery) or an **arteriovenous malformation** (a tangle of abnormal and poorly formed blood vessels (arteries and veins).

SOURCES: American Heart Association, 2017; American Stroke Association, 2017; Heart and Stroke Foundation of Canada, 2017b, 2017c.

FIGURE 10.10 Categories of Strokes

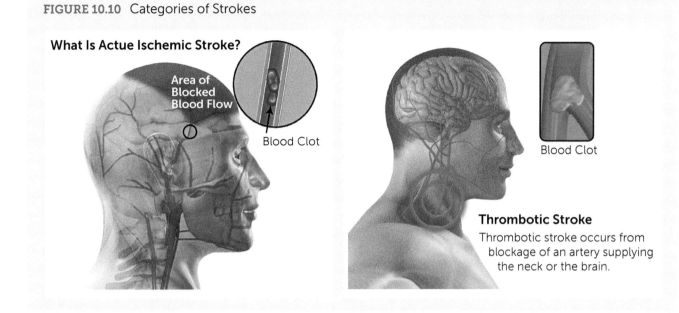

What Is Actue Ischemic Stroke?

Area of Blocked Blood Flow

Blood Clot

Blood Clot

Thrombotic Stroke
Thrombotic stroke occurs from blockage of an artery supplying the neck or the brain.

RECOGNIZING SIGNS OF A STROKE

The signs of a stroke are a medical emergency. Early recognition and treatment can sometimes reverse or prevent the effects of the stroke from getting worse. For an ischemic stroke, if the patient is given clot-busting drugs within three hours after symptoms start, it may prevent long-term effects from the stroke. See Table 10.2 for the ways to recognize the signs of someone having a stroke.

TABLE 10.2   FAST

F	FACE Ask the person to smile. Does one side of the face droop?
A	ARMS Ask the person to raise both arms. Does one arm drift downward?
S	SPEECH Ask the person to repeat a simple phrase. Is their speech slurred or strange?
T	TIME If you observe any of these signs, call 911 immediately.

SOURCES: American Heart Association, 2017; Health Canada, 2017c.

EFFECTS OF A STROKE

A stroke damages the brain and causes a sudden loss of brain function. Between one-third and two-thirds of stroke survivors will experience a loss of function in physical, cognitive, or communication skills that requires some form of rehabilitation (CIHI, 2009). Because your brain is divided into a number of sections, there are different effects for each. Figure 10.11 outlines the effects of a stroke, depending on its location.

DID YOU KNOW?
Strokes are the leading cause of disability in Canada and the third leading cause of death. For every minute of delay in treating a stroke, the average patient loses 1.9 million brain cells, 13.8 billion synapses, and 12 kilometres of axonal fibres (nerve fibres that conduct electrical impulses). A stroke survivor has a 20 percent chance of having another stroke within two years.

SOURCES: Cardiac Care Network of Ontario, 2016; Saver, 2006.

FIGURE 10.11 Effects of a Stroke

The effects of *right hemisphere strokes* include:

- weakness or paralysis on the left side of the body
- vision problems
- problems with depth perception, up and down, front and back
- inability to pick up objects, button a shirt, or tie a shoe
- inability to understand a map
- short-term memory loss
- forgetting or ignoring objects or people on your left side
- difficulty with judgment, including acting impulsively or not realizing your own limitations

The effects of *left hemisphere strokes* include:

- weakness or paralysis on the right side of the body
- trouble reading, talking, thinking, or doing math
- behaviour that is more slow and cautious than usual
- trouble learning or remembering new information
- requiring frequent instructions and feedback to finish tasks

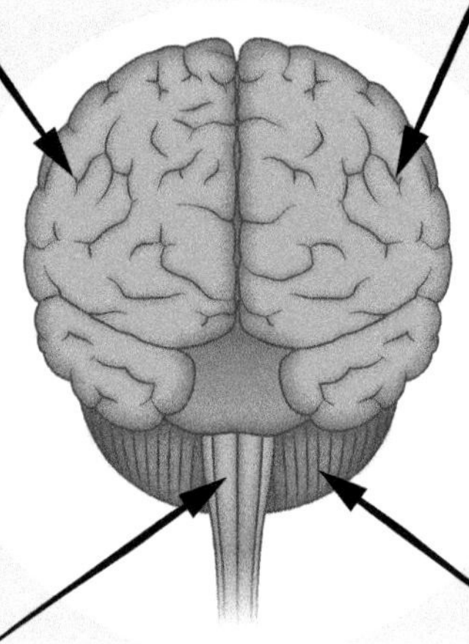

Brain stem strokes (at the base of brain), which are less common, include the following problems:

- difficulty with breathing and heart function
- body temperature control problems
- difficulties with balance and coordination
- weakness or paralysis of arms and legs on both sides of the body
- difficulty with chewing, swallowing, and speaking
- vision problems

Strokes in the cerebellum are also less common, but they have more severe effects, including:

- ataxia (inability to walk with coordination and balance)
- dizziness
- headache
- nausea and vomiting

PERSONAL PERSPECTIVE

NANCY: RECOGNIZING THE SIGNS OF A STROKE

In March 2017, my mother suffered from two transient ischemic attacks (TIA or mini strokes) and a stroke. In the case of the mini-strokes, she was sitting in a chair and failed to respond to my dad. When the clot had passed and the blood flow returned, she would insist that she was fine and that she didn't want my father calling an ambulance. Later in the month, she suffered a full stroke and my father, who recognized the signs and symptoms, called for the ambulance, getting her to the hospital and treatment so that she did not suffer from the physical effects of the stroke.

FACTS TO THINK ABOUT

STROKES

The severity of the stroke depends on factors such as:

- the type of stroke (ischemic or hemorrhagic)
- the side of the brain where the stroke occurred
- the lobes of the brain affected
- the size of the damaged area in the brain
- the body functions controlled by the affected area
- the amount of time the brain area had no blood flow
- the time it took to get to the hospital for treatment

THE RISK FACTORS FOR STROKE

As with heart attacks, there are risk factors for stroke that you cannot control, and others that you can.

UNCONTROLLABLE RISK FACTORS FOR STROKE

Risk factors for stroke that you *cannot* control include the following:

- *Age* Although strokes can occur at any age, most strokes occur in persons over 65.

- *Family history of stroke* Those with a parent or sibling who had a stroke before age 65 are at increased risk of having a stroke.

- *Ethnicity* Indigenous peoples and those of African or South Asian descent are more likely to have high blood pressure and diabetes, putting them at higher risk for strokes.

- *Gender* Until menopause, women have lower risk of stroke than men. After that, women take the lead.

- *Prior stroke or TIA* If you have had a previous stroke or a TIA, your risk is greater for another stroke.

- *Socio-economic status* Lower socio-economic levels increase the risk of a stroke due to poorer nutritional intake.

CONTROLLABLE RISK FACTORS FOR STROKE

Risk factors for stroke that you *can* control include the following:

- *High blood pressure* High blood pressure affects one in five Canadians and is the number one risk factor for stroke. Blood pressure that is consistently more than 140/90 is considered high, but if you are diabetic, 130/80 is high (Diabetes Canada, 2017; Leung et al., 2016). With high blood pressure, there is an increased risk of burst blood vessels, resulting in a stroke.

- *Smoking* Smoking, whether primary or second-hand, can contribute to plaque buildup in your arteries and increase the risk of blood clots, doubling the risk of an ischemic stroke (HSFC, 2006d).

- *High blood cholesterol* Increased levels of LDL cholesterol build up plaque in your arteries causing atherosclerosis, which can lead to a blockage in the brain.

- *Obesity* Those who carry extra weight are more at risk to suffer from high blood pressure, which places a great strain on the blood vessels of the brain.

- *Physical inactivity* Those who do not stay physically active increase their risk of unhealthy weight, high blood pressure, high cholesterol, and higher stress levels.

- *Excessive alcohol consumption* Those who drink too much alcohol can increase their blood pressure, which can lead to a stroke. A meta-analysis published in the *Journal of the American Medical Association* concluded that heavy alcohol consumption increases the relative risk of stroke, while light or moderate alcohol consumption may be protective against total and ischemic stroke (Reynolds et al., 2003).

- *Stress* Stress releases hormones that increase blood pressure and blood cholesterol, which leads to atherosclerosis.

- *Heart disease—atrial fibrillation* Atrial fibrillation affects approximately 200,000 to 250,000 Canadians. It is estimated that up to 15 percent of all strokes are due to atrial fibrillation. Caused by high blood pressure, atrial fibrillation can cause blood clots to form, leading to strokes (HSFC, 2006a).

- *Tumour, an infection, or brain swelling due to an injury or illness* In rare cases these can cause a stroke. Some people have irregularities in their arteries at birth that can cause a stroke later in life.

For information on treatments and rehabilitation of stroke patients go to Heart and Stroke Foundation of Canada at http://ww.heartandstroke.ca or Canadian Partnership for Stroke Recovery at http://www.canadianstroke.ca/en/.

Refer to **assignment 10.1** at www.emond.ca/fitness5e and assess your risk for cardiovascular disease.

HYPERTENSION

Hypertension (high blood pressure) is estimated to be the leading determinate of morbidity and mortality worldwide (Lim et al., 2010). It can narrow and block arteries, as well as strain and weaken the body's organs by placing too much pressure against your blood vessels as it circulates through the body, leading to health problems. Specifically, hypertension is a significant risk factor for a variety of cardiovascular diseases and kidney failure, including myocardial infarction, stroke, atherosclerosis, aortic aneurysm, hypertensive heart disease, heart failure, peripheral artery disease, and end-stage renal disease (Campbell et al., 2012; Rahimi, Emdin, & MacMahon, 2015). It also is related to dementia and sexual problems.

Known as the "silent killer," this health risk can be prevented by following an appropriate lifestyle that is relatively easy to manage. Most often, high blood pressure does not have symptoms and if people do not check their blood pressure regularly, there is no way to be sure that it is within a healthy range. In 2016, 7.5 million people in Canada lived with high blood pressure. Despite recent achievements, one in three people with hypertension have uncontrolled blood pressure (which means lifestyle and diet changes won't help and they must rely on medication) (Hypertension Prevention and Control, 2016).

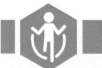

FYI

THE DASH EATING PLAN

The DASH (Dietary Approaches to Stop Hypertension) Eating Plan, supported through the National Heart, Lung, and Blood Institute (2012), was developed as an eating plan that is low in sodium, saturated fat, cholesterol, and total fat. It emphasizes fruits, vegetables, whole grain products, fish, poultry, nuts, and fat-free or low-fat milk and milk products that are rich in potassium, magnesium, and calcium, along with protein and fibre. It is a diet that limits the consumption of red meats, sweets, added sugars, and sugar-containing beverages. The emphasis of this diet is to lower blood pressure and decrease the risks of cardiovascular disease and diabetes. It also stresses losing weight, exercising regularly, and limiting consumption of alcohol. For more information about this plan, see US Department of Health and Human Services (2006, in the References).

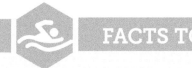

FACTS TO THINK ABOUT

BLOOD PRESSURE

We measure blood pressure using two numbers (e.g., 116/76 millimetres of mercury [mmHg]). The first number is the systolic pressure, which varies dramatically throughout the day depending on factors such as stress, exercise, diet, and sleep. The second number is the diastolic pressure, which stays pretty consistent throughout the day.

FIGURE 10.12 Effects of a Stroke

What Does My Blood Pressure Reading Mean?

Systolic Blood Pressure is the top (higher) number that measures arterial pressure when the heart beats measured in millimetres of mercury (mmHg).

Diastolic Blood Pressure is the bottom (lower) number that measures arterial pressure when the heart is at rest between beats in millimetres of mercury (mmHg).

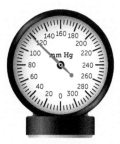

Blood Pressure Category	Systolic mmHg		Diastolic mmHg
Normal Blood Pressure	≤ 120	and	≤ 80
Prehypertension	120–139	or	80–89
High Blood Pressure (Mild Hypertension) Stage 1	140–159	or	90–99
High Blood Pressure (Moderate Hypertension) Stage 2	160–179	or	100–109
High Blood Pressure (Severe Hypertension) Stage 3	≥ 180	or	≥ 90

CAUSES OF HYPERTENSION

There are two forms of high blood pressure: essential (or primary) and secondary. Essential hypertension is a common condition that accounts for 90 to 95 percent of hypertension and originates within the body and is not a result of disease. Secondary hypertension develops as the result of disease and accounts for approximately 5 percent of cases. Table 10.3 lists the risk factors of hypertension.

TABLE 10.3   Risk Factors of High Blood Pressure

Essential Hypertension (linked to genetics, poor diet, lack of exercise, obesity)	• family history of hypertension. • gender (men are more likely to have hypertension at a younger age, but women's risk increases significantly after menopause). • age (more often in people over 35). • ethnicity (the risk is higher for South Asians, Indigenous peoples, and blacks than for whites). • obesity (if you are 20 percent or more above your ideal body weight, your blood must pump through more body tissue to supply necessary oxygen and nutrients, therefore increasing the pressure). • smoking (nicotine causes blood vessels to constrict, and other chemicals in burning tobacco damage the lining of the arteries). • high levels of salt or sodium in your diet. • heavy alcohol consumption (raises blood pressure by interfering with the flow to and from the heart). • use of oral contraceptives (hormonal supplements may increase blood pressure, and this tendency increases with age [over 35], obesity, and smoking). • physical inactivity (the less fit you are, the faster your heart pumps). • stress (your reaction to stress can cause elevated blood pressure).
Secondary Hypertension (develops as a result of disease, such as abnormalities of the kidneys, adrenal gland tumours, some congenital heart defects, pregnancy, and certain medications)	• narrowing of the renal arteries, which causes hypertension in the kidneys. • tumours of the adrenal glands (glands that sit right on top of the kidneys), which can cause other conditions, such as hyperaldosteronism, Cushing's syndrome, and pheochromocytoma. • coarctation of the aorta (a rare hereditary disorder characterized by the narrowing of the aorta above the renal arteries, causing lack of sufficient blood flow to the kidneys and influencing the release of a number of hormones to boost blood pressure to the kidneys). • pregnancy and pre-eclampsia (commonly called toxemia), an increase in blood pressure that can lead to kidney damage, convulsions, and coma in the mother, as well as eye or brain damage in the fetus. • metabolic syndrome and obesity, which characteristically exhibit insulin resistance, hyperinsulinemia and volume congestion, relative elevated heart rates, and cardiac outputs.

It is important to have regular checkups with your doctor to ensure that your blood pressure is normal and your general health is good. If you have high blood pressure, you will not be able to perform a BFOR test (see Chapter 1 and the Appendix) without medical clearance. Because the test is a means of screening for law enforcement recruits, you should be aware of your blood pressure.

Some people experience "white coat syndrome"—elevated blood pressure that is caused by anxiety about the tester who is taking your blood pressure or anxiety over the result of the test. For those people, it is important to understand what blood pressure is and to have their blood pressure tested repeatedly. Some individuals who are being tested for a BFOR and require medical clearance will bring documentation from a doctor.

REDUCING THE RISKS OF A CARDIOVASCULAR EVENT

By taking ownership of your health and well-being, you can significantly reduce your risk of heart attack and stroke.

The Heart and Stroke Foundation (HSFC, 2016a) makes the following recommendations:

- Have your blood pressure taken by a health-care professional at least once every two years and discuss your readings together. You can self-test at your local drug store to monitor your blood pressure on a more regular basis. If it is above the high–normal ranges make an appointment to talk to your health-care professional. Make sure to bring in the readings that you have been monitoring.

- Exercise. Be physically active for 30 to 60 minutes every day of the week, four to seven times a week. You need to work at an intensity of 70 to 85 percent (see Chapter 5 for more information).

- Maintain a healthy weight. If you are overweight, losing about 5 kilograms (11 pounds) may help you get within a healthy range (see Chapter 7).

- Choose foods such as fruits, vegetables, and whole grains, and those lower in saturated and trans fats and salt. Limit fast foods, canned foods, and prepared foods (especially those high in salt, sugar, saturated and trans fats) (see Chapter 8). Eat potassium-rich foods to help reduce blood pressure in those who are not high risk for hyperkalemia (Anderson et al., 2016). Reduce your intake of sugars, especially if you are diabetic.

- Reduce your intake of sodium. The goal of the Sodium Reduction Strategy for Canada (Sodium Working Group, 2010) is to reduce sodium intake to no more than 2,300 milligrams (less than a teaspoon of salt) per day by 2016. Read labels and limit the amount of salt you add while cooking and eating. Eat foods with less than 120 mg of sodium and choose not to eat foods with 360+ mg of sodium. Use less sauces on your food.

- Try to limit or quit smoking.

- Reduce consumption of alcohol. Follow the Canadian low-risk drinking guidelines (two or fewer standard drinks per day, with consumption not exceeding 14 standard drinks per week for men and 9 standard drinks per week for non-pregnant women).

- Avoid medication that increases blood pressure, which may put you at risk for stroke. Check with your doctor and/or pharmacist before taking medication if you are unsure.

- Make sure to follow your physician's directions around lifestyle changes and medication if you have cardiovascular disease, diabetes, truncal obesity (high amounts of abdominal fat), or abnormally high LDL cholesterol levels.

- Reduce your stress (see Chapter 12).

- Those with symptoms may consider surgical intervention (such as carotid stenting, which is the opening of the carotid arteries to allow better blood flow to the brain).

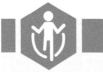

FYI

FURTHER INFORMATION

Further information on cardiovascular disease is available from the website of the Heart and Stroke Foundation of Canada (http://www.heartandstroke.ca) and through the local offices of the Ontario Heart and Stroke Foundation. The following topics might be of special interest to you or your family:

- blood clots
- aneurysms
- congestive heart failure
- congenital heart defects
- stress testing
- surgical procedures (including intrauterine surgery to correct heart defects before birth)
- drug therapy
- pacemakers

FINAL THOUGHTS

Although heart health is tied to heredity and diet, it is also linked to your lifestyle choices. You ultimately have the choice to ensure you keep your heart healthy throughout your lifetime. Make sure to eat healthy, manage your blood sugars and blood pressure, reduce your stress, and get enough exercise to ensure you maintain a healthy weight to reduce your chances of suffering from cardiovascular diseases.

KEY TERMS

aneurysm
a weak or thin area in a blood vessel that causes it to expand and fill with blood; aneurysms may occur as a result of a disease, an injury, or a congenital abnormality in the vessel

angina
severe chest pains associated with advanced cases of coronary heart disease

arrhythmia
irregular heartbeat or rhythm

arteriosclerosis
a blanket term for a group of ischemic cardiovascular diseases characterized by a narrowing or hardening of the arteries

arteriovenous malformation
a malformation of the blood vessels of the brain, usually present at birth; an AVM can increase the risk of stroke

atherosclerosis
a common type of arteriosclerosis; a slow, progressive disease in which arterial blockage results from fatty deposits collecting in the arteries

automated external defibrillator (AED)
a portable device the size of a laptop computer that checks the heart rhythm and can send an electric shock to the heart to try to restore a normal rhythm, aiding in rescuing people having sudden cardiac arrest

cardiac arrest
the heart stops pumping

cardiopulmonary resuscitation (CPR)
an emergency procedure that supports circulation and ventilation through chest compressions and artificial ventilation for a short period of time

coronary heart disease
a type of ischemic heart disease in which fatty deposits block one or more coronary arteries (arteries supplying the heart)

embolic stroke
a stroke caused by a blood clot or plaque debris that develops elsewhere in the body and travels through the bloodstream until it becomes stuck in the blood vessel in the brain

hemorrhagic stroke
a stroke that occurs when a blood vessel in the brain ruptures and bleeds

hypertension
high blood pressure—the term "essential hypertension" is used for cases in which the cause is unknown

intracerebral hemorrhage
bleeding in the brain resulting from the rupture of a blood vessel

ischemic heart disease
blockage of the coronary arteries resulting in lack of oxygen, angina, and dyspnea

ischemic stroke
occurs when a blood vessel that supplies the brain becomes blocked or clogged, impairing the blood flow

myocardial infarction
a heart attack

stroke
paralysis and a sudden loss of consciousness caused by an interruption of blood flow to the brain; a thrombotic or thromboembolic stroke occurs when blood flow is interrupted by a blood clot that travels to the brain; a hemorrhagic stroke occurs when very high blood pressure causes a weakened blood vessel near the brain to break

subarachnoid hemorrhage
hemorrhage that occurs when a blood vessel on the surface of the brain bleeds into the space between the brain and the skull

thrombotic stroke
stroke caused by a blood clot that develops in the blood vessels of the brain

transient ischemic attack (TIA)
a temporary interference with the blood supply to the brain

EXERCISES

MULTIPLE CHOICE

1. The condition where artery walls become thickened, hard, and non-elastic is
   a. arteriosclerosis
   b. atherosclerosis
   c. coronary embolism
   d. coronary thrombosis
   e. high blood pressure

2. Which of the following are considered controllable risk factors for heart disease?
   a. family history of heart disease, stress, obesity
   b. gender, high blood pressure, obesity
   c. inactivity, gender, high blood pressure
   d. high cholesterol levels, stress, inactivity
   e. diabetes, family history of heart disease, obesity

3. Which of the following is considered a major risk factor for heart disease that you can change?
   a. age
   b. gender
   c. family history
   d. genetics
   e. smoking

4. A myocardial infarction is caused by
   a. high blood pressure
   b. diabetes
   c. a clot in the brain
   d. weakness in the heart muscle
   e. a blockage in one of the coronary arteries

5. What is the main benefit of good blood supply and circulation in the coronary arteries?
   a. they strengthen heart valves by moving more blood through the heart
   b. they nourish the heart
   c. they help to prevent blood pooling in the lower limbs
   d. they increase blood pressure in the heart

6. Which of the following lifestyle practices may help control or prevent hypertension?
   a. maintaining a healthy body weight
   b. exercising regularly
   c. not drinking alcohol, or doing so only in moderation
   d. practising stress management
   e. all of the above

7. A stroke can be caused by
   a. a blood clot in the coronary artery
   b. a severe headache
   c. a blood clot in the brain
   d. a blood clot in the leg
   e. hardening of the arteries

8. Atherosclerosis is a term for
   a. angina
   b. myocardial infarction
   c. plaque buildup in the arteries
   d. hardening of the arteries
   e. blood clot

9. High blood pressure is, most directly, a measure of
   a. potential pain
   b. heart stress
   c. pressure within blood vessels
   d. cholesterol levels
   e. advanced aging

10. AED stands for
    a. arterial external defibrillator
    b. automated energy device
    c. arterial emergency dialysis
    d. automated external defibrillator
    e. atrial emergency device

11. The two upper chambers of the heart are called the
    a. atria
    b. ventricles
    c. aortic valves
    d. sinoatrial nodes
    e. aortic branches

12. The two lower chambers of the heart are called the
    a. atria
    b. ventricles
    c. aortic valves
    d. sinoatrial nodes
    e. aortic branches

13. A cardiac arrest is when
    a. you suffer a heart attack
    b. you suffer from angina
    c. plaque forms in your heart, leading to a clot blocking an artery
    d. your heart stops
    e. you suffer an aneurysm of the aorta

14. The upper limit of high–normal blood pressure, which is considered a moderate risk of CVD is
    a. 120/80
    b. 160/110
    c. 140/90
    d. 139/89
    e. 150/100

15. The reduction in oxygen flow to the heart causing chest pain is known as
    a. ischemia
    b. angina
    c. arrhythmia
    d. myocardial infarction
    e. atrial fibrillation

16. An irregular heartbeat is called
    a. tachycardia
    b. fibrillation
    c. arrhythmia
    d. bradycardia
    e. atrial flutter

17. Which of the following risk factors for cardiovascular disease is uncontrollable?
    a. heredity
    b. smoking
    c. physical inactivity
    d. drinking
    e. consuming large quantities of fat

18. Which of the following risk factors for cardiovascular disease is controllable?
    a. gender
    b. age
    c. high cholesterol level
    d. family history
    e. ethnicity

19. A mild form of a stroke, leaving only temporary symptoms, is called a(n)
    a. embolism
    b. thrombosis
    c. subarachnoid hematoma
    d. transient ischemic attack
    e. atrial flutter

20. Premenopausal women may have lower rates of heart attacks compared with men due to
    a. pregnancy
    b. the ability to cope with stress
    c. hormone replacement therapy
    d. eating better
    e. estrogen

21. Normal blood pressure is considered to be
    a. 120/90
    b. 120/80
    c. 130/90
    d. 130/80
    e. 110/60

22. Hypertension is known as the silent killer because
    a. people don't know how to take their blood pressure
    b. people don't pay attention to the symptoms
    c. people are unaware that they have high blood pressure
    d. people don't understand what their blood pressure means
    e. people ignore their symptoms in order to do things they want to do

SHORT ANSWER

1. What is arteriosclerosis? What is atherosclerosis?

2. What is coronary heart disease?

3. What are some possible signs of a heart attack?

4. How does hypertension affect the heart and arteries?

5. What special concerns surround women and cardiovascular disease?

6. Drawing on what you have learned so far, list five ways that people can lower their risk of cardiovascular disease. Include explanations of how these lower the risk.

7. What causes strokes?

8. What are the typical symptoms of an impending stroke?

9. Why is hypertension known as the silent killer?

10. Describe four different types of cardiovascular diseases.

11. Why is it important to learn about CPR and how to use an AED?

REFERENCES

American Heart Association. (2017). Warning signs. Retrieved from http://www.strokeassociation.org/STROKEORG/WarningSigns/Stroke-Warning-Signs-and-Symptoms_UCM_308528_SubHomePage.jsp

American Stroke Association. (2017). Types of strokes. Retrieved from http://www.strokeassociation.org/STROKEORG/AboutStroke/TypesofStroke/Types-of-Stroke_UCM_308531_SubHomePage.jsp

Anderson et al. (2016). Canadian Cardiovascular Society guidelines for the management of dyslipidemia for the prevention of cardiovascular disease in the adult. *Canadian Journal of Cardiology, 32*(11), 1263–1282. Retrieved from http://dx.doi.org/10.1016/j.cjca.2016.07.510

Campbell, N., Young, E., Drouin, D., Legowski, B., Adams, M.A., Farrell, J., … Tobe, S. (2011). A framework for discussion on how to improve prevention, management and control of hypertension in Canada. *Canadian Journal of Cardiology, 28*, 262–269.

Canadian Cancer Society. (2010). *Canadian cancer statistics 2010*. Toronto: Author.

Canadian Institute for Health Information (CIHI). (2009). *Factors predicting discharge home from inpatient rehabilitation after stroke*. Analysis in brief. Retrieved from https://secure.cihi.ca/estore/productFamily .htm?pf=PFC1334&lang=en&media=0

Canadian Institute of Health Information (CIHI). (2011). *A snapshot of health care in Canada as demonstrated by top 10 lists, 2011*. Ottawa: Author. Retrieved from https://secure.cihi.ca/free_products/Top10ReportEN -Web.pdf

Cappuccio F.P., Stranges, S., Kandala, N., Miller, M.A., Taggart, F.M., Kumari, M., … Marmot, M.G. (2007). Gender-specific associations of short sleep duration with prevalent and incident hypertension. The Whitehall II study. *Hypertension, 50*, 694–701.

Cardiac Care Network of Ontario. (2016). Stroke stats & facts. Retrieved from http://ontariostrokenetwork.ca/ information-about-stroke/stroke-stats-and-facts/

Centers for Disease Control and Prevention. (2011). *National diabetes fact sheet: National estimates and general information on diabetes and prediabetes in the United States, 2011*. Atlanta: US Department of Health and Human Services.

Chowdhury R., Warnakula, S., Kunutsor, S., Crowe, F., Ward, H.A., Johnson, L., … Di Angelantonio, E. (2014). Association of dietary, circulating, and supplement fatty acids with coronary risk: A systematic review and meta-analysis. *Annals of Internal Medicine, 160*(6), 398–406.

Cohen, B.E., Edmondson, D., I.M., & Kronish, I.M. (2015). State of the Art Review: Depression, stress, anxiety, and cardiovascular disease. *American Journal of Hypertension, 28*(11), 1295–1302. doi: 10.1093/ajh/ hpv047

Committee on Physical Activity and Physical Education in the School Environment; Food and Nutrition Board; Institute of Medicine. (2013). Physical activity and physical education: Relationship to growth development and health. Washington, D.C. National Academies Press (U.S.).

D'Elia, L., Barba, G., Cappuccio, F.P., & Strazzullo, P. (2011). Potassium intake, stroke and cardiovascular disease a met analysis of prospective studies. *Journal of the American College of Cardiology, 57*(10), 1210-1219.

Diabetes Canada. (2017). High blood pressure. Retrieved from https://www.diabetes.ca/diabetes-and-you/ complications/high-blood-pressure

Elmslie, K. (2012). *Against the growing burden of disease*. Ottawa: Centre for Chronic Disease Prevention, Public Health Agency of Canada. Retrieved from http://www.ccgh-csih.ca/assets/Elmslie.pdf

Government of Canada. Heart disease–heart health. (2017). Retrieved from https://www.canada.ca/en/ public-health/services/diseases/heart-disease-heart-health.html

Hall, M.E., do Carmo, J.M., da Silva, A.A., Juncos, L.A., Wang, Z., & Hall, J.E. (2014). Obesity, hypertension, and chronic kidney disease. *International Journal of Nephrology and Renovascular Disease, 7*, 75–88. http://doi.org/10.2147/IJNRD.S39739

Hazinski, M.R., Markenson, D., & Neish, S. (2004). American Heart Association Scientific Statement: Response to cardiac arrest and selected life-threatening medical emergencies. *Circulation, 109*, 278–291.

Health Canada. (2010). Sodium reduction strategy for Canada. Cat.: H164-121/2010E. Retrieved from http://www.hc-sc.gc.ca/fn-an/nutrition/sodium/ related-info-connexe/strateg/reduct-strat-eng.php

Health Canada. (2012). Start your new year right by following Canada's food guide. Retrieved from http://www.hc-sc.gc.ca/ahc-asc/media/advisories -avis/_2012/2012_01-eng.php

Heart and Stroke Foundation of Canada (HSFC). (2001). Risk factors. Retrieved from http://www .heartandstroke.ca

Heart and Stroke Foundation of Canada (HSFC). (2003, May). *The growing burden of heart disease and stroke in Canada*. Ottawa: Author.

Heart and Stroke Foundation of Canada (HSFC). (2006a). Heart disease—Atrial fibrillation. Retrieved from http://www.heartandstroke.ca

Heart and Stroke Foundation of Canada (HSFC). (2006b). Ischemic stroke & TIA (mini-stroke). Retrieved from http://www.heartandstroke.ca

Heart and Stroke Foundation of Canada (HSFC). (2006c). Mini strokes: What you need to know! Retrieved from http://www.heartandstroke.ca

Heart and Stroke Foundation of Canada (HSFC). (2006d). Smoking, heart disease and stroke. Retrieved from http://www.heartandstroke.ca

Heart and Stroke Foundation of Canada (HSFC). (2012). Statistics. Retrieved from http://www.heartandstroke.ca

Heart and Stroke Foundation of Canada (HSFC). (2016a). Heart risk and prevention. Retrieved from https://www.heartandstroke.ca/heart/risk-and-prevention

Heart and Stroke Foundation of Canada (HSFC). (2016b). High blood pressure. Retrieved from https://www.heartandstroke.ca/heart/risk-and-prevention/condition-risk-factors/high-blood-pressure

Heart and Stroke Foundation of Canada (HSFC). (2016c). Know any women. Then you need to know this. Retrieved from http://www.heartandstroke.ca/articles/know-any-women

Heart and Stroke Foundation of Canada (HSFC). (2016d). Saturated fat and your health. Retrieved from http://blog.heartandstroke.ca/2015/09/saturated-fat-and-your-health/ - respond

Heart and Stroke Foundation of Canada (HSFC). (2016e). What is cardiac arrest? Retrieved from https://www.heartandstroke.ca/heart/conditions

Heart and Stroke Foundation of Canada (2017a). Risk factors you cannot change. Retrieved from http://www.heartandstroke.ca/heart/risk-and-prevention/risk-factors-you-cannot-change

Heart and Stroke Foundation of Canada (2017b). Stroke/ Signs of stroke. Retrieved from https://www.heartandstroke.ca/stroke/signs-of-stroke

Heart and Stroke Foundation of Canada (2017c). What is a stroke? Retrieved from http://www.heartandstroke.ca/stroke/what-is-stroke

Heart and Stroke Foundation of Manitoba. (2011, October). Automated external defibrillators (AEDs)—Getting started. http://www.heartandstroke.mb.ca/site/c.lgLSIVOyGpF/b.3674275/k.F274/Automated_External_Defibrillators_AEDs.htm

Hypertension Prevention and Control. (2016). Hypertension in Canada fact sheet. Retrieved from http://www.hypertensiontalk.com/wp-content/uploads/2016/05/HTN-Fact-Sheet-2016_FINAL.pdf

Kaur, J. (2014). A comprehensive review on metabolic syndrome. *Cardiology Research and Practice, 2014*, 943162. Retrieved from http://doi.org/10.1155/2014/943162

Lee, D.S., Chiu, M., Manuel, D.G., Tu, K., Wang, X., Austin, P.C., ... Tu, J.V. (2009). Trends in risk factors for cardiovascular disease in Canada: Temporal, socio-demographic and geographic factors. *Canadian Medical Association Journal, 181*, 3–4. doi:10.1503/cmaj.081629

Leung, A.A., Nerenberg, K., Daskalopoulou, S.S., McBrien, K., Zarnke, K.B., Dasgupta, K., ... CHEP Guidelines Task Force. (2016). Hypertension Canada's 2016 CHEP Guidelines for blood pressure measurement, diagnosis, assessment of risk, prevention and treatment of hypertension. *Canadian Journal of Cardiology, 32*, 569–588. doi: 10.1016/j.cjca.2016.02.066

Lim, S.S., Vos, T., Flaxma, A.D., Danaei, G., Shibuya, K., Adair-Rohani, H., ... Memish, Z.A. (2010). A comparative risk assessment of burden of disease and injury attributable to 67 risk factors and risk factor clusters in 21 regions, 1990–2010: A systematic analysis for the Global Burden of Disease Study. *Lancet, 380*, 2224–2260.

Maas, A.H.E.M., & Appelman, Y.E.A. (2010). Gender differences in coronary heart disease. *Netherlands Heart Journal, 18*(12), 598–602.

McGinley, M., Morales-Vidal, S., Biller, J., & Levine, S. (2015). Hormonal contraception and stroke. *MedLink Neurology, September 2015*.

McSweeney, J., Cody, M., O'Sullivan, P., Elberson, K., Moser, D., & Garvin, B.J. (2003). Women's early warning symptoms of acute myocardial infarction. *Circulation, 108*, 2619–2623.

Miller, M.A., & Cappuccio, F.P. (2007). Inflammation, sleep, obesity and cardiovascular disease. *Current Vascular Pharmacology, 5*(2), 93–102.

Mozaffarian, D., et al. (2015). Heart disease and stroke statistics—2015 update: A report from the American Heart Association. American Heart Association Statistics Committee and Stroke Statistics Subcommittee. *Circulation*, e29–322.

National Heart, Lung, and Blood Institute. (2012). What is heart failure? Retrieved from http://www.nhlbi.nih.gov/health/health-topics/topics/hf

Public Health Agency of Canada (PHAC). (2009). *Tracking heart disease and stroke in Canada*. Retrieved from http://www.phac-aspc.gc.ca/publicat/2009/cvd-avc/index-eng.php

Public Health Agency of Canada (PHAC). (2010). Hypertension facts and figures. Retrieved from http://www.phac-aspc.gc.ca/cd-mc/cvd-mcv/hypertension_figures-eng.php

Public Health Agency of Canada (PHAC). (2016). Chronic disease and injury indicator framework. Edition 2016, using data from the Canadian Community Health Survey 2014. Retrieved from http://infobase.phac-aspc.gc.ca/cdiif/

Rahimi, K., Emdin, C.A., & MacMahon, S. (2015). The epidemiology of blood pressure and its worldwide management. Hypertension Compendium. *Circulation, 116*, 925–936.

Reynolds K., Lewis, B., Nolen, J.D.L., Kinney, G.L., Sathya, B., & He, J. (2003). Alcohol consumption and risk of stroke: A meta-analysis. *Journal of the American Medical Association, 289*, 579–588.

Roger V.L. et al. (2012). Heart disease and stroke statistics —2012 update: A report from the American Heart Association. *Circulation, 125*(1), e2–220. Retrieved from http://circ.ahajournals.org/content/125/1/e2.short?rss=1&ssource=mfr

Samis, A. (2016). Saturated fats and cardiovascular disease: Then and now webcast. Dairy Nutrition and Health Symposium 2016—November 8, 2016, Toronto, Ontario. Retrieved from https://webcast2016.dairynutrition.ca

Saver, J.L. (2006). Time is brain—Quantified. *Stroke, 37*, 263–266.

Sodium Working Group. (2010, July). *Sodium reduction strategy for Canada. Recommendations of the Sodium Working Group*. Retrieved from http://www.hc-sc.gc.ca/fn-an/nutrition/sodium/related-info-connexe/strateg/reduct-strat-eng.php

Stampfer, M.J., Hu, F.B., Manson, J.E., Rimm, E.B., & Willett, W.C. (2003). Primary prevention of coronary heart disease in women through diet and lifestyles. *New England Journal of Medicine, 343*, 16–22.

Statistics Canada. (2011). *Mortality, summary list of causes, 2008*. Catalogue no. 84F0209XWE. Retrieved from http://www.statcan.gc.ca/pub/84f0209x/84f0209x2008000-eng.pdf

Statistics Canada. (2012). Leading causes of death in Canada. Catalogue no. 84-215-X. Retrieved from http://www5.statcan.gc.ca/olc-cel/olc.action?ObjId=84-215-X&ObjType=2&lang=en&limit=0

Statistics Canada. (2015a). High blood pressure. Catalogue no. 82-625-X. Retrieved from http://www.statcan.gc.ca/pub/82-625-x/2015001/article/14184-eng.htm

Statistics Canada. (2015b). Overweight and obese adults (self-reported), 2014. Catalogue no. 82-625-X. Retrieved from http://www.statcan.gc.ca/pub/82-625-x/2015001/article/14185-eng.htm

Statistics Canada. (2015c). Smoking, 2014. Catalogue no. 82-625-X. Retrieved from http://www.statcan.gc.ca/pub/82-625-x/2015001/article/14190-eng.htm

Statistics Canada. (2015d). The 10 leading causes of death, 2011. Vital Statistics Death database, CANSIM Table 102-0561. Retrieved from http://www.statcan.gc.ca/pub/82-625-x/2014001/article/11896-eng.htm

Terry, D.F., Pencina, M.J., Vasan, R.S., Murabito, J.M., Wolf, P.A., Hayes, M.K., … Benjamin, E.J. (2005). Cardiovascular risk factors predictive for survival and morbidity-free survival in the oldest-old Framingham Heart Study participants. *Journal of the American Geriatric Society, 53*, 1944–1950.

US Department of Health and Human Services. (2006). *Your guide to lowering your blood pressure with DASH*. NIH publication no. 06-4082. Washington, DC: National Institutes of Health and National Heart, Lung, and Blood Institute. Retrieved from http://www.nhlbi.nih.gov/health/public/heart/hbp/dash/new_dash.pdf

US Department of Health and Human Services (2014). Let's make the next generation TOBACCO-FREE: Your guide to the 50th anniversary Surgeon General's Report on Smoking and Health. Retrieved from https://www.surgeongeneral.gov/library/reports/50-years-of-progress/consumer-guide.pdf

Weisfeldt, M.L., Sitlani, C.M., Ornato, J.P., Rea, T., Aufderheide, T.P., Davis, D., … ROC Investigators. (2010). Survival after application of automatic external defibrillators before arrival of the emergency medical system: Evaluation in the resuscitation outcomes consortium population of 21 million. *Journal of the American College of Cardiology, 55*, 1713–1720.

Women's Heart Foundation. (2007). Women and heart disease facts. Retrieved from http://www.womensheart.org/content/heartdisease/heart_disease_facts.asp

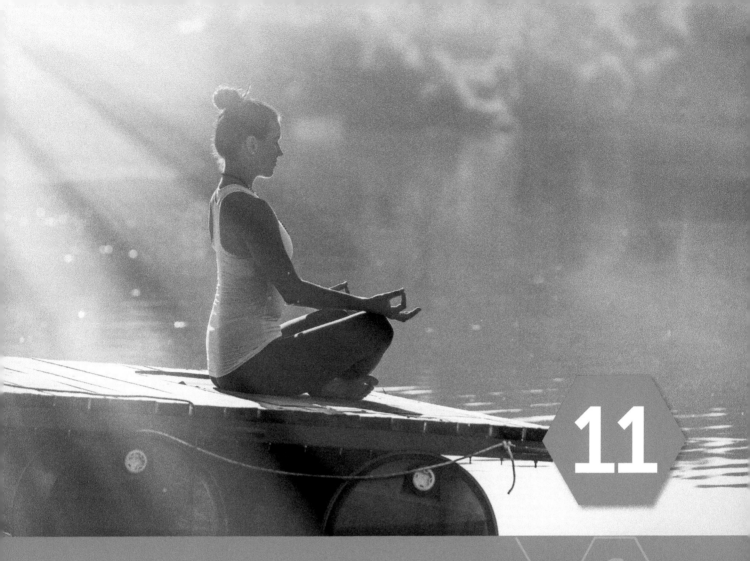

BACK
HEALTH

LEARNING OUTCOMES

After completing this chapter, you should be able to:

• Describe the prevalence of back pain and back injuries in policing.

• Describe the functions of the spine.

• Recognize the causes of back pain, and identify the special risks to a healthy back posed by policing.

• Examine how arthritis, osteoporosis, and repetitive strain injuries have a potential impact on a law enforcement officer.

• Explain how to maintain a healthy back.

• Describe how back injuries are treated and prevented.

• Identify proper posture techniques for sitting in a car or desk and standing.

Back pain, most of which occurs in the lower back, is one of the most common health complaints among Canadian adults. Four out of five Canadians experience at least one episode of low-back pain (LBP) at some point in their life (Canadian Physiotherapy Association, 2012). In most cases the pain subsides within a couple of days or weeks (acute pain). On average, 90 percent of people with acute low-back pain will recover within four weeks (Canadian Physiotherapy Association, 2012). However, for some it may occur repeatedly, and in some cases it may never go away (chronic pain). For some people it has a major impact on their ability to do regular chores around the house and perform simple daily tasks. More than 70 percent of back problems begin during routine daily activities. Accidents and other forms of trauma account for only 30 percent of back problems (Canadian Physiotherapy Association, 2012). Next to the common cold, low-back pain is the most common reason for missing work.

Low-back pain (LBP) is a common disorder involving the muscles, nerves, and bones of the back, resulting in pain. Low-back pain can be the result of inactivity. More than 70 percent of low-back pain problems are caused by inadequate muscular development (NINDS, 2014). Low-back pain usually makes its first appearance between the ages of 30 and 50, at a point in life when people are spending more time on family and job-related activities and are less physically active (National Institute for Neurological Disorders and Stroke, 2017). Routine activities such as housework, taking out the garbage and recycling bins, gardening, or reaching for an object may trigger an episode of acute back pain, which may last for hours, days, or even years. Pain can vary from a dull constant ache to a sudden sharp feeling.

FACTS TO THINK ABOUT

- Nearly one-third of female adults suffer from chronic lower-back pain, compared to one-quarter of males.
- LBP can have a negative impact on daily tasks (39 percent), exercise (38 percent), and sleep (37 percent).
- More than half (54 percent) of those who experience low-back pain spend the majority of their workday sitting. Prolonged sitting negatively affects your muscles and joints and leads to deconditioning (decline in physical functioning), fatigue, and stress on the spinal discs, causing LBP.
- Research shows a correlation between elevated body mass index (BMI) and a greater risk of suffering LBP. Since our rates of obesity are growing, the greater the risk that Canadians will develop low-back pain. Obesity rates tripled in Canada between 1985 and 2011.
- In terms of recovery and recurrence of LBP, 90 percent of cases resolve within six weeks, 60 to 80 percent have recurrences within two years, and 7 percent develop chronic back pain.

SOURCES: Choiniére et al., 2010; Lis, Black, Korn, & Nordin, 2007; Meucci, Fassa, & Faria, 2015; Seaman, 2013; Twell, Gregory, Reddigan, & Midodzi, 2014.

This chapter looks at the impact back pain and repetitive injuries have on law enforcement officers, the causes of low-back pain including the special risks faced by law enforcement officers, and conditions associated with these injuries. It also discusses how to prevent and manage back pain, including proper sitting and standing techniques.

The unpredictable and wide-ranging physical demands of law enforcement officers include running varied distances with or without loads, restraining non-compliant offenders, carrying injured or unconscious people, self-defence manoeuvres, and manual handling tasks (Bonneau & Brown, 1995; Brown, Wells, Trottier, Bonneau, & Ferris, 1998; Pryor, Colburn, Crill, Hostler, & Suyama, 2012). Back, shoulder, and neck pain are all too common in law enforcement. Sudden external forces when controlling a suspect or offender who is resisting arrest, trips and falls, and strains and sprains can all contribute to the high risk of injury (Achterstraat, 2008; Lyons, Radburn, Orr, & Pope, 2017). In addition to these demands, there is an ever increasing responsibility to drive longer at work in addition to commuting times. These have shown an increased risk for lower-back pain and other musculo-skeletal disorders from prolonged sitting in vehicles and having compromised pos-ture, pressure, and discomfort from the duty belt (Donnelly, Callaghan, & Durkin, 2009; Holmes, McKinnon, Dicerson, & Callaghan, 2013).

Due to the prevalence of back pain in our society, there have been many studies done to determine cause, prevention, and treatment in law enforcement. A study done in the late 1990s on a random sample of RCMP officers concluded that their prevalence of back problems was similar to that of the general public (Brown et al., 1998). So we know that it is not specifically law enforcement that causes back pain, but it may be related to the ergonomics of the job. Researchers found that the duty belt did not have significant effects on an officer's flexibility and range of motion, but it did increase the metabolic cost of wearing the equipment, which could tire individuals by the end of the day and predispose them to the onset of low-back pain (Kumar & Narayan, 2001). Other studies found that wearing heavy body armour, combined with exposure to vehicles with poor ergonomics and vibration for over two hours per day, did increase the risk of low-back pain (Arts, 2006; Burton, Tillotson, Symonds, Burke, & Mathewson, 1996). In another study, officers who drove and sat in a vehicle or at a desk all day were at greater risk than those whose daily tasks were varied, such as officers who spent part of their day walking. High discomfort levels were associated with computer use, duty belt, sidearm/radio, body armour, and lack of lumbar support (Donnelly, Callaghan, & Durkin, 2009; Gruevski, Holmes, Gooyers, Dickerson, & Callaghan, 2016; Lis et al., 2007). In the province of Ontario, many services have gone to load bearing vests (LBV) for their tactical units, which improves equipment distribution; however, since most have a policy prohibiting use of force equipment be placed on the vest, it has not solved the problem entirely. Some services have provided suspenders to help distribute the weight; however, there have been complaints of the shoulders being pulled forward and leading to upper back pain (Sgt. T. Conroy, personal communications, April, 7, 2017).

Wearing a vest and firearms or carrying an overloaded backpack may lead to poor posture, overstretching of the soft tissue of the neck and back, and excessive strain on muscles and joints. Over time, the physical strain of carrying heavy loads may lead to the following problems:

- Harmful strain and fatigue in the muscles and soft tissues of the back from overuse. Constantly carrying the weight on one side may cause the spine to develop an adaptive curve, and leaning forward too much may affect the natural curve of the lower back and increase the curve of the upper back and shoulders.

- Spinal compression, improper alignment, or both may hamper the proper functioning of the discs between the vertebrae that provide shock absorption, which in turn leaves the back more vulnerable to injury.

- Stress to or compression of the shoulders and arms can compress the nerves, resulting in tingling, numbness, or weakness in the arms or hands.

Preparing for a career in law enforcement, you will need to consider that there will be extra weight and bulk added to your uniform, as well as entire shifts spent walking, or sitting in a car or at a desk. It will be vital to ensure that you are coming into the job with a strong core, proper spine flexibility and range of motion, and an excellent grasp of what conditions await you.

THE SPINE

To understand back pain, you first need to understand the spine. The spine has 33 bones, called **vertebrae**. These extend from the base of the skull to the end of the trunk (see Figure 11.1). The spine has three natural curves—cervical, thoracic, and lumbar—which ensure proper balance and weight bearing. The spine has the following functions (AAOS, 2013):

- It provides structural support for the body, especially the thorax (chest). It supports the upper body and head and withstands external forces.

- It surrounds and protects the spinal cord (a column of nervous tissue that acts as a continuation of the brain and connects the brain to the rest of the nervous system).

- It serves as an attachment site for a large number of muscles, tendons, and ligaments. These trunk muscles and ligaments act on individual vertebrae for postural control and spinal stability. (See Chapter 4 for information on muscles, tendons, and ligaments.)

- It allows movement of the neck and back in all directions.

Each vertebra is made up of a large bone, called the body, and a bony ring including the spinous process (see Figure 11.2). The vertebrae link together to form a "tunnel" that protects the nerves and spinal cord. The spinal cord is a column of nerve fibres that transmit and receive messages from the brain to the rest of the body, controlling movement and organ function. There are 31 pairs of nerve roots that branch out into nerves that travel to the rest of the body.

FIGURE 11.1 The Spine

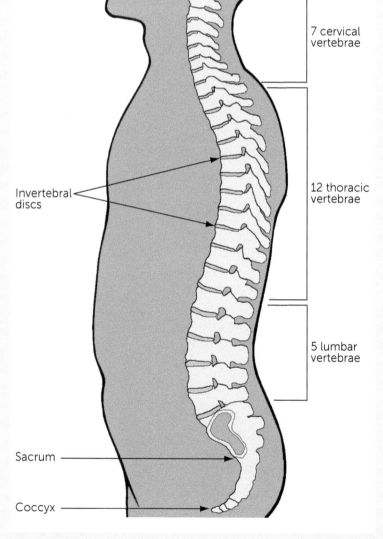

7 cervical vertebrae

12 thoracic vertebrae

5 lumbar vertebrae

Invertebral discs

Sacrum

Coccyx

FIGURE 11.2 Vertebra

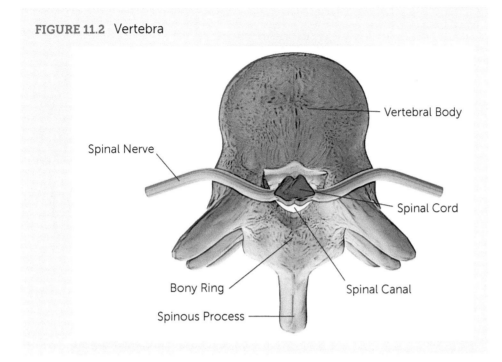

The lumbar vertebrae are under constant pressure from the weight of the upper body. The vertebra are separated by flexible, gelatinous, shock-absorbing pads called intervertebral discs. The discs act as shock absorbers for the spine. In young people, intervertebral discs are approximately 90 percent water, but are only 70 percent water in older persons (we lose water as we age) (Greenberg & Dintiman, 1997). As a result, as you age there is an inherent increased risk of injury.

THE CAUSES OF BACK PAIN

Although some people have a weak back for genetic reasons, inadequate muscular development is the major cause of back pain. The strength of a muscle is directly related to the amount of work it does. In physically inactive people, the large muscle groups are not worked enough and therefore lack sufficient strength. For the back, insufficient muscle strength means that correct body alignment is compromised. Poor posture is the result of musculoskeletal distortion in the neck, and lower and upper back. Rounded shoulders and postural neck problems result from the excessive anterior curve of the cervical and thoracic spine (see Figure 11.3).

The back is supported, and its movement is controlled, by 140 muscles. Typically, a muscle, ligament, or tendon strain or sprain causes nearby muscles to spasm (involuntarily contract) in an attempt to support the back. The most frequently documented cause of back pain is muscle strain, with overexertion and irregular (fast, awkward) movements such as lifting, twisting, turning, bending, pushing, and pulling being typical underlying factors (Bonneau, Stevenson, & Gledhill, 2001). It is estimated that 70 percent of back problems are due to improper alignment of the spine and pelvic girdle (hip bones) caused by inflexible and weak muscles (NINDS, 2014).

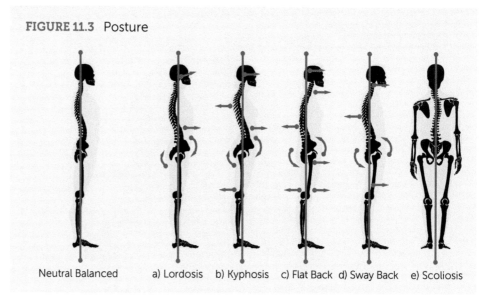

FIGURE 11.3 Posture

Neutral Balanced   a) Lordosis   b) Kyphosis   c) Flat Back   d) Sway Back   e) Scoliosis

There are key areas of imbalance that increase the risk of spinal injury: lower-back muscles which are too tight, too strong, and overused; abdominal muscles which are too weak, extended, and underused; hip muscles which are too tight, weak, and underused; and hamstrings that are too tight, shortened, and underused. Specifically:

- Poor flexibility and weak muscles in the abdominals, glutes, back, pelvis, and thighs may increase the curve of the lower back and cause the pelvis to tilt too far forward. This in turn causes the vertebrae in the lower back to become slightly displaced and press against one another, producing an ache in the lower back and putting pressure on the spinal nerves and vertebrae.

- The hamstring muscles are another muscle group implicated in low-back pain. This group consists of three large muscles, located at the back of each thigh, which are associated with movement at the hip and knee joints. The difficulty most people face in trying to touch their toes with their fingertips without bending their knees is largely due to the hamstrings' inability to stretch far enough. This inability stems from an inflexibility or shortening of the hamstrings caused by physical inactivity or long periods of sitting. The hamstrings' inflexibility or shortening may cause pain in the hamstrings themselves and referred pain to the lower back. Considering that forward bending is one of the most common daily activities, short hamstrings may increase the risk of injury of the spine from mechanical stresses (e.g., lifting with straight legs or trying to touch your toes with straight legs).

RISK FACTORS FOR BACK PAIN

Although we know that anyone can experience back pain, there are a number of factors that increase your risk. Several of these factors are not under your control:

- growing older
- having a family history of back pain

- those that work physically demanding careers
- having a congenital birth defect
- having a degenerative disease of the spine, such as osteoporosis or arthritis
- child bearing pre- and post-partum
- misalignment of spine
- joint dysfunction (wear and tear on the joint cartilage due to poor posture)

Factors that you *can* control include the following:

- lack of exercise including strength/muscular development
- sitting for long periods of time with poor posture (including driving, exposure to constant vibration)
- lifting or pulling heavy objects, and/or bending or twisting repetitively, without using proper form (see Figure 11.4)
- poor posture resulting in misalignment of the spine
- backpack overload—carrying more than 15 to 20 percent body weight, especially in children
- smoking—you are twice as likely to have low-back pain if you smoke or are exposed to second-hand smoke. Lorentzon and colleagues (2007) have shown that adolescent smokers have significant loss in bone mass density resulting in a lower peak bone mass, mainly as a consequence of reduced cortical thickness (the density of the outer layer of the bone).

FIGURE 11.4 Improper and Proper Techniques for Lifting Heavy Objects

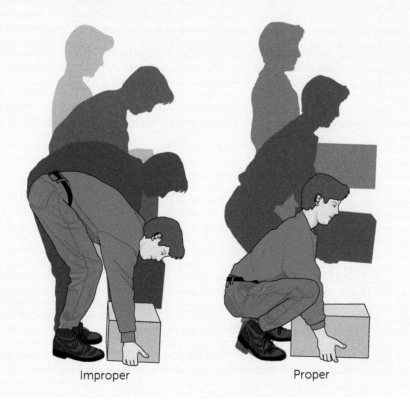

Improper   Proper

- being overweight—weighing more than 20 percent over your ideal body weight increases your risk of back problems. However, Zhao and colleagues (2006) and NIH (2016) believe that excessive weight loss to reduce back problems may increase the risk of osteoporosis in those over 50 years old
- having a mental health problem, such as severe anxiety or depression—the stress leading to chronic back pain (Matsudaira, Konishi, Miyoshi, Isomura, & Inuzuka, 2014; Pinheiro et al., 2015)
- participation in sports that involve contact, forceful twisting, or a high degree of risk of injury

ETIOLOGY OF BACK PAIN

Spondylosis is a broad term that refers to the general degeneration of the spine associated with normal wear and tear that occurs in the joints, discs, and bones of the spine as people get older. Repeated heavy lifting or a sudden awkward movement may strain back muscles and spinal ligaments and damage the components of the back (vertebrae, discs, and nerves).

Spondylosis can also be caused by an arthritic degenerative disorder called osteoarthritis (see below), which causes pain and loss of normal function of the vertebrae, facet joints, ligaments, and muscles.

DEGENERATIVE DISC DISEASE

Degeneration of the intervertebral discs is called degenerative disc disease (DDD). As we age (typically, age 40 onward), the normal gelatin-like centre of the discs loses fluid and begins to thin, making the spaces between the vertebrae narrow. Age, repetitive strain, improper spine alignment and movement, and possibly genetics cause disc wear and tear. Because there is little blood supply to the discs, they cannot repair themselves if injured. Over time, this degeneration can contribute to the development of back pain. And in older individuals, the spine will become more vulnerable to injury as the discs thin and the vertebrae are compressed together.

Disc degeneration in the neck is called cervical disc disease; in the mid-back it is known as thoracic disc disease, and in the lumbar spine it is called lumbago.

- Cervical disc disease affects the hand, shoulder, and arm, resulting in pain, numbness or tingling, and weakness. One possible cause of cervical disc degeneration is whiplash. Whiplash is the traumatic hyperextension of cervical vertebra resulting in damage to the soft tissue and may fracture spinous processes and rupture disks.
- Thoracic disc disease affects the area between the end of the neck and just above the waistline, resulting in limited or painful movement of the upper back, numbness or tingling, and weakness in the legs. It can be painful when coughing, sneezing, or taking a deep breath.
- Lumbago is pain in the lumbar region of the spine that can be caused by factors such as injury, arthritis, back strain, abuse of the back muscles (poor posture, sagging mattress, or ill-fitting shoes), or by a number

of disc degeneration disorders, resulting in numbness and tingling in the lower back and legs, weakness in the legs, loss of bowel or bladder control, fevers or chills, and unexplained weight loss.

- Disc degeneration may lead to other disorders such as spinal stenosis (narrowing of the spinal canal that houses the spinal cord and nerve roots), spondylolisthesis (forward slippage of a disc and vertebra), and retrolisthesis (backward slippage of a disc and vertebra).

CONDITIONS ASSOCIATED WITH DISC DEGENERATION

HERNIATED DISC

One common injury is a herniated disc, which occurs when sudden pressure causes the disc to rupture and its gelatinous interior to protrude through the outer coating of the disc (see Figure 11.5). The protruding material may put pressure on adjoining nerves. There are multiple risk factors for herniated discs including family history, heavy lifting, repetitive rounding of the spine, and obesity (Schroeder, Guyre, & Vaccaro, 2016). As we grow older, the discs become flatter, and if stressed or weakened, the outer part (annulus) may bulge or tear. Cummins et al. (2016) reported that the average age of patients with a herniated disc was 41 years, and the diagnosis was slightly more common in males than females (57 percent versus 43 percent, respectively). The location of the pain depends on where the disc is pressing on the nerve; individuals with low-back herniation may experience pain that radiates down the legs.

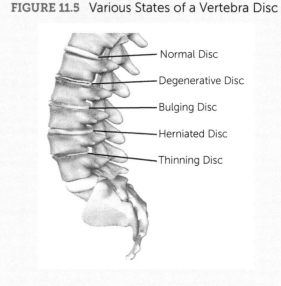

FIGURE 11.5 Various States of a Vertebra Disc

- Normal Disc
- Degenerative Disc
- Bulging Disc
- Herniated Disc
- Thinning Disc

SCIATICA

Sciatica, or sciatic neuritis, is a common back condition. The sciatic nerve exits the spinal column between the lowest vertebra and the sacrum. This nerve supplies sensation to the back of the thighs and buttocks, knee flexors, and foot muscles. It also supplies connectivity to the muscles in the back of the leg. When it is compressed, inflamed, or irritated anywhere along its length, pain may result. It may result from poor posture, disc degeneration, a bulging disc, or pregnancy where the fetus is pushing on the nerves. Symptoms range from a sensation of "pins and needles" or numbness to a burning feeling in the leg or foot. Sciatica may result in wasting of the muscles of the lower leg. The pain from sciatica is usually worse when you are active, and feels better when you are resting. Coughing, sneezing, sitting, driving, and bending forward may make the pain worse because these movements put more pressure on the nerve.

This problem is especially hard on individuals who must sit in their vehicles for long periods of time. With extended sitting in a vehicle, many people feel their legs burn or go numb, making it very difficult to get out of the vehicle quickly and respond to emergencies. Sciatica is most common in the right leg of police officers, as the right leg is extended and the officer has to twist to the right to access their computer.

ARTHRITIS

Arthritis is a group of conditions that affect the joints of the body. It involves inflammation of the joint(s) causing joint pain and swelling, and can interfere with the ability to manage daily activities. Over 4.6 million Canadian adults (one in six Canadians aged 15 years and older) report having arthritis. By 2036, this number is expected to grow to an estimated 7.5 million Canadian adults (one in five) (Arthritis Society, 2015). Arthritis is comprised of more than 100 conditions, including osteoarthritis, rheumatoid arthritis, gout, lupus, and fibromyalgia.

FACTS TO THINK ABOUT

THE COSTS OF ARTHRITIS IN CANADA

- The cumulative economic burden to Canadian society since 2010 resulting from the impact of arthritis on presenteeism (working while sick), absenteeism, and leaving the workforce has surpassed an estimation of $142.1 billion.
- The impact of arthritis on the Canadian economy in health care costs and lost productivity is estimated to be $33 billion each year.
- The cumulative economic burden to Canadian society since 2010 resulting from direct health care costs and indirect costs related to arthritis is estimated to have exceeded $233.5 billion.

SOURCE: Arthritis Society, 2015.

OSTEOARTHRITIS

Osteoarthritis is a chronic condition characterized by the breakdown of the cartilage that cushions the ends of the bones where they meet to form joints. Osteoarthritis is the most common type of arthritis in Canada (see Figure 11.6), and affects 10 percent of all Canadians (PHAC, 2012). In the spine, this occurs in the cartilage of the facet joints, where the vertebrae join, resulting in irritation and pain. As the cartilage begins to break down, extra movement occurs in the facet joints. The body compensates for this movement by forming bone spurs, which inhibit range of motion and further wearing of the joint. The bone spurs press on nerves resulting in pain or cause narrowing of the spinal canal, known as spinal stenosis (Arthritis Foundation, 2017). Osteoarthritis of the vertebrae is sometimes confused with, or may be associated with, degenerative disc disease. This is because osteoarthritis and degenerated discs are commonly found together; however, they are separate conditions.

FIGURE 11.6 Osteoarthritic Spine

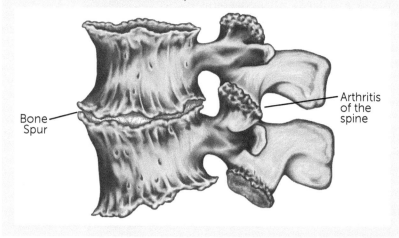

Bone Spur

Arthritis of the spine

RHEUMATOID ARTHRITIS

Rheumatoid arthritis (RA) is an autoimmune disease (that is, when the body attacks itself) specifically attacking healthy joints, resulting in damage to cartilage, bone, tendons, and ligaments. Rheumatoid arthritis is the second most common type of arthritis. Three times as many women as men get rheumatoid arthritis, and it most commonly appears between the ages of 25 and 50 (Arthritis Society, 2011b). Within ten years of the onset of the disease, if left untreated, up to 50 percent of people living with RA are work disabled. For those living with RA, related inflammation in the arteries results in an increased risk of mortality (Arthritis Alliance of Canada, 2011). In a 2006 survey, rheumatism was the most commonly reported chronic condition among Metis adults; at 21 percent, it was more prevalent among this population than for Canadians as a whole (13 percent) (Janz, Seti, & Turner, 2009).

ARTHRITIS TREATMENTS

Chronic pain and reduced mobility/function are the most common side effects of arthritis. Treatment of the pain depends on the history and when it started, how many joints are affected, how long the pain lasts, what aggravates the inflammation, and what helps to relieve the pain. Physical examinations and MRI/CT scans can assess the state of the condition, and blood tests confirm the diagnosis. Physical therapy, nutritional therapy, warm baths/showers, cold and warm-pack applications, paraffin wax, and surgery may help with the pain. There are medications that you may discuss with your doctor regarding treatment (anti-inflammatory drugs, pain medications, immune-altering medications). Early diagnosis of arthritis may help prevent irreversible joint damage.

OSTEOPOROSIS

Osteoporosis is a condition in which bones lose so much mass that they become brittle and prone to break. Osteoporosis commonly affects the spine. Approximately 1.4 million Canadians suffer from osteoporosis (H & K Perspectives, 2015). The vertebrae become weak and can break (compression fracture) and can lose about one-half their height. Osteoporosis is known as the "silent thief" because bone loss often occurs without symptoms until they break, resulting in severe back pain. One of the signs of osteoporosis is a substantial decrease in height and a stooped appearance.

FIGURE 11.7 Comparison of Bone Density

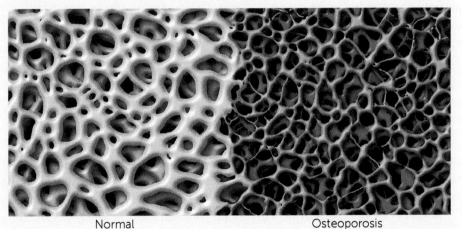

Normal   Osteoporosis

> **DID YOU KNOW?**
>
> Gout is a form of arthritis characterized by repeated flare-ups of intensely painful swelling. It's caused by a buildup of uric acid in the fluid around the joints. This can be due to genetic predisposition, some diseases, or consuming too much meat, seafood, fructose-sweetened drinks, or alcohol. The bunion joint—the joint that connects the big toe to the foot—is often affected first in people who have gout. Less commonly, gout can affect the spine, causing extreme pain, numbness, and tingling.
>
> SOURCE: Arthritis Society, 2011a.

> **DID YOU KNOW?**
>
> You can use paraffin wax to apply moist heat to your hands or feet to ease the pain and stiffness of osteoarthritis. Paraffin especially helps to reduce pain and loosen up your hand and finger joints before exercise.
>
> SOURCE: Healthwise, 2016.

FACTS TO THINK ABOUT

- Twenty-five percent of women over age 50, and 50 percent over age 70, develop osteoporosis. Seven in ten fractures in women over the age of 45 are due to this disease.
- One in three women and one in five men will suffer a fracture due to osteoporosis during their lifetime.
- The overall yearly cost to the Canadian health care system of treating osteoporosis and the fractures it causes was over $2.3 billion as of 2010. This cost includes acute care costs, outpatient care, prescription drugs, and indirect costs. This cost rises to $3.9 billion if a proportion of Canadians were assumed to be living in long-term care facilities because of osteoporosis.

SOURCES: Osteoporosis Canada, 2017a; PHAC, 2007; Tarride et al., 2012.

There are three main factors that are attributed to osteoporosis (Osteoporosis Canada, 2011; Osteoporosis, 2017a):

1. *Suboptimal bone growth* during childhood, adolescence, or early adulthood, not allowing for peak bone mass to be achieved. Peak bone mass density is achieved at an early age (16 to 20 in girls, 20 to 25 in boys). If there are nutritional concerns or lack of physical activity, peak bone mass density will be less.

2. *Accelerated bone loss* during adulthood, usually due to a drop in sex hormone levels associated with aging (that is, delayed onset of menstruation, absence of menstruation, an abnormal menstrual cycle, or menopause in women; low testosterone levels in men). Women and men alike begin to lose bone in their mid-30s; as they approach menopause, women lose bone at a greater rate, from 2 to 5 percent per year.

3. *Bone loss secondary to disease conditions* (celiac and Crohn's), including eating disorders (Mills, 2006), medications (including corticoid steroids), and medical treatments, which affect calcium and vitamin D absorption.

Osteoporosis Canada has recommended that everyone over the age of 65, and those who are over 50 and have at least one major risk factor or two minor risk factors, should have a bone densitometry test, which assesses density of the hip and spine, on a yearly basis (Mills, 2006; Osteoporosis, 2017b). Bone densitometry allows accurate and precise skeletal assessment, and enables detection of osteoporosis prior to actual fractures. It can also determine if there is any onset of fractures in the spine and limbs. With information about a patient's risk factors and the results of bone densitometry, a physician can determine diagnosis of mineral loss in the bone. For more information, go to the www.osteoporosis.ca website.

Osteoporosis may be prevented by eating foods rich in calcium, taking calcium supplements, hormone replacement, or bisphosphonates to improve the body's uptake of calcium, and by doing weight-bearing exercises. Research indicates that calcium loss may begin as early as 25 to 30 years old (Boskey & Coleman, 2010); the onset of calcium loss may depend on hormone imbalance, so those who do not have as much of the hormones may be affected sooner.

REPETITIVE STRAIN INJURY

Repetitive strain injuries (RSI) are injuries that result from doing the same motion repeatedly without adequate breaks or when the body is put in awkward positions during repetitive work or when exerting high forces. Repetitive activity damages tendons, affects circulation, and causes biomechanical stresses on soft tissue by not allowing enough recovery time between movements. Symptoms include pain, numbness, and tingling in the affected body parts (Tjepkema, 2003). Repetitive strain injuries take a toll not only physically but mentally. An RSI may affect work with functional and activity limitations, and may cause sleep disturbances.

In 2013–2014, 15 percent of Canadians (4.5 million people) reported an injury due to repetitive strain, with males and females equally likely to report this type of injury. For 55.4 percent of those with RSI, their injury was serious enough to limit their normal activities. Shoulders (22.6 percent) were the most common body part affected by repetitive strain injuries, followed by elbows (15.0 percent), wrists (12.8 percent), lower back (12.4 percent), and knees (12.3 percent) (Statistics Canada, 2015).

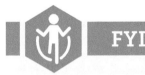

FYI

REPETITIVE STRAIN INJURIES OF THE ARMS

There are two broad groupings of repetitive strain injuries:

1. *tendon-related disorders* which involve the inflammation of the tendon and sheath or injuries to them, include tendinitis (inflammation of the tendon), tenosynovitis (inflammation of the tendon sheath), epicondylitis, and rotator cuff tendinitis.

2. *peripheral nerve entrapment disorders* which involve compression of a nerve. The most common is carpal tunnel syndrome (compression of the medial nerve), and the second most common is cubital tunnel syndrome (compression of the ulnar nerve).

SOURCES: Choi et al., 2015; Neal & Fields, 2010; Tjepkema, 2003.

Work-related repetitive strain injuries are among the most common ways of being injured on the job. Many workers have jobs in which they have little or no control over how the job is done or the rate at which the job must be completed. Often these jobs involve rapid, repetitive tasks. Law enforcement officers, for example, are often required to perform repetitive tasks that adversely affect their back and shoulder muscles and tendons. Anderson, Zutz, and Plecas (2011) and Calder, Stashuk, and McLean (2008) identify several features of law enforcement equipment and tasks that are conducive to RSI and back problems generally:

- Law enforcement may require individuals to perform the same task for a long time without a chance to rest or exercise a different set of muscles. Sitting in a vehicle for hours is an example. Studies have found that individuals are sitting in their vehicles for approximately half their shift (Cohen, Plecas, & McCormick, 2011).

- Law enforcement tasks and emergency circumstances may require substantial muscular force—for example, when an individual must restrain a person or remove him or her from a volatile situation.

- Employers may require officers to maintain an awkward posture that is difficult to hold for even a short time. For example, officers are sometimes required to stand for long periods of time (possibly an entire shift) in boots that provide inadequate foot support.

- Officers may require training on the use of firearms for extended periods of time, which may result in non-specific arm, shoulder, and/or neck pain from holding up their firearm (loaded weight 0.99 kg [2.2 lb.]) and the repetitive isometric contraction of the forearm to fire the gun.

- The equipment belt that officers wear weighs 4.2–7 kg (9.3–15.4 lb.) and puts strain on the lower back whether one is sitting or standing. Most duty belts are typically 5.5–5.7 cm (2.25 in.) wide (see Figure 11.8). Slowly, services are replacing leather ones (which were stiff and inflexible) with nylon ones. However, with the addition of a radio, flashlight, latex gloves, baton, taser, pepper spray canister, handcuffs, handgun, and spare magazines, this can place uncommon pressure on the front of the pelvis and abdomen. In addition, the equipment attached to the belt may cause an individual to sit in an awkward position while at a desk or in a vehicle.

- Patrol vehicle seats can be another factor in belt discomfort. Raised sides on seats can produce pressure on the sidearm and radio, causing the individual to push forward to reduce the amount of low-back support. Worn seats cause individuals to sink lower in the middle of the seat, causing additional discomfort. Similarly, vehicle seat design does not address the needs of different body types. If a seat has been damaged by excessive use and has not been repaired, individuals are forced to sit in a position that does not allow them to maintain proper posture, which puts additional strain on the back. Many are sitting in a twisted position for nearly 30 percent of their shift to use the equipment in the vehicle (Plecas, McCormick, & Cohen, 2011).

- Individuals who work outdoors in winter face a higher risk of back injuries. If they have to respond quickly to an altercation or other incident, their cold, stiff muscles and joints are more likely to suffer damage.

FIGURE 11.8   Wearing an Equipment Belt

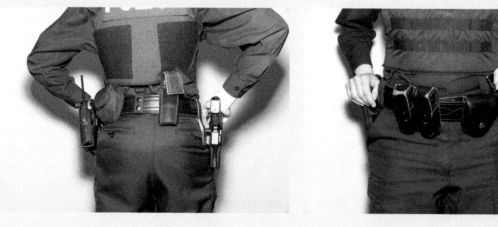

TREATING BACK INJURIES

Although prevention is the key to keeping your back healthy, almost everyone will experience low-back pain at some point. Treatment usually involves the following:

- One to two days of bedrest on a firm mattress. Remember that excessive rest can increase sickness behaviour through deconditioning of body muscles (Al-Otaibi, 2015; U.S. Preventive Services Task Force, 2005).

- Moderate application of heat and cold, switching between 20 mins of cold and 20 mins of heat. After 48 hours, cold is no longer recommended and a warm bath with Epsom salts may help relax a strained back.

- Gentle massage until muscle spasms are eliminated or significantly reduced.

- If pain persists, you may need to consult your doctor, who can refer you to an appropriate professional for help—physiotherapist, chiropractor, massage therapist, osteopath, athletic therapist, sports physician, certified exercise professional.

- For patients with a new episode of low-back pain, prompt access to physiotherapy is cost- and time-effective. More than 70 percent of patients require only a single clinic visit, and less than 5 percent need to be referred to a specialist (Al-Otaibi, 2015; Pinnington, Miller, & Stanley, 2004).

In the longer term, you are encouraged to do the following:

- Exercise aerobically for 30 minutes three or four times a week, working toward 30 minutes every day.

- Reduce abdominal fat by changing your dietary habits; abdominal fat strains the lower back.

- Get enough sleep to rest your spine (approximately 8 hours).

- Daily back and abdominal exercises (examples listed below, under "Exercises for a Healthy Back").

- Incorporate proper techniques when lifting, sitting, and standing (tips/advice listed below).

- Surgery is rarely needed to correct low-back problems, but be sure to consult a physician for diagnosis and treatment in all cases of back pain. Do not take your back's health lightly.

PREVENTING BACK PAIN

Physical conditioning is the key to preventing back injury. In addition to getting regular aerobic exercise, officers need to develop strong back and stomach muscles, which are necessary to support the spine. Law enforcement personnel also need to learn the proper ways to stand, bend, lift, sit, rest, and sleep. They must regularly perform exercises that stretch and strengthen the major muscles affecting the back, and be as active as possible. Flexibility is a major factor in back health. Without it, many individuals suffer back strain.

Both abdominal and back muscles require adequate exercise to maintain strength and tone. Although we use our thigh muscles whenever we walk or climb stairs, deep abdominal and back muscles are usually left unconditioned and inactive. It is important to strengthen the flexor, extensor, and oblique muscles to support the spine. Lack of such exercises can lead to muscle atrophy (wasting), which can cause back pain from the inability of the muscles to hold up the spine. Under stress, our muscles tighten. This means that when we have a physical altercation or fight-or-flight response, we tighten and may injure the lower back.

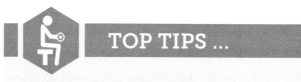

TOP TIPS ...

FOR A HEALTHY BACK

In addition to exercising, the following tips will help you keep your back strong and flexible and prevent low-back pain.

1. To warm up for an activity, swing any tool you will be using (such as a rake, shovel, axe, or golf club) lazily back and forth around your head and shoulders in different positions, gradually working up to a full range of motion. Work your way up to the effort required to do the activity.

2. When lifting an object, warm up the muscles first. Then stand close to the load, facing the direction you want to go. Bend at the knees and hips rather than keeping your legs straight and bending at the waist. Your feet should be shoulder-width apart. Ensure that you have a good grip on the load. Lift gradually, keeping your arms straight and pushing up with your leg muscles. Keep the object close to your body. If you must turn, do not twist at the waist; ensure that you have enough space for your entire body to turn before lifting. Also, be aware that lowering objects causes less strain than lifting; pulling them is easier than carrying; and pushing is less demanding than pulling.

3. Leaning against a solid support when you are sitting, such as sitting on a chair rather than a bench with no back, helps reduce fatigue. Make sure that you have a lumbar support fitted into the natural curve of your lumbar spine while you are sitting, so that you keep your spine aligned. This could be a small pillow, rolled up towel, or even a shirt or jacket if you are in the car.

4. Once a day, make sure that you relieve the stress on your back by lying down or doing some back stretches.

5. Try sleeping on your side with your knees and hips bent and a pillow between your knees. If you lie on your back, place a pillow under your knees. Do not lie on your stomach; this hyperextends the back and puts a twist in your neck. Your mattress should be firm enough to support your spine in its neutral position. The mattress should not sag. Consider adding a layer of foam for extra support.

6. When walking, keep your toes pointed straight ahead. Keep your back flat, your head up, and your chin in. If you walk while looking at your smartphone, your neck will be flexed forward immensely.

For specific proper sitting posture, see Figure 11.20.

For specific proper standing posture, see "Proper Standing Posture."

EXERCISES FOR A HEALTHY BACK

Exercises for the lower back should spare the spine, enhancing the muscle challenge and the motor control system to ensure that spine stability is maintained in all other activities. Here is some practical information to be aware of prior to exercising your back (McGill, 2003):

1. While there is a common belief among some 'experts' that exercise sessions should be performed at least three to five times per week, it appears low-back exercises have the most beneficial effect when performed daily.

2. The 'no pain-no gain' axiom does not apply when exercising the low back. In pained individuals, particularly when applied to weight training, the scientific and clinical wisdom would suggest the opposite is true.

3. While there are specific low-back exercises, general exercise programs that also combine cardiovascular components (like walking) have been shown to be more effective in both rehabilitation and for injury prevention.

4. Intervertebral discs are more hydrated in the morning after rising from bed, and lose fluid throughout the day. You are at the highest risk for disc injury when your discs are fully hydrated. So this means that it is not sensible to perform full-range spine motion while under load, shortly after rising from bed.

5. There is no doubt that back injury can occur during seemingly low level demands (such as picking up a pencil) and that the risk of injury from motor control error can occur (i.e., the more fatigued you are, the greater the risk of injuring your back). Given that endurance has more protective value than strength, strength gains should not be overemphasized at the expense of endurance.

6. Remember that there is no one specific program for all individuals. Each individual's training objectives must be identified and the exercises, sets, and reps should be chosen appropriately. If you experience pain or discomfort, stop what you are doing and refer to an expert to determine what is appropriate for you.

7. Be patient and stick with the program. Increased function and/or reduction of pain may not occur for three months.

RECOMMENDED EXERCISES

The following is a list of exercises that are designed to help develop and strengthen the core muscles, while keeping the spine stabilized. Each exercise can be performed daily, starting with 1 set and working up to 3 sets (Briggs & Buchbinder, 2009; McGill, 2010, McGill 2016):

- *Modified curl up* This exercise focuses on the front abdominal region. Lie on your back with one knee bent and one leg flat on the floor. Using your hands or a towel, place them under the lumbar spine to maintain neutral spinal posture. Brace your core, as you ever so slightly lift your head and shoulders off the ground. The movement should be minimal. Don't tuck your chin or let your head fall back. Hold yourself up for no longer than 10 seconds. Begin with 5 to 8 repetitions. See Figure 11.9.

FIGURE 11.9   Modified Curl Up

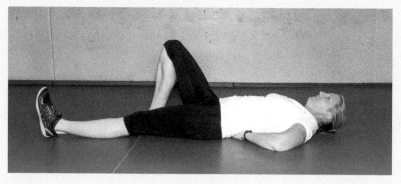

- *Bird-dog* This is a stabilizer exercise of the core, back, and glutes muscles. By lifting an alternate leg and arm at the same time the load of the spine is reduced by 50 percent. This exercise helps you train for the core endurance test (modified Sorenson's back extension test listed in the *Fit for Duty, Fit for Life* training guide). Starting on your hands and knees, make sure your back is flat. Raise your right arm out in front while extending your left leg straight back, keeping them in line with your torso. Try to keep the back completely still while performing the exercise, so that there is no bending, twisting, or rotating of the spine. Complete the exercise slowly, and hold your arm and leg out for maximum 7 to 8 seconds. Lower your arm and leg and bring your elbow and knee together under your body. Begin with 5 repetitions and then switch to the other side. See Figure 11.10.

FIGURE 11.10   Bird-dog

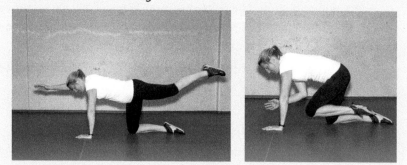

- *Plank* The plank is an isometric exercise that develops strength in the core, shoulders, arms, and glutes. Lie facedown with legs extended and elbows aligned directly below your shoulders. Plant your toes on the floor and press up through your hips, so that your body forms a straight line from head to heels. Focus on activating your core muscles. Hold for as long as you can staying in correct form. See Figure 11.11.

FIGURE 11.11 Plank

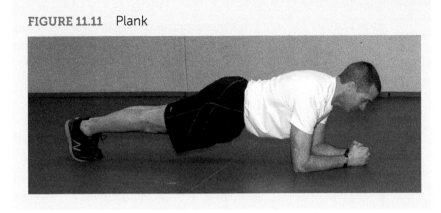

- *Side bridge* While the standard plank targets the connection between the lower back and the abdominals, this most common variation targets the obliques and helps stabilize the spine from side to side. Lie down on your side, leaning on your elbow with your chest facing out. Make sure your elbow is aligned with your shoulder. Lift your hips off the ground, so that you are supported by your elbow and feet. Your body should be a straight line from your shoulders through your hips to your feet. Your top arm can point toward the ceiling or rest on your top hip. Hold the position for as long as you can, then lower the hips back down. See Figure 11.12.

FIGURE 11.12 Side Bridge

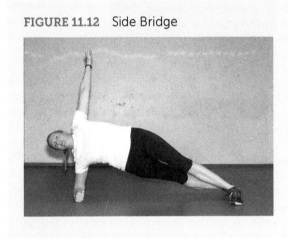

- *Hip bridge* This exercise is designed to stimulate the use of gluteal muscles and reduce hamstring involvement in hip extension. Lying on the ground with your knees bent, feet flat on the floor, and arms at the side, contract your gluteal muscles as you raise your hips off the ground. Make sure you don't drive the head of the femur forward; instead activate your core muscles and use your hips as the hinge moving up and down. Hold for 5 seconds at the top for 5 to 8 repetitions. When you can maintain a level spine, you can try a one leg lift. See Figure 11.13.

FIGURE 11.13 Hip Bridge

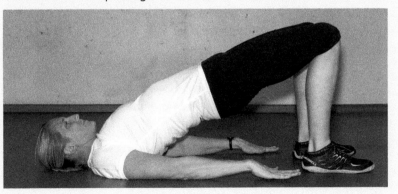

FIGURE 11.14 Suitcase Carry

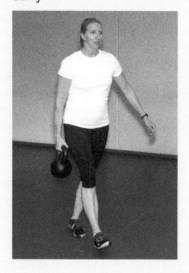

• *Suitcase carry* An asymmetrical carry challenges the lateral abdominal musculature. This is a great functional exercise for those that need to carry loads regularly. Using a kettlebell (or dumbbell) that is heavy enough to create tension in your abdominals, walk 30 to 50 steps while concentrating on using your core muscles to stay in a straight upright position so you don't lean to the weighted side. Switch arms. See Figure 11.14.

• *Stir the pot* An exercise that challenges the core muscles especially the rectus abdominus and obliques. Kneel on the floor behind a stability ball with your knees hip-width apart. Place your hands on the ball with your palms together. Keep your spine in neutral alignment as you roll the ball away from you until your elbows are on top of the ball. Move your elbows on the ball to simulate stirring a big pot, while maintaining a stable plank. Pull your abs toward your lower back to initiate the return to your starting position. To add more challenge, lift the knees and perform the exercise from the toes. Note that the size of the circle in your "stirring" motion directly affects the intensity—a larger circle is more challenging. Do 5 to 10 reps in one direction and repeat in the other direction. See Figure 11.15.

FIGURE 11.15 Stir the pot

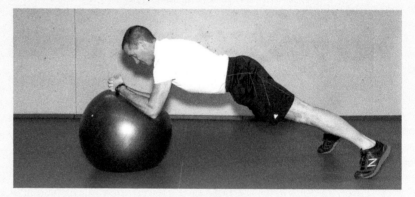

EXERCISES TO AVOID

A number of exercises that were popular in the 1960s and 1970s and are still recommended by some people put too much strain on the spine and should be avoided. Here are a few examples:

• standing toe touch while keeping the legs straight with knees locked (which puts strain on your lumbosacral joints)

• prone arch (aka, Superman)—lying on your stomach and trying to bring your head to your feet (the compression can put 1300 lb. of force on the spine)

• back extensions past 90 degrees on a Roman chair—your upper body is over a bench with your feet braced while you pull your trunk back up over the bench (this exercise puts a lot of stress on your back [approximately 890 lb. of compression] plus any additional weight you are holding)

- yoga plow—lying on your back and trying to put your feet up behind your head (which strains the neck and back)
- sit-ups, especially where you put your hands behind your head and pull on your neck to assist the sit-up (which may also pull your vertebrae out of alignment). Although it trains your abdominals and hip flexors, it imposes extremely large compression forces (more than 730 lb.) on the discs of your spine.

If you are involved in a fitness program and believe an exercise you are asked to do may harm your back, speak to the instructor and ask for an alternative. Do not do anything that causes pain. Protecting your back is more important than adhering strictly to a fitness program, and you are the person most aware of your body's limitations.

STRETCHING A HEALTHY SPINE

Regular stretching exercises help keep muscles and ligaments flexible. Stretches can also reduce stress on joints and improve the flow of blood and nutrients throughout the body. Without stretching, stiffness, limitation of movement, and pain can occur or increase. Stretching is important to prepare the muscles for physical activity, exercise, and job-related work. Stretching can prevent muscle strain and soreness, improve posture, improve range of motion, and help avoid injuries (National Institute of Arthritis and Musculoskeletal and Skin Diseases, 2016). See the *Fit for Duty, Fit for Life* training guide for instructions of an active warm-up with dynamic stretching and a cool-down with static stretching. Here are four examples of specific stretches for the back and legs:

- *Cat-cow stretch* Kneel on the floor, resting on your hands and knees. Lift your chest and tailbone to the ceiling while curving your spine down toward the floor. Raise your head up and hold for a few seconds. Slowly bring your spine back to the starting position and then arch your back like a cat as high as possible. Drop your head toward the floor and hold this position for a few seconds. Slowly bring your spine back to the starting position. Repeat 10 to 20 times. See Figure 11.16.

FIGURE 11.16 Cat-Cow Stretch

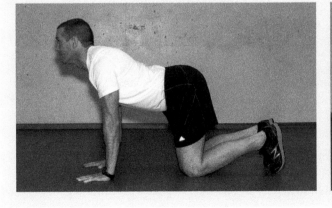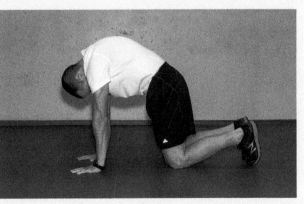

- *Modified back extensions* Lie on your stomach. Prop yourself up on your elbows extending your back. If there is no pain, slowly begin to straighten your elbows, further extending your back, until you feel a mild stretch. Hold for 20 to 30 seconds. Return to the starting position. See Figure 11.17.

FIGURE 11.17   Modified Back Extensions

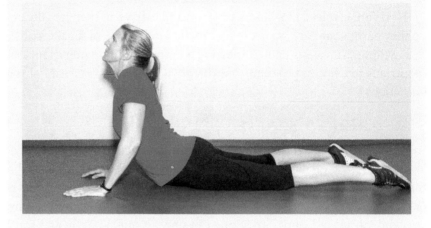

- *Hamstring stretch (lying down)* Lie flat on your back and put one leg straight up in the air. Keeping your leg as straight as possible, grasp behind your thigh and slowly bring your leg toward your chest until a gentle stretch is felt. Hold for 20 to 30 seconds. Repeat with other leg. A partner can assist you with this stretch by holding your leg straight and helping you stretch. See Figure 11.18.

FIGURE 11.18   Hamstring Stretch

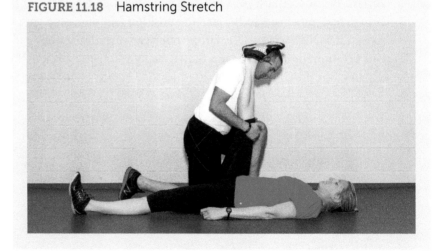

- *Piriformis stretch* Lie flat on your back with your knees bent. Lift one ankle up and place it across the opposite knee. Reach underneath the bottom leg and pull it up toward your chest until you feel a gentle stretch. Hold for 20 to 30 seconds. Repeat with other leg. See Figure 11.19.

FIGURE 11.19 Piriformis Stretch

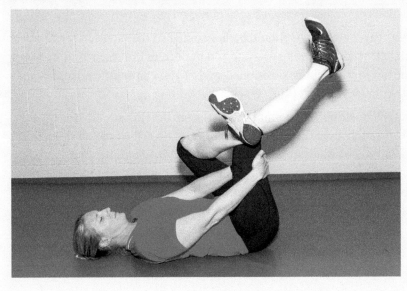

TIPS ON PROPER POSTURE
PROPER SITTING IN A VEHICLE

It is essential to sit properly, especially when driving. Because law enforcement officers may spend a great deal of time in vehicles, it is important that they look after their backs. Law enforcement officers complain of low-back pain and general backaches as the result of sitting in vehicles that are damaged and uncomfortable. Whether you are on the job or enjoying a drive, here are some guidelines to assist you in sitting correctly (CCHOS, 2009; Kumar & Narayan, 2001; Mack, 2002):

- Initially set up the seat properly by having the steering wheel fully up and forward, and the seat at its lowest height with the cushion tilted so the front edge is in the lowest position so there is no pressure on your knees or strain on your back and shoulder muscles. Have the back rest in upright position with the torso at approximately 100-degrees so it provides continual lumbar support but is not too far back that you bend your neck and head (don't slide forward on the cushion). The head restraint should be in middle back of head to prevent whiplash, and have your seat fully rearwards when first getting in.

- Then, raise your seat as high as is comfortable to improve your vision of the road. Ensure roof clearance. Adjust your seat so that there is about two to three fingers' width in the space between the front of the seat cushion and the back of the driver's knee. If it is too long, it will exert pressure on the back of the knees, be uncomfortable, and may impede proper blood circulation in the legs and feet.

- Adjust the steering wheel for height or tilt and pull it back downwards (facing your chest) for easy reach. The centre of the steering wheel should be about 25 to 30 cm (10 to 12 in.) from the driver's breast bone. Shorter individuals may require seat cushions and pedal extenders to depress the break and accelerator pedals. The closer you are to the air bag, the higher the possibility of injury if the air bag deploys, even if you are wearing a seat belt.

- Your rear-view mirror should be positioned so that you can see the two rear pillars as well as the roofline and bottom of the rear window. Your side mirrors should be positioned so that you can see the adjacent lane rather than the side of the vehicle.

- Seatbelt position is very important. The lap portion should be pulled down snugly over the hipbones to prevent the belt from riding up in a crash (which could cause internal injuries). The shoulder belt should be high enough to ensure that the belt does not fall off your shoulder (to prevent your hitting the steering wheel or windshield). Purchase a shoulder strap cushion to help reduce discomfort.

- When getting in the vehicle, sit and then rotate your legs in as one unit to prevent twisting of the spine. When exiting, make sure to rotate your legs as one unit to the door, place your feet on the ground, and then stand up.

- Redistribution of the components in your duty belt can help you sit properly. Some suggestions include moving the baton to a pocket on the thigh and the radio or phone to a pocket on the chest in a designed uniform. The bullet magazine, handcuffs, and pepper spray should all be placed on the front of the duty belt to ensure that the back is fully supported by the car's backrest. A soft pouch like the one containing latex gloves could be placed on the lumbar spine.

- Remove items from your pockets including wallet and keys. The compression on your soft tissue can reduce circulation and press on nerves. Position items that you may need while driving close to you (e.g., sunglasses, tissues, mints). Take time to pull over if necessary to access these items instead of reaching awkwardly for them while seated.

- Individuals should consciously and periodically change their posture, move around, or change physical activity. It is recommended that every 50 minutes of continuous work of one type should be followed by a 10-minute period of another activity.

PROPER SITTING AT A DESK

Low-back pain is associated with awkward sitting postures. In addition to the tips in Figure 11.20, here are a few things to consider:

- Your torso should be an arm's length away from the monitor, which should be at eye level. If you use a laptop, you may have to prop it up on some books or a box to be at the proper height.

- If you are using a mouse, make sure it is right next to your keyboard so you don't overreach or twist your shoulders, arm, or wrist.

- Keep both feet flat on the floor. If they don't touch, use a foot rest. Sitting cross-legged twists your spine, no longer keeps your shoulder square, overstretches the pelvic muscles, and increases your risk for varicose veins by interrupting blood flow.

FIGURE 11.20   Sitting at Work

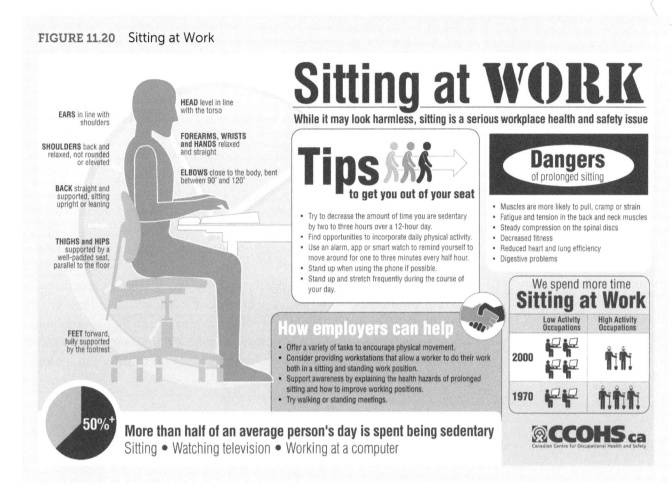

PROPER STANDING POSTURE

It is likewise important to have good posture while standing, which law enforcement officers may have to do for long stretches of time. Here are some tips:

- Stand with most of your weight on the balls of the feet, not the heels.

- Keep feet slightly apart, about shoulder width. Avoid locking your knees.

- Be sure that your head is square on top of the spine, not pushed forward. Stand straight and tall with shoulders upright. Sometimes rolling your shoulders backwards helps to align you. A way to determine if your head is in the correct alignment is to stand against a wall with your shoulders and bottom touching the wall. If your head is not also touching the wall then you are carrying your head too far forward (anterior head carriage).

- If you are standing for long periods of time, shift your weight from side to side and rock from heels to toes.

NUTRITIONAL CONSIDERATIONS FOR A HEALTHIER BACK

The mineral calcium helps your muscles, nerves, and cells work normally. Your body also needs calcium (as well as phosphorus) to make healthy bones. Our bodies continually remove small amounts of calcium from our bones and replace it with new calcium. If the body removes more calcium from bones than it replaces, they slowly become weaker and more prone to breaking (see information above on osteoporosis). Eating a diet rich in calcium allows the body to deposit calcium in bones so they stay strong (see Chapter 8 for more information). It is also important to know that calcium absorption can be affected by caffeine, and excessive amounts of protein, refined sugars, and fats.

Vitamin D, the "sunshine vitamin," is also necessary to bone health and is essential in helping to absorb and use calcium. It helps maintain serum calcium (the amount of calcium found in the bloodstream) and phosphate concentrations in the body (Ross et al., 2011). It improves muscle strength, and reduces fracture rates and rates of falling (Bischoff-Ferrari et al., 2004a, 2004b, 2005). In some cases, it plays a role in the prevention of certain cancers and protection against autoimmune diseases (Garland et al., 2006).

Although exposure to sunlight helps the body produce vitamin D, increased sun exposure is not recommended because it increases the risk for skin cancer (Health Canada, 2012). Many people do not get enough vitamin D from food sources alone. Health Canada recommends that everyone consume 400 to 2,000 IU of a vitamin D supplement daily (depending on health status) (Health Canada, 2012; Health Canada, 2015).

FINAL THOUGHTS

With increasing evidence that we need to spend less time sitting down (whether it's commuting, sitting at a desk, or in a work vehicle), it is important to move around, exercise your core muscles for a strong back, and seek prompt medical assistance if you have any back pain.

Refer to **assignment 11.1** (at www.emond.ca/fitness5e) to complete an assessment of your own back health.

KEY TERMS

arthritis
a group of conditions in which there is a degeneration of a joint following trauma to the joint (as a result of an infection or aging)

degenerative disc disease (DDD)
degeneration of the intervertebral discs, the result of aging and mechanical wear and tear

herniated disc
the rupture and protrusion of the gelatinous interior through the outer coating of the disc due to sudden pressure

intervertebral discs
flexible, gelatinous, shock-absorbing pads that separate the vertebrae

low-back pain (LBP)
a common disorder involving the muscles, nerves, and bones of the back, resulting in pain

osteoarthritis
arthritic degenerative disorder which causes pain and loss of normal spinal structure and function including vertebrae, facet joints, ligaments, and muscles

osteoporosis
a condition where bones become increasingly soft and porous, thinner, and more brittle, making them susceptible to risk of fracture, particularly of the hip, spine, and wrist

repetitive strain injury (RSI)
an injury that arises when soft tissue is subjected to repeated trauma (such as may be caused by typing or using a computer mouse) without the chance to recover from each trauma

rheumatoid arthritis
an autoimmune disease where the body attacks healthy joints, resulting in damage to cartilage, bone, tendons, and ligaments

sciatica
nerve pain down the leg as a result of nerves being compressed, inflamed, or irritated

spondylosis
a term that refers to the general degeneration of the spine associated with normal wear and tear that occurs in the joints, discs, and bones of the spine as people get older

vertebrae
the bones of the spine (singular: vertebra)

EXERCISES

TRUE OR FALSE?

1. Back flexibility and strengthening exercises should be done daily to maintain a healthy back.

2. When lifting the 36-kg (80-lb.) bag in the PARE test, it is best to keep your knees straight and lift primarily with your arms to prevent back strain.

3. Sharp muscle pain in the back is an indication that you should stop the activity you are engaged in.

4. Numbness, tingling, or burning in your legs can be a symptom of a cervical injury.

5. Lumbago is a term used for low-back pain.

6. It is important to do only work on your abdominals when you have a sore back.

7. Your intervertebral discs have more fluid in them at the end of the day.

8. The most common cause of a repetitive strain injury in law enforcement is an altercation with a non-compliant offender.

MULTIPLE CHOICE

1. The solution for reducing muscular imbalances is to _____ tight back muscles and _____ weak abdominal muscles.
   a. strengthen, stretch
   b. strengthen, rest
   c. stretch, strengthen
   d. shorten, strengthen
   e. rest, exercise

2. Which of the following is true of posture?
   a. a rigid posture is desirable
   b. muscle weakness does not influence posture
   c. alignment of one body part may affect another
   d. good posture requires additional muscular effort
   e. poor posture has not been linked to any health problems

3. The most common health complaint in people under the age of 50 is
   a. headache
   b. neckache
   c. backache
   d. leg problems
   e. foot problems

4. Which of the following is recommended for lifting a heavy load?
   a. lift with the leg muscles
   b. push or pull an object instead of carrying it
   c. carry the load in one arm to keep the other arm free
   d. let the arm muscles do most of the work
   e. bend over the object with a straight back and lift up with your arms

5. What is least likely to lead to back problems?
   a. aging
   b. lack of strength
   c. poor flexibility
   d. poor coordination
   e. protruding abdomen

6. When directing traffic, what standing position should you avoid?
   a. back arched
   b. knees locked
   c. knees bent
   d. one foot forward
   e. back straight

7. The most common cause of low-back pain is
   a. a slipped disc
   b. a herniated disc
   c. weak back muscles and strong stomach muscles
   d. weak stomach muscles
   e. weak stomach muscles and lack of back flexibility

8. Which of the following factors can contribute to low-back pain or increase the risk for low-back pain?
   a. being between the ages of 50 and 64
   b. depression, apathy, inattentiveness, boredom, emotional upsets, and lack of focus when doing your job
   c. tight muscles due to stress

   d. all of the above put an individual at higher risk for low-back pain
   e. there are no known factors that contribute to back pain

9. Pain that radiates down the back of the leg is known as
   a. osteoarthritis
   b. sciatica
   c. osteoporosis
   d. fibromyalgia
   e. repetitive strain injury

10. Which statement is true of arthritis?
    a. it is a rare condition
    b. it includes a variety of joint problems
    c. flexibility makes arthritis worse
    d. it is typically better at night
    e. it is characterized by good range of motion of a joint

11. If you lift an object, you should
    a. bend forward from the waist
    b. bend to the side
    c. lift as heavy a weight as you can
    d. bend at the knees and hips
    e. pay someone to do it for you

SHORT ANSWER

1. Describe the functions of the spine.

2. Summarize the causes of low-back pain.

3. What is a herniated disc? What are some of the causes of this type of injury?

4. What is arthritis and what impact does it have on your joints?

5. What is an RSI? What are some of the symptoms associated with RSI?

6. What is osteoporosis and what can you do to prevent the disease?

7. What special risks to a healthy back do law enforcement officers' duties create?

8. Describe some techniques for preventing low-back pain.

9. How are back injuries treated?

REFERENCES

Achterstraat, P. (2008). Managing injured police: NSW Police Force. Auditor-General, Ed.; Audit Office of New South Wales, Sydney Australia. Retrieved from http://www.audit.nsw.gov.au/ArticleDocuments/140/184_Managing_Injured_Police.pdf.aspx?Embed=Y

Al-Otaibi, S.T. (2015). Prevention of occupational back pain. *Journal of Family & Community Medicine, 22*(2), 73–77. Retrieved from http://doi.org/10.4103/2230-8229.155370.

American Association of Orthopaedic Surgeons (AAOS). (2013). Spine basics. Retrieved from http://orthoinfo.aaos.org/topic.cfm?topic=A00575

Anderson, G.S., Zutz, A., & Plecas, D.B. (2011). Police officer back health. *Journal of Criminal Justice Research, 2*(1), 1–17.

Arthritis Alliance of Canada (2011). The impact of arthritis in Canada: Today and over the next 30 years. Retrieved from http://www.arthritisalliance.ca/en/

Arthritis Foundation. (2017). Arthritis and diseases that affect the back. Retrieved from http://www.arthritis.org/about-arthritis/where-it-hurts/back-pain/causes/back-arthritis.php

Arthritis Society. (2011a). *Arthritis in the workplace.* Toronto: Author. Retrieved from http://www.arthritis.ca

Arthritis Society. (2011b). Rheumatoid arthritis—Know your options. Retrieved from http://www.arthritis.ca/document.doc?id=87 (offline as of September 2017)

Arthritis Society. (2015). Arthritis in Canada. Facts & figures. Retrieved from https://arthritis.ca/getmedia/43e83e3e-1a54-4fda-81d5-042ffaf9983f/Arthritis-Facts-Figures-EN.pdf

Arts, J.G., (2006). Low back pain in police officers. *Masters Theses.* 641. Retrieved from http://scholarworks.gvsu.edu/theses/641

Bischoff-Ferrari, H.A., et al. (2004a). Effect of vitamin D on falls: A meta-analysis. *Journal of the American Medical Association, 291*, 1999–2006.

Bischoff-Ferrari, H.A., et al. (2004b). Higher 25-hydroxyvitamin D concentrations are associated with better lower-extremity function in both active and inactive persons aged 60 years. *American Journal of Clinical Nutrition, 80*, 752–758.

Bischoff-Ferrari, H.A., et al. (2005). Fracture prevention with vitamin D supplementation: A meta-analysis of randomized control trials. *Journal of the American Medical Association, 295*, 2257–2264.

Bonneau, J., & Brown, J. (1995). Physical ability, fitness and police work. *Journal of Clincal Forensic Medicine, 2*, 157–164.

Bonneau, J., Stevenson, J.M., & Gledhill, N. (2001). Back fitness and back health assessment considerations for the Canadian physical activity, fitness and lifestyle appraisal. *Canadian Journal of Applied Physiology, 26*(3), 291–317.

Boskey, A.L., & Coleman, R. (2010). Aging and bone. *Journal of Dental Research, 89*(12), 1333–1348. Retrieved from http://doi.org/10.1177/0022034510377791

Briggs, A.M., & Buchbinder, R. (2009). Back pain: A national health priority area in Australia. *Medical Journal of Australia, 190*(9), 499–502.

Brown, J.J., Wells, G.A., Trottier, A.J., Bonneau, J., & Ferris, B. (1998). Back pain in a large Canadian police force. *Spine, 23*(7), 821–827.

Burton, A.K., Tillotson, K.M., Symonds, T.L., Burke, C., & Mathewson, T. (1996). Occupational risk factors for the first-onset and subsequent course of low back trouble: A study of serving police officers. *Spine, 21*(22), 2612–2620.

Calder, K.M., Stashuk D., & McLean L. (2008). Physiological characteristics of motor units in the brachioradialis muscle during fatiguing isometric contractions. *Journal of Electromyography and Kinesiology, 18*(1), 2–15.

Canadian Centre for Occupational Health and Safety (CCOHS). (2009). Driving and ergonomics; OSH answers fact sheets. Retrieved from https://www.ccohs.ca/oshanswers/ergonomics/driving.html

Canadian Physiotherapy Association. (2012). Low back pain. Retrieved from https://physiotherapy.ca/sites/default/files/valuePT/cpa_valuept_lowbackpain-en.pdf

Choi, S.-J., Ahn, J.H., Ryu, D.S., Kang, C.H., Jung, S.M., Park, M.S., & Shin, D.-R. (2015). Ultrasonography for nerve compression syndromes of the upper extremity. *Ultrasonography, 34*(4), 275–291. Retrieved from http://doi.org/10.14366/usg.14060

Choiniére, M., et al. (2010) The Canadian STOP-PAIN Project—Part 1: Who are the patients on the waitlists of multidisciplinary pain treatment facilities? *Canadian Journal of Anesthesia, 57*, 539–548.

Cohen, I.M., Plecas, D., & McCormick, A.V. (2011). *Getting a break in general duty police work: The Case of the Surrey RCMP*. Centre for Public Safety and Criminal Justice Research. University of the Fraser Valley.

Cummins, J., Lurie, J.D., Tosteson, T.D., Hanscom, B., Abdu, W.A., Birkmeyer, N.J.O., Herkowitz, H. (2016). Descriptive epidemiology and prior healthcare utilization of patients in the spine patient outcomes research trial's (SPORT) Three obeservational cohorts: Disc herniation, spinal stenosis and degenerative spondylolisthesis. *SPINE, 31*(7), 806–814.

Donnelly, C.J., Callaghan, J.P., & Durkin, J.L. (2009). The effect of an active lumbar system on the seating comfort of officers in police fleet vehicles. *International Journal of Occupational Safety and Ergonomics, 15*(3), 295–307.

Garland, C.F., et al. (2006). The role of vitamin D in cancer prevention. *American Journal of Public Health, 96*, 252–261.

Greenberg, J.S., & Dintiman, G.B. (1997). *Wellness: Creating a life of health and fitness*. Needham Heights, MA: Allyn and Bacon.

Gruevski, K.M., Homes, M.W., Gooyers, C.E., Dickerson, C.R., & Callaghan, J.P. (2016). Lumbar postures, seat interface pressures and discomfort responses to a novel thoracic support for police officers during prolonged simulated driving exposures. *Applied Ergonomics, 52*, 160–168.

H & K Perspectives. (2015). Bone health: A survey of Canadians, June 4–14, 2015.

Health Canada. (2012, March 22). Vitamin D and calcium: Updated dietary reference intakes. Retrieved from https://www.canada.ca/en/health-canada/services/food-nutrition/healthy-eating/vitamins-minerals/vitamin-calcium-updated-dietary-reference-intakes-nutrition.html

Health Canada. (2015, June 12). Health Canada's proposed changes to the daily values (DVs) for use in nutritional labelling. Retrieved from https://www.canada.ca/en/health-canada/services/food-nutrition/public-involvement-partnerships/technical-consultation-proposed-changes-daily-values-use-nutrition-labelling/consultation.html

Healthwise. (2016). Parafin wax for arthritis. Retrieved from https://www.healthlinkbc.ca/health-topics/zt1153

Holmes, M.W.R., McKinnon, C.D., Dicerson, C.R., & Callaghan, J.P. (2013). The effects of police duty belt and seat design changes on lumbar spine posture, driver contact pressure and discomfort. *Applied Ergonomics, 56*(1).

Janz, T., Seti, J., & Turner, A. (2009). Aboriginal Peoples Survey, 2006: An overview of the health of the Métis population. Statistics Canada; Cat. No. 89-637 no. 004.

Kumar, S., & Narayan, Y. (2001). Low back pain among RCMP officers: An investigation into vehicles, duty belts, and boots. *Canadian Police Research Centre (CPRC) Technical Report*, September, 1999. TR-01-99.

Lis, A.M., Black, K.M., Korn, H., & Nordin, M. (2007). Association between sitting and occupational LBP. *European Spine Journal, 16*(2), 283–298.

Lorentzon, M., Mellstrom, D., Haug, E., & Ohlsson, C. (2007). Smoking is associated with lower peak bone mineral density mainly as a result of reduced cortical thickness in young adult men. *Journal of Clinical Endocrinology & Metabolism, 92*(2), 428–429.

Lyons, K., Radburn, C., Orr, R., & Pope, R. (2017). A profile of injuries sustained by law enforcement officers: A critical review. *International Journal of Environmental Research and Public Health, 14*(2), 142.

Mack, T. (2002, February–March). Health news: Just sit right here. *Leisureways*. Oakville, ON: Formula.

Matsudaira, K., Konishi, H., Miyoshi, K., Isomura, T., & Inuzuka, K. (2014). Potential risk factors of persistent low back pain developing from mild low back pain in urban Japanese workers. *PLoS ONE, 9*(4), e93924. Retrieved from http://doi.org/10.1371/journal.pone.0093924

McGill, S. (2003). Enhancing low back health through stabilization. *ACE Certified News*. February/March. Retrieved from http://citeseerx.ist.psu.edu/viewdoc/download?doi=10.1.1.601.9172&rep=rep1&type=pdf

McGill, S. (2010). Core training: Evidence translating to better performance and injury prevention. *Strength & Conditioning Journal, 32*(3), 33–46.

McGill, S. (2016). *Low back disorders: Evidence-based prevention and rehabilitation*. 3rd Edition. Champaign, IL: Human Kinetics.

Meucci, R.D., Fassa, A.G., & Faria, N.M.X. (2015). Prevalence of chronic low back pain: Systematic review. *Revista de Saúde Pública, 49*, 1. Retrieved from http://doi.org/10.1590/S0034-8910.2015049005874

Mills, K. (2006). Standards for bone mineral density testing. Retrieved from http://www.osteoporosis.ca

National Institute of Arthritis and Musculoskeletal and Skin Diseases. (2016). Back pain. Retrieved from https://www.niams.nih.gov/health_info/back_pain/

National Institute of Health (NIH). (2016). Osteoporosis and related bone diseases handout on health: Osteoporosis. Retrieved from https://www.niams.nih.gov/health_info/bone/osteoporosis/osteoporosis_hoh.asp

National Institute for Neurological Disorders and Stroke (NINDS). (2014). Low back pain fact sheet. NID Publication No. 15-5161. Retrieved from https://www.ninds.nih.gov/Disorders/Patient-Caregiver-Education/Fact-Sheets/Low-Back-Pain-Fact-Sheet

National Institute for Neurological Disorders and Stroke. (2017). Low-back pain fact sheet. Retrieved from https://www.ninds.nih.gov/Disorders/Patient-Caregiver-Education/Fact-Sheets/Low-Back-Pain-Fact-Sheet

Neal, S.L., & Fields, K.B. (2010). Peripheral nerve entrapment and injury of the upper extremity. *American Family Physician, 81*(2), 147–155.

Osteoporosis Canada. (2011). Facts and statistics. Retrieved from http://www.osteoporosis.ca/index.php/ci_id/8867/la_id/1.htm

Osteoporosis Canada. (2017a). Osteoporosis Facts & Statistics. Retrieved from http://www.osteoporosis.ca/osteoporosis-and-you/osteoporosis-facts-and-statistics/

Osteoporosis Canada. (2017b). Testing. Retrieved from http://www.osteoporosis.ca/osteoporosis-and-you/diagnosis/testing/

Pinheiro, M.B, Ferreira, M.L., Refshauge, K., Ordonana, J.R., Machado G.C., Prado, L.R., Maher, C.G., & Ferreira, P.H. (2015). Symptoms of depression and risk of new episodes of low back pain. A systematic review and meta-analysis. *Arthritis Care & Research, 67*(11), 1591–1603.

Pinnington, M.A., Miller, J., & Stanley, I. (2004). An evaluation of prompt access to physiotherapy in the management of low back pain in primary care. *Family Practice, 21*(4), 372–380.

Plecas, D., McCormick, A.V., & Cohen, I.M. (2011). *An Analysis of police officer vehicle time: The case of Surrey RCMP officers*. Centre for Public Safety and Criminal Justice Research, University of the Fraser Valley: Abbotsford, BC. Retrieved from http://www.ufv.ca/CPSCJR.htm

Pryor, R.R., Colburn, D., Crill, M.T., Hostler, D.P., & Suyama, J. (2012). Fitness characteristics of a suburban special weapons and tactics team. *Journal of Strength and Conditioning Research, 26*, 752–757.

Public Health Agency of Canada (PHAC). (2007). Trends and impact: The basis for investment decisions. Trends related to health spending and prevention strategies. Retrieved from http://www.phac-aspc.gc.ca/alw-vat/trends-tendances/index-eng.php

Public Health Agency of Canada (PHAC). (2012). Life with arthritis in Canada: A personal and public health challenge. 2011. Retrieved from http://www.phac-aspc.gc.ca/cd-mc/arthritis-arthrite/lwaic-vaaac-10/index-eng.php

Ross, A.C., et al. (Eds.). (2011). Institute of Medicine (US) Committee to Review Dietary Reference Intakes for Vitamin D and Calcium; Dietary Reference Intakes for Calcium and Vitamin D. Washington (DC): National Academies Press (US); 2, Overview of Calcium. Retrieved from https://www.ncbi.nlm.nih.gov/books/NBK56060/

Schroeder, G.D., Guyre, C., & Vaccaro, A. (March 2016). The epidemiology and pathophysiology of lumbar disc herniations. *Seminars in Spine Surgery, 28*(1), 2–7. Lumbar Disc Herniation. doi:10.1053/j.semss.2015.08.003

Seaman, D.R. (2013). Body mass index and musculoskeletal pain: Is there a connection? *Chiropractic & Manual Therapies, 21*,15. doi: 10.1186/2045-709X-21-15

Statistics Canada. (2015). 2014 Canadian Community Health Survey. Cat. No. 11-001-X. Retrieved from http://www.statcan.gc.ca/daily-quotidien/150617/dq150617b-eng.htm

Tarride, J.-E., Hopkins, R.B., Leslie, W.D., Morin, S., Adachi, J.D., Papaioannou, A., Bessette, L., Brown, J.P., & Goeree, R. (2012). The burden of illness of osteoporosis in Canada. *Osteoporosis International, 23*(11), 2591–2600. Retrieved from http://doi.org/10.1007/s00198-012-1931-z

Tjepkema, M. (2003). Repetitive strain injury. Ministry of Industry. *Health Reports, 14*(4). Statistics Canada Catalogue no. 0040282-003-XIE. Ottawa: Statistics Canada.

Twell, L.K., Gregory, D.M., Reddigan, J., & Midodzi, W.K. (2014). Current and predicted prevalence of obesity in Canada: A trend analysis, *Canadian Medical Association Journal, 2*(1).

U.S. Preventative Services Task Force. (2005 June 15). Primary care interventions to prevent low back pain in adults: Recommendation statement. *American Family Physician. 71*(12), 2337–2338.

Zhao, L.J., Liu, Y.J., Hamilton, J., Recker, R.R., & Deng, H.W. (2006). Interventions decreasing obesity risk tend to be beneficial for decreasing risk to osteoporosis: A challenge to the current dogma. *Osteoporosis International, 17*(Suppl. 2), S37 (Abstract P152SU).

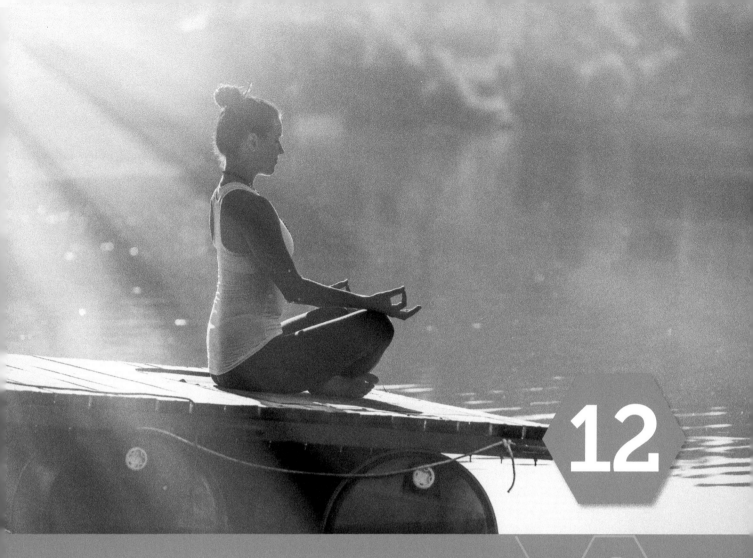

STRESS

LEARNING OUTCOMES

After completing this chapter, you should be able to:

- Explain the differences among neutral, good, and bad stress.

- Describe the health effects of stress.

- Describe the stressors that we face in daily life and that law enforcement personnel face.

- Explain what a critical incident is, what are the causes and symptoms for law enforcement personnel, and how to assist someone suffering from a critical incident.

- Explain what post-traumatic stress disorder is, how to recognize someone suffering from it, and what you can do to help an individual.

- Explain what resiliency and mindfulness are when dealing with operational stress injuries.

- Develop and implement coping techniques to deal with stress.

Stress is part of life. You can feel stress when you have too much to do, when too many expectations are put on you, or when you haven't slept well. Everyone lives with stress; it is an equal-opportunity destroyer, affecting people in all demographics. The World Health Organization has described stress as "a global epidemic" (WHO, 2003, p. 7). Stress itself is neither positive nor negative. How you handle or react to what you perceive as stress is what determines its effect on your life. This chapter examines what stress is; its causes, effects, and symptoms; and how it can be managed. More specifically, it looks at stress in law enforcement, with a special focus on critical incidents and post-traumatic stress disorder. We will also look at strategies for managing stress.

DEFINING STRESS

Dr. Hans Selye (1974) was the first to define **stress**, which in his words is the "non-specific response of the body to any demands made upon it" (p. 14). Shafer (1996) explains stress as the arousal of the mind and body in response to demands made on them. Experts in the field of psychoneuroimmunology suggest that as much as 85 percent of all disease and illness—from the common cold to cancer—can be linked to stress (Kiecolt-Glaser, 1999; Seaward, 2005).

Stress is a reaction to a stressor (stimulus or demand) that produces an elevated state of readiness or arousal. The greater the stimulus, the greater the stress reaction. Too much stress can lead to physical and emotional health issues. Emergency personnel benefit from a moderate amount of stress arousal, which makes a person more alert to his or her surroundings and helps the individual respond to the stress. A stressor can be a physical, psychological, social, biological, or chemical factor or force that puts real or perceived demands on the body, emotions, mind, or spirit of an individual.

TYPES OF STRESS

There are three types of stress response to a stressor (Le Fevre, Gregory, & Matheny, 2006; Morse & Furst, 1979; Selye, 1974; Sivasubramanian, 2016; see Figure 12.1):

1. *Neutral stress* (**neustress**) With this kind of stress, the mind and body are aroused but the stress is neither harmful nor helpful (Morse & Furst, 1979). An example is observing that traffic is slowing down in front of you, but you aren't in a hurry.

2. *Good stress* (**eustress**) This kind of stress is caused by the factors that initiate emotional and psychological growth. Eustress provides pleasure, adds meaning to life, and fosters an attitude that tries to find positive solutions to problems. It encourages optimal performance and can improve health. An example is competing with classmates to win a race or climbing Mount Kilimanjaro. Eustress is related to self-efficacy. Self-efficacy is one's judgment of how they can carry out a required task, action, or role. Having the belief that you can perform a task successfully will allow you to view stress as a positive challenge. High self-efficacy (optimistic, proactive, and confident) increases one's ability to set their goals higher and be motivated to achieve them.

3. *Bad stress* (distress) This kind of stress results in negative responses both in a person's career and in life. Unchecked negative stress can interfere with the physiological and psychological functioning of the body and may ultimately give rise to a hypokinetic disease or disability (Selye, 1974). Distress causes anxiety or concern and elicits the perception that an individual may not have the coping skills to deal with the situation. An example would be being faced with a challenge you cannot or have difficulty accomplishing (such as passing a BFOR test to meet job requirements or not having enough money to pay for next month's rent).

Figure 12.1 shows the relationship between stress and performance. Not enough stress will keep you from reaching your potential goals. Too much stress (distress) can harm your mental and physical health. Eustress challenges you in a positive way. Just the right amount of stress allows you to perform at your optimal level.

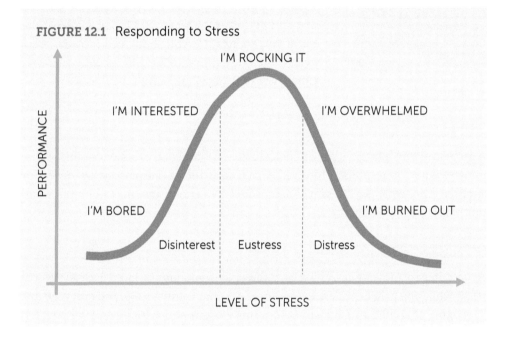

FIGURE 12.1 Responding to Stress

Refer to **assignment 12.1** (at www.emond.ca/fitness5e) to fill out a life experience survey and rate how experiences in your life are impacting your stress level.

THE STRESS RESPONSE

Hans Selye concluded that the body reacts to good and bad stress in the same way. He labelled the stress response—the body's reaction to stress—the general adaptation syndrome (GAS). It includes three stages: the fight-or-flight response, the stage of resistance, and the stage of exhaustion (Selye, 1956, 1976).

The fight-or-flight response (or alarm stage) is the stage when the body prepares itself to cope with a stressor. The response is a warning signal that a stressor is present (whether real or imagined). The body prepares for fight or flight by releasing cortisol and adrenaline. These two powerful hormones increase heart rate, blood pressure, and breathing rate. They redirect blood from the stomach and digestive organs to muscles, activating and tensing them, preparing them for action.

It's important to be aware of your fight-or-flight response and that it gives you an appropriate response for an appropriate event. If you are in a state of alarm all the time (for real or imagined events), then it may be time to seek professional help.

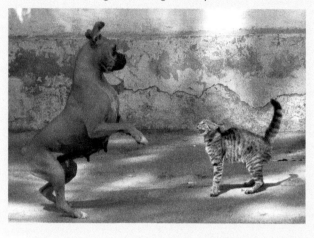

FIGURE 12.2 Fight-or-Flight Response

In the **stage of resistance**, the body actively resists and attempts to cope with the stressor. If you are able to channel that energy, your body returns to normal. However, being aroused for too long and too often may lead to fatigue. Headaches, forgetfulness, constipation, diarrhea, asthma, anxiety attacks, and high blood pressure are all signs of prolonged arousal.

The **stage of exhaustion** is the phase in which the body is subjected to continual stress and fatigue for days and weeks and the body begins to shut down, usually resulting in illness. You may notice at the end of exam period you always tend to get a cold or the flu. If you are healthy, your body will recover; however, if the body cannot cope, disease and malfunction of organ systems may result.

STRESSORS

A **stressor** is any physical, psychological, or environmental event or condition that initiates the stress response. However, what is stressful for one person may not be for another. Also, what is a stressor for someone at a certain time may not be stressful for that same person later.

STRESSORS IN DAILY LIFE

As you prepare for your career in law enforcement, you may be faced with additional stress while you gain experience through education, volunteering, and everyday life. Teen stress is similar to adult stress in terms of signs and symptoms. However, the transition period into adulthood has unique stressors, such as the following:

- school stressors (academic responsibilities or pressures for good grades, finances or debt, anxiety, poor work/school–life balance, discrimination (El-Ghoroury, Galper, Sawaqdeh, & Bufka, 2012))

- physical changes/stressors (increases in weight and height, menarche (onset of menstruation), and pubertal changes, as well as poor diet, lack of sleep, and lack of exercise resulting in fatigue or illness)

- mental changes/stressors (issues with independence, sexual attraction, aggressive behaviour, and exposure to experimenting with new things (such as substance abuse))

- emotional issues (changing relationships with peers, responsibilities to family, separation or divorce of parents, romantic relationships, and getting along with siblings and other family members)

- feelings of being **overloaded** (excessive time pressure, excessive responsibility, and excessive expectations to succeed)

- changes and transitions (starting or ending a relationship, death of a loved one, moving, job change or loss, going to school away from home or for the first time in a number of years)

- money problems (finding a part-time or full-time job, paying tuition/rent/bills, learning how to save money, support a family)

- loss of self-esteem (falling behind academically or professionally, failing to meet personal standards and goals or others' expectations).

FACTS TO THINK ABOUT

STRESS AND MENTAL HEALTH STATISTICS

In 2016, the National College Health Assessment (Ontario Canada Reference Group) found:
- The majority (65 percent) of students reported experiencing overwhelming anxiety in the previous year (up from 57 percent in 2013).
- Almost half (46 percent) of students reported feeling so depressed in the previous year it was difficult to function (up from 40 percent in 2013).
- Students who had seriously considered suicide in the previous year increased from 10 percent in 2013 to 13 percent in 2016.
- Students reporting a suicide attempt within the previous year also increased: 2.2 percent (or 558 students), up from 1.5 percent in 2013. Additionally, 9 percent of students (or 2,245 students) indicated that they had attempted suicide, but not in the previous year.

Regarding overall mental health:
- In any given year, one in five Canadians experiences a mental health or addiction problem.
- By the time Canadians reach 40 years of age, one in two has—or have had—a mental illness.
- Mental illness is a leading cause of disability in Canada.
- Most (70 percent) mental health problems have their onset during childhood or adolescence.
- Young people aged 15 to 24 are more likely to experience mental illness and/or substance use disorders than any other age group.
- Men have higher rates of addiction than women, while women have higher rates of mood and anxiety disorders.
- Mental and physical health are linked. People with a long-term medical condition such as chronic pain are much more likely to also experience mood disorders. Conversely, people with a mood disorder are at much higher risk of developing a long-term medical condition.
- Regarding the stigma of mental health, in 2014, 64 percent of Ontario workers would be concerned about how work would be affected if a colleague had a mental illness and 39 percent of Ontario workers indicate that they would not tell their managers if they were experiencing a mental health problem.
- The economic burden of mental illness in Canada is estimated at $51 billion per year. This includes health care costs, lost productivity, and reductions in health-related quality of life.

SOURCES: ACHA, 2016; Boak, Hamilton, Adlaf, Beitchman, Wolfe, & Mann, 2016; Dewa, 2014; Government of Canada, 2006; Pearson, Janz, & Ali, 2013; Smetanin, Stiff, Briante, & Khan, 2011.

STRESSORS FACED BY LAW ENFORCEMENT

Evidence shows that law enforcement officers such as police officers, correctional officers, custom officers, and Canadian military are at least twice as likely as the general population to suffer from post-traumatic stress disorder (PTSD), due to the risk of routine exposure to traumatic stressors (Ontario Ministry of Labour, 2016). Added to these stressors are the issues of dealing with ever-changing technology, cultural diversity, and the imperative of "political correctness." Below is a summary of the stressors that various law enforcement agencies are facing.

STRESSORS FACED BY PROVINCIAL AND FEDERAL CORRECTIONAL OFFICERS

In corrections, guarding inmates in overcrowded facilities can be dangerous and thankless work, fuelling stress that impacts an officer both at work and at home. Many correctional officers feel isolated and alienated from society and over time they become cynical or hypervigilant to the point where they cannot relax. Stress levels continue to increase because, in spite of statistics indicating a general decline in violent crime in Canada since 1991, public perception, public scrutiny, and adverse media publicity suggest otherwise. While Ontario's incarceration rate has fallen, it has not dropped as dramatically as the province's crime rate (Statistics Canada, 2015, 2016). Among the offences that have increased in recent years are homicides, sexual offences against children, and child pornography, including exploitation of children over the Internet (Statistics Canada, 2012). More than one in four officers have been physically assaulted by an inmate, more than 80 percent have responded to a serious injury to an inmate, and almost 20 percent have witnessed the death of an inmate (Boyd, 2011). The main stressors facing correctional officers are shown in Table 12.1.

TABLE 12.1   Stressors Faced by Provincial and Federal Correctional Officers

Operational Stressors	• Exposure to occupational violence (overcrowding, gang involvement, and inmates' mental-health issues). • Verbal and physical abuse from inmates, confrontational individuals. • Negative work environment (co-workers who may be bringing in contraband, getting too friendly with inmates, using unnecessary force). • Burned out co-workers venting their frustrations. • Custodial responsibilities (maintaining security, preventing escapes and inmate fights, and victimization) while maintaining treatment functions (confinement issues and rehabilitation). • Harassment issues (sexist, racist, and homophobic). • Extensive paperwork, reports, segregation reviews.
Organizational Stressors	• Staffing issues (rotating shift work, mandatory overtime, understaffed, rapid staff turnover, lack of appropriate backup, competition for assignments and favouritism). • Capacity issues (overcrowding and limited resources). • Weak leadership (officers feeling vulnerable, scrutinized, and unsafe). • Lack of adequate resources (e.g., programming and services for inmates with mental-health issues). • Scrutinized over quick decisions on life and death situations.
Public View Stressors	• Perception of negative treatment of inmates. • Poor support from friends and family (feelings of isolation and estrangement). • Unrealistic expectation of what correctional services can do for rehabilitation to address a lifetime of trauma and dysfunction while incarcerated.

SOURCES: Brower, 2013; Finn, 2000; MCSCS, 2015, 2016a; Sapers, 2017; ToersBijns, 2012.

FYI

ASSAULTS IN CORRECTIONAL INSTITUTIONS

Recent statistics from Correctional Service of Canada (CSC)'s Offenders Management System state an average of 310 recorded assaults on staff in federal institutions every year across the country. Of the ones that occurred from 2011 to 2016, roughly two-fifths were physical assaults, while the others involved less harmful actions like spitting, throwing or swinging objects, lunging, or making threats. Although most of these physical assaults were punches, hits, or kicks, more than 40 entailed the use of weapons. Out of all of the reported assaults over the same five-year period, about 30 percent occurred in situations involving prison security intervention, roughly one-quarter during escorts and/or handcuffing, and more than 10 percent during kitchen meal service.

SOURCE: Cottrill, 2017.

STRESSORS FACED BY CANADIAN CUSTOM OFFICERS

The Canadian Border Services Agency (CBSA) is responsible for administrating the legislation that governs the admissibility of people and goods into and out of Canada. They must identify, detain, and remove people who are inadmissible, bar illegal goods, administer and enforce trade legislation and agreements, protect food safety, plant and animal health, and collect duties and taxes on imported goods. Table 12.2 is a composite of stressors faced by custom officers.

TABLE 12.2   Stressors Faced by Canadian Custom Officers

Operational Stressors	• Potential risk at border crossings (weapons, contraband, infectious diseases, organized crime, and terrorism).
	• Dealing with sophisticated criminal activity and concealment risks around contraband crossing the border.
	• Dealing with individuals crossing borders illegally.
	• Dealing with refugee claims.
	• Safety concerns of working alone in rural areas.
	• Repetitive and mundane tasks (administrative and booth work).
	• Doing secondary searches (potentially angry or non-compliant individuals).
	• Language barriers.
	• Welcoming and resettling refugees from conflict areas around the world.
Organizational Stressors	• Out-of-date management strategies.
	• Limited opportunities for advancement.
	• Responsible for knowing and administrating over 90 acts of legislation.
	• Inadequate resources for security and detainment.
Public View Stressors	• Perception that individuals are targeted for secondary searches.
	• Criticism on how they handle firearms, arrest, and detention.

SOURCES: CBSA, 2016, 2017; Côté-Boucher, 2015; Hopkins, 2017; Kalman, 2016.

STRESSORS FACED BY POLICE AND PUBLIC/PRIVATE SECURITY

The complexities of policing have changed drastically in the last 20 years. We have seen a decline in the number of police officers in Canada years while the proportion of police officers aged 40 years and older has grown to 55 percent, which potentially increases the number of exposures to critical incidents (Greenland & Alam, 2017). Given the financial and personnel investments associated with training police officers, officer retention is an emerging area of research. Some research suggests that turnover can lead to disruption in the workplace, can have a negative impact on police work and crime control, and may hinder the development of leadership within the ranks (Scheer, 2014). There is an increased demand for greater transparency over situations involving officers, a continual need to keep up with cultural and mental health currency, and the perception that 'serve' is being emphasized over 'serve and protect' with safety consequences to officers.

Community policing has come to the forefront of the job in policing. Working directly with the community can provide job satisfaction and overall departmental efficiency. However, the transition to community policing has caused apprehension on the part of officers who must implement this fundamental shift in policing philosophy on a day-to-day basis. At times, the stress to perform to both service and community standards can be overwhelming.

With communities grappling with increasing economic costs of policing and fiscal challenges, since the late 2000s, there has been an increase in the hiring of private security to fill in the gaps and/or replace what public policing used to cover, especially in service-oriented duties and social events. Private security is growing at a faster pace than the public police, almost doubling in numbers in the past 20 years (Canadian Broadcasting Corporation, 2013). In some provinces, these special constables provide court security, prisoner transportation, or other security services that had once been done by sworn officers. Educational institutions, health care facilities, housing, and transit authorities employ special constables. Although required to provide the same level of security as public policing, many private policing/security agencies, while patrolling communities, waterfront, business and housing developments, colleges and universities, transit, etc., are not equipped in terms of resources, training, or equipment resulting in safety issues like assaults, break and enters, domestic violence, and drug trafficking (Ruddell & Jones, 2014). The stressors for policing and security are listed below in Table 12.3.

STRESSORS FACED BY THE CANADIAN MILITARY

Canada is home to a significant military population per capita: close to 70,000 regular force members in the Canadian Armed Forces, 27,000 reserve force members, 54,000 military families, and more than 600,000 veterans. These Canadians require unique standards of health protection, prevention, and care (CIMVHR, 2016). In addition to stressors faced by law enforcement, they face combat stressors. **Combat stress** is a common experience for military personnel in a war zone and can be seen as a healthy adaptation to a potentially life-threatening environment. For instance, being hypervigilant during a dangerous combat exposure is important and necessary. But it may be problematic in a safe environment, such as one's home or in a restaurant (Kelly, 2016). This stress, described by terms like 'shell shock,' 'battle fatigue,' and 'combat stress reaction,' takes a tremendous toll on individuals who risk their lives for our freedom. Some stressors and traumatic events unique to the military are presented in Table 12.4.

TABLE 12.3   Stressors Faced by Police, Public and Private Security, and Other Protective Agencies

Operational Stressors	• Threats to officers' safety (entering an unfamiliar building, responding to a weapons call, pursuing vehicles at high speeds, and responding to disturbances). • Responsibility of protecting the lives of others. • Exposure to criminals and people in pain/distress (dangers involved, language barriers, conflict resolution, and being lied to). • Excessive computer and paperwork. • Boredom alternating with sudden alertness/energy/excitement. • Issues of not being in control of a situation.
Organizational Stressors	• Staffing issues (rotating shift work, work overload, understaffing, promotional issues, paramilitary nature of the job, complying with rules and procedures). • Leadership issues (lack of support, lack of rewards, poor communication, being second guessed or punished for minor infractions, and top-down decisions). • Lack of funding (out-of-date equipment, having to adopt a "band-aid" approach to problems). • Court issues (unfavourable court decisions, attending during time off). • Stigma attached to disclosing psychological, emotional, and physical issues at work.
Public View Stressors	• Expectations of the public to do what they ask. • Women and minorities discrimination. • Isolation from friends and family. • Being recorded on someone's smartphone while working.

SOURCES: Anderson, Litzenberger, & Plecas, 2002; Andersen, Papazoglou, Koskelainen, Nyman, Gustafsberg, & Arnetz, 2015; Andersen, Gustafsberg, Papazoglou, Nyman, Koskelainen, & Pitel, 2015; Amaranto, Steinberg, Castellano, & Mitchell, 2003; Duxbury & Higgins, 2012; Malm, 2005; Violanti, 2014.

TABLE 12.4   Stressors Faced by the Canadian Military

Operational and Organizational Stressors	• Working in a paramilitary structure (hierarchy, lack of freedom in decision making, imposed dress/hygiene conditions, directed physical training, imposed living locations in Canada and abroad). • Deployments (detachment from family/partner, operation prep, decompression and reintegration, living in countries with different cultures, going between safe and unsafe zones). • Gender, racial, or sexual orientation biases. • Fear of release from service due to occupational unfitness (musculoskeletal disorders and injuries and unsure of another career). • Transition from military to civilian life.
Combat Stressors	• Continual sound of long-range artillery and surface-to-surface missiles. • Dangers (search-and-rescue operations, disaster aid, training accidents, front-line missions). • Witnessing horrific events (violence, disasters, genocide, handling injured bodies). • Realistic fears (dying on tour, being captured and tortured, getting injured).
Public Perception Stressors	• Failure to recognize, understand, and support those with PTSD. • Isolation and lack of support from friends and family. • Lack of support for family while on tour.

SOURCES: CIMVHR, 2016; El-Gabalawy et al., 2016; Kelly, 2016,

STRESSORS FROM WORKPLACE HEALTH AND SAFETY HAZARDS

Law enforcement officers encounter many occupational health and safety risks on a daily basis or at some point in their career. These are grouped into five categories, as shown in Table 12.5.

TABLE 12.5   Stressors from Workplace Health and Safety Hazards

Physical Hazards	• Confrontation with a suspect or inmate with a weapon. • Physical threats and assaults when arresting and transporting suspects and prisoners. • Exposure to ambient environmental factors (low or high temperatures, rain, wind, snow) resulting in acute or chronic diseases. • Excessive exposure to sunshine (UVA/UVB) being linked to cancers. • Exposure to high noise level from emergency alarms/sirens and firearms training.
Chemical Hazards	• Second-hand smoke, furnace fumes, car exhaust (carbon monoxide), subway iron particles, or carcinogens. • Exposure to radio frequencies (e.g., the use of police traffic radar). • Officers who carry OC spray are at risk of suffering the effects of its use especially in confined spaces (jail, interview room, vehicle).
Biological Hazards	• Exposure to micro-organisms in the air (bacteria, virus, fungi, mould). • Exposure to communicable diseases like HIV/AIDS, tuberculosis, hepatitis A, B, or C, rabies. • Infected needle stick injuries. • Human or animal bites.
Ergonomic Hazards	• Injuries to the musculoskeletal system from uncomfortable working positions, heavy physical tasks, altercations with suspects. • Back problems related to seatbelt use and riding in vehicles all day, vibrations from vehicles, wearing body armour and duty belt, and working on a computer in a confined space (such as car computers). • Injuries to the back and lower extremities from standing/walking all day in improper footwear and poor posture.
Psycho-Social Hazards	• Difficulties with supervisors or fellow workers, sexual harassment, discrimination, or dealing with issues like suicide. • Stress from exposure to violent and life-threatening situations (critical incidents). • Stress from departmental politics, inadequate resources to do the job, and lack of support. • Increase in requirements of the job with less resources and more accountability.

SOURCES: Boyd, 1995, 2011; Brown, Wells, Trottier, Bonneau, & Ferris, 1998; CDC, 2015; Cottrill, 2017; Czarnecki & Janowitz, 2003; Ellis, Choi, & Blaus, 1993; ILO, 2012; Kohan & O'Connor, 2002; Loo, 2003; Parsons, 2004; Public Service Foundation of Canada, 2015; Van Netten, Brands, Hoption, Cann, Spinelli, & Sheps, 2003; Wirth, Vena, Smith, Bauer, Violanti, & Burch, 2013.

IMPACT OF STRESS ON THE FAMILY

Stress can cause major difficulties within the family. The demands placed on law enforcement officers and ongoing threats of and exposure to violence can seep into their family life. Divorce due to stress from the job is higher than other occupations (Galatzer-Levy et al., 2013; Russell, 2014). Shift work, conflict with personality, and family roles (wanting to keep their family safe) can all take their toll on the family (Karaffa et al., 2015). Like any injury, the symptoms of critical incidents/trauma can make it difficult to cope and get along with sufferers. Reactions include (Carlson & Ruzek, 2014; CIMVHR, 2016; Meis, Erbes, Polusny, & Compton, 2010; Veterans Affairs Canada, 2006):

- although sympathy may be helpful initially, over time it may lead to low expectations of the sufferer, eroding confidence in the ability to recover from the trauma.

- changes in how the family functions may lead to feelings of pain or loss or feelings of isolation, from changes in family communications to alienation or depression.

- fear and worry experienced by the one suffering from this negative stress may make others feel unsafe or feel they have to walk on eggshells.

- expressions of anger and aggression may produce fear or fear of violence toward family members.

- family members may avoid talking about the traumatic event to avoid further pain or because they are fearful of the person's reaction.

- family members may feel anger about the trauma and how it affected their lives; children may react to concerns over their parent's safety by having nightmares, regressive behaviour (temper tantrums, whining, thumb sucking), lack of emotion, anxiety, aggressive and inappropriate outbursts.

- the person with stress who cannot sleep may make it more difficult for family members to sleep as well.

- partners/adult children must assume the role of both parents, rearrange their agendas to fit duty schedules (especially in specialized units), or simply learn to function independently.

THE EFFECTS OF STRESS

Most people look after their cars better than their bodies. They fill their gas tank with proper fuel, get regular oil changes, check the air pressure, and rotate their tires, but can the same be said for looking after themselves?

Stress has the ability to wear your body down. Stress can have short- or long-term effects on your body. When your body responds negatively to stress, such responses often manifest as psychosomatic symptoms (physical symptoms resulting from mental conflict).

Refer to **assignment 12.2** (at www.emond.ca/fitness5e) to take a test to determine whether you recognize stress in your life and assess your coping strategies.

SHORT- AND LONG-TERM EFFECTS OF STRESS

Table 12.6 outlines some of the short- and long-term effects of stress and their physical, mental, and emotional consequences.

Not understanding that these changes in the body are due to stress, some individuals turn to their doctor to treat the symptoms rather than the problem. For example, a doctor may prescribe medication for blood pressure, irritable bowel syndrome, or depression, rather than suggesting counselling, meditation, or time off for coping with stress.

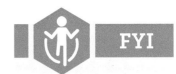

FYI

EXPOSURE TO HUMAN BIOWASTE

More than 90 percent of correctional officers had been exposed to blood, and more than 75 percent to feces, spit, and urine. Notably, more than 90 percent had responded to requests for staff assistance and to medical emergencies, two-thirds had received a credible threat of harm from an inmate, and almost 40 percent had been hit by feces, urine, vomit, or spit.

SOURCE: Boyd, 2011.

TABLE 12.6   Effects of Stress

Short-Term Effects	<ul><li>Muscle tension</li><li>Rapid breathing</li><li>Increased heart rate and blood pressure</li><li>Reduced digestive activity and urine output</li><li>Increased mental alertness</li><li>Bronchiole dilation</li><li>Increased metabolic rate</li><li>Headaches, fatigue</li><li>Helps create new memories, improves mood, and encourages creative thinking</li></ul>
Long-Term Effects	<ul><li>Increased blood pressure (retention of water and sodium by kidneys)</li><li>Suppresses immune system</li><li>Severe headaches, depression, anxiety, and fatigue</li><li>Weight control problems</li><li>Digestive issues like constipation, diarrhea, inflammation of the intestines</li><li>Sleep issues</li><li>Impairs memory formation</li><li>Interferes with performance, impairs efforts to be physically active, makes us uncomfortable</li><li>Increased risk of metabolic syndrome</li></ul>

SOURCES: Kim & McKenzie, 2014; Stults-Kolehmainen & Sinha, 2014; Vogel & Schwabe, 2016.

Some individuals will turn to drugs, alcohol, caffeine, or supplements to cope with their symptoms of fatigue, depression, and weight gain, instead of consulting with a professional and they may wind up with even more health issues due to the effects of those substances on the body.

CHRONIC STRESS

Over time, chronic stress can also have emotional consequences. Ignored or poorly managed chronic stress can have serious consequences, including:

- depression, leading to an inability to function normally at work and at home
- cynicism and suspiciousness
- emotional detachment from daily life
- excessive aggressiveness (which may trigger citizen complaints)
- marital or family problems
- alcoholism and other substance abuse
- suicide

It is important to recognize these symptoms, determine what stressors are impacting you, and find healthy coping techniques to deal with your circumstances, whether it be your lifestyle, thoughts, and/or emotions. Physical or mental stresses may cause physical illness as well as mental or emotional problems. Figure 12.3 shows the parts of the body most affected by stress.

FIGURE 12.3 The Effects of Chronic Stress

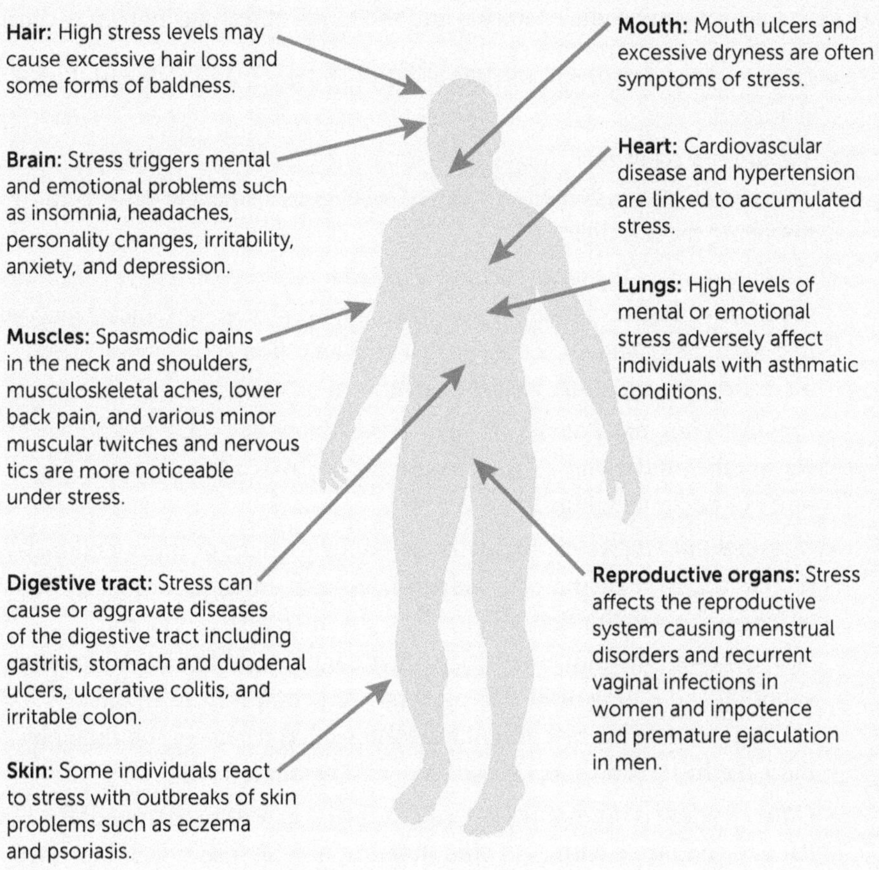

Hair: High stress levels may cause excessive hair loss and some forms of baldness.

Brain: Stress triggers mental and emotional problems such as insomnia, headaches, personality changes, irritability, anxiety, and depression.

Muscles: Spasmodic pains in the neck and shoulders, musculoskeletal aches, lower back pain, and various minor muscular twitches and nervous tics are more noticeable under stress.

Digestive tract: Stress can cause or aggravate diseases of the digestive tract including gastritis, stomach and duodenal ulcers, ulcerative colitis, and irritable colon.

Skin: Some individuals react to stress with outbreaks of skin problems such as eczema and psoriasis.

Mouth: Mouth ulcers and excessive dryness are often symptoms of stress.

Heart: Cardiovascular disease and hypertension are linked to accumulated stress.

Lungs: High levels of mental or emotional stress adversely affect individuals with asthmatic conditions.

Reproductive organs: Stress affects the reproductive system causing menstrual disorders and recurrent vaginal infections in women and impotence and premature ejaculation in men.

CRITICAL INCIDENTS

A critical incident (traumatic event) is a situation faced by an individual that causes unusually strong emotional reactions, which may interfere with their ability to function at the scene (current stress) or later (residual stress). Critical incidents are sudden and unexpected; disrupt one's sense of control; disrupt beliefs and values, as well as assumptions about the world in which we live, the people in it, and the work we do; involve the perception of a life-damaging threat; and may involve emotional or physical loss. How a given person will react to a particular event on a particular day cannot be predicted.

In law enforcement it is inevitable that you will be exposed to various critical incidents/traumatic events. For individuals who are used to being in control of their emotions and their surroundings, the debilitation caused by a critical incident may be surprising, embarrassing, frustrating, or overwhelming. Your response to a critical incident may have to do with what type of event it is and how relatable or catastrophic it may be.

TYPES OF CRITICAL INCIDENTS

Law enforcement personnel are often faced with critical incidents related to life and death. The following are some examples and the kinds of feelings they may cause:

- *Death/injury/shooting in the line of duty* The myth of invulnerability is shattered.

- *Suicide of a co-worker* Job and personal life pressures, and the pressure of balancing the two, come into focus. Colleagues also experience guilt over not being there to help.

- *Death of a child* The innocence represented by children can have a profound impact on officers, sometimes pushing them over the edge. Officers may feel that what they stand for is useless. Whether an officer should have a family of his or her own and other factors of identification can add even more stress.

- *Prolonged but failed rescue attempt* If the officer has come to know the victim, the officer may exhibit symptoms of stress arising from a deep sense of personal failure.

- *Mass-casualty incidents* Incidents involving carnage or mass fatalities— such as the 2011 earthquake, tsunami, and ensuing nuclear meltdowns in Japan, the Alberta flooding of 2013, the 2016 Prince Alberta, Saskatchewan medium-security penitentiary riot, or the 2014 Moncton shooting and killing of RCMP officers—can compromise an officer's ability to cope. This reaction may be intensified when compounded by mass confusion and shortages of staff and resources.

- *Officer's safety is unusually jeopardized* Daily exposure to potential danger, combined with a specific situation in which an officer becomes unusually vulnerable and lacks control, can trigger a stress reaction. An example is the York Regional Police officer who died during a routine traffic stop in 2011 or the 2016 fire in Fort McMurray, Alberta, which destroyed 1,500,000 acres and over 2,400 homes and businesses were lost.

- *Responding officer knows the victim* Arriving on the scene and discovering that you know the victim can trigger a critical stress reaction of the "if only I had driven faster" variety.

- *Officer responding to an abused individual* Officers must respond to incidents involving serious physical assault, including sexual assault, incest, molestation, and gang assaults that go beyond comprehension of human decency.

- *Events with excessive media coverage* In addition to dealing with the situation, officers must deal with crowd control and onlookers' morbid interest in seeing what has happened.

FACTORS AFFECTING RESPONSES TO CRITICAL INCIDENTS

Some officers are better able than others to cope with the stress of critical incidents. The following are some factors that affect coping (Connor & Butterfield, 2003):

- *Nature of the event* Has the officer witnessed this type of incident before? How severe is the incident?

EXPOSURE TO CRITICAL INCIDENTS

In the Ombudsmen report *In the Line of Duty*, Mr. Marin wrote "Police officers are often exposed to brutal murders, assaults, and shocking accidents; horrific sights, smells, and sounds. They put themselves in the line of fire and risk attack by knives, guns and ramming cars. This is the stuff of nightmares. Sometimes those nightmares stick, and sometimes they accumulate, wearing down even those with the strongest of constitutions."

SOURCE: Marin, 2012.

- *Degree of warning* Was the officer dispatched to the scene with an appropriate warning, or did the officer happen upon the scene?
- *Ego strength/coping style* Does the officer cope with tragic situations more easily than others do by accepting those situations as "fate"?
- *Prior mastery of the experience* How many times has the officer been exposed to a similar situation?
- *Proximity* How close does the officer feel to the person or incident? For example, if a child is involved, has the officer a child of the same age?
- *The amount of stress in the officer's life at the time* Is there already a great deal of stress in the officer's life, either at work or at home? If so, the incident may have a stronger impact.
- *The nature and degree of social support available to the officer after the critical incident* The more support an officer receives, the better are his or her chances of coping with the stress of a critical incident. The reactions of those supporting the officer may or may not be appropriate, and thus may further affect the individual.

SYMPTOMS OF STRESS ARISING OUT OF CRITICAL INCIDENTS

While most individuals recover from critical incident stress and remain healthy and productive, some critical incidents can be overwhelming. Each individual will respond differently, and what may be easy to cope with one day is impossible to cope with the next. Recognizing the symptoms of stress can allow us to help them. Developing symptoms is never a sign of weakness. Symptoms should be taken seriously. Symptoms that last for more than four weeks may indicate a much more serious problem. If you are suffering from any of the symptoms listed below, it is possible that you are suffering from post-traumatic stress disorder (PTSD). The symptoms of stress exhibited after a critical incident can be divided into four types: physical, cognitive, emotional, and behavioural (Table 12.7).

These symptoms can lead to an operational stress injury (OSI), which is a non-medical term that is generally defined as "persistent, psychological difficulties resulting from operational duties" (Public Safety Canada, 2017b). Within the broad category of operational stress injuries related to public safety officers and other operational personnel, a number of mental health issues can be described as post-traumatic stress injuries (PTSI), including depression, substance abuse, and clinically diagnosed PTSD (Public Safety Canada, 2017b).

POST-TRAUMATIC STRESS DISORDER (PTSD)

For some, symptoms from a critical incident can be overwhelming to every part of their being. For others, the effect takes weeks, months, or possibly years to be totally felt (cumulative effect of many events). These overwhelming responses to stress can result in post-traumatic stress disorder (PTSD). PTSD can be defined as a condition where symptoms evolve in the aftermath of an extreme traumatic stressor that overwhelms the individual's coping capacities (Gupta, 2013).

PTSD is a mental illness that is diagnosed after experiencing symptoms for at least a month. It changes the way the body responds to stress, probably as a result of chemical imbalances that increase the levels of stress hormones and alter the reactions of the nervous system.

TABLE 12.7   Symptoms Exhibited After a Critical Incident

PHYSICAL	COGNITIVE	EMOTIONAL	BEHAVIOURAL
• aches, pains, muscle tension, trembling, poor coordination • jumpiness • startled by sudden sounds or movements • cold sweats, dry mouth, pale skin, difficulty focusing the eyes • feeling out of breath, hyperventilating • upset stomach, vomiting, diarrhea, constipation, frequent urination • chronic fatigue and pain • a distant, haunted, faraway stare • substance abuse • sexual dysfunction • insomnia	• difficulty making decisions • confusion • detachment and withdrawal • disorientation • poor concentration and loss of interest in activities • memory loss, (recent events or the trauma itself) • inability to perform multiple tasks • flashbacks (visual or auditory) • daydreams, nightmares/bad dreams • avoidance of reminders of the event • contemplation of suicide • compulsive behavioural patterns • symptoms of attention deficit hyperactivity disorder (ADHD)	• grief, including spontaneous crying • numbness • guilt • feelings of hopelessness and being overwhelmed • depression, extended periods of sadness • anxiety, fear, edginess • panic attacks • self-doubt • irritability, anger, resentment • hyper-startled responses • feeling detached from reality • vigilance to the point of paranoia • intrusive thoughts • flashbacks or nightmares • sudden floods of emotions or images related to the initial event • a loss of previously sustained beliefs	• decreased job performance • increased absenteeism • detachment and increased isolation from colleagues, friends, family • increased premature departure from work or social gatherings • outbursts of laughter or tears • changes in normal humour patterns • excessive silence or talkativeness • low morale • hostile tone of voice • destructive changes in relationships with family, friends, colleagues • hypervigilance, jumpiness, or an extreme sense of being "on guard" • curling up and rocking continuously • body tremors, hand-wringing, facial tics • running without purpose • substance abuse • taking up reckless, sometimes life-threatening hobbies • obsession with death

SOURCE: American Psychiatric Association, 2013.

Although research is not conclusive on why trauma causes PTSD in some people but not others, it is linked to many different factors including length of time the trauma lasted, the number of other traumatic experiences in their reaction to the event, and the kind of support they received after the event. Research suggests that first responders are twice as likely as the general population to experience PTSD due to exposure to traumatic events in the course of duty (Ferguson, 2016; Ontario Ministry of Labour, 2016). Critical incident stress may be thought of as a continuum of severity, with PTSD at the most extreme pole.

COMMON SIDE EFFECTS OF PTSD

Some of the common side effects of PTSD include (APA, 2013; Kelly, 2016; Veterans Affairs Canada, 2017):

1. *Intrusion* unwanted and obsessive thoughts, feelings, sensory experiences, or a combination of these symptoms, including:

   • involuntary, recurrent, and intrusive memories

- flashbacks, re-experiencing, or re-living the event
- strong reactions to daily events (exaggerated startled responses or angry outbursts)
- vivid dreams and nightmares

2. *Avoidance* the individual makes an effort to avoid distressing trauma-related stimuli including:
   - avoiding trauma-related thoughts, feelings, or external reminders such as persons, places, activities, situations, or objects
   - social isolation from family, friends, and colleagues

3. *Negative changes in cognitions and mood* including:
   - inability to recall the event (dissociative amnesia)
   - negative outlook and inability to experience positive emotions
   - gaps in memory
   - losing interest in normal and previously enjoyed activities

4. *Alterations in arousal and reactivity* including:
   - as the result of physical injury or assault some suffer from effects similar to mild traumatic brain injury (difficulty with attention, concentration, moodiness, agitation, sleep disturbances)
   - irritability or aggressive behaviour
   - self-destructive or reckless behaviour
   - hypervigilance

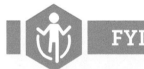

FYI

HYPERVIGILANCE

Hypervigilance is the enhanced state of sensory sensitivity along with an exaggerated intensity of behaviours. This heightened state of awareness is part of the fight-or-flight response but it is locked in a permanent 'battle stations' mode. This narrowed focus is helpful when there is a real threat (while on duty), however when the individual is constantly alert (even off duty), it causes inappropriate or even aggressive reactions to everyday situations. Hypervigilant officers are known to suspect regular people of being criminals, never sit with their back to the door, and always be on high alert when walking crowded city streets. Some become agitated in crowded spaces and want to escape or avoid the threat that isn't there. Long-term effects can include severe depression, generalized anxiety disorder, and various debilitating physical ailments. Hypervigilance may trigger panic attacks and flashbacks. It is important to be able to switch off the fight-or-flight response when off duty and develop appropriate coping skills including exercise and relaxation techniques.

SOURCES: Andersen & Papazoglou, 2015; O'Hara & Violanti, 2009.

PTSD prevalence rates are high for individuals who serve in the military, corrections, police, firefighters, and paramedics. Figure 12.4 illustrates the lifetime PTSD prevalence rates in Canada. The variance in numbers is due to actual diagnosis (dark blue) versus responses on a self-assessment questionnaire (light blue). The bottom line is that based on 2010 statistics, we could have between 25,000 and 46,000 full-time first responders and 12,000 to 23,000 volunteer first responders who have experienced PTSD in their lifetime (Wilson, Guliani, & Boichev, 2016), and that number will increase with the passing of the *Ontario's First Responders Act* (MCSCS, 2016b) in 2016.

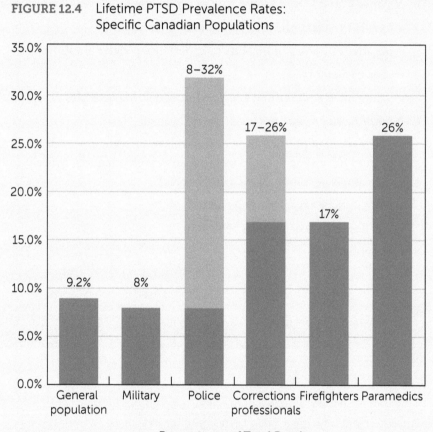

FIGURE 12.4 Lifetime PTSD Prevalence Rates: Specific Canadian Populations

FYI

ONTARIO'S FIRST RESPONDERS ACT

The *Ontario's First Responders Act* was passed in April 2016 to assist individuals with faster access to WSIB benefits, resources, and timely treatment. Once a first responder is diagnosed with PTSD by either a psychiatrist or a psychologist, the claims process to be eligible for WSIB benefits will be expedited, without the need to prove a causal link between PTSD and a workplace event. It also allows the minister of labour to request and publish PTSD prevention plans from employers of workers who are covered by the presumption.

SOURCE: Ontario Ministry of Labour (2016).

SUICIDE

Unresolved stress can sometimes lead to suicide. In Canada, suicide is the second highest cause of death for youths aged 10 to 24, following motor vehicle collisions (see Figure 12.5 for more statistics). Aboriginal teens and lesbian, gay, bisexual, and transgender young persons may be at particularly high risk, depending on the community in which they live, family support, and their own self-esteem. Mental health issues like depression and PTSD are commonly associated with suicide. And although some individuals may show signs of distress, others may show no signs of contemplating suicide. For many people, it is the overwhelming desire to escape the pain rather than the desire to die that leads to suicide attempts. Learning effective coping techniques to deal with stressful situations can help.

It is important to listen to people. Talking calmly about suicide, without showing fear or making judgments, can bring relief to someone who is feeling terribly isolated. Asking them if they are suicidal will not cause them to become suicidal. Ask them if they would like some help, because they may want assistance, but just don't know how to ask for it. Be willing to listen, show sincere concern, and encourage someone to speak about their feelings. The person will often feel relieved that there is someone who will talk honestly with them about their feelings and this may help reduce the risk of a suicide attempt (Canadian Children's Rights Council, 2016).

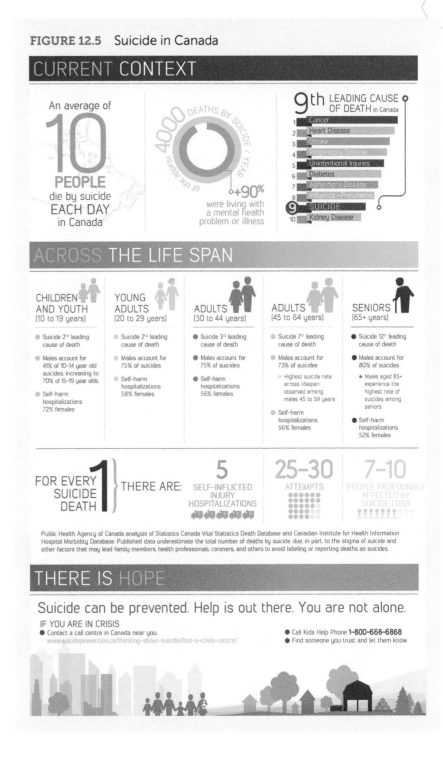

FIGURE 12.5 Suicide in Canada

CURRENT CONTEXT

An average of **10** PEOPLE die by suicide EACH DAY in Canada

4000 DEATHS BY SUICIDE / YEAR or the approx. +90% were living with a mental health problem or illness

9th LEADING CAUSE OF DEATH in Canada

1 Cancer
2 Heart Disease
3 Stroke
4 Respiratory Disease
5 Unintentional Injuries
6 Diabetes
7 Alzheimer's Disease
8 Influenza + Pneumonia
9 SUICIDE
10 Kidney Disease

ACROSS THE LIFE SPAN

CHILDREN AND YOUTH (10 to 19 years)
- Suicide 2nd leading cause of death
- Males account for 41% of 10-14 year old suicides, increasing to 70% of 15-19 year olds
- Self-harm hospitalizations 72% females

YOUNG ADULTS (20 to 29 years)
- Suicide 2nd leading cause of death
- Males account for 75% of suicides
- Self-harm hospitalizations 58% females

ADULTS (30 to 44 years)
- Suicide 3rd leading cause of death
- Males account for 75% of suicides
- Self-harm hospitalizations 56% females

ADULTS (45 to 64 years)
- Suicide 7th leading cause of death
- Males account for 73% of suicides
- Highest suicide rate across lifespan observed among males 45 to 59 years
- Self-harm hospitalizations 56% females

SENIORS (65+ years)
- Suicide 12th leading cause of death
- Males account for 80% of suicides
- Males aged 85+ experience the highest rate of suicides among seniors
- Self-harm hospitalizations 52% females

FOR EVERY **1** SUICIDE DEATH THERE ARE: **5** SELF-INFLICTED INJURY HOSPITALIZATIONS **25–30** ATTEMPTS **7–10** PEOPLE PROFOUNDLY AFFECTED BY SUICIDE LOSS

Public Health Agency of Canada analysis of Statistics Canada Vital Statistics Death Database and Canadian Institute for Health Information Hospital Morbidity Database. Published data underestimate the total number of deaths by suicide, due, in part, to the stigma of suicide and other factors that may lead family members, health professionals, coroners, and others to avoid labeling or reporting deaths as suicides.

THERE IS HOPE

Suicide can be prevented. Help is out there. You are not alone.

IF YOU ARE IN CRISIS
- Contact a call centre in Canada near you: www.suicideprevention.ca/thinking-about-suicide/find-a-crisis-centre/
- Call Kids Help Phone **1-800-668-6868**
- Find someone you trust and let them know

SUICIDE WARNING SIGNS

A change in behaviour or presence of entirely new behaviours, especially if related to a painful event, loss, or change, may be warning signs that an individual is not managing their mental health and may be contemplating suicide. Table 12.8 includes some common warning signs.

TABLE 12.8   Suicide Warning Signs

Talk If a person talks about:	• Being a burden to others • Feeling trapped • Experiencing unbearable pain • Having no reason to live • Killing themselves
Behaviour Specific things to look for in someone's behaviour include:	• Increased use of alcohol or drugs • Looking for a way to kill themselves, such as searching online for materials or means • Acting recklessly • Withdrawing from activities • Isolating themselves from family and friends • Sleeping too much or too little • Visiting or calling people to say goodbye • Giving away prized possessions • Aggression
Mood People may display one or more of the following moods:	• Depression • Loss of interest • Rage • Irritability • Humiliation • Anxiety

SOURCE: Adapted from Lifeline Canada Foundation. Suicide Warning Signs. Retrieved from https://thelifelinecanada.ca/help/warning-signs.

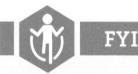

FYI

SUICIDE IN LAW ENFORCEMENT

Over the past few years, more than 200 Canadian public safety (police, corrections, customs, firefighters, and paramedics) and military personnel have died by suicide (TEMA, 2017). Twice as many officers die by their own hand as do in the line of duty. Suicide among law enforcement officers occurs at a rate of almost twice that of the general population. Officers going through a divorce are five times more likely to die by suicide, and if they are in serious trouble on the job, suspended, or facing termination, they are seven times more likely to die by suicide.

There is a great concern that law enforcement work provides a fertile ground for suicide-precipitating factors, including relationship problems, culturally approved alcohol use, and maladaptive coping mechanisms. In addition, the availability of firearms and exposure to psychologically adverse incidents may contribute to this causal chain of suicide.

SOURCES: O'Hara & Violanti, 2009; TEMA, 2017; Violanti, 2014.

PERSONAL PERSPECTIVE

IN MEMORY OF DOUG MARSHALL

On the evening of April 10, 2012, I received a call from an OPP officer. He wanted to be the one to let me know that after a courageous battle with PTSD, Sgt. Doug Marshall took his own life. He was a former student of mine, a graduate of Georgian College's Law and Security Program and a great ambassador for our program. He was a 23-year veteran of policing. He was a dedicated community volunteer, accomplished triathlonist, and had the opportunity to run the Boston Marathon. More importantly, he was a proud father and dedicated husband to his college sweetheart. He would drop by the college to visit, talk to students, and share with me how much he loved his family and his job.

When he got back from Moosonee he had promised to come see me. He never made it. Unknown to me, he had been diagnosed with post-traumatic stress disorder. His wife, Rachel, reflected that she believed that the depression associated with PTSD heightened his feelings of isolation, loneliness, and fear of people's perception, and robbed him of his relationships at work and home. She feels it is important, even though it is difficult, to share their story, so that the stigma of this illness is removed and those that need help will seek it.

One of the officers that Doug served with and who is a close family friend, eloquently shared:

> When you first started teaching Mike, Kerry, Tony and me, you always instilled in us the passion to stay fit throughout our careers. I am still out running and doing pushups with the recruits and holding my own. I believe strongly that the young recruits need to see a senior Sgt. still staying fit. Fitness has been my physical and mental outlet to get me through long shifts, arrests, and long murder trials.
>
> When Doug died, I often went for runs just trying to clear my head and sort out life. There were many times I cried during my runs. Doug was such a strong independent person that I never dreamed someone like him would succumb to PTSD. He was the last cop in the world I would have worried about. I felt so much guilt that I didn't do more to help him. It was Doug, he will bounce back in no time, and be going full out on our next ski trip to Quebec. I didn't get to say goodbye to him. I miss him. Doug's family are still very much in our personal life.
>
> Your friend, Dan

It is important to know that PTSD is an illness and not a weakness. With help, education, and proper treatment, people can recover. In 2014, as part of a program run by United by Trauma (http://ubyt.ca), the organization donated their first service dog, 'Marshall,' a chocolate lab, in memory of Sgt. Doug Marshall. Marshall resides with a former Toronto police officer who is healing from PTSD. Doug would be honoured.

COPING WITH STRESS
AFTER A CRITICAL INCIDENT

In the aftermath of a critical incident, it is important that everyone involved (victims, first responders, and bystanders) receives proper support and coping strategies. In law enforcement, this is done through debriefing, which is the provision of assistance by a qualified mental health professional after a traumatic incident. Debriefing is intended to help alleviate the trauma felt by the officers and to help speed up the recovery process. The point is not to deal with blame or the cause of the incident, but rather its emotional and psychological consequences, such as guilt, sadness, or anger. Whether debriefing is done on an individual basis or with all those on your shift, it is important that supervisors ensure it is done in a timely fashion (Everly & Mitchell, 2000).

In addition to debriefing, just being aware of the physical, cognitive, emotional, and behavioural responses that one might have following a critical incident is important (see Table 12.7). Identifying a friend or colleague who is at risk for PTSD and providing early intervention for them is paramount. According to the Ontario

Ombudsman's report, *In the Line of Duty* (Marin, 2012), police services are far from providing what current and former officers and their families need to deal with operational stress injuries and prevent suicide.

The emergency services and law enforcement subculture holds on to many myths that can lessen an individual's ability to cope with the aftermath of a critical incident. A law enforcement officer's recovery can be hampered by beliefs such as "If you can't deal with it, you need to find a new line of work" and "Officers should keep their problems to themselves." Attempting to deny their reactions to stress can cause officers to suffer in silence and not seek help, and in some instances, to disrupt their lives and the lives of their families. It is important that everyone is educated on how to cope with their stress.

Here are some ways you can help others when you see that someone is suffering the effects of stress after a critical incident:

1. *Manage the situation* by staying calm, removing the individual from the scene, and encouraging them to talk and validating their reactions.

2. *Mobilize support* by notifying their family and providing medical and emotional support.

3. *Follow up* with the individual and ensure that they are aware and have access to the support networks in place.

Do *not* do the following:

- Second-guess the individual.

- Say, "I understand how you feel." (You may think you do, but to a victim, his or her pain is unique.)

- Say, "Everything is going to be fine." Acknowledge that things may never be the same but they will get better over time.

- Try to protect the individual by withholding information (but use your judgment in this regard, and seek legal advice if necessary).

- Say things like, "It could have been worse," "You can always get another (pet, house, car)," "It's best if you just stay busy," and "You need to get on with your life."

- Say, "When this happened to me …" Even if you had an identical experience, the victim's need to talk about his or her own trauma is probably greater than the need to listen to another person's experience.

- Give too much advice or make promises you can't keep.

The majority of people return back to normal after one month, but 30 percent of individuals will have symptoms that last longer. For many, the symptoms generally subside and normal function gradually returns. For some, symptoms may appear to be gone, but can surface again in another stressful situation. It is in the best interest of the individual and the organization to follow up, especially around the anniversary of the event (U.S. Department of Veteran Affairs, 2016).

Some individuals will find that moving on to another career is appropriate, but law enforcement is as much of a calling as medicine or the clergy. Make sure you have exhausted all methods of support before letting someone—possibly yourself—make such a monumental decision.

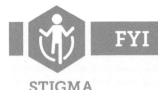

FYI

STIGMA

In law enforcement, a stigma is a marked disgrace or disapproval associated with a particular circumstance or person resulting in the individual feeling diminished, devalued, and fearful. For example, many officers suffer in silence rather than addressing mental illness so they aren't labelled as weak.

RESILIENCY AND MINDFULNESS

The *In the Line of Duty* Ombudsman report Marin (2012) recommended that services needed to confront the stigma of PTSD, increase the availability of psychological services, and develop province-wide programs aimed at preventing and dealing with operational stress injuries and suicide. As a result, in 2017, the Ministerial Roundtable on Post-Traumatic Stress Disorder in Public Safety Officers (Public Safety Canada, 2017a) directed public safety organizations to offer support to their officers.

Resilience is the process of adapting well in the face of adversity, trauma, tragedy, threats, or significant sources of stress—such as family and relationship problems, serious health problems, or workplace and financial stressors. It means "bouncing back" from difficult experiences and/or developing coping skills to deal with the stressful event (APA, 2017). Part of the strategy, in a psychologically safe, stigma-free environment, is to create a positive work environment for law enforcement that prioritizes mental health, addresses stigma, and provides psycho-education on PTSD (Ferguson, 2016). Providing these strategies may prevent PTSD from becoming worse, possibly prevent suicides, promote a healthy recovery, and support a successful return to work or maintenance at work.

Resiliency training speaks to the need to build PTSD and other OSIs into the everyday dialogue of public safety organizations by ensuring officers have the tools to recognize early symptoms, are aware of coping mechanisms, and know when to seek professional support. This could include things like stigma reduction through educational campaigns or access to evidence-based training tools. The military developed a program called the Road to Mental Readiness (R2MR). This program provides resilience training before, during, and after deployment to improve short-term performance and long-term mental health outcomes (CAF, 2015). It involves the mental health continuum model and teaches the "Big 4"—positive self-talk, visualization, tactical breathing, and SMART goal setting to cope with stress. Law enforcement services have adopted this model to assist their employees and their families.

At the foundation of the resiliency model is "mindfulness." Mindfulness is a mental state achieved by focusing one's awareness on the present moment, while calmly acknowledging and accepting one's feelings, thoughts, and bodily sensations. Mindfulness training helps with sleep management, stress management, and depression so officers can thrive rather than just survive. It is important to develop keen self-awareness to understand how your body is affected by stress. One of the methods of mindfulness incorporates focusing on breathing while being in the present moment and being non-judgmental (Kabat-Zinn, 1991). Another method focuses on developing self-awareness skills to have better grounded compassion and skillful action (Strozzi-Heckler, 2003).

STRATEGIES FOR COPING WITH STRESS

Remember that it is important to stay away from unhealthy and unproductive coping strategies. Examples include smoking, binge eating, drinking too much, using pills or drugs to try to relax, withdrawing from friends and family, taking stress out on others, sleeping too much, zoning out for hours on your smartphone, avoiding the problem by being busy, and procrastination. Below are a number of strategies that you might consider to help you cope, become more resilient and mindful of the stressors you are facing. It is helpful if you practise the 4 A's: Avoid, Alter, Adapt, or Accept (Robinson, Smith, & Segal, 2017).

THE "FOUR A'S" WHEN DEALING WITH STRESS

1. *Avoid* unnecessary stress
   - Learn to say no, avoid people who stress you out, control your environment, and pare down your to-do list.
   - Decide which battles are worth fighting. Don't stress over issues that are relatively unimportant. Learn to take a stand, or learn to decline—and stick by it.
   - Keep away from poor nutrition habits and substance abuse.

2. *Alter* the situation
   - Manage self-talk (how you perceive and express yourself) by avoiding self-blame and guilt.
   - Reframe your point of view and accentuate the positive with effective communication skills.
   - Engage in hobbies like reading, writing, drawing, or playing a musical instrument; watching a funny show, being in nature, or playing with pets can also have a significant impact on stress management.
   - Develop satisfying relationships and friendships outside of work to get a different perspective and support.
   - Exercise to lower blood pressure, improve sleep, and prepare yourself for emergency situations.
   - Seek professional help if needed from a social worker, grief counsellor, psychologist, psychiatrist, mentor, or clergy.

3. *Adapt* to the stressor
   - Change your expectations and attitude by reframing the problem, looking at the big picture, adjusting your standards, and appreciating what you have.
   - Manage your situations as opportunities rather than setbacks, taking things less seriously, finding humour where you can, and learning to laugh at yourself.
   - Set realistic goals and work on your time management skills to balance work and play.

4. *Accept* the things you can't change
   - Learn that you cannot control everything (e.g., illness, injury, or critical incident).
   - Find the positive under the circumstances, learn from mistakes, learn to forgive and move on, and share your feelings.

RELAXATION TECHNIQUES

Let's look at how stress responses can be controlled by relaxation techniques.

BREATHING

Breathing is affected by the stress response. When you are stressed, your breathing becomes more rapid and shallow, and your heart rate increases. To elicit a relaxation response, you must slow down your breathing and learn to take deeper breaths. By breathing correctly, you will oxygenate your blood more efficiently, and this will trigger the parasympathetic "quieting response" (a sense of control over the body and its reactions to stressors).

Try the following breathing exercise:

1. Monitor your heart rate for 15 seconds and then multiply by 4 to obtain beats per minute.

2. Sit up straight with your spine against a chair back.

3. Put your left hand over your chest and your right hand over your abdomen.

4. Breathe normally. You will probably notice that your chest expands more than your abdomen.

5. Now practise a new way of breathing by briefly holding in your breath and then slowly releasing the air. To do this most effectively, breathe through your nose. When you take a deep breath, you should feel your diaphragm (the muscle that separates the thoracic cavity from the abdominal cavity) push down and your abdomen expand outward as you get oxygen into the lower third of the lungs. Diaphragmatic breathing focuses on the expansion of the abdomen rather than the chest when breathing.

6. Continue to breathe slowly for about 5 minutes while attempting to relax and slow your breathing. At the end of 5 minutes, you should feel relaxed and be able to resume normal activities.

7. Monitor your heart rate again. If you are more relaxed, your heart rate should be lower than when you started.

Diaphragmatic breathing is a skill that takes practise. Once you become familiar with the technique, you will be able to do it almost anywhere you are, at any time.

MEDITATION

Meditation can involve focusing the mind, and thereby quieting the body, by sitting or lying down comfortably and quietly with eyes closed for 10 to 20 minutes once or twice a day (see Figure 12.6). It does not involve thinking, though you will probably find that turning off thoughts is almost impossible. Rather than fight your thoughts, simply try not to get caught up in them. Some people find that listening to the sound of the wind or ocean waves helps them to quiet their thinking. Ideally, you should not fall asleep when you meditate, although this may happen if you are extremely tired.

FIGURE 12.6   Meditation

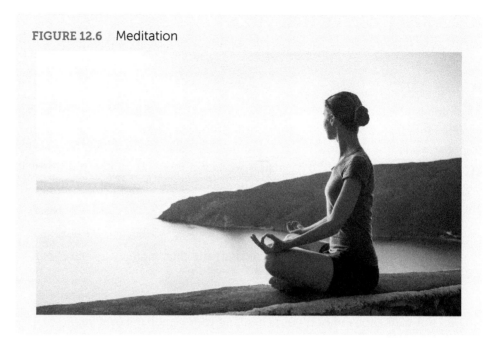

Meditation methods include the following:

- Mindful meditation is simply noting internal thoughts and bodily processes, such as your breathing (Kabat-Zinn, 1991).
- Transcendental meditation involves inducing a meditative state twice a day by closing your eyes and repeating a mantra (a sound without meaning).
- Zen meditation focuses on breathing.
- Benson's (1975) meditation technique for relaxation involves focusing on a word or phrase associated with your beliefs. The idea is to turn to your inner self to find harmony. He used a quiet environment, a mental device (sound of waves), a passive attitude (relax), and a comfortable position.

PROGRESSIVE MUSCLE RELAXATION

This technique requires you to alternately tense and relax your muscles. Systematically you release the tension and notice how your muscles feel as you relax them. This should help lower your overall tension and stress levels and help you relax when you are feeling anxious.

1. While lying on your back or sitting in a comfortable position, monitor your heart rate for 15 seconds and then multiply by 4 to obtain beats per minute. Concentrate on relaxing and slowing your breathing.
2. Moving from toe to head, concentrate on tensing muscles for 10 seconds and then release. For example curling your toes, flexing your feet up toward your head, tightening your calves, thighs, abdominals, lower back, shoulders, hands, arms, neck, and facial muscles.
3. Monitor your heart rate again to see whether it has gone down.

VISUALIZATION

Also called mental imagery, guided imagery, or guided daydreaming (Samuels & Samuels, 1975), visualization involves imagining yourself in a quiet and peaceful place, usually a natural setting. Known as Jacobson's method of relaxation, the objective of this technique is to work on the peripheral nervous system to reduce the physiological symptoms of anxiety (Jacobson, 1938) by progressive relaxation of the body and the use of mental imagery to achieve relaxation. It can be done entirely on your own or with the help of instructors or recordings (such as sounds of ocean waves or birds). In a recent cardiology study, Paul-Labrador and colleagues (2006) found that patients who used visualization improved their blood pressure and insulin-resistance components of metabolic syndrome, as well as cardiac autonomic nervous system tone (including heart rate, the heart's ability to contract, and tolerance to physical activity), thereby reducing the physiological response to stress and improving coronary heart disease risk factors.

PERSONAL PERSPECTIVE

NANCY'S BEACH

The following exercise is based on memories of locations that have had special meaning for me. Feel free to visualize a setting of your own once you have tried this technique.

You will probably need someone to read these instructions to you the first time you try this. I usually do this exercise immediately after doing the progressive muscle relaxation technique described above.

Find a quiet, comfortable spot in which to sit or lie down. Begin by monitoring your heart rate for 15 seconds.

Take a deep breath and relax. Concentrate on how relaxed you are becoming and how comfortable you are. Close your eyes and concentrate on your breathing. Relax your back, arms, and legs. Concentrate on releasing the tension stored in your body. Feel your chest go up and down with your breathing. Relax and concentrate on your breathing.

Now imagine that you are getting up from your spot to walk down a corridor toward a door. Open that door and walk through it to an escalator. Together, let's go down the escalator: 1, 2, 3, 4, 5, 6, 7, 8, 9, 10. Now step off the escalator and go to the door.

When you reach that door, imagine that you are taking off your shoes, picking up a towel lying beside the door, and then walking through the door. On the other side of the door is a beach and you can feel the warmth of the sun on your body and the white sand under your feet. Close the door behind you.

As you walk toward the dark blue ocean on the right, you can feel the sun on your face and back. You are able to hear the waves and feel a slight breeze on your face. You can feel the cool sand under your feet. Above you, the sky is a clear blue. Find a place to sit or lie down. Remember that you have a towel to use if you need it. You will continue to feel the warmth of the sand and sun. You will hear the waves and the birds in the distance. You are relaxed and quiet. For the next several minutes, allow your mind to relax and continue to enjoy the beach. Enjoy the stillness, warmth, and quiet you are experiencing.

Next, imagine that you are getting up and walking to the water's edge. Dip your hand in the water and splash it on your face. You can now return to the door, feeling refreshed, alert, and at peace. Open the door and take one last look at the beach. Close the door. Lock the door with the key that's hanging by the door, and put the key in your pocket. Know that the imaginary key to this location is yours alone, so that no one but you can gain access to this special place.

You are now going back up the escalator to the first door. Together, let's go back up the escalator: 10, 9, 8, 7, 6, 5, 4, 3, 2, 1. Step off the escalator. Open the door, walk down the corridor, and return to the spot where you began your journey. Take a moment to remember the peaceful time you spent at the beach.

Bring your attention back to the here and now. Take a deep breath. Before you get up, check whether you were able to slow your heart rate. You should feel refreshed and alert.

HYPNOSIS/SELF-HYPNOSIS

Hypnosis and self-hypnosis act as stress reducers by having you concentrate on key words and images. It is a scientifically verified and effective technique that can promote accelerated human change.

With self-hypnosis, you can create desired changes in behaviour and encourage mental and physical well-being including anxiety reduction (Bryant, Moulds, Guthrie, & Nixon, 2005). People use it to lose weight, quit smoking, reduce physical pain, and deal with traumatic events. Consultation with a clinical hypnotherapist can help individualize goals and specific techniques.

BIOFEEDBACK

Biofeedback is a form of alternative medicine that assesses bodily processes such as blood pressure, heart rate, skin temperature, galvanic skin response (sweating), eye movement, and muscle tension to raise a person's awareness and conscious control over physiological responses. It involves a physiological feedback monitor such as an electrocardiograph for monitoring heart activity. It allows you to learn appropriate relaxation responses (Choe et al., 2007; Institute of Medicine, 2014).

MUSIC

Music conjures up images and memories, and can be relaxing and renewing. The music you choose will depend on your own preferences, although music that is quiet, slower, lower pitched, and with a constant beat is usually more effective. Music in a group setting can reduce isolation and feelings of detachment, and increase pleasurable emotions (Garrido, Baker, Davidson, Moore, & Wasserman, 2015). Drumming can be used to express rage and anger about trauma (Sorensen, 2015). Music has been shown to trigger the release of chemicals to distract the body and mind from pain. For access to this type of music look up "healing meditation music" on the Web.

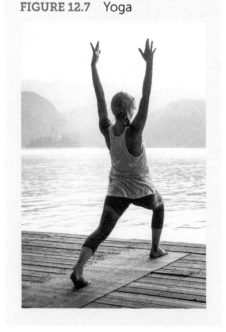

FIGURE 12.7 Yoga

YOGA

Yoga is a discipline that seeks to unite the mind, body, and soul (Figure 12.7; Seaward, 2005). The practice of hatha yoga combines breathing, stretching, and balance exercises to achieve a spiritual focus. It helps to improve posture, balance, coordination, range of motion, proprioception, core strength, and neuromuscular integration, and lowers anxiety. A recent study in the Canadian Armed Forces found yoga helped to reduce the severity of physical and psychological conditions of those suffering from PTSD (Groll, Charbonneau, Bélanger, & Senyshyn, 2016). The Ontario Police College integrated a yoga program into their fitness components for recruits, senior staff, and employees. The beneficial effects are from focused breathing and being present while increasing your knowledge of your internal state so that you can control your thoughts and physical stress.

T'AI CHI CH'UAN

Known as the "softest" martial art (Seaward, 2005), this discipline brings the body and mind together through the *chi*, or life force, when you do a series of graceful martial arts movements. T'ai chi ch'uan attempts to achieve deep relaxation and as much softness in the musculature as possible. It is characterized by the leverage through the joints based on relaxing the muscles to enhance and increase breathing, body heat, the lymph system, and peristalsis, working toward homeostasis (returning your internal circulation to a healthier, balanced state). This discipline can help you keep calm and steady under pressure. Many community centres offer programs in T'ai chi ch'uan.

MASSAGE

Massage stimulates blood flow and improves muscle tone. It relaxes the muscles and thereby creates a calming effect. Now more popular than ever, massage can be performed by registered massage therapists, chiropractors, physiotherapists, reflexologists, acupuncturists, and other professionals. Non-professionals can also learn massage. Some types of therapies include deep tissue massage, Swedish massage, lymphatic massage, cranial massage, reflexology, and aromatherapy.

ACUPUNCTURE

Acupuncture stems from traditional Chinese medicine practices in which trained practitioners stimulate specific points on the body by inserting thin needles into the skin to release endorphins and activate natural pain killers to help treat depression, anxiety, and pain.

HYDROTHERAPY

Hydrotherapy—soaking in a hot tub, warm bath, or hot shower—is a great way to relax at the end of the day. Warm water (about 38 °C) appears to quiet and soothe the body while slowing down the activity of internal organs. Whirlpool baths appear to have higher stress-relief benefits, including reducing anxiety. Herbal baths scented with lavender, linden, passionflower, and chamomile also appear to be effective.

FINAL THOUGHTS

Ultimately, it is up to you to discover what helps you relax and brings your stress levels down. You may need to try several methods, or a particular method a few times, before you find something that suits your needs and personality. Take time for yourself, mentally and physically, so that you do not become consumed by stress.

❝ You can't stop the waves, but you can learn to surf. ❞

—Jon Kabat-Zinn

KEY TERMS

combat stress
an expected and predictable reaction to combat experiences where you are under constant physiological stress (poor diet, extreme temperatures, poor hygiene, etc.) and psychological stress (concern over explosive devices, snipers, or death of service members or civilians, etc.)

critical incident or traumatic event
a situation faced by law enforcement that causes them to experience unusually strong emotional reactions that have the potential to interfere with their ability to function at the scene (current stress) or later (residual stress)

debriefing
the provision of assistance, by a qualified mental health professional, to officers who have been involved in a traumatic incident

diaphragmatic breathing
deep breathing focusing on the contraction of the diaphragm and expansion of the abdomen rather than the chest

distress
a type of stress that results in negative responses both in a person's career and in life

eustress
a type of good stress that is caused by the factors that initiate emotional and psychological growth

fight-or-flight response
the alarm stage when the body prepares itself to cope with a stressor and you either decide to take on the challenge or back away from it

general adaptation syndrome (GAS)
the body's reaction to stress

hypervigilance
an enhanced state of sensory sensitivity along with an exaggerated intensity of behaviours

meditation
focusing on the mind while quieting the body

mild traumatic brain injury
difficulties with attention, concentration, moodiness, and agitation that an individual may suffer from as a result of physical trauma

mindfulness
a mental state achieved by focusing one's awareness on the present moment, while calmly acknowledging and accepting one's feelings, thoughts, and bodily sensations; used as a therapeutic technique

neustress
a type of stress where the mind and body are aroused but the stress is neither harmful nor helpful

operational stress injury (OSI)
a non-medical term that is generally defined as "persistent, psychological difficulties resulting from operational duties" (Public Safety Canada, 2017b) and can include post-traumatic stress injuries and post-traumatic stress disorder

overload
feelings of being burdened by excessive time pressure, excessive responsibility, and excessive expectations to succeed

post-traumatic stress disorder (PTSD)
a mental illness where symptoms evolve in the aftermath of an extreme traumatic stressor that overwhelms the individual's coping capacities

post-traumatic stress injury (PTSI)
a number of mental health issues, including depression, substance abuse, and clinically diagnosed PTSD, within the broad category of operational stress injuries (OSIs)

psychosomatic symptoms
physical symptoms resulting from mental conflict

resilience
the process of adapting well in the face of adversity, trauma, tragedy, threats, or significant sources of stress

stage of exhaustion
when the body is subjected to continual stress and fatigue for days and weeks, and begins to shut down, usually resulting in illness

stage of resistance
when the body actively resists and attempts to cope with the stressor

stress
a "non-specific response of the body to any demands made upon it" (Selye, 1974)

stressor
any physical, psychological, or environmental event or condition that initiates the stress response

visualization
a technique that involves imagining yourself in a quiet and peaceful place; also referred to as guided imagery

EXERCISES

MULTIPLE CHOICE

1. Which of these statements about stress is *incorrect*?
   a. Stress can be self-induced.
   b. Stress can be pleasurable.
   c. Stress can cause psychological disorders.
   d. Individuals differ in what they find stressful.
   e. Your ability to handle stress is hereditary and fixed.

2. A technique of relaxation that uses a machine to monitor body processes is called
   a. yoga
   b. autogenic feedback
   c. biofeedback
   d. transcendental meditation
   e. progressive relaxation

3. Which of the following is the *least* healthy way to relieve tension?
   a. taking a brisk walk after sitting for a long time
   b. doing slow stretching exercises
   c. doing rhythmical exercises
   d. drinking alcohol
   e. getting a massage

4. How did Selye label the negative level of stress?
   a. neustress
   b. distress
   c. eustress
   d. burnout
   e. hypervigilance

5. What is the first step in managing stress?
   a. Use a relaxation technique.
   b. Recognize symptoms and causes.
   c. Be as fit and healthy as possible.
   d. Get eight hours of sleep a night.
   e. Control lifestyle and avoid stressors.

6. Which is a good way to manage stress?
   a. Allow more time for work.
   b. Avoid talking about your problems.
   c. Think positively.
   d. Insist that things should go your way.
   e. Pretend that the problem will just go away.

7. Why might those in law enforcement be more likely to suffer from critical incident stress?
   a. They don't suffer from stress any different than the general population.
   b. They haven't been given the proper tools to deal with the stress.
   c. Their job involves facing dangerous situations potentially on a daily basis.
   d. They are more sensitive than the general population.
   e. They enjoy the "buzz" of constant stress.

8. Which behaviour is not the result of a mild traumatic brain injury?
   a. having difficulty concentrating
   b. being more considerate
   c. being more moody
   d. being more agitated
   e. being more stressed

9. Jacobson's method of relaxation emphasizes
   a. imagery
   b. visualization
   c. yoga
   d. meditation
   e. progressive relaxation

10. Post-traumatic stress disorder refers to
    a. a positive ability to handle stress
    b. the result of completing all your credits in first year
    c. a mental illness where symptoms overwhelm the individual's coping capacities
    d. the response to completing an assignment on time
    e. none of the above

11. Any physical, social, or psychological event or condition that causes our body to have to adjust to a specific situation is known as
    a. an obstacle
    b. PTSD
    c. a stressor
    d. a strain
    e. a road block

12. During which stage of general adaptation syndrome does the brain prepare the body to respond to a stressor?
    a. resistance stage
    b. adaptation stage
    c. exhaustion stage
    d. alarm stage
    e. homeostasis stage

13. Working out when stressed can help by
    a. increasing energy
    b. improving mental alertness
    c. allowing you to step back from the situation to view it in a different way
    d. reducing hostility
    e. all of the above

14. General adaptation syndrome explains
    a. the pattern followed by our physiological responses to stress
    b. the path of our autonomic nervous system when we are aroused by a stressful situation
    c. a means of dealing with post-traumatic stress disorder
    d. how to achieve homeostasis
    e. how well we adapt to new situations

15. With a full load of college courses and a part-time job, Steve suffers from excessive time pressure, excessive responsibility, and excessive expectations to succeed. Steve is suffering from

a. neustress

b. burnout

c. eustress

d. overload

e. inconsistent goals and behaviours

16. The physiological arousal response in which the body prepares to combat a real or perceived threat is called

a. the response stage

b. the resistance stage

c. homeostasis

d. the fight-or-flight response

e. distress response

SHORT ANSWER

1. Define stress.

2. What are the differences among neustress, eustress, and distress?

3. What are some of the general symptoms of stress?

4. List five stressors associated with law enforcement work.

5. What is a critical incident?

6. Describe post-traumatic stress disorder (PTSD).

7. What are some of the signs and symptoms of PTSD?

8. What is hypervigilance? What are some of the effects on the individual?

9. What can you do for a colleague who is suffering from critical incident stress or PTSD?

10. Explain what an operational stress injury is.

11. Briefly explain five relaxation techniques for coping with stress.

REFERENCES

Amaranto, E., Steinberg, J., Castellano, C., & Mitchell, R. (2003). Police stress interventions. *Brief Treatment and Crisis Interventions, 3*(1), 47–53.

American College Health Association (ACHA). (2016). National college health assessment 2016. Ontario Canada Reference Group

American Psychiatric Association (APA). (2013). *Diagnostic and statistical manual of mental disorders.* 5th ed. Washington, D.C: Author.

American Psychiatric Association (APA). (2017). The road to resilience. Retrieved from http://www.apa.org/helpcenter/road-resilience.aspx

Andersen, J.P., Gustafsberg, H., Papazoglou, K., Nyman, M., Koskelainen, M., & Pitel, M. (2015). A potentially lifesaving psychophysiological intervention for special forces officers. Poster presented at the annual conference of the American Psychosomatic Society, Savannah, GA.

Andersen, J.P., & Papazoglou, K. (2015). Compassion fatigue and compassion satisfaction among police officers: An understudied topic. *International Journal of Emergency Mental Health and Human Resilience, 17*(3), 661–663. ISSN:1522-4821. Retrieved from https://www.omicsonline.com/open-access/compassion-fatigue-and-compassion-satisfaction-among-police-officers-an-understudied-topic-1522-4821-1000259.pdf

Andersen, J.P., Papazoglou, K., Koskelainen, M., Nyman, M., Gustafsberg, H., & Arnetz, B.B. (2015). Applying resilience. Promotion training among special forces police officers. *Journal of Police Emergency Response, 5*(2).

Anderson, G.S., Litzenberger, R., & Plecas, D. (2002). Physical evidence of police officer stress. *Policing: An International Journal of Police Strategies and Management, 25*(2), 399–420.

Benson, H. (1975). *The relaxation response.* New York: Morrow.

Boak, A., Hamilton, H.A., Adlaf, E.M., Beitchman, J., Wolfe, D., & Mann, R.E. (2016). *The mental health and well-being of Ontario students, 1991–2015: Detailed OSDUHS findings*. CAMH Research Document Series no. 43. Toronto: Centre for Addiction and Mental Health. Retrieved from https://www.camh.ca/en/research/news_and_publications/ontario-student-drug-use-and-health-survey/Documents/2013 OSDUHS Docs/2013OSDUHS_Detailed_MentalHealthReport.pdf

Boyd, N. (1995). Violence in the workplace in British Columbia: A preliminary investigation. *Canadian Journal of Criminology, 37*(4), 491–519.

Boyd, N. (2011). *Correctional officers in British Columbia, 2011: Abnormal working conditions* (p. i). School of Criminology, Simon Fraser University. Retrieved from http://former.bcgeu.ca/sites/default/files/FINAL Boyd-Report-2011_0.pdf

Brower, J. (2013). Correctional officer wellness and safety literature review. *U.S. Department of Justice Office of Justice Programs Diagnostic Centre*. Retrieved from https://www.ojpdiagnosticcenter.org/content/correctional-officer-wellness-and-safety

Brown, J.J., Wells, G.A., Trottier, A.J., Bonneau, J., & Ferris, B. (1998). Back pain in a large Canadian police force. *Spine, 23*, 821–827.

Bryant, R.A., Moulds, M.L., Guthrie, R.M., & Nixon, R.D.V. (2005). The additive benefit of hypnosis and cognitive-behavioural therapy in treating acute stress disorder. *Journal of Consulting and Clinical Psychology, 73*(2), 334–340. DOI: 10.1037/0022-006X.73.2.334

Canada Border Services Agency (CBSA). (2016). 2016–17 report on plans and priorities. Government of Canada. Retrieved from http://www.cbsa-asfc.gc.ca/agency-agence/reports-rapports/rpp/2016-2017/rpp-2016-2017-eng.pdf

Canada Border Services Agency (CBSA). (2017). 2018–2018 Part III—Departmental expenditure plans: Departmental plans. Government of Canada. Catalogue No. PS35-6E-PDF. Retrieved from http://www.cbsa-asfc.gc.ca/agency-agence/reports-rapports/rpp/2017-2018/report-rapport-eng.html

Canadian Armed Forces (CAF). (2015). Road to mental readiness (R2MR). National Defence and the Canadian Armed Forces. Government of Canada. Retrieved from http://www.forces.gc.ca/en/caf-community-health-services-r2mr/index.page

Canadian Broadcasting Corporation. (2013). Surge in private security raises concerns over rights. Retrieved from http://www.cbc.ca/news/canada/story/2013/01/15/policing-private-security-industry.html

Canadian Children's Rights Council. (2016). Child and teen suicides in Canada. Retrieved from http://www.canadiancrc.com/Youth_Suicide_in_Canada.aspx

Canadian Institute for Military and Veterans Health Research (CIMVHR). (2016). Annual report 2016. Serving those who serve us. Retrieved from https://cimvhr.ca/documents/cimvhr-annual-2016-en.pdf

Carlson, E.B., & Ruzek, J. (2014). PTSD and the family. Retrieved from http://www.ptsd.va.gov

Centers for Disease Control and Prevention. (CDC). (2015, December 4). CDC Grand Rounds: Prevention and control of skin cancer. *Morbidity and Mortality Weekly Report (MMWR), 64*(47), 1312–1314. Retrieved from https://www.cdc.gov/mmwr/preview/mmwrhtml/mm6447a2.htm

Choe, H.M., et al. (2007). Treatment and control of blood pressure in patients with diabetes mellitus. *American Journal of Health System Pharmacy, 64*(1), 97–103.

Connor, K.M., & Butterfield, M.I. (2003). Posttraumatic stress disorder. *Focus, 1*(30), 247–263.

Côté-Boucher, K. (2015). The paradox of discretion: Customs and the changing occupational identity of Canadian border officers. *British Journal of Criminology*, April, azv023. doi:10.1093/bjc/azv023

Cottrill, J. (2017). Trouble in the big house. OHS Canada. *Canada's Occupational Health & Safety Magazine, January/February 2017*, 20–25. Retrieved from https://issuu.com/glaciermedia/docs/02_ohs__jan_feb_2017_final_mar

Czarnecki, F., & Janowitz, I. (2003). Ergonomics and safety in law enforcement. *Clinics in Occupational and Environmental Medicine, 3*(3), 399–417. Retrieved from http://www.theppsc.org/Staff_Views/Czarnecki/ergonomics_and_safety_in_law_enforcement.htm

Dewa, C.S. (2014). Worker attitudes towards mental health problems and disclosure. *International Journal of Occupational and Environmental Medicine, 5*, 175–186.

Duxbury, L., & Higgins, C. (2012). Caring for and about those who serve: Work-life conflict and employee well-being within Canada's police departments. Ottawa, ON: Sprott School of Business. Retrieved from http://sprott.carleton.ca/wp-content/files/Duxbury-Higgins-Police2012_fullreport.pdf

El-Ghoroury, N.H., Galper, D.I., Sawaqdeh, A., & Bufka, L.F. (2012). Stress, coping, and barriers to wellness among psychology graduate students. *Training and Education in Professional Psychology, 6*(2), 122–134. doi:10.1037/a0028768.

El-Gabalawy, R., Thompson, J.M., Sweet, J., Erickson, J., Mackenzie, C.S., Pietrzak, R.H., … Sareen, J. (2016). Comorbidity and functional correlates of anxiety and physical conditions in Canadian veterans. *Journal of Military, Veteran and Family Health, 2*(1). http://jmvfh .utpjournals.press/doi/abs/10.3138/jmvfh.2014-03

Ellis, D., Choi, A., & Blaus, C. (1993). Injuries to police officers attending domestic disturbances: An empirical study. *Canadian Journal of Criminology, 35*(2), 149–168.

Everly, G.S., & Mitchell, J.T. (2000). The debriefing "controversy" and crisis intervention: A review of lexical and substantive issues. *International Journal of Emergency Mental Health, 2*(4), 211–225.

Ferguson, D. (2016). Standing Committee on Public Safety and National Security (SECU). *Evidence,* Number 008 1st Session, 42nd Parliament, 22 March 2016. Retrieved from http://www.parl.gc.ca/ HousePublications/Publication.aspx?Mode=1&Parl= 42&Ses=1&DocId=8166643&Language=E

Finn, P. (2000). Addressing correctional officers stress: Programs and strategies. *Issues and Practices in Criminal Justice.* National Institute of Justice. Retrieved from https://www.ncjrs.gov/pdffiles1/ nij/183474.pdf

Galatzer-Levy, I.R., Brown, A.D., Henn-Haase, C., Metzler, T.J., Neylan, T.C., & Marmar, C.R. (2013). Positive and negative emotion prospectively predict trajectories of resilience and distress among high-exposure police officers. *Emotion, 13*(3), 545-553. doi:10.1037/ a0031314

Garrido, S., Baker, F.A., Davidson, J.W., Moore, G., & Wasserman, S. (2015). Music and trauma: The relationship between music, personality, and coping style. *Frontiers in Psychology, 6,* 977. Retrieved from http://doi.org/10.3389/fpsyg.2015.00977

Government of Canada. (2006). *The human face of mental health and mental illness in Canada.* Ottawa: Minister of Public Works and Government Services Canada. Cat.: HP5-19/2006E. Retrieved from http://www.phac-aspc.gc.ca/publicat/human -humain06/index-eng.php

Greenland, J., & Alam, S. (2017). Police resources in Canada. Statistics Canada. Jusistat 85-002-x. Retrieved from http://www5.statcan.gc.ca/olc-cel/ olc.action?objId=85-002-X&objType=2&lang=en &limit=0

Groll, D., Charbonneau, D., Bélanger, S., & Senyshyn, S. (2016). Yoga and Canadian Armed Forces members' well-being: An analysis based on select physiological and psychological measures. *Journal of Military, Veteran and Family Health, 2*(2).

Gupta, M.A. (2013). Review of somatic symptoms in PTSD. *International Review of Psychiatry, 161,* 1370–1376.

Hopkins, A. (2017, March 5). 'Swiss cheese border': Canadian border patrol union calls for hundreds more workers as it struggles to cope with wave of immigrants fleeing to the country on foot from Trump's America. Retrieved from http://www.dailymail.co.uk/news/article-4284086/ Canada-border-control-union-suggests-increased -patrols.html - ixzz4f5q3UuKH

Institute of Medicine. (2014). *Treatment for posttraumatic stress disorder in military and veteran populations: Final assessment* (p. 203). Washington, D.C.: The National Academies Press. Retrieved from https://doi.org/10.17226/18724

International Labor Organization (ILO). (2012). Officer, police/law enforcement: International hazard datasheet on occupation. Retrieved from http://www.ilo.org/safework/cis/WCMS_192426/ lang--en/index.htm

Jacobson, E. (1938). *Progressive relaxation.* Chicago: Chicago University Press.

Kabat-Zinn, J. (1991). *Full catastrophe living.* New York: Delacorte.

Kalman, I. (2016). "Don't blame me, it's just the computer telling me to do this": Computer attribution and the discretionary authority of Canada Border Services Agency officers. Max Planck Institute for Social Anthropology Working papers. Retrieved from https://www.eth.mpg.de/3958110/mpi-eth-working -paper-0166.pdf

Karaffa, K., Openshaw, L., Koch, J., Clark, H., Harr, C., & Stewart, C. (2015). Perceived impact of police work on marital relationships. *Family Journal, 23*(2), 120. doi:10.1177/1066480714564381

Kelly, J. (2016). Understanding invisible wounds: Post traumatic stress. George W. Bush Institute. Retrieved from http://www.bushcenter.org/publications/ articles/2016/02/invisible-wounds-pts.html

Kiecolt-Glaser, J.K. (1999). Stress, personal relationships and immune function: Health implications. *Brain Behavior Immunology, 13,* 61–72.

Kim, J.-H., & McKenzie, L.A. (2014). The impacts of physical exercise on stress coping and well-being in university students in the context of leisure. *Health, 6,* 2570–2580. Retrieved from http://dx.doi.org/10.4236/health.2014.619296

Kohan, A., & O'Connor, B.P. (2002). Police officer job satisfaction in relation to mood, well-being and alcohol consumption. *Journal of Psychology, 136,* 307–318.

Le Fevre, M., K., Gregory S., & Matheny, J. (2006). Eustress, distress and their interpretation in primary and secondary occupational stress management interventions: Which way first? *Journal of Managerial Psychology, 21*(6), 547–565. doi: 10.1108/02683940610684391

Loo, R. (2003). A meta-analysis of police suicide rates: Findings and issues. *Suicide and Life Threatening Behaviour, 33*(3), 313–325.

Malm, A., Pollard, M., Brantingham, P., Tinsley, P., Plecas, D., Brantingham, P., … Kinney, B. (2005). *A 30 year analysis of police service delivery and costing: "E" division: Research summary.* Centre for Criminal Justice Research (CCJR). Retrieved from https://www.ufv.ca/media/assets/ccjr/ccjr-resources/ccjr-publications/30_Year_Analysis_(English).pdf

Marin, A. (2012). *In the line of duty: Investigation into how the Ontario Provincial Police and the Ministry of Community Safety and Correctional Services have addressed operational stress injuries affecting police officers.* Ombudsman Report. Retrieved from http://www.ombudsman.on.ca/Resources/Reports/In-the-Line-of-Duty.aspx

Meis, L.A., Erbes, C.R., Polusny, M.A., & Compton, J.S. (2010). Intimate relationships among returning soldiers: The mediating and moderating roles of negative emotionality, PTSD symptoms, and alcohol problems. *Journal of Traumatic Stress, 23*(5), 564–572.

Ministry of Community Safety & Correctional Services (MCSCS). (2015). *Facility and service delivery options, analysis and recommendations report—Executive summary.* Toronto: Queen's Printer for Ontario. Retrieved from http://www.mcscs.jus.gov.on.ca/sites/default/files/content/mcscs/docs/ec168135.pdf

Ministry of Community Safety & Correctional Services (MCSCS). (2016a). Corrections. Ottawa-Carleton Detention Centre Task Force Action Plan. Retrieved from http://www.mcscs.jus.gov.on.ca/english/Corrections/OttawaCarletonDetentionCentreTaskForce/OCDCTaskForceActionPlan.html

Ministry of Community Safety & Correctional Services (MCSCS). (2016b). Minister's statements. Supporting Ontario's First Responders Act (posttraumatic stress disorder), 2016. Retrieved from http://www.mcscs.jus.gov.on.ca/english/Ministryinformation/MinistersNewsandStatements/FirstRespondersAct.html.

Morse, D.R., & Furst, M.L. (1979). *Stress for success: A holistic approach to stress and its management.* New York: Van Nostrand Reinhold.

O'Hara, A.F., & Violanti, J.M. (2009). Police suicide—A web surveillance of national data. *International Journal of Emergency Mental Health, 11*(1), 17–23.

Ontario Ministry of Labour. (2016). Ontario passes legislation to support first responders with PTSD. Retrieved from https://news.ontario.ca/mol/en/2016/04/ontario-passes-legislation-to-support-first-responders-with-ptsd.html

Parsons, J. (2004). *Occupational health and safety issues of police officers in Canada, the United States and Europe: A review essay.* International Council of Police Representative Associations. Retrieved from https://www.mun.ca/safetynet/library/OHandS/OccupationalHS.pdf

Paul-Labrador, M., et al. (2006). Effects of a randomized controlled trial of transcendental meditation on components of the metabolic syndrome in subjects with coronary heart disease. *Archives of Internal Medicine, 166*(11), 1218–1224.

Pearson, C., Janz, T., & Ali, J. (2013). Health at a glance: Mental and substance use disorders in Canada. Statistics Canada. Catalogue no. 82-624-X. Retrieved from http://www.statcan.gc.ca/pub/82-624-x/2013001/article/11855-eng.pdf

Public Safety Canada. (2017a). Ministerial roundtable on post-traumatic stress disorder in public safety officers. Retrieved from https://www.publicsafety.gc.ca/cnt/rsrcs/pblctns/mnstrl-rndtbl-ptsd/index-en.aspx?wbdisable=true

Public Safety Canada. (2017b). Post-traumatic stress injuries and support for public safety officers. Retrieved from https://www.publicsafety.gc.ca/cnt/mrgnc-mngmnt/mrgnc-prprdnss/ptsi-en.aspx

Public Service Foundation of Canada. (2015). Crisis in Correctional Services: Overcrowding and inmates with mental health problems in provincial correctional facilities. Retrieved from https://publicservicesfoundation.ca/sites/publicservicesfoundation.ca/files/documents/crisis_in_correctional_services_april_2015.pdf

Robinson, L., Smith, M., & Segal, R. (2017). Stress management. Simple tips to get stress in check and regain control of your life. Helpguide.org. Retrieved from https://www.helpguide.org/articles/stress/stress-management.htm - resources

Ruddell, R., & Jones, N.A. (2014). *The economics of Canadian policing five years into the great recession.* Collaborative Centre of Justice and Safety. Retrieved from http://www.justiceandsafety.ca/rsu_docs/the-economics-of-canadian-policing—-june-2014_1.pdf

Russell, L. M. (2014). An empirical investigation of high-risk occupations: Leader influence on employee stress and burnout among police. *Management Research Review, 37*(4), 367-384. doi:10.1108/MRR-10-2012-0227

Samuels, M., & Samuels, N. (1975). *Seeing with the mind's eye: The history, techniques, and uses of visualization.* New York: Random House.

Sapers, H. (2017). Segregation in Ontario. Independent Review of Ontario Corrections. March 2017. Ministry of Community Safety & Corrections. Retrieved from http://www.mcscs.jus.gov.on.ca/english/Corrections/IndependentReviewOntarioCorrections/IndependentReviewOntarioCorrectionsSegregationOntario.html - _edn10

Scheer, C. (2014). Current trends in police retention: Strategies for keeping good talent. *RCMP Gazette, 76*(3).

Seaward, B.L. (2005). *Managing stress* (5th ed.). Sudbury, MA: Jones and Bartlett Publishers.

Selye, H. (1956). *The stress of life.* New York: McGraw-Hill.

Selye, H. (1974). *Stress without distress.* Philadelphia: Lippincott.

Selye, H. (1976). *Stress in health and disease.* Boston-London: Butterworths.

Shafer, W. (1996). *Stress management for wellness* (3rd ed.). Fort Worth, TX: Holt, Rinehart, and Winston.

Sivasubramanian, P. (2016). Eustress vs Distress—A review. *International Journal of Research in Humanities & Social Sciences, 4*(5). Retrieved from http://raijmr.com/wp-content/uploads/2017/02/4_12-15-Sivasubramanian.pdf

Smetanin, P., Stiff, D., Briante, C., & Khan, M. (2011). Life and economic impact of hypothetical intervention scenarios on major mental illness in Canada: 2011 to 2041. Prepared for the Mental Health Commission of Canada. Toronto: RiksAnalytica. Retrieved from http://www.mentalhealthcommission.ca/sites/default/files/MHCC_Life_Economic_Impact_Scenarios_FINAL_ENG_0_0.pdf

Sorensen, M. (2015). The neurology of music for post-traumatic-stress disorder treatment: A theoretical approach for social work implications. *Master of Social Work Clinical Research Papers*, paper 528. Retrieved from http://sophia.stkate.edu/msw_papers/528

Statistics Canada. (2012). *Police reported crime statistics in Canada, 2011.* Retrieved from http://www.statcan.gc.ca/pub/85-002-x/2012001/article/11692-eng.pdf

Statistics Canada. (2015). Incident-based crime statistics, by detailed violations annual. Table 252-0051. Ottawa: Government of Canada. Retrieved from http://www5.statcan.gc.ca/cansim/a26?lang=eng&id=2520051

Statistics Canada. (2016). Adult correctional services, average counts of adults in provincial and territorial programs annual. Table 251-0005. Ottawa: Government of Canada. Retrieved from http://www5.statcan.gc.ca/cansim/a26?lang=eng&retrLang=eng&id=2510005&tabMode=dataTable&srchLan=-1&p1=-1&p2=9

Strozzi-Heckler, R. (2003). *In search of the warrior spirit: Teaching awareness disciplines to the Green Berets.* Berkeley, CA: North Atlantic Books.

Stults-Kolehmainen, M.A., & Sinha, R. (2014). The effects of stress on physical activity and exercise. *Sports Medicine (Auckland, N.Z.), 44*(1), 81–121. Retrieved from http://doi.org/10.1007/s40279-013-0090-5

TEMA. (2017). Mental health injury and suicide statistics. Retrieved from https://www.tema.ca/infographics-statistics

ToersBijns, C. (2012). Stress, the correctional officer's silent killer. Retrieved from http://www.corrections.com/news/article/31896-stress-the-correctional-officer-s-silent-killer

U.S. Department of Veteran Affairs (2016). PTSD: National Center for PTSD. Types of debriefings following disasters. Retrieved from https://www.ptsd.va.gov/ professional/trauma/disaster-terrorism/debriefing -after-disasters.asp

Van Netten, C., Brands, R.H., Hoption Cann, S.A., Spinelli, J.J., & Sheps, S.B. (2003). Cancer cluster among police detachment personnel. *Environment International, 28,* 567–572.

Veterans Affairs Canada. (2006). Post-traumatic stress disorder and post war-related stress. Ministry of Veteran Affairs. Cat. No.: V32-166/2006E. Retrieved from http://www.veterans.gc.ca/eng/services/ health/mental-health/publications

Veterans Affairs Canada. (2017). Learn about PTSD. Retrieved from http://www.veterans.gc.ca/eng/ services/health/mental-health/publications/ learn-ptsd

Violanti, J.M. (2014). Police suicide: A detrimental outcome of psychological work exposures. In *Dying for the job: Police work exposure and health* (pp. 115–123). Springfield IL: Charles C Thomas Publishers.

Vogel, S., & Schwabe, L. (2016). Learning and memory under stress: Implications for the classroom. *npj Science of Learning, 1,* 16011. doi:10.1038/ mjpscilearn.2016.11

Wilson, S., Guliani, H., & Boichev, G. (2016). Reviews: On the economics of post-traumatic stress disorder of first responders in Canada. *Journal of Community Safety and Well-Being.* Retrieved from https:// journalcswb.ca/index.php/cswb/article/view/6/30

Wirth, M., Vena, J.E., Smith, E.K., Bauer, S.E., Violanti, J., & Burch, J. (2013). The epidemiology of cancer among police officers. *American Journal of Industrial Medicine, 56*(4), 439–453. Retrieved from http://doi.org/10.1002/ajim.22145

World Health Organization (WHO). (2003). *The solid facts: The social determinants of health.* Retrieved from http://www.euro.who.int/__data/assets/pdf_ file/0005/98438/e81384.pdf

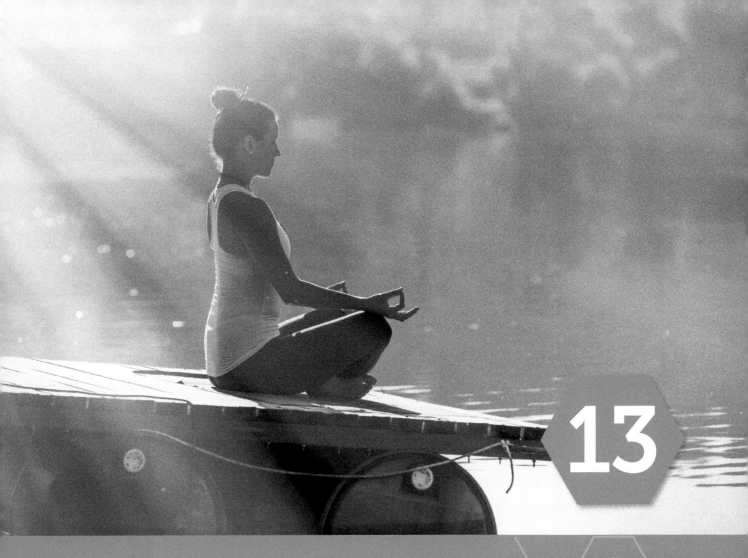

SHIFT WORK AND SLEEP

LEARNING OUTCOMES

After completing this chapter, you should be able to:

- Identify the physiological, psychological, and social effects of shift work.

- Identify the physiological stages of sleep.

- Explain the importance of proper sleep for shift workers.

- Describe the medical impact of shift work on your health.

- Describe healthy sleeping habits.

- Develop shift work coping strategies.

It is estimated that approximately 28 percent of employed Canadians work non-traditional hours (Williams, 2008). This non-standard schedule includes evening or night shifts, rotating shifts, flex time, and extended hours on the job. The mental, physical, and social implications can be challenging. The non-stop "24/7" nature of the world today results in working longer or nighttime work hours for many. While many jobs have "flex time" available, those in emergency services and law enforcement are required to provide continuous, non-interrupted service around the clock. We are seeing entertainment establishments open later, arrival of airplane flights at almost any hour, delivery of suspects to correctional institutes into the early morning, and highway traffic that never seems to ease. As a result, there is a greater chance of changes in schedules to fill shifts, complete a special assignment, continue into overtime to address an occurrence, or attend a court appearance after finishing up a night shift.

Some young people entering into law enforcement find the idea of working late into the night appealing. Many become "night owls" in their teenage years, finding it easier to do homework and study at night, sometimes into the early morning hours, and perhaps working nights at part-time jobs. Shift work allows individuals to do things during the day when conventional workers are working, such as doctor's appointments, shopping without long line-ups, or playing sports. Once an individual is on the job, however, the routines of daytime court appearances, family commitments, and rotating shifts pose a challenge to getting good-quality sleep.

FACTS TO THINK ABOUT

The impact of shift work on physical, mental, occupational, health, and social life:

- Approximately 20 percent of shift workers quit their job because they cannot adapt to the demands of shift work. Those who persevere even though they cannot adjust suffer the effects of ill health long after they stop working shifts.
- A higher incidence of serious illness, including heart disease and cancer, is found among police officers and correctional workers who work rotating shifts. Night shifts increase the risk of strokes and heart attacks, regardless of age.
- As individuals age, their ability to cope with shift changes diminishes. They find it more difficult to fall asleep and are less able to sleep without interruption.
- Lack of sleep has been shown to have a harmful impact on carbohydrate metabolism and endocrine function, which can contribute to metabolic disorders. Individuals working the night shift had elevated waist circumferences compared to those who worked non-midnight shifts.
- Shift work may cause fatigue, which leads to exhaustion, burnout, somatic anxiety, depersonalization, and may lead to cardiovascular and digestive symptoms.

- Rotating shifts that disrupt your sleep cycle and working more than 60 hours a week can also set you up for fatigued driving. Law enforcement personnel who work the night shift have more accidents. The mental and physical effects of night work have been shown to affect a worker's concentration, alertness, motivation, and memory. These factors can slow a person's reaction time. Fatigue also increases the risk of driver inattention, speeding, and running off the road.
- Car crashes (as the result of drowsiness or falling asleep while driving) are one of the top four causes of occupational fatalities in Canada and incurred the highest fatality rate in 2015 in Alberta. More than half of fatigued-related crashes are caused by drivers younger than 25.
- Some 60 to 70 percent of shift workers experience sleep disruption, including activity in the home, phone calls, social life away from work, court appearances, appointments that can only be made during the day, and so on.
- The demands and risks of shift work limit socialization with people outside the job as many feel that those in the job can relate to the stressors of the work. The job beomes his or her life. This isolation can also create a feeling of or lack of communication between family, co-workers, and supervisory staff.

SOURCES: Alberta Labour, 2015; American Academy of Sleep Medicine, 2007; Basinska & Wiciak, 2012; Brinkley, 2010; NIOSH, 2014; NOISH, 2017; Violanti et al., 2007; Violanti et al., 2009; Violanti et al., 2012; Waters & Ussery, 2007.

This chapter looks at shift work and its effects on your health. It also considers the importance of sleep and ways to get better-quality sleep, as well as strategies to alleviate the stress caused by shift work. See Figure 13.1.

FIGURE 13.1 Fatigue and Work

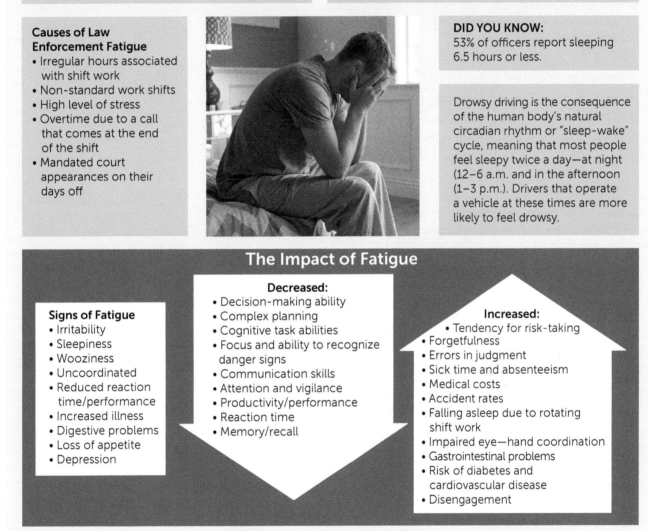

Fatigue is the state of feeling very tired, weary, or sleepy resulting from insufficient sleep, prolonged mental or physical work, shift work, or extended periods of stress or anxiety.

Not sleeping for 17 hours impairs motor skills, speech, balance, coordination, and mental judgment to an extent equivalent to having an alcoholic toxicity of 0.05%, and after 24 hours to a toxicity level of 0.10%.

Causes of Law Enforcement Fatigue
• Irregular hours associated with shift work
• Non-standard work shifts
• High level of stress
• Overtime due to a call that comes at the end of the shift
• Mandated court appearances on their days off

DID YOU KNOW:
53% of officers report sleeping 6.5 hours or less.

Drowsy driving is the consequence of the human body's natural circadian rhythm or "sleep-wake" cycle, meaning that most people feel sleepy twice a day—at night (12–6 a.m. and in the afternoon (1–3 p.m.). Drivers that operate a vehicle at these times are more likely to feel drowsy.

The Impact of Fatigue

Signs of Fatigue
• Irritability
• Sleepiness
• Wooziness
• Uncoordinated
• Reduced reaction time/performance
• Increased illness
• Digestive problems
• Loss of appetite
• Depression

Decreased:
• Decision-making ability
• Complex planning
• Cognitive task abilities
• Focus and ability to recognize danger signs
• Communication skills
• Attention and vigilance
• Productivity/performance
• Reaction time
• Memory/recall

Increased:
• Tendency for risk-taking
• Forgetfulness
• Errors in judgment
• Sick time and absenteeism
• Medical costs
• Accident rates
• Falling asleep due to rotating shift work
• Impaired eye—hand coordination
• Gastrointestinal problems
• Risk of diabetes and cardiovascular disease
• Disengagement

UNDERSTANDING THE IMPORTANCE OF SLEEP

We need sufficient sleep to work effectively, sustain emotional health, and resist stress. We spend a third of our lives sleeping. Sleep experts say the average amount of sleep we need is eight hours a night, although some individuals require ten hours while others seem to get by on six hours. While you sleep, your brain is hard at work forming the pathways necessary for learning and creating memories and new insights. Without enough sleep, you can't focus and pay attention or respond quickly.

FYI

CANADIAN STATISTICS ON SLEEP

Here are some Canadian statistics on sleep (Canadian Sleep Society, 2016):

- The majority (74 percent) of Canadians claim to sleep less than seven hours a night.
- In terms of priority to become healthier, Canadians indicate exercise and nutrition are more important than sleep.
- Women are more affected by their partners' sleeping habits than men, with almost half (47 perecnt) of women reporting that their partner's snoring disrupts their sleep versus one-quarter (26 percent) of men reporting the same thing.

As shown in Figure 13.2, young adults (18 to 34 years old) may require more sleep than adults. Here are some statistics specifically regarding young adults:

- Many (56 percent) will sacrifice sleep in order to gain time for other activities.
- They are more likely (41 percent) to sleep more while on vacation.
- Many (58 percent) will sleep less in the spring/summer (more daylight hours).
- About one-quarter (27 percent) report that working extra hours and sacrificing sleep is championed in their workplace (compared with 15 percent of total Canadians).
- Only some (13 percent) realize that screens (e.g., phones and computers) have an adverse effect on their sleep.
- Most (71 percent) believe that lack of sleep increases aging and signs of aging but it's the first thing that they sacrifice when running short of time (compared to 57 percent of Canadians overall).

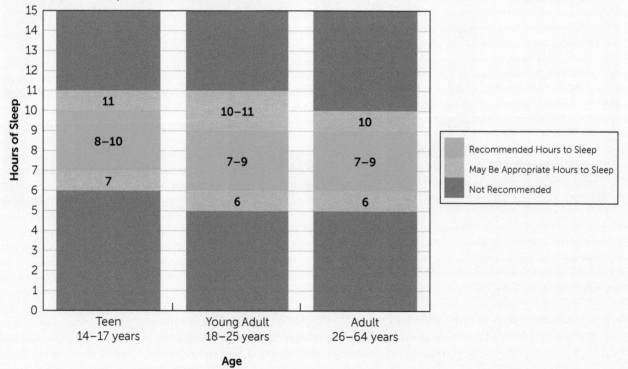

FIGURE 13.2   Sleep Duration Recommendations

Each individual has a different time of day when they are more alert or tired. An individual's tolerance toward shift work has been found to be related to his or her chronotype, which is the scientific name given to an individual's particular circadian rhythm. Circadian rhythm is the 24-hour cycle on which the human biological clock is based. While some people are morning types (up and alert early in the morning), others are evening types (wake up later and stay up later), and some are in between (indifferent).

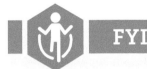

FYI

DETERMINING YOUR CHRONOTYPE

Humans can be categorized as falling into three chronotypes, using such measures as the Horne-Östberg Morningness–Eveningness Scale. The three types are "morning" (Larks), "evening" (Owls), and "indifferents" (those that fall in between).

Morning and evening types each represent approximately 15 to 20 percent of the human population, while the remaining 60 to 70 percent of the population fall into the "indifferent" category.

- Morning-type individuals (Larks) can be described as those persons who naturally waken about two hours earlier than the majority of the population and are ready for sleep between 8 p.m. and 10 p.m. To them, midnight is the middle of the night. Larks cope more easily with early shifts.

- Evening-type individuals (Owls) can be described as those persons who naturally waken about two hours later than the majority of the population and don't feel sleepy until between midnight and 2 a.m. Owls cope more easily with late shifts.

- If you don't readily identify yourself as a Lark or an Owl, then you most likely fall into the "indifferent" category. If you have any doubts, then you can take the Morningness–Eveningness Self-Assessment found at http://www.ubcmood.ca/sad/MEQ.pdf.

Studies show that in the short term, Larks have greater difficulty coping with night shifts than Owls, as their natural tendency to wake early reduces their daytime sleep after a night shift. If you identify yourself as a Lark, then napping in the evening is one strategy to help boost mental alertness on a night shift, although this does not replace good-quality sleep time.

SOURCE: Horne & Östberg, 1976.

Many Canadians are functioning with chronic sleep debt, a pervasive issue and a significant health concern. Sleep debt is the cumulative effect of not getting enough sleep (sleep deprivation). It can occur from just a few days of getting less than six hours of sleep. Sleep deprivation sets up a vicious cycle: fatigue decreases your ability to deal with stress and stress decreases your ability to deal with fatigue (Martin-Doto, 2011; Vila, 2000). One sleep deprivation study (Dawson & Reid, 1997) found that not sleeping for 17 hours can impair a person's motor skills to an extent equivalent to having an alcohol toxicity of 0.05 percent; not sleeping for 24 hours was equivalent to a toxicity level of 0.10 percent. This level of deprivation would impair speech, balance, coordination, and mental judgment. In Canada it is a criminal offence to drive with a blood alcohol concentration (BAC) of 0.08. In another study, Vila (2000) found that half the officers involved with on-the-job accidents and injuries were considered impaired because of fatigue. They found that accidents were caused by impaired hand–eye coordination and propensity to nod-off behind the wheel as well as impaired balance and coordination.

HOW DOES THE SLEEP CYCLE WORK?

Think of sleep as a slow elevator ride down to the bottom floor. At the bottom is where you sleep deeply, and halfway up is where you dream. Usually, we ride the elevator about five times each night—every 70 to 90 minutes—as we cycle through the three ever-deeper stages of non-dreaming sleep, then shift into rapid-eye movement (REM) sleep. This is the stage of sleep during which we dream. In this intensely cerebral stage, muscle paralysis keeps the body from acting out the dreams that occur.

Each of the four stages of sleep (known as the non-REM [NREM] and REM stages) provide different resources for recovery from the day's demands (Moser et al., 2009). Each night you typically go through the same sequence of sleep stages. Your body begins to slow down and muscle tension decreases. As you enter stage N1 of non-REM sleep, mundane thoughts go through your head. If you are awakened at this stage, you may not know you were asleep. Your brain waves at this stage are smaller and irregular. As you enter N2, your eye movement stops and your brain waves become larger with an occasional burst of electrical activity. We spend almost 50 percent of our night sleeping in N2. In N3, you start to enter your deep sleep, where your brain waves are much larger and slower (known as delta waves). You are in such a deep sleep that it can be hard to wake you. If you are woken up during slow wave delta sleep you can suffer from what is called "sleep inertia." This is when your body continues to feel groggy and sleepy upon waking and your motor functions are diminished. Sleep inertia can take up 15 to 30 minutes to lessen, but has been known to last hours. See Figures 13.3 and 13.4.

FIGURE 13.3 Stages of Sleep

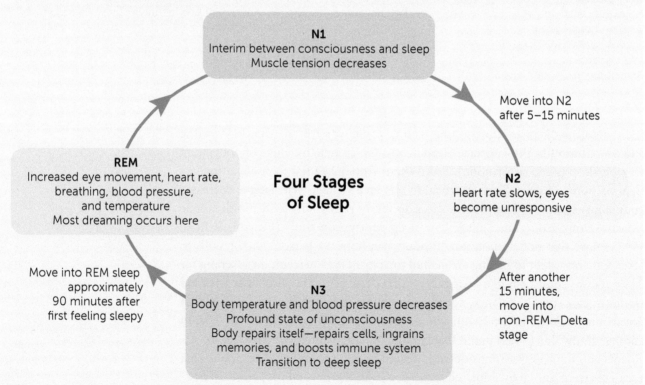

N1
Interim between consciousness and sleep
Muscle tension decreases

Move into N2
after 5–15 minutes

**Four Stages
of Sleep**

N2
Heart rate slows, eyes
become unresponsive

REM
Increased eye movement, heart rate,
breathing, blood pressure,
and temperature
Most dreaming occurs here

After another
15 minutes,
move into
non-REM—Delta
stage

Move into REM sleep
approximately
90 minutes after
first feeling sleepy

N3
Body temperature and blood pressure decreases
Profound state of unconsciousness
Body repairs itself—repairs cells, ingrains
memories, and boosts immune system
Transition to deep sleep

We then go back up through the stages to REM sleep. REM sleep is when your brain becomes active and your eyes dart back and forth, your pulse and breathing quicken, and your temperature and blood flow increase. If you are woken up during REM sleep, you are usually able to remember the dream you were experiencing.

N3, the deepest stage of sleep, is necessary for recovery from physical fatigue. It is believed that non-REM sleep helps repair cells, rests the body and mind, and boosts the immune system. REM stage sleep allows the body to recover from mental fatigue. It helps to store memories and consolidate learning.

The first two or three full sleep cycles of the night contain relatively short REM periods and longer periods of deep, delta wave sleep. As the sleep progresses, more time is spent in REM sleep, while deep sleep decreases. Most individuals experience about five to six cycles per night. All stages of sleep are important for recovery, which is why it is so crucial to be getting the full recommended seven to nine hours of sleep.

FIGURE 13.4   Sleep Hypnogram

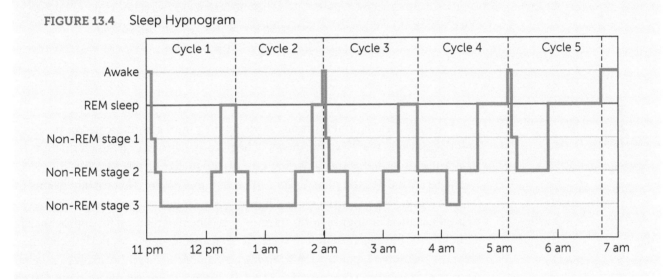

THE EFFECTS OF SHIFT WORK ON SLEEP

Let's look more closely at some effects of shift work and lack of sleep.

PHYSIOLOGICAL AND PSYCHOLOGICAL EFFECTS

The human biological clock is based on a 24-hour circadian rhythm. We are diurnal animals, which means that we are most active during the day and sleep at night, as opposed to nocturnal animals that are active at night and sleep during the day. Exposure to light and dark helps establish these rhythms. The organ that appears to be responsible for this is the suprachiasmatic nuclei (SCN), a small cluster of nerve tissue connected to the point where the optic nerves meet the brain. Stimulated by nerve impulses triggered by exposure to light and dark, this photosensitive nerve centre sets and resets the biological clock. At regular intervals each day, the body becomes hungry and tired, active or lethargic. Body temperature, blood pressure, heart rate, glandular activity, digestion, and brain waves rise and fall in a rhythmic pattern. Interference with this cycle, such as working a night shift, creates chaos to a very sophisticated balance and body rhythm. See Figure 13.5.

FIGURE 13.5 Normal Circadian Rhythm Cycle for a Day

The word "circadian" derives from the Latin "circa," meaning "approximately" and "dies," meaning "day." The circadian clock (as shown below) synchronizes with cycles of light/dark, eating, and activity.

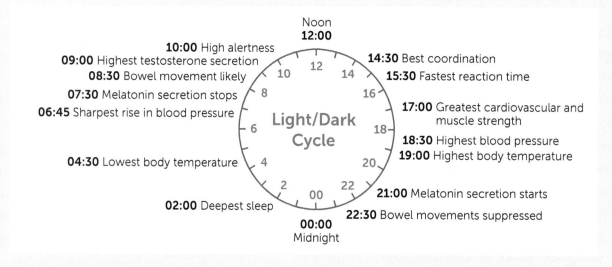

Noon
12:00

10:00 High alertness
09:00 Highest testosterone secretion
08:30 Bowel movement likely
07:30 Melatonin secretion stops
06:45 Sharpest rise in blood pressure

04:30 Lowest body temperature

02:00 Deepest sleep

Light/Dark Cycle

14:30 Best coordination
15:30 Fastest reaction time

17:00 Greatest cardiovascular and muscle strength
18:30 Highest blood pressure
19:00 Highest body temperature

21:00 Melatonin secretion starts
22:30 Bowel movements suppressed

00:00
Midnight

Melatonin is a natural hormone made by the pineal gland (located in the midbrain). Known as the "sleep hormone," it helps to synchronize circadian rhythms by increasing drowsiness and lowering body temperature in preparation for sleep. Darkness stimulates the pineal gland to secrete melatonin. This usually begins to happen around 9 p.m., when natural light is gone. Unless an individual is subjected to bright artificial indoor lighting, melatonin is generally released for approximately 12 hours. As you age, the amount secreted decreases. People with flexible circadian rhythms are more adaptable to shift work when young, but are more likely to develop intolerance to shift work later in life (Arendt, 2010). Decreased melatonin is linked to an increased risk of cancer, diabetes, metabolic syndrome, obesity, and heart disease as well as an impaired immune system (Brum, Filho, Schnorr, Bottega, & Rodrigues, 2015; Canuto, Gracez, & Olinto, 2013; Karlsson, 2001; Pan, Schernhammer, Sun, & Hu, 2011; Van Drongelen, Boot, Merkus, Smid, & van der Beek, 2011).

Working a night shift interferes with your circadian rhythm because it forces you to be awake when your body wants to be asleep. When individuals switch from working a day shift to a night shift, they need time to adjust to this new body clock. Biologically, it takes one day for each hour of adjustment, meaning that it would take close to two weeks to adjust from days to nights; however, some jobs ask that you do this in one or two days. This means that you are usually starting a night shift having already been awake for many hours.

When dayworkers move to the night shift, they sleep an average of five-and-a-half hours a day, not the seven or eight hours required. As the sleep debt builds, we see indications of decreased efficiency in reasoning and reaction time. The sleep debt can lead to brief periods of dozing or micro-sleeping, where you fall in and out of sleep for only seconds at a time. One of the serious results of rotating shift work is that 15 to 40 percent of these shift workers report falling asleep on the job at least once a week or driving while sleepy (Rajaratnam, et al., 2011; Tefft, 2014).

Some individuals may be too sleep-impaired (impaired mental or physical functions due to lack of sleep) to drive, putting themselves and others at risk. Some may actually drive faster to try to compensate for their sleepiness by doing riskier, more stimulating things. Some may experience temporary partial paralysis and temporary memory loss. Some experience peripheral hallucinations and see phantom runners out of the corners of their eyes. Others find it hard to keep their thoughts straight and difficult to speak in complete sentences. It is almost as if they are sleep-drunk. These symptoms usually occur during the early morning hours. For those driving or carrying firearms, fatigue and reduced alertness can become a life-threatening problem (Vila, 2000).

With reduced resources, many individuals are having to work overtime into the day. Whether it is covering a shift, completing paperwork, or going to court, an individual may have to come in during his or her day off or have to work a night shift and then stay awake to work the overtime and get as little as four hours sleep before being required to go in for the next night shift. Inevitably, night shift individuals reduce their sleep time to take advantage of daytime activities on the days they are off duty. This throws the body's sleep adjustment processes into disarray, and the readjustment period must start all over again.

Because the hours that shift workers have for sleep do not coincide with natural and social rhythms, they must make a special effort to ensure that they get enough uninterrupted sleep. If their sleep is interrupted, they may not pass through all four stages of sleep and may suffer health problems as a result. Socially, night shift routines also affect dating opportunities, marriage, child care, and dining routines.

Just turning clocks forward by one hour in the spring can disrupt circadian rhythms and influence the duration and quality of sleep, and the effects can last for several days after the time change. This transition has been statistically shown to increase the incidence of acute myocardial infarction (Janszky & Ljung, 2008). Consideration must be made when individuals have to rotate shifts or wake up early to go to work, thus depriving themselves of necessary sleep.

Tied to our circadian rhythm, our body becomes used to metabolizing foods (especially carbohydrates) during the day. At night, our digestive system slows down. Many individuals tend to eat too fast (based on call volume) and rely on fast foods or snacks, which contain a high percentage of sugars and fat. A growing trend for police is drinking "energy drinks." These are loaded with caffeine and sugars. Enlarged waist circumferences are a direct result. Gastrointestinal and digestive problems such as indigestion, heartburn, stomach ache, and loss of appetite are more common among rotation shift workers and night workers than among day workers (CCOHS, 2010).

Increasing evidence links disruptions in the body's various circadian timekeepers to obesity and malfunctions in metabolism. It is generally accepted that light exposure can reset the main clock in the suprachiasmatic nucleus of the brain, and that cues from the main clock as well as from eating and activity can reset peripheral clocks that operate in almost all the body's cells (Bray & Young, 2009). In addition, those with chronic stress (occupational) and acute stress (major traumas and/or a succession of minor psychological traumas in everyday work with the potential of leading to post-traumatic stress disorder) have an increased risk of suffering from metabolic syndrome symptoms (Garbarino & Magnavita, 2015).

DID YOU KNOW?

Five Signs It's Time to Pull Over

1. Feeling restless or irritable.
2. Frequent blinking or yawning or having trouble keeping your head up and eyes open.
3. Missing exits or traffic signs.
4. Drifting into another lane.
5. Daydreaming or not knowing how you got to that location.

SHIFT SCHEDULES

There are typically two types of shift schedules for law enforcement officers (although there are many variations):

- Three eight-hour shifts, usually beginning at 7 a.m. (the day shift), 3 p.m. (the afternoon shift), and 11 p.m. (the night or "graveyard" shift).
- Two 12-hour shifts, usually beginning at 7 a.m. and 7 p.m.

Most shift work schedules involve four to seven days on and two to four days off. Each service has its own arrangement. Some arrangements are tailored to times of peak demand for services (such as rush hour, number of individuals crossing the border, overcrowding in correctional facilities).

The various shift schedules have different benefits and drawbacks for law enforcement officers:

- Fixed shifts offer the least amount of disruption to the circadian rhythm; however, if you are working straight night shifts it may be hard to revert back to normal hours to participate in family or social events.
- Working rapidly rotating shifts (two days/two nights) keeps the circadian rhythm day-oriented, because there is insufficient time to adjust and there is less sleep debt; however, individuals may feel "out of sync," and their alertness may be affected.

Research has resulted in recommendations for devising healthier shift work routines (Wedderburn & King, 1996) based on physical and psychological effects of long-term shift work:

- Minimize permanent night shifts.
- Minimize the sequence of night shifts: only two to four night shifts in succession should be worked. Working four to seven night shifts in a row has been condemned by experts.
- Consider shorter night shifts (a maximum of seven or eight hours will minimize errors and accidents).
- Plan rotations with some free weekends.
- Avoid overlong work shifts.
- If you have an early shift, adjust your sleep accordingly (reduced sleep leads to fatigue and increased risk of errors and accidents on morning shifts).
- Rotate forward (clockwise rotation from mornings to afternoons to nights).

Ultimately, it is up to the individual agency, in consultation with the professional associations, to address what works most effectively for employees.

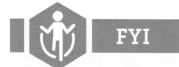

FYI

ISSUES WITH FALLING ASLEEP

Individuals who work 3 p.m. to 11 p.m. and 7 p.m. to 3 a.m. shifts generally find it very difficult to fall asleep right away. Many are still alert after hours of trying to fall asleep.

SOURCE: Akerstedt, Nordin, Alfredsson, Westerholm, & Kecklund, 2010.

SOCIAL EFFECTS

As mentioned earlier, most of the world operates during daytime hours. Society disregards shift workers in planning its schedules. This, of course, poses special problems for shift workers, especially those who work only at night. Most shift workers restrict their work week activities to sleeping and eating, and do everything else on their days off. This affects leisure activities, volunteer work, and time with family and friends. Thirty percent of police divorces are related to shift work stress. Reduced family time, mismatched energy levels for intimacy, and domestic violence are spillovers from the effects of the stress of working in law enforcement (Anderson, 2011).

Scheduling is a must if significant others are to cope with shift work. Planning your days and keeping each other informed of family activities are very important. The parent who works shifts misses school functions, birthday parties, sporting events, and family outings. It becomes difficult to explain to a child why you are constantly missing his or her soccer games. Young children find it difficult to understand why a parent has to sleep during the day and why they must play quietly in the house; similarly, they cannot understand why a parent must work weekends. The parent who is not a shift worker has to compensate for the other, and at times feels overloaded.

Single individuals can find the social aspect difficult. They have a hard time meeting people during their off hours. Because of the time spent at work, shift workers as a whole fall into the trap of socializing only with their co-workers for the majority of time. They tend to lose touch with dayworkers, who in turn have a difficult time understanding shift workers. However, with the trend toward service industries' offering more hours (for example, fitness facilities that are open 24 hours), shift workers today may not miss out as much.

There can be a positive side to shift work. Individuals who get four consecutive days off have time for chores and activities around the house that a dayworker may not have. Having days off during the week allows you to go shopping without having to stand in line, to play a round of golf in short order, to walk your child to school and to bring school-aged children home for lunch. Some weekends can be extended to four days, and during the week you can go to a fitness facility during off-peak hours. Those individuals with hectic family schedules get some quiet time for themselves while their children are at school.

PERSONAL PERSPECTIVE

CHALLENGES AND OPPORTUNITIES

Shift work can offer opportunities that those working day shifts can't enjoy. Shift work can afford time to get to appointments and complete errands (e.g., shopping) without long wait times. One of the perks that my husband (who served as a police officer for 34 years) enjoyed was walking our children to school on the first day of school. I shared the moment only through pictures because it was always the first day of college classes. However, there were many times I had to organize birthday parties and juggle two soccer or hockey games alone. Many times I felt like a single parent and it was a bonus when he was there.

Shift work not only robs the individual of precious family moments, it also affects his or her family. We had to reschedule our 20th anniversary for a homicide and our 25th anniversary because of the G8 conference. For my girls, many birthdays and activities were spent without Dad.

Interestingly enough, when we discussed this issue in class, I was surprised by the number of my students who had had similar experiences yet never discussed the situation as a family.

Feeling robbed of special moments and memories can be hard for all concerned. It is really important to maintain open dialogue about the challenges and to set time aside for both your significant other and family in order to ensure that all feel included.

MEDICAL CONDITIONS ASSOCIATED WITH SHIFT WORK

SLEEP DISORDERS

There are a number of sleep disorders that can be triggered by lack of sleep. These conditions must be assessed and treated. For more information, see National Sleep Foundation (2017a).

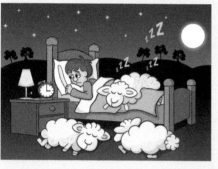

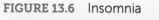
FIGURE 13.6 Insomnia

INSOMNIA

Insomnia is a disorder where an individual has trouble falling or staying asleep (see Figure 13.6). Causes are varied from poor sleep habits, anxiety, life transitions, and medication. If you have insomnia, you are more likely to have trouble working shifts and more likely to develop shift work disorder.

SHIFT WORK DISORDER

Shift work disorder is a circadian rhythm disorder where there is a misalignment or desynchronization in sleep patterns (National Sleep Foundation, 2017d). Shift work disorder can look like insomnia but it is directly linked to a person's work schedule. If they were to stop shift work their symptoms would disappear. Approximately 10 percent of shift workers have this disorder (National Sleep Foundation, 2017d). Symptoms include:

- excessive sleepiness when you need to be awake, alert, and productive
- trouble falling asleep or waking up before you've slept sufficiently
- sleep that feels unrefreshing or insufficient
- difficulty concentrating
- lack of energy
- irritability or depression
- difficulty with personal relationships, work, or family life

Even if you get enough hours of sleep, you may still experience some symptoms of shift work disorder. This is because your internal clock continues to send you drowsy-making signals during the night (as it is naturally programmed to do), even if you've technically slept enough during the day.

NARCOLEPSY

Narcolepsy is a sleep disorder that is characterized by excessive sleepiness, sleep attacks, sleep paralysis, hallucinations, and for some, sudden loss of muscle control (cataplexy). It affects 1 in 2,000 people and can go undiagnosed for years. It is a malfunction in the part of the brain that decides whether you're awake or asleep. People with narcolepsy suddenly fall asleep without warning while carrying on their usual daytime activities. They may experience sudden loss of muscle control, and this may be triggered by strong emotions and vivid dreams. Some of the symptoms include the following (National Sleep Foundation, 2017b):

- Excessive sleepiness.
- Cataplexy, which is a sudden loss in muscle tone and deep tendon reflexes, leading to muscle weakness, temporary paralysis, or a complete

postural collapse. Cataplexy is usually brought on by an outburst of emotion—notably laughter, anger, or being startled.

- Sleep paralysis, which is the temporary inability to move or talk during the episode.
- Hypnagogic hallucinations, which are sensory dream-like experiences during the transition from wakefulness to sleep. These can be vivid, bizarre, and frightening to the individual.
- Disrupted sleep (disruption of the longest sleep episode that occurs on a daily basis), which involves frequent awakening and increased body movement.
- Automatic behaviour, which is unaware behaviour when fluctuating between sleep and wakefulness, such as irrelevant words, lapses in speech, and being unable to explain how you got somewhere.

RESTLESS LEGS SYNDROME

Restless legs syndrome (RLS) is a common and distressing condition that is characterized by an overwhelming urge to move the legs when they are at rest. Symptoms are more profound at night and during sleep (National Sleep Foundation, 2017c), and include:

- uncomfortable feeling in the legs (such as cramps and numbness, tingling, creeping, itching, or aching).
- involuntary jerking of limbs that is relieved by movement.
- difficulty falling or staying asleep due to the symptoms.

SLEEP APNEA

Sleep apnea is a chronic sleep disorder that can potentially be life threatening. It occurs when you have pauses in your breathing while you sleep that last anywhere from ten seconds to one minute. These pauses are often accompanied by snoring and can happen as often as 20 to 60 times per hour. Often a gasp or choke will momentarily wake you and you will resume breathing.

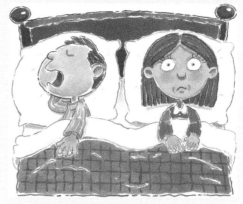

FIGURE 13.7 Snoring

There are two types of sleep apnea:

- *Central sleep apnea,* which occurs when the brain fails to send the appropriate signals to the breathing muscles to initiate respiration.
- *Obstructive sleep apnea,* which is far more common, occurs when the throat muscles fail to keep the airway open and air cannot flow into or out of the nose or mouth.

Public Health Agency of Canada (2010) funded a study that showed that 3 percent of Canadian adults reported being told by a health professional that they have sleep apnea. In addition to those individuals, one in four Canadian adults reported having three or more of the seven symptoms and risk factors associated with having obstructive sleep apnea. Symptoms and risk factors include (National Sleep Foundation, 2017e):

- snoring loud enough to be heard through closed doors.
- often feeling tired, fatigued, or sleepy during the daytime.

- having been observed to stop breathing during their sleep.
- having been diagnosed with high blood pressure.
- having a body mass index (BMI) greater than 35.
- being a male over the age of 50 years.
- being a smoker.
- having a small upper airway.

Canadians with sleep apnea are also more prone to develop other chronic conditions such as diabetes, hypertension, heart disease, mood disorders, and memory problems. If you feel as though you may have sleep apnea, or your snoring is affecting your partner's sleep, your first step would be to assess the risk factors and see if you can reduce your sleep apnea with some lifestyle changes. Examples of changes include avoiding alcohol before bed, losing weight, quitting smoking, and/or sleeping on your side to keep your airway open.

There are sleep diaries and apps that can help you track your sleep, allowing you to see habits and trends that you are experiencing so you can discuss them with your health professional. Otherwise, your doctor may wish to have you complete a sleep study, where they can properly observe and monitor your sleep and breathing patterns. Some treatments available for sleep apnea include mouthpieces, breathing training, breathing devices such as CPAP (continuous positive airway pressure) machines, and even surgery.

CANCER AND SHIFT WORK

Shift work that involves circadian disruption may be carcinogenic (having the potential to cause cancer) to humans (IARC, 2017; Saunders, 2010). This disruption causes insomnia or non-restorative sleep, and a change in hormonal levels which can influence cell growth and division. Specifically,

- Compared to regular day shift workers, there is a modest increased risk for lung cancer mortality (Fangyi et al., 2015).
- Women who work on rotating night shifts with at least three nights per month in addition to days and evenings in that month appear to have a moderately increased risk of breast cancer after extended periods of working rotating night shifts (IARC, 2017; Schernhammer et al., 2001, Schernhammer et al., 2006).
- There is evidence of elevated risk of colorectal cancer for those working rotational shifts (Schernhammer et al., 2003).
- Those working rotating shifts had a significantly higher risk of prostate cancer than dayworkers, but there was no significant increase in risk for those on fixed night shifts. Some of the causes postulated include polycyclic aromatic hydrocarbons in exhausts, occupational whole body vibration from driving in a vehicle, and sitting in a vehicle much of the shift (Kubo et al., 2006).

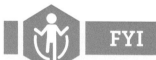

REPRODUCTIVE RISKS

The constant disruption of hormonal balances from shift work may cause elevated reproductive risks including irregular menstrual cycles, spontaneous premature births, and lower birth weights, as well as infertility issues.

SOURCE: Gamble, Resuehr, & Johnson, 2013.

DIABETES AND SHIFT WORK

Within 10 to 15 years of service, 30 to 40 percent of law enforcement officers become obese and many are less fit than the general population (Girard, 2013). These are two risk factors for diabetes. We are aware that shift work affects your appetite, leading to weight loss or gain. Many individuals find themselves with digestive problems like constipation, diarrhea, indigestion, and heartburn. Shift work forces you to eat and sleep at different times than you normally would and this greatly affects your blood glucose levels, especially if you can't make healthy choices or don't feel like eating. There is also the additional factor that mental and physical stressors affect your blood glucose levels.

It is not uncommon for people living with diabetes to conceal their disease from their employers and fellow workers. Many do not want to deal with negative reactions or discrimination. As a result, blood glucose tests are forgotten, insulin injections are missed, and meals are postponed, jeopardizing overall health and safety on the job (Diabetes Canada, 2017).

Human rights legislation directs employers that they must accommodate an individual with diabetes up to the point of "undue hardship." Reasonable accommodations means having the ability to have regular breaks so you can monitor blood sugar, administer medication, and eat when needed. It is prudent that you make your employer, co-workers, and family members aware of the process you must go through and how to treat you for hypoglycemia (low blood sugar). Refer to the publication *A Place for All: A Guide to Creating an Inclusive Workplace* (CHRC, 2006) for more information. Whether you are diabetic or not, it is important to keep regular meals and have healthy snacks available to keep your blood glucose levels from dropping quickly (for more information, refer to Chapter 8). It is also important to exercise regularly and take active breaks during your shift.

> **DID YOU KNOW?**
> It wasn't until 2006 that the RCMP adopted a policy of individual assessment and implemented the Royal Canadian Mounted Police Diabetes Mellitus Medical Guidelines so type 1 diabetics could be hired as RCMP officers.

COPING STRATEGIES FOR SHIFT WORK

The following suggestions will help you cope with the stress of shift work in your professional and personal life.

EATING NUTRITIOUS FOOD

Following *Eating Well with Canada's Food Guide* (Health Canada, 2012) is very important (see Chapter 8). Fruits, vegetables, yogurt, seeds, nuts, and water should replace snacks such as chocolate bars, chips, pop, and candy, which are high in fat and sugar. Consuming light to moderate amounts of protein (meat, fish, low-fat dairy products) is recommended for the beginning of the shift, and complex carbohydrates (whole grains, fruits, vegetables, and legumes) can help get you through the shift. Make sure to get your daily requirement of water intake (McCormick, Cohen, & Plecas, 2011).

You should eat the same for a night shift as you would for a day shift. So, breakfast when you wake, and meals and snacks throughout the shift as you would normally eat. Having a regular eating schedule for the shift you are on will reduce the risk of developing gastrointestinal disorders and diabetes.

Tryptophan and melatonin help improve sleep and promote a calm mind. Tryptophan (found in nuts, fish, chicken, turkey, eggs, cheese, and tofu) is an amino acid that synthesizes serotonin, a neurotransmitter that primarily affects mood regulation. Melatonin is a hormone that helps regulate your circadian rhythm for healthy sleep patterns. Although most people take it in the form of a supplement, there are foods (oats, rice barley, pineapple, tart cherry juice, tomatoes, and oranges) that contain melatonin and can help bring your levels back to where they should be.

Don't go to bed hungry or overly full. Have a light snack about one hour before you hit the pillow. Avoid sugary snacks, which may cause your blood sugar to plummet later, causing you to wake up. Also, avoid drinking excessive amounts of liquids right before bed as it may increase the likelihood of needing to go to the bathroom during your sleep time.

Avoid caffeinated soft drinks, tea, coffee, chocolate, and ASA (Aspirin®, Entrophen®) within five hours of going to sleep. Caffeine affects some people for up to 12 hours. Tobacco should also be avoided because nicotine acts as a stimulant. Alcohol and sleep aids interfere with the depth and quality of sleep. Although alcohol may help you fall asleep quicker, it disrupts your REM sleep and suppresses breathing (precipitating sleep apnea), and therefore creates a more disrupted sleep (Ebrahim, Shapiro, Williams, & Fenwich, 2013). One or two standard drinks before bed seems to have minimal effects, but the more a person drinks, the stronger the disruption. Alcohol should not be used as a sleep aid, as it may result in alcohol dependence. Most sleeping pills contain antihistamines, which have a sedative side effect, inducing light sleep but robbing you of deep sleep. Stimulants to counter listlessness and sleepiness create an unhealthy stimulant–depressant cycle. Recreational drugs can cause restlessness and interfere with sleep.

THE ROLE OF LIGHT

Some people are prone to depression in winter, when natural light levels are low. Seasonal affective disorder (SAD) is a syndrome associated with decreased light due to climate, latitude, and changes in neurotransmitter function as a result of seasonal changes. If you experience moodiness or depression during winter, getting some sunlight (for example, by taking brisk walks on sunny days, or going south for a holiday) could get you back on track. Artificial light—through the use of full-spectrum lighting in your home or office, or with a phototherapy light box—can replicate the effects of sunlight.

Darkness, on the other hand, is conducive to promoting sleep. When you have to sleep during the day, reduce as much of the light coming into your room as possible. Use dark blinds for your windows, or sleep in a room without windows. It has been found that light that has blue wavelengths, which is beneficial to us during the daylight hours because it increases alertness, is most disruptive at night. Blue light emitted from device screens (phones, televisions, computer monitors) affects our ability to fall asleep. Blue light suppresses the production of melatonin in our bodies by making it seem like it is still daytime. Make sure that for the hour before sleep, you eliminate any screen time and resist the temptation to fall asleep with the television or computer on in the bedroom. If you need to turn on a light at night, keep it dim, indirect, and/or use a red light, which does not affect the production of melatonin. Sleeping masks may help as well.

To help you wake up, use a bright lamp with a timer. Set the timer to go off about half an hour before you need to wake up. The light from the lamp will help you wake up by stimulating your body, and is more effective than waking up to the blare of a radio. This should help trick your body into resetting its wake–sleep cycle so you can better cope with changing shifts.

IMPORTANCE OF BREAKS WHILE ON DUTY

It is important to take breaks during your shift, whether to release the tension in your back, have a bathroom break, help with sleepiness, or get a healthy meal and adequate amount of water. With unpredictable workloads (due to sickness, vacation time, or understaffing) and ever-changing workflow, it can be difficult to ensure you take regular breaks (Cohen, Plecas, & McCormick, 2011; McCormick, Cohen, & Plecas, 2011; Vila, 2006).

If you are in a vehicle, get out and walk around. If you are working at a monitor or doing computer work, it is important that you take a five- to ten-minute break every hour. Many agencies are being proactive about encouraging officers to come off the road, for their one-hour lunch break. Make sure that you use that time wisely. Spend the time eating a nutritious meal and catching up with friends or working out. This also could be a good time for a 15-minute power nap. Many workplaces offer dark rooms with a bed, so that you can rest if you need to.

Similarly, while you are studying or working on your computer, it is important to get up from your desk and move around. Get a glass of water, chat, or take a lap around your residence. It is also important to do some gentle exercises and stretches to help relieve muscle fatigue.

PHYSICAL ACTIVITY

Increase your physical activity to increase energy, alertness, balance, appetite, and stamina, and to facilitate sleeping. Beware of prolonged or high-exertion exercise, which can actually increase fatigue. You should engage in physical activity every day.

For those working afternoon shifts, it may be effective to work out at the end of the shift, when you are still keyed up. Make sure that you have a warm (not hot) shower and a light meal to help you relax when you are done working out.

Most night shift workers find it extremely difficult to work out in the morning. A more appropriate time for them is the evening before beginning a shift, or if the employer allows it, during a lunch period. The only difficulty with an early evening workout is that it can interfere with family time, including meals and children's activities.

There are times when you need to stay awake, whether it is to do a double shift or make it through the night shift. Ways to help you stay alert include:

- exercising, walking outside in the cold air,
- turning up the light to ease fatigue,
- splashing your face with cold water,
- having an interesting conversation, singing,
- giving your eyes a break to avoid fatigue, and
- switching tasks to stimulate your mind.

DID YOU KNOW?

Sleepidemic

According to Dr. Mark Tremblay (participACTION, 2016), sedentary lifestyles are connected to a creeping "sleepidemic" in Canada with our young people. Sleep deprivation creates an insidious threat to individuals' mental and physical health. Many are too tired to get enough physical activity during the day and not active enough to be tired at night, creating a vicious cycle. Studies (Mah, Mah, Kerzirian, & Dement, 2011; Samuels, 2008) have shown that sleep will reduce the risk of overtraining/under-recovery, enhance resistance to illness, and improve recovery from injury in athletes. The same applies to physically demanding careers.

PERSONAL PERSPECTIVE

LETTER FROM A FORMER STUDENT

Hey Nancy,

It has been just over 3.5 years since I graduated from the police studies degree program at Georgian, and since then I have enjoyed a career with the OPP. Policing and shift work have been everything that you promised they would be: long, drawn-out hours followed by minutes of heart-pumping adrenaline rushes. The work has been difficult, yet rewarding. And it has challenged me both mentally and physically.

The fitness aspect is what I wanted to write to you about. Since joining the force, I have had first-hand experience with the challenges of maintaining a healthy lifestyle while working bizarre hours. I had no idea how draining shift work and poor nutrition can be on a person's physical and mental health. Strangely, in my first year on the force, the motivation and pleasure that I once had in hitting the gym waned drastically. And it was all too easy to buy a sub or a slice of pizza every day for lunch.

But your lessons reinforced the importance of fitness and nutrition, even when maintaining these is not convenient. And am I ever grateful to you. Not only has my fitness helped me in physical confrontations on the job, but it has also helped me to deal effectively with the many stresses of policing and shift work.

Today I am still leading an active, healthy lifestyle, enjoying sports like hockey, baseball, and mountain biking, on top of weight training 3–5 times a week with my wife. Also, I am watching my nutrition, always trying to pack and buy healthy options. All of this contributes to a much happier life off the job.

So here I am, sitting in my cruiser under an overpass running some radar, thinking about how grateful I am for the dedication of teachers such as yourself, and the great example you set for your students.

I hope all is well with you. I will have to stop by one day to catch up over a cup of green tea.

Take care,

Dave

KEEPING HEALTHY RELATIONSHIPS

Balancing relationships, family, and friends can be more difficult when you work shifts. Here are some suggestions to help:

- Be proactive about setting up times to do things with people you care about (e.g., meet for breakfast instead of dinner, invite them along to run errands so you have a chance to talk, opt for short coffee dates to get caught up, plan activities weeks in advance so everyone can be included based on your schedule).

- Cultivate friendships with other shift worker families for social enjoyment as well as for a support system to help you cope with the unique stresses of shift work with a different perspective.

- Join a fitness centre or volunteer for an organization so that you can meet new people.

- Create a visual schedule or calendar for your children/significant other so they know what to expect and incorporate activities (routine and special) into the schedule so that they have things to look forward to.

- Keep small rituals in place, such as handwritten notes in someone's lunchbox or phone calls or live video calls before bed, after a game, or during a special event that you can't attend.

HEALTHY SLEEP TIPS

Having healthy sleep habits can make a big difference in your quality of life. Here are some practices to consider:

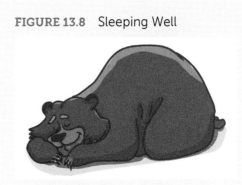

FIGURE 13.8   Sleeping Well

- Meditation and other relaxation techniques (see Chapter 12) help combat high blood pressure (Dickinson et al., 2008), asthma, high cholesterol, sleep disturbances, irritability, and muscle jumpiness (Gooneratne, 2008).

- Learn to wind down from work by reading or listening to music. It is important for shift workers to "leave work at work." All too often, individuals take unresolved issues home.

- Stick to a sleep schedule of the same bedtime and wake up time, especially on your days off. This helps regulate your internal clock.

- Develop a bedtime routine that does not involve bright lights (phone, computer, TV), as these can interfere with your production of melatonin and can cause excitement, stress, or anxiety, making it more difficult to get to and stay asleep. Turn off your phone so you are not interrupted by text messages or calls.

- Add a relaxing bath to your routine. Going from a warm (not hot) bath to a cool room (between 16 and 19 °C) will cause you to release heat, lowering your internal body temperature, which is a key step in inducing sleep.

- Make your bedroom a sleep-friendly zone. Sleep on a comfortable mattress and pillow. Life expectancy of a comfortable and supportive mattress is about ten years. Make sure you have the appropriate blinds to block out light. Keep your room cool, the optimal sleeping temperature is approximately 17 °C. During the summer months, consider sleeping in the basement when on night shifts, as it is always much cooler and can get quite dark during the day.

- Find ways to cope with noise during sleep time. Loud noises interrupt deeper sleep and bring individuals back to lighter sleep, which means they do not get the proper physical and mental restoration. Ways to reduce noise during the day so that you can have an effective sleep include adding sound barriers to your bedroom and building a sleeping area in the basement that keeps you secluded from the rest of the family. An alternative is to create white noise. A fan or white noise machine can mask noises inside and outside the house and should help you fall asleep. Ear plugs may also help.

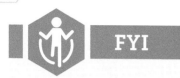

SLEEP ISSUES

For more information on sleep issues, including sleep disorders and treatments, try the following websites:

- Canadian Sleep Society (CSS) https://css-scs.ca
- National Sleep Foundation http://www.sleepfoundation.org
- National Center on Sleep Disorders Research (National Heart, Lung, and Blood Institute) https://www.nhlbi.nih.gov/about/org/ncsdr/index.htm
- Center for Advanced Research in Sleep Medicine http://www.ceams-carsm.ca/en/

- Use your circadian rhythm to your advantage. Shift workers need to monitor their body temperature. Body temperature passes through two cycles a day. From about 3 a.m. to 6 a.m. there is a trough, or low point. Body temperature rises from 8 a.m. to 10 a.m., when it reaches a peak. After that it falls until reaching a trough around 2 p.m. to 4 p.m., followed by a steady rise until reaching another peak between 7 p.m. and 9 p.m. If you can determine your peaks and troughs, you may be able to cope better with shift work. Do highly skilled tasks and complex thinking when your body temperature reaches its peak and menial tasks and paperwork when body temperature is falling.

- Learn to nap effectively. The goal is a nap of 10 to 20 minutes at least 8 hours before going to bed (any longer can make you more tired and interfere with REM sleep). A 20-minute nap allows you to stay in stages 1 and 2 sleep. If you sleep longer (45 to 60 minutes), you will go into your deep sleep and you will risk having sleep inertia when you wake, feeling more tired than you did before the nap. If you are able to, it is recommended to nap for 90 to 100 minutes and complete a full sleep cycle, as you will wake up feeling more refreshed.

- It is important to learn your body's sleep cycles, so that while on shift work you can set your alarm for the perfect amount of time. There are now apps on your phone that can track your sleep by monitoring your movement in bed and advise you on when is the best time to wake up.

FINAL THOUGHTS

Remember that shift work will become a part of your life and your family's life. You will have to make an effort not to let its physical impact interfere with your quality of life. Be aware of what your body is telling you, and learn to take care of yourself. It is important to get enough sleep for boosting your mood and immune system while reducing the risk of various diseases.

Your task is to determine how you will cope with the effects of shift work and rotating shifts based on your ability to handle different sleep patterns/times. Refer to **assignment 13.1** (at www.emond.ca/fitness5e) to assess your sleep habits and strategies for improving your sleep.

Refer to **assignment 13.2** (at www.emond.ca/fitness5e) to assess and devise some strategies for coping with shift work.

KEY TERMS

cataplexy
a sudden loss in muscle tone and deep tendon reflexes, leading to muscle weakness, temporary paralysis, or a complete postural collapse usually brought on by an emotional outburst

chronic sleep debt
a pervasive issue and a significant health concern where you begin to feel the cumulative effect of not getting enough sleep (sleep deprivation); it can occur from just a few days of getting less than six hours of sleep

chronotype
a person's individual circadian rhythms, including body temperature, cognitive faculties, and eating and sleeping patterns

circadian rhythm
the 24-hour cycle on which the human biological clock is based

diurnal
awake during the day, asleep at night

fatigue
the state of feeling very tired, weary, or sleepy resulting from insufficient sleep, prolonged mental or physical work, shift work, or extended periods of stress or anxiety

insomnia
a disorder where an individual has trouble falling or staying asleep

jet lag
a disruption to your circadian rhythm based on crossing time zones

melatonin
a hormone, realized in the absence of light, that helps us sleep better by increasing drowsiness and lowering body temperature

micro-sleeping
falling asleep for seconds or milliseconds

narcolepsy
a disorder that causes brain malfunction, leading to one's falling asleep without warning

non-REM sleep
stages of sleep, including N1, N2, and N3, where your body has increasingly slower heart rates, eye movement, and brain wave activity

peripheral hallucinations
seeing things out of the corner of your eye that aren't really there

rapid-eye movement (REM) sleep
a stage of sleep that allows your body to recover from mental fatigue and helps to store memories and consolidate learning

restless legs syndrome (RLS)
a condition characterized by an overwhelming urge to move the legs when they are at rest

seasonal affective disorder (SAD)
a syndrome associated with decreased light due to climate, latitude, and changes in neurotransmitter function as a result of seasonal changes

shift work disorder
a circadian rhythm disorder where there is a misalignment or desynchronization in sleep pattern as a result of shift work

sleep apnea
a breathing-related sleep disorder in which inappropriate brain signals do not tell the breathing muscles to initiate respiration

sleep-impaired
impaired mental or physical function due to lack of sleep

sleep inertia
when your body feels groggy and sleepy upon waking, and motor functions are diminished

EXERCISES

MULTIPLE CHOICE

1. What amount of sleep do shift workers get compared with non-shift workers?
   a. the same
   b. more
   c. less
   d. none of the above

2. How does the most effective shift work rotate?
   a. from days to nights to afternoons
   b. from days to afternoons to nights
   c. from afternoons to days to nights
   d. from nights to afternoons to days
   e. from nights to days to afternoons

3. Which of the following happens during REM sleep?
   a. Your body repairs cells and boosts your immune system.
   b. You don't get a restful sleep.
   c. You recover from mental fatigue.
   d. You don't easily wake up.
   e. Your brain waves become larger.

4. The long-term effects of shift work can include
   a. sleep disorders
   b. eating disorders
   c. cardiovascular disorders
   d. reproductive disorders
   e. all of the above

5. Circadian rhythm refers to
   a. your heartbeat
   b. your biological clock
   c. your reproductive clock
   d. a method of birth control
   e. the amount of blood flowing through your heart

6. The possible symptoms experienced by sleep-deprived shift workers do *not* include
   a. temporary partial paralysis
   b. poor appetite
   c. peripheral hallucination
   d. difficulty speaking
   e. staying awake easily around sunrise

7. Coping strategies for shift work include
   a. eating healthy foods
   b. getting regular exercise
   c. creating a sleep friendly environment
   d. avoiding alcohol to fall asleep
   e. all of the above

8. To try to sleep during the day with other people around, *avoid*
   a. putting sound barriers around your bedroom to keep noise out
   b. using white noise to reduce sounds
   c. sleeping in the basement when kids are playing in the house
   d. using relaxation techniques to fall asleep
   e. consuming coffee or chocolate before going to sleep

9. The hormone that helps you feel tired is
   a. serotonin
   b. melatonin
   c. tyroxine
   d. adenosine
   e. cryprochrome

10. Many people have a clear reduction in task performance around which time of day?
    a. midday
    b. early morning
    c. post-lunch
    d. late afternoon
    e. early evening

11. Which type of work is most disruptive in terms of causing harmful effects through major changes to the circadian rhythm?
    a. permanent night work
    b. slowly rotating shift work
    c. rapidly rotating shift work
    d. non-rotating shift work
    e. permanent day work

12. In which stage of sleep does dreaming occur?
    a. N1
    b. N2
    c. N3
    d. REM
    e. non-REM

13. Under which condition is melatonin released, and what is the effect of the release of this hormone?
    a. Melatonin is released when light levels are high, making a person feel sleepy.
    b. Melatonin is released when light levels are high, increasing body temperature and making a person feel awake.
    c. Melatonin is released when light levels are low, decreasing body temperature and making a person feel sleepy.
    d. Melatonin is released when light levels are low, decreasing body temperature and making a person feel awake.
    e. Melatonin is released when a person wakes up, increasing body temperature and making a person feel sleepy.

SHORT ANSWER

1. List five negative physiological effects of shift work.

2. List some positive aspects of shift work.

3. How can shift work affect your social life?

4. List six ways to cope with shift work.

5. Describe the differences between insomnia and shift work disorder.

6. Describe the difference between the causes of central sleep apnea and obstructive sleep apnea.

7. Describe some nutritional ways to deal with shift work.

8. Describe some ways to sleep more effectively.

9. What is seasonal affective disorder and how can you reduce its affects?

10. In terms of fatigue, why is it important to take breaks at work?

REFERENCES

Akerstedt, T., Nordin, M., Alfredsson, L., Westerholm, P., & Kecklund, G. (2010). Sleep and sleepiness: Impact of entering or leaving shift work—A prospective study. *Chronobiology International, 27*(5), 987–996.

Alberta Labour. (2015). 2015 Workplace injury, disease and fatality statistics provincial summary. Retrieved from https://work.alberta.ca/documents/2015-ohs-data.pdf

American Academy of Sleep Medicine. (2007, June 13). Sleep disorders highly prevalent among police officers. *Science Daily*. Retrieved from http://www.sciencedaily.com/releases/2007/06/070612075008.htm

Anderson, A. (2011). Intimate partner violence within law enforcement families. *Journal of Interpersonal Violence, 26*(6), 1176–1193.

Arendt, J. (2010). Shift work: Coping with the biological clock. *Occupational Medicine (London), 60*(1), 10–20. doi:10.1093/occmed/kqp162

Basinska, B.A., & Wiciak, I. (2012, July). Fatigue and professional burnout in police officers and firefighters. *Internal Security, 4*(2), 267–275.

Bray, M.S., & Young, M.E. (2009). The role of cell-specific circadian clocks in metabolism and disease. *Obesity Review, 10*(2), 6–13.

Brinkley, M. (2010). Effects on health for the night shift worker. Retrieved from http://www.livestrong.com/article/112321-effects-health-night-shift-worker

Brum, M.C.B., Filho, F.F.D., Schnorr, C.C., Bottega, G.B., & Rodrigues, T.C. (2015). Shift work and its association with metabolic disorders. *Diabetology & Metabolic Syndrome, 7*, 45. Retrieved from http://doi.org/10.1186/s13098-015-0041-4

Canadian Centre for Occupational Health and Safety (CCOHS). (2010). Rotational shift work. Retrieved from http://www.ccohs.ca/oshanswers/ergonomics/shiftwrk.html

Canadian Human Rights Commission (CHRC). (2006). *A place for all: A guide to creating an inclusive workplace*. Minister of Public Works and Government Services. Cat. No. HR21-62/2006. ISBN 0-662-49503-9. Retrieved from http://www.chrc-ccdp.gc.ca/eng

Canadian Sleep Society. (2016). Canadian sleep review 2016: Current issues, attitudes and advice to Canadians.

Canuto, R., Garcez, A.S., & Olinto, M.T.A. (2013). Metabolic syndrome and shift work: A systematic review. *Sleep Medicine Review,17*, 425–431. doi:10.1016/j.smrv.2012.10.004

Choy, M., & Salbu, R.L. (2011). Jet lag: Current and potential therapies. *Pharmacy and Therapeutics, 36*(4), 221–224, 231.

Cohen, I.M., Plecas, D., & McCormick, A.V. (2011). *Taking breaks in general duty police work: The case of Surrey RCMP officers*. Centre for Public Safety and Criminal Justice Research. University of the Fraser Valley. Retrieved from https://www.ufv.ca/media/assets/ccjr/reports-and-publications/Surrey_-_Break_Time.pdf

Dawson, D., & Reid, K. (1997). Fatigue, alcohol and performance impairment. *Nature, 388*, 235.

Diabetes Canada. (2017). *Diabetes in the workplace: A guide for employers and employees*. Retrieved from http://www.diabetes.ca/diabetes-and-you/know-your-rights/employment-discrimination-your-rights/diabetes-in-the-workplace-a-guide-for-employers

Dickinson, H., et al. (2008). Relaxation therapies for the management of primary hypertension in adults: A Cochrane review. *Journal of Human Hypertension, 22*(12), 807–808.

Ebrahim, I.O., Shapiro, C.M., Williams, A.J., & Fenwich, P.B. (2013). Alcohol and sleep I: Effects on normal sleep. *Alcohol Clinical and Experimental Research, 37*, 539–549. doi:10.111/acer.12006

Fangyi G., Han, J., Laden, F., Caporaso, N.E., Stampfer, M.J., Kawachi, I., … Schernhammer, E.S. (2015). Total and cause-specific mortality of U.S. nurses working rotating night shifts. *American Journal of Preventive Medicine, 48*(3), 241–252. doi:10.1016/j.amepre.2014.10.018

Gamble, K.L., Resuehr, D., & Johnson, C.H. (2013). Shift work and circadian dysregulation of reproduction. *Frontiers in Endocrinology, 4*, 92. Retrieved from http://doi.org/10.3389/fendo.2013.00092

Garbarino, S., & Magnavita, N. (2015). Work stress and metabolic syndrome in police officers. A prospective Study. *PLoS ONE, 10*(12), e0144318. Retrieved from http://doi.org/10.1371/journal.pone.0144318

Girard, G. (2013). Obesity in law enforcement. *Canadian Journal of Diabetes, 37*, S243. Retrieved from http://dx.doi.org/10.1016/j.jcjd.2013.03.159

Gooneratne, N.S. (2008). Complementary and alternative medicine for sleep disturbances in older adults. *Clinical Geriatric Medicine, 24*(1), 121–138.

Health Canada. (2012). *Eating well with Canada's Food Guide*. Retrieved from https://www.canada.ca/en/health-canada/services/food-nutrition/canada-food-guide/get-your-copy.html

Horne, J.A., & Östberg, O. (1976). A self-assessment questionnaire to determine morningness–eveningness in human circadian rhythms. *International Journal of Chronobiology, 4,* 97–100.

International Agency for Research on Cancer (IARC). (2017). IARC mongraphs on the evaluation of carcinogenic risks to humans. Retrieved from http://monographs.iarc.fr/ENG/Classification/

Janszky, I., & Ljung, R. (2008). Shifts to and from Daylight Saving Time and incidence of myocardial infarction. *New England Journal of Medicine, 359,* 1966–1968.

Karlsson B. (2001). Is there an association between shift work and having a metabolic syndrome? Results from a population based study of 27 485 people. *Occupational and Environmental Medicine, 58,* 747–752. doi: 10.1136/oem.58.11.747

Kubo, T., Ozasa, K., Mikami, K., Wakai, K., Fujino, Y., Watanabe, Y., … Tamakoshi, A. (2006). Prospective cohort study of the risk of prostate cancer among rotating-shift workers: Findings from the Japan collaborative cohort study. *American Journal of Epidemiology, 164*(6), 549–555. Retrieved from https://doi.org/10.1093/aje/kwj232

Mah, C.D., Mah, K.E., Kerzirian, E.J., & Dement, W.C. (2011). The effects of sleep extension on the athletic performance of collegiate basketball players. *Sleep, 34*(7), 943–950.

Martin-Doto, C. (2011). Anti-fatigue measures could cut cop deaths 15%, researcher claims. *Force Science News, 172* (February). Retrieved from http://www.forcescience.org/fsnews/172.html

McCormick, A.V., Cohen, I.M., & Plecas, D. (2011). *Nutrition and general duty police work: The case of Surrey RCMP members*. Centre for Public Safety and Criminal Justice Research. University of the Fraser Valley.

Moser, D., Anderer, P., Gruber, G., Parapatics, S., Loretz, E., Boeck, M., … Dorffner, G. (2009). Sleep classification according to AASM and Rechtschaffen & Kales: Effects on sleep scoring parameters. *Sleep, 32*(2), 139–149.

National Institute for Occupational Safety and Health (NIOSH). (2014). NIOSH Center for Motor Vehicle Safety: Strategic plan for research and prevention, 2014-2018. Cincinnati, OH: U.S. Department of Health and Human Services, Centers for Disease Control and Prevention, National Institute for Occupational Safety and Health, DHHS (NIOSH) Publication 2014–122.

National Institute for Occupational Safety and Health (NIOSH). (2017). Center for Motor Vehicle Safety. Retrieved from https://www.cdc.gov/niosh/docs/2017-157/CMVS-PPOP-2017-157.pdf

National Sleep Foundation. (2017a). Homepage. Retrieved from http://www.sleepfoundation.org

National Sleep Foundation. (2017b). Narcolepsy. Retrieved from https://sleepfoundation.org/narcolepsy/homeward

National Sleep Foundation. (2017c). Restless Legs Syndrome (RLS) and sleep. Retrieved from https://sleepfoundation.org/sleep-disorders-problems/restless-legs-syndrome

National Sleep Foundation. (2017d). Shift work disorder. Retrieved from https://sleepfoundation.org/shift-work/what-is-shift-work-disorder

National Sleep Foundation. (2017e). Sleep apnea. Retrieved from https://sleepfoundation.org/sleep-disorders-problems/sleep-apnea

Pan, A., Schernhammer, E.S., Sun, Q., & Hu, F.B. (2011). Rotating night shift work and risk of type 2 diabetes: Two prospective cohort studies in women. *PLoS Medicine, 8.* doi: 10.1371/journal.pmed.1001141

ParticipACTION. (2016). Are Canadian kids too tired to move? The ParticipACTION Report Card on Physical Activity for Children and Youth. Toronto, ON.

Public Health Agency of Canada (PHAC). (2010). Fast facts from the 2009 Canadian community health survey—Sleep apnea rapid response. Public Health Agency of Canada. Cat.: HP35-19/1-2010E-PDF. ISBN: 978-1-100-17359-7. Retrieved from http://www.phac-aspc.gc.ca/cd-mc/sleepapnea-apneesommeil/ff-rr-2009-eng.php

Rajaratnam, S.M.W., Barger, L.K., Lockley, S.W., Shea, S.A., Wang, W., Landrigan, C.P., … Czeisler, C.A. (2011). Harvard work hours, health and safety group FT. Sleep disorders, health, and safety in police officers. *Journal of the American Medical Association, 306*(23), 2567–2578. doi:10.1001/jama.2011.1851

Samuels, C. (2008). Sleep, recovery, and performance: The new frontier in high-performance athletics. *Neurologic Clinics, 26*(1), 169–180.

Saunders, R. (2010). Shift work and health. Issue Briefing. *Institute for Work & Health*. Retrieved from https://www.iwh.on.ca/system/files/documents/iwh_briefing_shift_work_2010.pdf

Schernhammer, E.S., Laden, F., Speizer, F.E., Willett, W.C., Hunter, D.J., Kawachi, I., & Colditz, G.A. (2001). Rotating night shifts and risk of breast cancer in women participating in the nurses' health study. *Journal of National Cancer Institute, 93*(20), 1563–1568.

Schernhammer, E.S., et al. (2003). Night-shift work and risk of colorectal cancer in nurses' health study. *Journal of the National Cancer Institute, 95*, 825–828.

Schernhammer, E.S., Kroenke, C.H., Laden, F., & Hankinson, S.E. (2006). Night work and risk of breast cancer. *Epidemiology, 17*, 108–111.

Tefft, B.C. (2014). AAA Foundation for Traffic Safety. Prevalence of motor vehicle crashes involving drowsy drivers, United States, 2009–2013. Washington, DC: AAA Foundation for Traffic Safety. Retrieved from https://www.aaafoundation.org/sites/default/files/AAAFoundation-DrowsyDriving-Nov2014.pdf

Van Drongelen, A., Boot, C.R.L., Merkus, S.L., Smid, T., & van der Beek, A.J. (2011). The effects of shift work on body weight change a systematic review of longitudinal studies. *Scandinavian Journal of Work Environment & Health, 37*, 263–275. doi: 10.5271/sjweh.3143

Vila, B. (2000). *Tired cops: The importance of managing police fatigue.* Washington, DC: Police Executive Research Forum.

Vila, B. (2006). Impact of long work hours on police officers and the communities they serve. *American Journal of Industrial Medicine, 49*(11), 972–980.

Violanti, J.M., et al. (2007). Post-traumatic stress symptoms and cortisol patterns among police officers. *Policing: An International Journal of Police Strategies & Management, 30*(2), 189–202.

Violanti, J.M., et al. (2009). Atypical work hours and metabolic syndrome among police officers. *Archives of Environmental & Occupational Health, 64*(3), 194–201.

Violanti J.M., Fekedulegn, D., Andrew, M.E., Charles, L.E., Hartley, T.A., Vila, B., & Burchfiel, C.M. (2012). Shift work and the incidence of injury among police officers. *American Journal of Industrial Medicine, 55*, 217–227. Retrieved from http://dx.doi.org/10.1002/ajim.22007

Waters, J., & Ussery, W. (2007). Police stress: History, contributing factors, symptoms and interventions. *Policing: An International Journal of Police Strategies & Management, 30*(2), 169–189.

Wedderburn, A.A.I., & King, C. (1996). *Shift workers' health: Evaluation of a self-help guidebook. The shift worker's guide.* Edinburgh: Heriot-Watt University.

Williams, C. (2008). Work-life balance of shift workers. Perspectives on labour and income. Statistics Canada; Catalogue no. 75-001-X. vol. 9 no. 8. Retrieved from http://www.statcan.gc.ca/pub/75-001-x/2008108/pdf/10677-eng.pdf

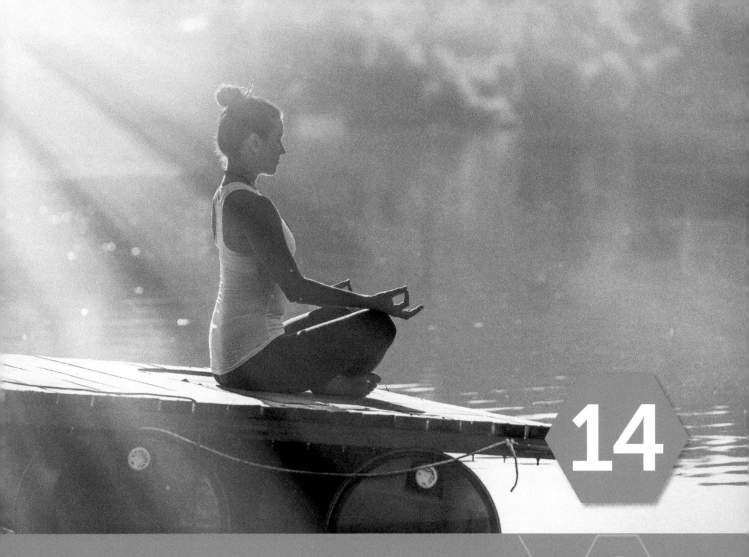

COMMON INJURIES

LEARNING OUTCOMES

After completing this chapter, you should be able to:

- Identify the causes, signs, symptoms, and treatments of common musculoskeletal injuries.

- Describe delayed-onset muscle soreness (DOMS), its prevention, and its treatment.

- Describe the signs, symptoms, treatments, and prevention of a concussion.

- Identify the causes, signs, symptoms, treatments, and prevention of heat- and cold-related injuries.

Advances in technology, changing demographics, and emerging trends in law enforcement combine to create unique ergonomic challenges to keep law enforcement officers safe and effective. Approximately 50 percent of total work safety claims between 1997 and 2005 for law enforcement officers were attributed to MSI (musculoskeletal injuries) or motor vehicle incidents (Hovbrender, 2009). Equipment on the duty belt impacts the ability of an officer to move, work, and sit. Specifically, it results in MSI around the lumbar spine when sitting or twisting to work. There are also sudden external forces when controlling a suspect or offender who is resisting arrest, trips or falls, and strains and sprains, which can contribute to the high risk of injury within the law enforcement occupations (Achterstraat, 2008). The most common body site of injury for an officer on duty is the upper extremity as a result of a non-compliant offender, often involving an assault (Lyons, Radburn, Orr, & Pope, 2017).

Exercise-related injuries can also be painful and frustrating. They always seem to happen when we're the most motivated to participate in an exercise program. It's no secret why this happens—people who have not exercised for a long time try to push their body past a safe level in an attempt to get back what they had. Many people try to achieve their training goals in too short a period of time. Some people leave training for the BFOR test to just weeks before it is scheduled to take place. Overtraining has resulted in many injuries.

Here are some statistics on common injuries (Billette & Janz, 2015; Weisenthal, Beck, Maloney, DeHaven, & Giordano, 2014):

- Over the last 15 years, 15 percent of Canadians aged 12 or older suffered an injury severe enough to limit their usual activities on an annual basis.

- Thirty-five percent of injuries occurred during participation in some type of sport or exercise. The main causes of injuries were falls and overexertion. Sports accounted for three in five falls among adolescents.

- Sprains and strains were the most common type of injury (51 percent), followed by fractures and broken bones (17 percent).

- Shoulder and back injuries are the most common with gymnastic style and power lifting movements, especially without trainer supervision and proper form.

This chapter looks at various injuries, their causes, and treatments for them.

MUSCULOSKELETAL INJURIES

Musculoskeletal injuries are injuries of the muscles, nerves, tendons, ligaments, joints, cartilage, or spinal discs. These happen over time and are more chronic in their development rather than being caused by an instantaneous or acute event (such as a slip, trip, or fall) (CDC, 2016).

MUSCULOSKELETAL INJURY RISK FACTORS

The main risk factors that contribute to musculoskeletal injuries include (Infrastructure Health & Safety Association, 2017; Lyons, Radburn, Orr, & Pope, 2017):

- Forceful exertion—the more force exerted, the greater the stress on the body. Lifting, pushing, pulling, and gripping an object are all examples of activities that require muscular force.

- Awkward postures—where joints are held or moved away from the body's natural alignment. The closer the joint is to its end of range of motion (e.g., bending forward to reach something on the floor), the greater the stress placed on soft tissues around the joint including muscles, tendons, and ligaments. It also can injure the nerves in that area.

- Repetitive movements—where the person is in proper alignment but doing the task or activity for long periods of time such as computer use, sitting in/driving a car, and twisting at a work station. This continual stress may result in injury if the body isn't given enough recovery time.

Some secondary risk factors include:

- Contact pressure—pressure exerted on soft tissue (e.g., holding a shield or baton for extended periods of time for crowd control or lockdown).

- Vibration—which can cause damage to nerves as well as soft tissue (e.g., riding a dirt or mountain bike).

- Temperature—can affect muscles. In cold temperatures tissues are stressed by reduction in range of motion and flexibility, while in hot temperatures muscles fatigue sooner and are slower to recover.

Due to the unpredicted, varied, and physical nature of law enforcement, risk factors include:

- running various distances with and without loads
- restraining non-compliant individuals
- external forces when controlling a suspect or offender who has resisted arrest
- self-defence manoeuvres
- trips and falls while chasing a suspect or offender

GENERAL TREATMENTS FOR MUSCULOSKELETAL INJURIES

Many sport injuries are the result of doing too much, too soon, too fast. By overdoing it, you increase your risk for sprained joints, strained muscles, and other minor musculoskeletal injuries. One important but simple way to decrease your risk of injury is to make sure that you warm up properly before exercising or doing sports and cool down afterward. A good warm-up consists of performing your regular activity at a lesser intensity. (Refer to the *Fit for Duty, Fit for Life* training guide, which accompanies this textbook, for more information.) Remember that there is a difference between feeling uncomfortable because you are out of shape and being in pain. Don't believe that "no pain, no gain" is true. Trying to exercise through pain will likely just cause an injury or make an existing injury worse.

General treatment for a musculoskeletal injury involves resting. Proper care during the first day or two after the injury may reduce the time it takes to heal. Remember that even though something may hurt only slightly while you are exercising, it may get worse when you stop. Endorphins, a chemical released by the brain during exercise, tend to dull the sensation of pain. After an injury occurs, the damaged area may bleed (internally or externally) and become inflamed. Healing starts as collagen, the primary component of scar tissue, replaces the damaged tissue. In order for an individual to return to the activity, ideally, the scar tissue should be completely repaired. In the case of acute musculoskeletal injuries, follow the RICE principle.

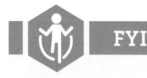

INFLAMMATION

Inflammation is our body's biological response to an injury. It involves a protective response of various immune, endocrine, and neurological mediators to clear the pathogen and begin a repair process. It is characterized by five signs: pain, redness, immobility (loss of function), swelling, and heat.

THE RICE PRINCIPLE

The RICE principle (rest, immobilize, cool, elevate) is an immediate, simple treatment for a musculoskeletal injury. You can ease pain and assist the healing process if you act quickly. If you are unsure of the extent of your injury, follow the RICE principle, and seek medical help as soon as possible.

REST

Reduce regular exercise or daily activities as needed. Rest is important to protect the injured muscle, tendon, ligament, or other tissue from further damage. Rest is also important in order to conserve the energy needed to heal the injury most effectively. Depending on the severity of the injury, do not use the injured area for 48 hours. If you cannot put weight on an ankle or knee, crutches may help.

IMMOBILIZE

Keep the affected part of your body immobilized, and generally reduce your movement. If you need to move an individual, immobilize the injured area in the position in which it was found. Otherwise keep the person still so movement doesn't cause further damage.

COOL

To reduce swelling, apply an ice pack (a gel pack, a plastic bag of ice or snow, or a bag of frozen peas) wrapped in a towel to the injured area for 20 minutes every hour for up to 48 hours. Never put ice directly on the tissue, as it may damage your skin.

ELEVATE

If possible, keep the injured part elevated on a pillow, above the level of your heart, to help decrease swelling.

SORTING OUT MUSCLE SORENESS

Aside from the pain of muscle injuries such as strains, there are two common kinds of exercise-related muscle soreness: acute muscle soreness, which occurs during or immediately after exercise, and delayed-onset muscle soreness (DOMS), which develops 12 hours or more after exercise.

Acute muscle soreness during and immediately after exercise usually reflects simple fatigue caused by a buildup of chemical waste products (lactic acid and hydrogen ions). The discomfort will often subside after a minute or two of rest when the muscles can replace energy substrates and oxygen. Once the soreness goes away, you can usually continue exercising with no residual effects. If discomfort persists despite a rest period, stop your activity and rest the part of the body that is hurting. Don't proceed with your workout until you're able to exercise that area without pain.

DOMS after a workout is common, particularly if you aren't used to the activity. If, for example, you haven't exercised for six months, and then you suddenly jump on the treadmill for 5 kilometres and do some push-ups and sit-ups, you may feel soreness throughout much of your body the next morning. You may also notice muscle stiffness and weakness. Such symptoms are a normal response to unusual exertion and are part of an adaptation process that leads to greater strength once the muscles recover. The soreness generally produces the greatest pain between 24 to 48 hours after the exercise has been performed (ACSM, 2011).

DOMS is thought to be a result of microscopic tearing of the muscle fibres. The amount of tearing depends on how hard and long you exercise and what type of exercise you do. Exercises in which muscles forcefully contract while they are lengthening tend to cause the most soreness. These eccentric contractions (explained in Chapter 4) provide a braking action. Examples include running down stairs, running downhill, lowering weights, and performing the downward movements of squats, chin-ups, and push-ups.

In addition to microscopic tearing, swelling may take place in and around a muscle, which can contribute to delayed soreness. Such swelling increases pressure on the neighbouring structures, resulting in greater muscle pain and stiffness.

TREATMENT FOR DOMS

Treatment for DOMS consists of

- gentle stretching to relieve tightness and diffuse the pain,
- foam rolling or gentle massage on the affected muscles,
- cold and hot treatment (alternating every 20 minutes) to promote circulation and muscle recuperation,
- analgesics (acetaminophen) and non-steroidal anti-inflammatory drugs (acetylsalicylic acid or ibuprofen) to reduce pain and enhance analgesia,
- yoga—there is some evidence that yoga may reduce DOMS (Boyle, Sayers, Jensen, Headley, & Manos, 2004),
- rest—let your muscles heal before you attempt to go back to the activity.

TOP TIPS ...

FOR PREVENTING DOMS

- Warm up by doing a few minutes of a light, low-impact aerobic activity such as walking or biking. This should help to increase blood flow to the affected muscles and help to reduce soreness. An emphasis on dynamic stretching can be done prior to a workout while static stretching is more appropriate after a workout.

- Build up slowly in terms of intensity, duration, and frequency of the exercise. In weight lifting, for example, start with lighter weights, fewer sets, and fewer repetitions.

- Avoid the weekend warrior approach, where you only play a pickup game of football or basketball on the weekends without a proper warm-up and some type of aerobic activity during the week.

COMMON SPORT-RELATED MUSCULOSKELETAL INJURIES

Certain types of injuries plague sport participants. Although most are minor, knowing the early signs, symptoms, and how to treat them properly can help prevent them from becoming chronic conditions.

SPRAIN

A sprain is the stretching or tearing of a ligament. A ligament is a short band of connective tissue that connects two bones or cartilage across a joint. The severity of the injury depends on the extent of the tear to a single ligament (whether the tear is partial or complete) and the number of ligaments involved. A sprain can result from a fall, a sudden twist, or a blow to the body that forces a joint out of its normal position. This results in overstretching or tearing of the ligament supporting that joint. Typically, sprains occur when people fall and land on an outstretched arm, slide into base, land on the side of their foot, or twist a knee with the foot planted firmly on the ground when involved in an altercation with a suspect. The most common site of sprains is ankles.

There are three grades of sprains (see Figure 14.1):

- *Mild sprains* (Grade I) happen when ligaments are stretched excessively or torn slightly. They are somewhat painful, especially with movement. There is not a lot of swelling, and you can put weight on the joint.

- *Moderate sprains* (Grade II) occur when there is partial rupture of the fibres. The area is painful and tender. There is swelling and discoloration, and it is hard to move and bear weight on the joint.

- *Severe sprains* (Grade III) take place when one or more ligaments are completely torn. You can't put weight on the joint or move it easily. There is swelling, discoloration, and pain. It is hard to distinguish a severe sprain from a fracture or dislocation. You may need a brace to stabilize the joint, and surgery may be required to repair the ligaments.

FIGURE 14.1   Grades of Sprains

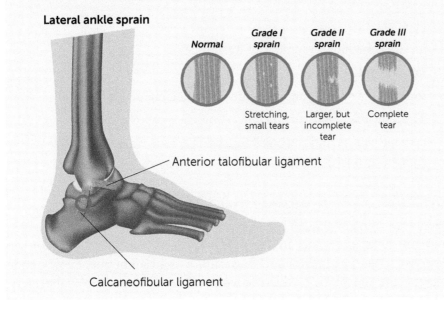

SIGNS AND SYMPTOMS

The usual signs and symptoms of a sprain include the following:

- varying degrees of pain
- swelling
- bruising
- inability to move and use the joint
- may hear or feel a pop

STRAIN

A strain is the stretching, pulling, or tearing of a muscle or tendon (see Figure 14.2). There are two types of strains: acute and chronic. An acute strain is caused by trauma or an injury such as a blow to the body; improperly lifting heavy objects or overstressing the muscles can also cause it. Chronic strains are usually the result of overuse—prolonged, repetitive movement of the muscles and tendons.

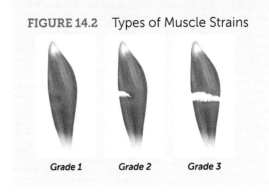

FIGURE 14.2   Types of Muscle Strains

Grade 1   Grade 2   Grade 3

The two most common sites for a strain are the back and the hamstring muscle (located in the back of the thigh). Law enforcement officers risk injury when they go from prolonged sitting in a vehicle and then are faced with a physical confrontation or other demand on their body. Altercations with suspects and inmates also put officers at risk for injury. Contact sports such as soccer, football, hockey, boxing, and wrestling put people at risk for strains. Gymnastics, tennis, rowing, golf, and other sports that require extensive gripping can increase the risk of hand and forearm strains. Elbow strains sometimes occur in people who participate in racquet sports, throwing, and contact sports.

SIGNS AND SYMPTOMS

Signs and symptoms of a strain include the following:

- pain, muscle spasm
- localized swelling, cramping, or inflammation
- muscle weakness
- some loss of muscle function (minor or moderate strain)
- complete loss of muscle function (if muscle is completely torn)
- extreme pain, significant bleeding, swelling and bruising, if muscle is completely torn

TREATMENT FOR SPRAINS AND STRAINS

You should see a doctor about a sprain or strain if you have severe pain, you cannot move the joint, it is tender to touch, there are lumps and bumps (other than swelling), you are experiencing numbness, and/or you cannot put any weight on the injured joint. You may see redness or red streaks spreading out from the injury.

Treatment for sprains and strains is similar and can be thought of as having two stages. The goal during the first stage is to reduce swelling and pain. At this stage, doctors usually advise patients to follow the RICE formula (rest, immobilize, cool, elevate) for the first 24 to 48 hours after the injury. A doctor may prescribe a nonsteroidal anti-inflammatory drug, such as acetylsalicylic acid (Aspirin®, Entrophen®) or ibuprofen (Advil®, Motrin®), to help decrease pain and inflammation.

For people with a moderate or severe sprain, particularly of the ankle, a hard cast or air cast may be applied (NIAMS, 2017). An X-ray may be needed to determine whether a fracture is causing the pain and swelling. Severe sprains and strains may require surgery to repair the torn ligaments, muscles, or tendons.

The second stage of treating a sprain or strain is rehabilitation, where the overall goal is to improve the condition of the injured part and restore its function. An exercise program designed to prevent stiffness, improve range of motion, and restore the joint's normal flexibility and strength is key.

TENDINITIS

Tendinitis is inflammation (redness, soreness, and swelling) of a tendon. Tendinitis injuries are more common in the upper shoulder and lower section of the elbow including the rotator cuff attachments (examples include tennis elbow, wrist, and bicep tendinitis). Lower body tendinitis (including achilles and patella tendinitis) are common injuries from sports with a lot of jumping, running, and lunging such as basketball and volleyball. Shin splints are a type of tendinitis that runners can acquire from repeated trauma to the connective muscle tissue surrounding the tibia.

Chronic diseases may also weaken the tendon as they potentially disrupt blood supply. Chronic diseases which may weaken tendons include chronic renal failure, rheumatoid arthritis, systemic lupus erythmatosus (SLE), diabetes mellitus, and metabolic disease. Medications like corticosteroids and anabolic steroids have been linked to muscle and tendon weakness.

TENDINITIS OF THE ELBOW AND WRIST

Tennis elbow is the inflammation of the tendon on the outside of the elbow connecting the bone to the muscle that allows extension of the wrist and finger. Golfer's elbow involves the tendons on the inside of the arm. When you constantly use your arm in a repetitive motion, the tendons at the elbow end develop small tears. These lead to inflammation and put stress on the rest of your arm making it painful to lift and grip things. The cause is poor technique and repetitive movements such as playing racket sports, painting, tree-cutting, shaking hands, and lifting weights.

Wrist tendinitis is caused by the irritation of tendons that surround the wrist. Repetitive motions of the wrist and/or fingers, such as typing on a keyboard, playing a musical instrument, using vibrating equipment or tools, or playing sports like baseball, bowling, golf, or tennis, can lead to tenderness, pain, swelling, and inflammation. As noted in Koder (2005), "It is recognized that keyboard work, while it entails a minimum of forceful exertion, can have injurious effect on the finger control tendons because of rapid, frequent and sustained activation of the tendons. Sustained periods of frequent finger activity even with low force can be consistent with the development of carpal tunnel syndrome and tendinitis" (p. 5).

TENDINITIS OF THE SHOULDER

In tendinitis of the shoulder, the rotator cuff (the group of muscles that surround the shoulder) and/or biceps tendon become inflamed, usually as a result of being pinched by surrounding structures. Tendinitis occurs over a long period of time from performing repetitive activities. The injury may vary from mild to severe inflammation.

When the rotator cuff tendon becomes inflamed and thickened, it may get trapped under the outer edge of the shoulder blade, where the collarbone is attached. Squeezing of the rotator cuff muscles is called shoulder impingement syndrome (see Figure 14.3) when the tendons of the rotator cuff become irritated and inflamed as they pass through the subacromial space, the passage beneath the acromion. This can result in pain, weakness, and loss of movement at the shoulder. If left untreated, the muscle can actually tear in two.

FIGURE 14.3   Shoulder Impingement Syndrome

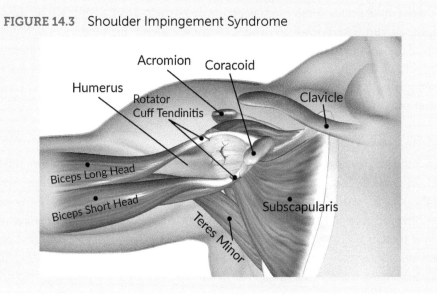

Tendinitis and impingement syndrome are often accompanied by inflammation of the bursa sacs (sacs of fluid near joints) that protect the shoulder. An inflamed bursa is called bursitis. Inflammation caused by a disease such as rheumatoid arthritis may cause rotator cuff tendinitis and bursitis. Sports that involve overuse of the shoulder and occupations that require frequent overhead reaching are other potential causes of irritation to the rotator cuff or bursae, and may lead to inflammation and impingement.

SIGNS AND SYMPTOMS

Signs and symptoms of tendinitis, impingement syndrome, and bursitis of the shoulder include the following:

- the slow onset of discomfort and pain in the upper shoulder or upper third of the arm
- difficulty sleeping on the shoulder
- pain when the arm is lifted away from the body or overhead (such as when trying to put on a coat)
- if tendinitis involves the biceps tendon (the tendon located in front of the shoulder that helps bend the elbow and turn the forearm), pain in the front or side of the shoulder that may travel down to the elbow and forearm (pain may also occur when the arm is forcefully pushed upward)
- significant weakness and difficulty lifting the arm

TENDINITIS OF THE LOWER LEG

Achilles tendinitis is a common condition that causes pain along the back of the leg near the heel. This condition is the result of repetitive stress on the tendon caused by sudden increase in the amount or intensity of the exercise activity (e.g., increasing your running mileage too quickly) and tight calf muscles, which put additional strain on the tendon or a bone spur on the heel which rubs against the tendon. Symptoms include pain and stiffness (more often in the morning), pain along the tendon while exercising, swelling, and feeling a bone spur at the back of the ankle.

Patella tendinitis is common in people who participate in activities that require jumping or running. Sometimes called "jumper's knee," the tendon usually tears when the knee is bent and foot is planted. Symptoms include pain while jumping, instability of the knee, inability to straighten the knee, difficulty walking due to knee buckling or giving way, and hearing a tearing or popping sensation (when the tendon tears completely).

TREATMENT

These injuries are treated with rest, ice, and non-steroidal anti-inflammatory medicines. In some cases, the doctor or therapist will use ultrasound (gentle sound wave vibrations) to warm deep tissues and improve blood flow. Gentle stretching and strengthening exercises are added gradually, preceded or followed by use of an ice pack. If there is no improvement, the doctor may inject a corticosteroid medicine (these injections must be used with caution because they may lead to tendon rupture). Severe cases may need surgery to repair damage and relieve pressure on the tendons and bursae.

DISLOCATED SHOULDER

The shoulder comprises a large number of muscles, tendons, and bones that work together to provide movement, structure, and strength. Fifteen muscles move and stabilize the scapula. Nine muscles stabilize the gleno-humeral joint, and six muscles support the scapula on the thorax. The rotator cuff is made up of a group of four muscles (supraspinatus, infraspinatus, teres minor, and subscapularis) that support the shoulder joint. The muscles attach to the skeletal elements by tendons. The rotator cuff stabilizes the gleno-humeral joint to provide rotation, elevation, depression, protraction, and retraction.

A dislocation of the shoulder joint happens when the ball of the joint (the end of the arm bone, or humerus) and the socket (part of your shoulder blade, or scapula) move apart. When the ball part of the joint is dislocated in front of the socket, it is called an anterior dislocation. Anterior dislocations are the most common type of shoulder dislocation, making up 95 percent of cases (Bass & Kortyna, 2017). When it is dislocated behind the socket, it is called a posterior dislocation. (See Figure 14.4.) In severe cases, ligaments, tendons, and nerves also can be stretched and injured.

In young people, the cause of an anterior dislocation is usually sports-related. In older individuals, the cause is usually due to a fall on an outstretched hand. A posterior dislocation may occur as a result of a powerful direct blow to the front of your shoulder. A violent twisting of your upper arm, such as that caused by an electric shock or seizure, may also cause it. Dislocated shoulders are common in contact sports such as football, rugby, hockey, and lacrosse. Other sports that may cause the injury include downhill skiing, volleyball, and soccer. In law enforcement, officers sometimes deal with altercations where someone is pulling at their arms or aggressively pushing or punching.

SIGNS AND SYMPTOMS

Signs and symptoms of a dislocated shoulder include the following:

- pain in the shoulder and upper arm that is made worse by movement
- shoulder instability
- shoulder tenderness and weakness
- possible numbness in the shoulder area, arm, or hand
- significant deformity of the shoulder—may have abnormal bumps, ridges, or hollows.

FIGURE 14.4   Dislocations of Shoulder Joint

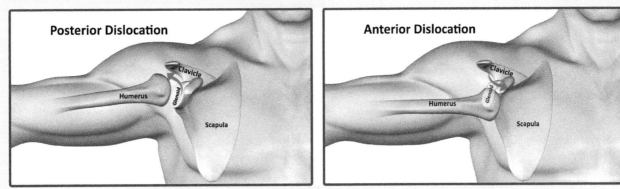

TREATMENT

Put ice on the shoulder immediately to reduce swelling caused by internal bleeding and the buildup of fluids in and around the injured area, and put the arm in a sling. See a doctor to reposition the head or ball of the joint back into the joint socket. The doctor may give you a prescription for pain, a muscle relaxant, and anti-inflammatory medication. If your shoulder joint becomes weak because of repeated dislocations, your doctor may recommend an operation to tighten the ligaments that hold the joint together. The healing process may take 4 to 12 weeks, depending on the extent of your injury. With proper healing and rehabilitation exercises, you should regain full movement of your shoulder. Delays in diagnosis remain the single biggest obstacle to optimum results. A significant proportion may require eventual surgery and up to a third of these patients will go on to develop long-term shoulder arthritis. Even patients who have experienced a single episode of dislocation may go on to develop long-term issues (Cutts, Prempeh, & Drew, 2009).

PATELLO-FEMORAL SYNDROME (CHONDROMALACIA PATELLA)

Patello-femoral syndrome, or chondromalacia patella refers to softening and deterioration of the cartilage underneath the kneecap (patella). This disorder occurs most often in young adults, especially females, and can be caused by injury, overuse, muscle tightness, or muscle weakness. Instead of gliding smoothly across the lower end of the thigh bone, the kneecap is pulled to the left or right and rubs against the bone, roughening the cartilage underneath the kneecap (see Figure 14.5). The damage may range from a slightly abnormal surface of the cartilage to a surface that has been worn away to the bone. The disorder is common in runners and is also seen in skiers, cyclists, and soccer players.

> **DID YOU KNOW?**
>
> In Ontario, common musculoskeletal injuries account for 38 percent of all lost-time claims, 39 percent of all lost-time claim costs, and 39 percent of all lost-time days on the job.
>
> SOURCE: WSIB, 2016.

FIGURE 14.5 Patello-Femoral Syndrome

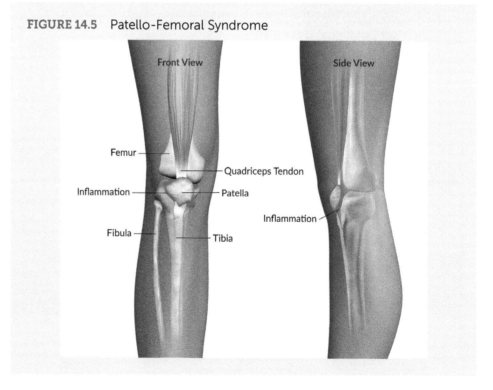

SIGNS AND SYMPTOMS

Signs and symptoms of patello-femoral syndrome include the following:

- dull pain around or under the kneecap
- pain that is made worse by prolonged sitting, or activities that load the patello-femoral joint, such as climbing or descending stairs, squatting, and running
- grinding, clicking, popping, or catching of the knee
- instability of the knee

TREATMENT

Apply the RICE formula (rest, immobilize, cool, elevate). Physical therapy is effective in treating patello-femoral syndrome, however there is no one program that will be effective for all patients. The rehabilitation program should focus on correcting maltracking of the patella by addressing the underlying cause (Dixit, DiFiori, Burton, & Mines, 2007). Perform low-impact exercises that strengthen muscles, particularly the muscles in the inner part of the quadriceps, without injuring joints and bending the knee more than 90 degrees. Tape the knee to keep the kneecap in line. Electrical stimulation may also be used to strengthen the muscles. Surgery is available to some individuals who do not progress with therapy to correct the alignment of the kneecap, and relieve friction.

SHIN SPLINTS (TIBIAL STRESS SYNDROME)

Shin splints are pain along the shin (tibia) and are commonly seen as an overuse injury in runners (see Figure 14.6). They usually develop gradually over a period of weeks to months, but may occur after a single excessive bout of exercise.

Shin splints can be caused by running on the insides of your feet. They often occur in both legs. This usually happens when someone is beginning a running program, doing excessive downhill running, landing on their heels when they run, or engaging in sports that require rapid starts and stops which cause damage to the muscle, resulting in pain.

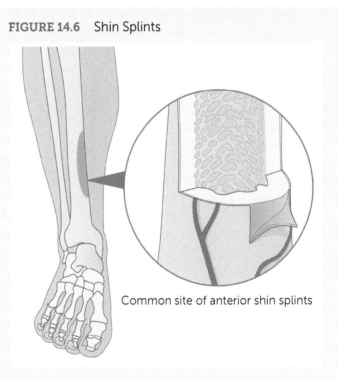

FIGURE 14.6 Shin Splints

Common site of anterior shin splints

SIGNS AND SYMPTOMS

Signs and symptoms of shin splints include the following:

- pain on the side and front of the shin (often experienced by runners)
- noticeable pain when exercise starts, which then decreases or goes away as exercise continues; worse after exercise stops or the following morning

TREATMENT

Rest. This means dramatically decreasing both the frequency and the duration of exercise and increasing (doubling or tripling) the time between workouts. Put ice directly on the sore area. Massage the muscles that are affected. A doctor may prescribe anti-inflammatory medications. If the shin splints are caused by the way your feet turn in when you walk or run (overpronation, or flat feet), you may need a good arch support in the form of an orthotic (a shoe insert that corrects the alignment of the foot), taping your shins, or a professional to look at your running technique. Changing your running shoes every 800 kilometres is another good idea.

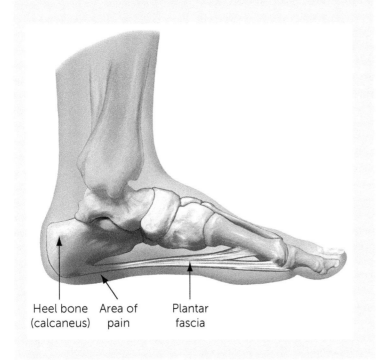

FIGURE 14.7 Plantar Fasciitis

Heel bone Area of Plantar
(calcaneus) pain fascia

PLANTAR FASCIITIS

Plantar fasciitis is the most common cause of pain on the bottom of the heel (see Figure 14.7). The fascia, a thin strip of tissue at the bottom of the foot, stretches to the point of developing small tears. Pain occurs with the onset of activity such as walking and running, or even the first few morning steps. The pain subsides as the activity progresses, and usually returns after resting and then resuming activity.

Plantar fasciitis is considered a chronic inflammatory response. It is common in runners, who repetitively flex their feet and toes. It is also common in people who experience sudden weight gain. Shoes with poor cushioning can contribute to the tearing of the fascia. People who work in occupations that require prolonged standing or weight-bearing activities may strain the fascia. Individuals working in law enforcement that have to stand all day, especially in work-designated shoes, are more at risk. Standing at an airport terminal, walking kilometres within a correctional facility, directing traffic, or walking the beat for extended periods of time can contribute to this condition.

SIGNS AND SYMPTOMS

Signs and symptoms of plantar fasciitis include the following:

- heel pain (especially when you get out of bed in the morning or after sitting for prolonged periods)
- pain worsens with exercise and weight-bearing activities (like walking)
- tight Achilles tendon
- sometimes a heel spur (a calcium deposit on the bottom of the heel), but it is typically not a cause

TREATMENT

Take non-steroidal anti-inflammatory drugs (ask a doctor). Avoid activities that cause pain, and avoid walking barefoot on hard surfaces. Lose weight if your weight is a cause of the injury. Stretch the calf muscle, Achilles tendon, and plantar fascia. Taping the heel and arch may also help to reduce pain. You may need to wear arch supports if you have flat feet. Massaging the fascia by rolling your foot over a 7- to 10-centimetre diameter tube, such as a rolling pin or soup can, has been an effective treatment. Strengthening exercises include scrunching up a hand towel with the toes or pulling a towel weighted with a soup can across the floor. After any physical activity, put ice on the fascia.

OSGOOD-SCHLATTER DISEASE

Osgood-Schlatter disease is caused by repetitive stress or tension on part of the growth area of the upper tibia (the leg bone between the knee and the ankle), especially from jumping and kneeling. As a result, there is inflammation of the tendon in the knee-cap and surrounding soft tissues at the point where the tendon is attached to the tibia (see Figure 14.8). The disease may also be associated with an injury in which the tendon is stretched so much that it tears away from the tibia and takes a fragment of bone with it. The body then repairs the bone by depositing calcium, which results in a buildup of bone.

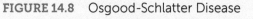

FIGURE 14.8 Osgood-Schlatter Disease

The bone is inflamed and broken up at the attachment of the patellar tendon to the tibia (shin bone).

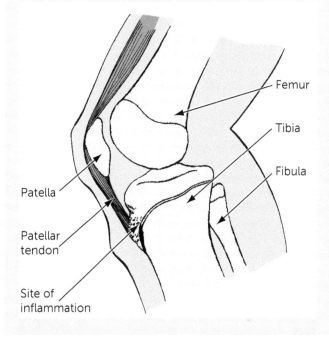

SIGNS AND SYMPTOMS

Signs and symptoms of Osgood-Schlatter disease include the following:

- pain is experienced just below the knee joint; the pain usually worsens with activity and is relieved by rest

- a bony bump that is particularly painful when pressed may appear on the upper edge of the tibia, below the kneecap. Although knee motion is usually not affected, it can be very difficult to kneel

- pain may last a few months and may recur until the individual's growth is completed. Teens are especially prone to the pain, which can carry on into their 20s

- x-rays show that there are microfractures on the growth plate.

TREATMENT

When pain begins, apply ice to the knee to help relieve inflammation. Do stretching and strengthening exercises, rest, and limit your participation in vigorous sports. Wear knee pads for protection when you are taking part in sports, and apply ice to the knee afterward.

ILIOTIBIAL BAND SYNDROME

The iliotibial (IT) band runs along the outside of the thigh, from the pelvis to the tibia, crossing both the hip and knee joints which stabilizes and moves the joint. Iliotibial band syndrome is an overuse condition typically caused by compression of the ligaments on the outer leg. The cause is due to an abnormal movement pattern of the femur, which is caused by weak gluteal muscles. (See Figure 14.9.) Although IT band syndrome may be caused by direct injury to the knee, it is most often caused by the stress of long-term overuse, such as sports training, toed-in cycling and running, and running on horizontally banked surfaces, and up-and-down hills.

SIGNS AND SYMPTOMS

Signs and symptoms of iliotibial band syndrome include the following:

- ache or burning sensation at the outer side of the knee during activity
  - pain at the side of the knee or radiating up the side of the thigh
  - a snap felt when the knee is bent and then straightened

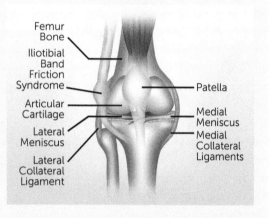

FIGURE 14.9 Iliotibial Band Syndrome (front view)

Femur Bone
Iliotibial Band Friction Syndrome
Articular Cartilage
Lateral Meniscus
Lateral Collateral Ligament
Patella
Medial Meniscus
Medial Collateral Ligaments

Note that there is usually no swelling and knee motion is normal.

TREATMENT

Reduce activity and do fascial stretching exercises followed by muscle-strengthening exercises. Strengthening the hips and glutes is the most valuable treatment strategy for IT band syndrome. These muscles will control rotation of the femur, position of the pelvis, and ensure the IT band is properly aligned. In rare cases, when the syndrome doesn't disappear, surgery may be necessary to split the tendon so that it isn't stretched too tightly over the bone.

LIGAMENT SPRAINS TO THE KNEE

Four ligaments connect the leg bones and give the knee joint strength and stability:

1. The medial collateral ligament (MCL) (see Figure 14.9) provides stability to the inner (medial) part of the knee. The MCL is more easily injured than the lateral collateral ligament (LCL). The cause is most often a blow to the outer side of the knee that stretches and tears the ligament on the inner side of the knee. Such blows frequently occur in contact sports like football or hockey. In law enforcement, they can occur during altercations or when performing self-defence manoeuvres.

2. The lateral collateral ligament (LCL) (see Figure 14.9) provides stability to the outer (lateral) part of the knee. This ligament is the least likely to be sprained. Injury is caused by a blow to the inside of the knee, which is usually protected by the other leg.

3. The anterior cruciate ligament (ACL) is in the centre of the knee and forms an 'X' with the posterior cruciate ligament (PCL) which limits

rotation and forward movement of the tibia (the shin bone). The ACL is most often stretched and/or torn by a sudden twisting motion (for example, when the feet are planted one way and the knees are turned another). This can happen when you stretch your upper torso while keeping your legs planted, such as when a law enforcement officer must drag a suspect or offender.

4. The posterior cruciate ligament (PCL), also in the centre of the knee, works with the ACL to limit backward movement of the tibia (behind the patella in Figure 14.9). The PCL is most often injured by a direct impact, such as in an automobile accident (trying to brake) or knee on the dashboard.

SIGNS AND SYMPTOMS

Signs and symptoms of ligament injuries of the knee include the following:

- a popping sound
- knee pain
- tenderness, swelling
- leg buckling when you try to stand
- top part of leg moves while lower leg remains stationary

TREATMENT

Immediate treatment includes the RICE approach. If there is an incomplete tear, an exercise program can strengthen the surrounding muscles. You may need to wear a brace to protect the knee during activity. You may also need surgery to reattach or reconstruct a ligament that is completely torn.

INJURIES TO THE MENISCUS

Separating the bones of the knee are pads of connective tissue called the menisci, or meniscus in the singular. The menisci are divided into two crescent-shaped discs positioned between the leg bones on the outer and inner sides of each knee. They act like shock absorbers, cushioning the lower part of the leg from the weight of the rest of the body, as well as enhancing stability. (The removal of all four of former hockey player Bobby Orr's menisci, one at a time, left his knees unstable, which eventually led to his retirement from hockey.)

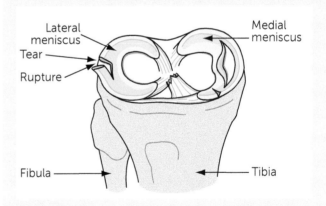

FIGURE 14.10 Injuries to the Meniscus

Through degeneration over time or too much concentrated force, the meniscus can be torn, as shown in Figure 14.10. The entire rim of the medial meniscus can be torn.

SIGNS AND SYMPTOMS

Signs and symptoms of injuries to the meniscus include the following:

- pain in the knee, especially when the leg is straight.
- severe pain if a fragment of the meniscus catches between the leg bones.

- swelling may occur as a response to the deterioration of the surface of the joint.
- the knee may click, lock, or feel weak.
- on examination, when the leg is rotated outward and inward while extended, there is pain and audible clicking, suggesting a tear; an MRI scan can confirm this.

TREATMENT

Immediate treatment includes the RICE approach. Muscle-strengthening programs for the knee (quadriceps and hamstrings) can help. Surgery may be needed to repair the tear if there is good blood supply to the area. If the blood supply is poor, parts of the meniscus, or the entire meniscus, may need to be removed. Artificial meniscus replacement has met with limited success to date.

CONCUSSIONS

Concussion (also sometimes called mild traumatic brain injury) is the most common form of traumatic brain injury (see Figure 14.11). A concussion is caused by a bump, blow, or jolt to the head or by a hit to the body that causes the head and brain to move rapidly back and forth. This sudden movement can cause the brain to bounce around or twist in the skull, creating chemical changes in the brain and sometimes stretching and damaging brain cells (CDC, 2017).

FIGURE 14.11 What Is a Concussion?

Concussion: A traumatic brain injury that changes the way your brain functions.

The brain is made up of soft tissue and is protected by blood and spinal fluid. When the skull is jolted too fast or is impacted by something, the brain shifts and hits against the skull.

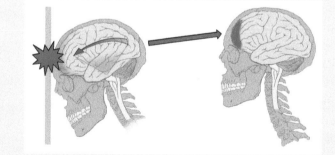

This can lead to bruising and swelling of the brain, tearing of blood vessels, and injury to nerves, causing the concussion.

Most concussions are mild and can be treated with appropriate care. But left untreated, it can be deadly.

Figure 14.12 looks at some of the statistics on sports-related concussions.

FIGURE 14.12   Heads-up on Sport-Related Brain Injuries

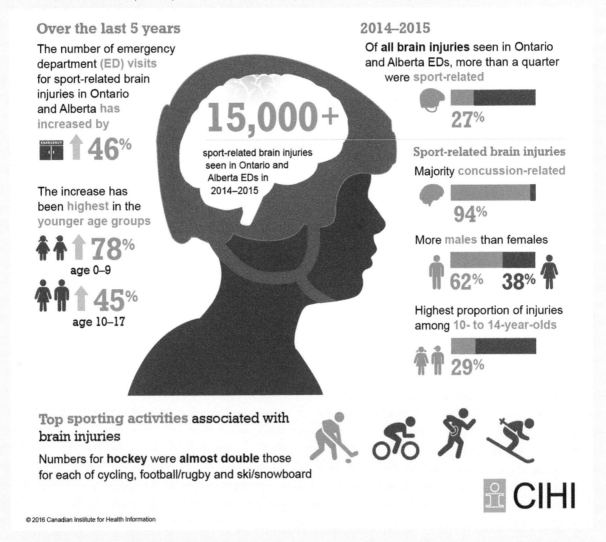

Most people will recover from a concussion, whether it takes one or several weeks; however, 15 to 20 percent of people who sustain a concussion have longer, potentially difficult and persistent symptoms that interfere with their functioning and daily lives (Ontario Neurotrauma Foundation, 2016). Known as the "invisible injury," diagnosis of concussion can be overlooked or downplayed resulting in increased risk of more damage to the brain. Due to lack of knowledge, some people still believe that the definition of a concussion includes loss of consciousness, although it is now known that about 95 percent of concussions occur without loss of consciousness. In addition, many sports participants still do not recognize that "dings" or "seeing stars" are likely to be concussions, and most importantly, there is still some uncertainty whether coaches, trainers, and parents recognize that concussions are brain injuries (Tator, 2009).

Table 14.1 lists the signs and symptoms of a concussion.

TABLE 14.1   Signs and Symptoms of a Concussion

PHYSICAL	EMOTIONAL	SLEEP	RED FLAGS*
• Dizziness • Nausea or vomiting • "Pressure in the head" • Headaches • Balance problems • Sensitivity to light • Neck pain • Seizure or convulsion • Blurred vision • Loss of consciousness	• Irritability • Nervous or anxious • More emotional • Feeling in a "fog" • "Don't feel right" • Sadness	• Insomnia—unable to sleep • Poor sleep quality • Sleeping too much	• Individual complains of neck pain • Deteriorating conscious state • Increasing confusion or irritability • Severe or increasing headache • Repeated vomiting • Unusual behavioural change • Seizure or convulsion • Double vision • Weakness or tingling/burning in arms or legs

*Seek medical attention immediately.
SOURCES: Davis et al., 2017; Mayo Clinic, 2017; Parachute, 2017.

SYNDROMES ASSOCIATED WITH A CONCUSSION

Post-concussion syndrome is a complex disorder in which various symptoms—such as headaches and dizziness—last for weeks and sometimes months after the injury that caused the concussion (Mayo Clinic, 2017).

Second impact syndrome describes rapid swelling of the brain which sometimes can be catastrophic if the person afflicted suffers a second head injury before the symptoms from the first have gone away. Although this condition is rare, it is very dangerous and can lead to death (Brain and Spinal Cord, 2017). The highest percentage is seen in teens and young adults.

DIAGNOSIS OF A CONCUSSION

At this time, no single test can prove that you have a concussion and/or post-concussion syndrome. The following steps may be required:

- A brain scan (MRI or CT scan) to check for brain abnormalities.
- See an ear, nose, and throat specialist if you are experiencing dizziness.
- See a psychologist or psychiatrist if you are experiencing symptoms including anxiety or depression or you're having problems with memory or problem solving.

TREATMENT

Most people recover from a concussion within days to a few weeks. However, due to the difficulty in prognosis, there are not simple guidelines about when/how to return to work/play as there is no way to determine if the person will have a recurrent concussion (Cancelliere et al., 2014).

After a concussion, you need to rest your body (physical rest) and your brain (mental rest) so you can return to the activities you want or need to participate in. Requirements include, for example, the need to sleep effectively, eat a healthy carbohydrate diet to feed your brain, reduce the amount of reading or watching screens, rest when needed, stay away from loud noises, learn relaxation techniques, and avoid stress. Individuals can be helped by physiotherapists, massage therapists, and chiropractors who specialize in concussion injuries. Individuals should not return to work/sports until they have been cleared by their physician.

FYI

Resources for more information:

- Concussions Ontario (Ontario Neurotrauma Foundation [ONF])
  http://concussionsontario.org
- Heads Up: Preventing Concussion (Centers for Disease Control and Prevention [CDC])   https://www.cdc.gov/headsup/index.html
- Parachute Canada   http://www.parachutecanada.org/thinkfirstcanada
- Concussion Awareness Training Tool   http://www.cattonline.com

HEAT- AND COLD-RELATED INJURIES AND ILLNESSES

HEAT-RELATED INJURIES

Heat-related injuries have become a huge issue in athletics. In recent summers, a number of athletes have died due to heat-related injuries. You need to be aware of the symptoms. If you do volunteer work with children's sports teams, be especially vigilant because children's body temperatures easily fluctuate and they can quickly suffer from heat-related injuries. Heat can affect law enforcement officers that have to work outside or in facilities without proper air flow and/or conditioning. Along with the protective equipment that must be worn, officers can be subjected to additional heat stress via the impairment of heat dissipation and sweat evaporation through the clothing ensemble (McLellan, Daanen, & Cheung, 2013). Table 14.2 outlines the basics on heat related disorders (Ministry of Labour, 2014; NIOSH, 2016).

FYI

HEAT AND HYDRATION

On a hot day, two to three hours before exercising or working, you should drink 500 to 600 millilitres of fluid, and then another 200 to 300 millilitres right before with another 200 to 300 millilitres every 10 to 15 minutes during exercise or work. Post-exercise hydration should contain water to restore hydration status, carbohydrates to replenish glycogen stores, and electrolytes to speed rehydration. When rehydration must be quick, you need to replace sweat and urine losses by drinking 25 to 50 percent more than what was lost to sweat. That means upward of 500 millilitres for every half-kilogram of weight loss within two hours of finishing to be at optimal hydration four to six hours after the event (Casa, Armstrong, & Hillman, 2000).

When body weight drops 1 to 2 percent (0.7 to 1.4 kg in a 70-kg person) due to sweating, exercise performance can be impaired and heat exhaustion becomes a possibility.

Under Ontario's *Occupational Health and Safety Act*, employers and employees are required to take every precaution reasonable in the circumstances for the protection of workers. For example, law enforcement officers are issued baseball caps and sunscreen to help reduce the effects of heat. For more information, see Ministry of Labour (2014) (in References).

TABLE 14.2   Heat-Related Injuries

CONDITION	CAUSE	SIGNS/SYMPTOMS	TREATMENT	PREVENTION
Heat rash (irritation of the skin that results from excessive sweating during hot and humid weather)	• Hot, humid weather • Plugged sweat glands	• Clear, fluid blisters, and bumps • Rash with red bumps, itching or prickly feeling • Thirst	• Avoid hot environments. • Change into dry clothes. • Rinse with cool water.	• Keep skin clean and dry. • Take appropriate fluid and breaks.
Heat cramps (brief muscle cramps that occur during or after exercise or work in a hot environment)	• Heavy sweating • Can't replace electrolytes with water	• Cramps from electrolyte imbalance • Cramps are a warning of a more serious condition (e.g., heat exhaustion) • Thirst	• Drink electrolyte beverage or 1.5–2.5 mL salt in 1 L water. • Massage and stretch cramps. • Seek medical aid if cramps don't go away.	• Reduce activity or heat exposure. • Take appropriate fluid and breaks. • Wear appropriate clothing.
Heat exhaustion (body overheats and core body temp raises to 38–40 °C)	• Fluid loss and inadequate salt intake • Body is unable to cool itself	• Paleness • Heavy sweating • Nausea, vomiting • Fatigue, irritability, headaches • Dizziness, light-headedness, fainting • Cool, clammy skin • Decreased performance	• Seek medical attention (condition can lead to death). • Move to cool shaded area. • Loosen/remove clothing. • Fan/cool rags/ice packs. • Replacement of electrolytes.	• Reduce activity or heat exposure. • Acclimatize to weather. • Take appropriate fluid and breaks. • Wear appropriate clothing.
Heat stroke (body overheats and effects the central nervous system while core body temp raises to +40 °C)	• Classic heat stroke—in adults where electrolytes and water are used up and temperature rises, and body is unable to cool itself • Exertional heat stroke—engaging in physical activity or work in a hot environment and body loses ability to dissipate heat	• Hot, dry, red skin (classic) • Profuse sweating (exertional) • Weak, confused, upset • Fast pulse • Headache or dizzy • Nausea, vomiting • Dyspnea (difficult or laboured breathing) • May pass out or go into convulsions	• Call an ambulance or seek medical treatment immediately (condition can lead to death). • Move to cool shaded area. • Loosen/remove clothing. • Fan/cool rags/ice packs.	• Reduce activity or heat exposure. • Acclimatize to weather. • Take appropriate fluid and breaks. • Wear appropriate clothing.

SOURCES: ACSM, 2007; CCOHS, 2016; Fortune, Mustard, Etches, & Chambers, 2013; Government of Canada, 2012; Health Canada, 2011; Ministry of Labour, 2014; Popkin, D'Anci, & Rosenberg, 2010.

COLD-RELATED INJURIES AND ILLNESSES

Under most conditions, your body is able to maintain a healthy temperature. But when you are exposed to a cold environment, if you are not dressed appropriately, more heat can escape from your body than you can produce. When the body's control mechanism can no longer maintain normal body temperature, hypothermia can set in. In law enforcement, prolonged exposure in cases such as directing traffic in January, overseeing an accident on the highway, or tracking a lost skier may lead to deadly results. Hypothermia can also happen on cool days when it is wet and windy, because evaporation from your skin lowers your core temperature.

Hypothermia usually comes on gradually. At first, your body shivers (muscles contract) in an attempt to generate heat. Then, as your nervous system is affected, you begin to mumble, fumble, grumble, and stumble. You may lose consciousness and experience loss of fine motor coordination. Additional signs and symptoms include slurred speech, slowed breathing, cold, pale skin, and fatigue that is accompanied by lethargy or apathy. If not dealt with, severe hypothermia can lead to cardiac and respiratory failure and, ultimately, death.

The following is a list of people who are more at risk for hypothermia:

- people who have spent prolonged periods of time in cold environments or cool, wet, and windy environments
- young children and older adults
- substance abusers
- those with impaired mental status
- those who have been immersed in cold water

One-sixth of Ontario's terrain is covered with lakes, rivers, and streams (Encyclopedia of Canadian Provinces, 2017). Many law enforcement officers are called upon to assist and rescue individuals who have fallen into the water. Immersion in cold water numbs the extremities quickly, causes shivering, and can lead to amnesia, unconsciousness, and death (US Search and Rescue Task Force, n.d.). Although it is imperative to get out of the water as soon as possible, physical exertion causes the body to lose heat at a fast rate, because blood is being sent to the extremities and quickly cooled. Survival time can be shortened by more than 50 percent (US Search and Rescue Task Force, n.d.). Learning to swim effectively is important.

Other cold-related injuries include frostnip and frostbite. Frostnip is a mild form of frostbite where only the top layer of skin freezes. There may be a painful tingling or burning sensation; skin appears yellowish or white, but feels soft to the touch. Frostbite is a more severe condition where both the skin and the underlying tissue (fat, muscle, bone) are frozen. The area is numb and the skin appears white and waxy, and is hard to the touch. At this point, medical attention is necessary.

When headed outdoors, you need to be aware of the wind chill index (WCI) instead of just consulting outside air temperatures. The wind chill represents how the temperature would feel on your skin if the wind were reduced to a walking pace of 4.8 kilometres per hour. As a general rule, if the WCI is less than −28 °C (−20 °F), caution must be taken when participating in outdoor activities. See Table 14.3 for wind chill and frostbite risk levels, health concerns, and their remedies.

TABLE 14.3   Wind Chill Hazards and What to Do

WIND CHILL (°C)	RISK OF FROSTBITE	OTHER HEALTH CONCERNS	WHAT TO DO
0 to −9	Low	• Slight increase in discomfort	• Dress warmly. • Stay dry.
−10 to −27	Low	• Uncomfortable • Risk of hypothermia if outside for long periods without adequate protection	• Dress in layers of warm clothing, with an outer layer that is wind-resistant. • Wear a hat, mittens or insulated gloves, a scarf, and insulated, waterproof footwear. • Stay dry. • Keep active.
−28 to −39	Risk: Exposed skin can freeze in 10–30 minutes	• Risk of frostnip or frostbite: Check face and extremities for numbness or whiteness • Risk of hypothermia if outside for long periods without adequate clothing or shelter from wind and cold	• Dress in layers of warm clothing, with an outer layer that is wind-resistant. • Cover exposed skin. • Wear a hat, mittens or insulated gloves, a scarf, neck tube or face mask, and insulated, waterproof footwear. • Stay dry. • Keep active.
−40 to −47	High risk: Exposed skin can freeze in 5–10 minutes*	• High risk of frostbite: Check face and extremities for numbness or whiteness • Risk of hypothermia if outside for long periods without adequate clothing or shelter from wind and cold	• Dress in layers of warm clothing, with an outer layer that is wind-resistant. • Cover all exposed skin. • Wear a hat, mittens or insulated gloves, a scarf, neck tube or face mask, and insulated, waterproof footwear. • Stay dry. • Keep active.
−48 to −54	Very high risk: Exposed skin can freeze in 2–5 minutes*	• Very high risk of frostbite: Check face and extremities frequently for numbness or whiteness • Serious risk of hypothermia if outside for long periods without adequate clothing or shelter from wind and cold	• Be careful—dress very warmly in layers of clothing, with an outer layer that is wind-resistant. • Cover all exposed skin. • Wear a hat, mittens or insulated gloves, a scarf, neck tube or face mask, and insulated, waterproof footwear. • Be ready to cut short or cancel outdoor activities. • Stay dry. • Keep active.
−55 and colder	Extremely high risk: Exposed skin can freeze in less than 2 minutes*	• DANGER! Outdoor conditions are hazardous	• Stay indoors

* In sustained winds over 50 km/h, frostbite can occur faster than indicated.

SOURCE: Environment Canada, 2012.

EXERCISING IN COLD TEMPERATURES

As long as we maintain core temperature, it is rarely too cold to exercise. In cold conditions, although we can wear scarves to warm inhaled air, most times the air will naturally warm up to a safe temperature by the time it reaches the lungs. Aerobic exercise helps to maintain core temperature by producing three-quarters of the energy in the form of heat. Aerobic capacity is not adversely affected as long as core temperature is maintained. If we stand around for long periods of time or stop exercising but stay outside, that's when the cold air begins to affect our body. Caution on running is indicated when wind chill warnings are greater than –27 degrees Celsius, risking frostbite injury (Castellani et al., 2006).

As core temperature drops, muscles set off a greater anaerobic metabolism, producing more lactic acid and associated muscle burn in an attempt to maintain core temperature. This results in an overall reduction in the strength and power that can be produced by the muscle tissue in severely cold weather. Combined with cold water in the form of rain, hail, or snow, along with fatigue, these factors can make law enforcement officers easy targets for hypothermia.

Proper apparel and common sense are key to preventing hypothermia. You can wear up to four layers of clothing, with a ventilation layer next to the skin. It is important to wear gloves and a hat, as large amounts of heat are lost through your head. Keep your neck and throat area covered. Change your socks if your feet get wet.

Turn to **assignment 14.1** at www.emond.ca/fitness5e and research an injury (chronic or acute) that you have experienced from working out or while playing sports, or research an injury that you are interested in knowing more about. Prevention and treatment are key to being able to successfully participate fully in sports you enjoy and maintaining a healthy career.

BIOLOGICAL AND CHEMICAL HAZARDS IN LAW ENFORCEMENT

Emergency response teams encounter hazardous products on a daily basis. Sources of biological hazards include bacteria, viruses, insects, plants, birds, animals, and humans. Methamphetamine laboratories in homes, drugs stashed on persons, hepatitis, tuberculosis, anthrax, Lyme disease (a bacterial infection acquired from the bite of an infected tick), and HIV/AIDS are just a few hazards that officers may face when they respond to a call, while inspecting vehicles, and dealing with the population they work with. Officers' health can be affected in ways ranging from skin irritation, allergies, and respiratory infections to contraction of diseases, including HIV/AIDS, and exposure to a mix of known or suspected agents or activities that may increase cancer risk.

Chemical hazards include individual chemicals, mixtures like petroleum solvents, and synthetic polymers (plastics). In 1988, the national Workplace Hazardous Materials Information System (WHMIS) was developed to familiarize workers with safety information about potentially hazardous products in the workplace (CCOHS, 2015). Workers are required to learn the WHMIS symbols and their meanings, the labels on products, and how to read and understand material safety data sheets. These sheets provide information about the physical, chemical, and environmental characteristics of a material, along with information regarding toxicity and potential hazards (such as whether it is reactive, flammable, combustible, or toxic). Data sheets will also include preparation and production information about the substance, as well as the appropriate first aid measures that should be taken upon exposure.

The Canadian Centre for Occupational Health and Safety (CCOHS) provides information on biological and chemical hazards. Each law enforcement service and community is required to develop an emergency response plan based on risk assessment (what is in a community that could expose its members to hazardous materials). Each community must develop a comprehensive emergency preparedness policy and response program to deal with each emergency in the safest and most efficient manner possible. For more information, see CCOHS (2015) (in References).

FINAL THOUGHTS

As you prepare for a physically demanding career, remember that injuries can have long-term effects on your ability to meet the bona fide occupational fitness requirements of the job. Make sure to be smart, train safely, and look after any injury that you may be faced with, so that you will enjoy the quality of your life being fit and healthy through to retirement.

KEY TERMS

acute muscle soreness
reflects simple fatigue caused by a buildup of chemical waste products (lactic acid and hydrogen ions) during or after exercise

bursitis
inflammation of a bursa (a sac of fluid near a joint)

concussion
a type of traumatic brain injury (TBI) caused by a bump, blow, or jolt to the head or by a hit to the body that causes the head and brain to move rapidly back and forth, which causes the brain to bounce around or twist in the skull, creating chemical changes in the brain and sometimes stretching and damaging brain cells

delayed-onset muscle soreness (DOMS)
soreness of muscles 12 hours or more after exercise

frostbite
severe condition where both the skin and the underlying tissue (fat, muscle, and bone) are frozen

frostnip
a mild form of frostbite, where only the top layer of skin freezes

heat cramps
illness caused by a water and sodium deficiency; painful, brief muscle cramps that occur during or after exercise or work in a hot environment

heat exhaustion
excessive heat and dehydration raising the body temperature to 38 to 40 °C (100 to 104 °F) resulting in symptoms that may include heavy sweating and a rapid pulse as a result of your body overheating

heat rash
an irritation of the skin that results from excessive sweating during hot and humid weather

heat stroke
illness caused by failure of the body's heat-regulating mechanism; may lead to permanent disability or death

hypothermia
condition occurring when the body's control mechanism can no longer maintain a normal body temperature, and the body's temperature drops to an abnormally low level

musculoskeletal injuries
injuries of the muscles, nerves, tendons, ligaments, joints, cartilage, or spinal discs

post-concussion syndrome
a complex disorder in which various symptoms—such as headaches and dizziness—last for weeks and sometimes months after the injury that caused the concussion

RICE principle
rest, immobilize, cool, elevate; an immediate, simple treatment for a musculoskeletal injury

second impact syndrome
describes rapid swelling of the brain which sometimes can be catastrophic if the person afflicted suffers a second head injury before the symptoms from the first have gone away

shoulder impingement syndrome
squeezing of the rotator cuff (the group of muscles that surrounds the shoulder)

sprain
a stretching or tearing injury to a ligament

strain
stretching, pulling or tearing of a muscle or tendon

tendinitis
inflammation of a tendon

wind chill index (WCI)
measure representing how the temperature would feel on your skin if the wind were reduced to a walking pace of 4.8 km/h

Workplace Hazardous Materials Information System (WHMIS)
a system that familiarizes workers with safety information about potentially hazardous products in their workplace

EXERCISES

TRUE OR FALSE?

1. Overuse problems are more common when someone is beginning a fitness program, and account for the majority of injuries.

2. Alternating a high-impact activity with a low-impact activity may prevent overuse of specific muscle groups.

3. Being fatigued during a workout will not make you more susceptible to developing an injury.

4. Mild muscle soreness that develops at the beginning of a new exercise program will usually disappear in one to three days.

MULTIPLE CHOICE

1. The most common preventable cause of exercise injury is
   a. overuse
   b. poor nutrition
   c. sudden trauma
   d. dehydration
   e. muscular endurance

2. To help prevent overuse of muscles, you should
   a. work through the soreness
   b. increase the length of your workout each day to toughen your muscles
   c. exercise seven days a week to toughen your muscles
   d. alternate days spent on aerobic and strength conditioning
   e. do two-a-day workouts to toughen your muscles

3. According to the RICE principle, for a mild ankle sprain you should
   a. apply heat immediately
   b. apply ice for 20 minutes after 24 hours
   c. apply tape and leave it wrapped for 12 hours
   d. keep exercising unless there is extreme pain
   e. raise the ankle up and apply ice

4. Injury to a ligament caused by a sudden force is called a
   a. cramp
   b. bursitis
   c. sprain
   d. strain
   e. plantar fasciitis

5. Injury to a tendon caused by a sudden force is called a(n)
   a. pull
   b. sprain
   c. strain
   d. inversion
   e. eversion

6. Which of the following activities can result in a repetitive stress injury?
   a. pitching a baseball
   b. playing a violin
   c. typing
   d. lifting weights
   e. all of the above

7. For people working with computers, which of these reduces the risk for a repetitive stress injury?
   a. taking short, frequent breaks
   b. using wrist pads
   c. using flat keyboards
   d. not typing for more than one hour without taking a break
   e. all of the above

8. In what age group is second impact syndrome most prevalent?
   a. toddlers and children
   b. teens and young adults
   c. middle age
   d. elderly
   e. stats show that they are all at similar risk

9. What is the best practice regarding an athlete returning to contact sports following a concussion?
   a. the day of injury if no symptoms persist
   b. the following day if no symptoms persist
   c. whenever a medical professional signs a release form validating that they are symptom free
   d. after gradual, stepwise evaluation with stress, even if symptoms persist
   e. whenever the parents feel the athlete is ready to play

10. Heat cramps may be treated by
    a. increased salt intake
    b. water, cool air, and rest
    c. alternating heat with ice on the affected area
    d. wrapping the affected muscle
    e. applying more clothes to keep the muscle warm

SHORT ANSWER

1. What are musculoskeletal injuries?

2. What are three of the risk factors associated with musculoskeletal injuries?

3. What is the RICE principle?

4. What does DOMS stand for and what is DOMS?

5. Why do people suffer from delayed-onset muscle soreness?

6. Differentiate between a sprain and a strain.

7. What is tendinitis? What are some common types of tendinitis in the body?

8. How do you treat a sprain or a strain?

9. What are shin splints? How do you prevent shin splints?

10. What is a concussion? What happens to the brain?

11. List five signs and symptoms of a concussion.

12. Name and briefly explain the three heat-related illnesses.

13. How do you treat heat-related illnesses?

14. What is hypothermia? What are some of its signs and symptoms?

15. How do you treat someone who has developed hypothermia?

16. What are some of the biological or chemical hazards that an officer may face while working?

REFERENCES

Achterstraat, P. (2008). *Managing injured police: NSW police force.* Auditor-General, ED. Audit Office of New South Wales, Sydney, Australia. Retrieved from http://www.audit.nsw.gov.au/ArticleDocuments/140/184_Managing_Injured_Police.pdf.aspx?Embed=Y

American College of Sports Medicine (ACSM). (2007). Exercise and fluid replacement. *Medicine and Science in Sports & Exercise, 39*(2), 377–390.

American College of Sports Medicine (ACSM). (2011). *Delayed Onset Muscle Soreness (DOMS).* Retrieved from https://www.acsm.org/docs/brochures/delayed-onset-muscle-soreness-(doms).pdf

Bass, A.B., & Kortyna, R. (2017). Shoulder dislocations. *Clinician Reviews, 27*(1), 32–35.

Billette, J.-M., & Janz, T. (2015). Health at a glance. Injuries in Canada: Insights from the Canadian community health survey. (Statistic Canada Catalogue no. 82-624-X).

Boyle, C.A., Sayers, S.P., Jensen, B.E., Headley, S.A., & Manos, T.M. (2004). The effects of yoga training and a single bout of yoga on delayed onset muscle soreness in the lower extremity. *Journal of Strength and Conditioning Research, 18*(4), 723–729.

Brain and Spinal Cord. (2017). Second impact syndrome. Retrieved from http://www.brainandspinalcord.org/second-impact-syndrome/

Canadian Centre for Occupational Health and Safety (CCOHS). (2015). *WHMIS 2015 fact sheets.* Retrieved from https://www.ccohs.ca/products/publications/whmis_ghs/

Canadian Centre for Occupational Health and Safety (CCOHS). (2016). Hot environments—Health effects and first aid. OSH answers fact sheets. Retrieved from https://www.ccohs.ca/oshanswers/phys_agents/heat_health.html

Cancelliere, C., et al. (2014). Systematic review of prognosis and return to play after sport concussion: Results of the International Collaboration on Mild Traumatic Brain Injury Prognosis. *Archives of Physical Medicine and Rehabilitation, 95*(suppl), S210–S229.

Casa, D.J., Armstrong, L.E., & Hillman, S.K. (2000). National Athletic Trainer's Association position statement: Fluid replacement for athletes. *Journal of Athletic Training, 35*(2), 212–224.

Castellani, J.W., Young, A.J., Ducharme, M.B., Giesbrecht, G.C., Glickman, E., Sallis, R.E., American College of Sports Medicine (ACSM). (2006). American College of Sports Medicine position stand: Prevention of cold injuries during exercise. *Medical Science and Sports Exercise, 38*(11), 2012–2029.

Centers for Disease Control and Prevention (CDC). (2016). *Work-related musculoskeletal disorders & ergonomics.* Retrieved from https://www.cdc.gov/workplacehealthpromotion/health-strategies/musculoskeletal-disorders/

Centers for Disease Control and Prevention (CDC). (2017). What is a concussion? Retrieved from https://www.cdc.gov/headsup/basics/concussion_whatis.html

Cutts, S., Prempeh, M., & Drew, S. (2009). Anterior shoulder dislocation. *Annals of The Royal College of Surgeons of England, 91*(1), 2–7. Retrieved from http://doi.org/10.1308/003588409X359123

Davis, G.A., Purcell, L., Schneider, K.J., Yeates, K.O., Gioia, G.A., Anderson, V., … Kutcher, J.S. (2017). The child sport concussion recognition tool 5. *British Journal of Sports Medicine, 0*, 1. Retrieved from http://bjsm.bmj.com/content/bjsports/early/2017/04/26/bjsports-2017-097508CRT5.full.pdf

Dixit, S., DiFiori, J.P., Burton, M., & Mines, B. (2007). Management of patellofemoral pain syndrome. *American Family Physician, 75*(2), 194–202.

Encyclopedia of Canadian Provinces. (2017). Ontario. Retrieved from http://www.nationsencyclopedia.com/canada/Nunavut-to-Yukon/Ontario.html

Environment Canada. (2012). Canada's wind chill hazards and what to do. Retrieved from http://www.ec.gc.ca/meteo-weather/default.asp?lang=en&n=5FBF816A-1-table1

Fortune, M.K., Mustard, C.A., Etches, J.J.C., & Chambers, A.G. (2013). Work-attributed illness arising from excess heat exposure in Ontario, 2004–2010. *Canadian Journal of Public Health, 104*(5), e420–e246.

Government of Canada. (2012). Extreme heat: Heat waves. In Sun Safety. Retrieved from https://www.canada.ca/en/health-canada/services/sun-safety/extreme-heat-heat-waves.html

Health Canada. (2011). Extreme heat events guidelines: Technical guide for health care workers. Cat. No.: H128-1/11-642E. Retrieved from https://www.canada.ca/en/health-canada/services/environmental-workplace-health/reports-publications/climate-change-health/extreme-heat-events-guidelines-technical-guide-health-care-workers.html

Hovbrender, A. (2009). Identification of potential risk factors for injury to police officers in using new technologies. Work Safe BC. Retrieved from https://www.worksafebc.com/en/resources/about-us/research/identification-of-potential-risk-factors-for-injury-to-police-officers-using-new-technologies

Infrastructure Health & Safety Association. (2017). What risk factors contribute to MSDs? Retrieved from https://www.ihsa.ca/topics_hazards/msd_faqs.aspx-what_are_msds

Koder, G. (2005). Ergonomics and the future of the police vehicle. Retrieved from http://www.fdle.state.fl.us/cms/FCJEI/Programs1/SLP/Documents/Full-Text/Koder-george-paper.aspx

Lyons, K., Radburn, C., Orr, R., & Pope, R. (2017). A profile of injuries sustained by law enforcement officers: A critical review. *International Journal of Environmental Research and Public Health.* Retrieved from http://www.mdpi.com/1660-4601/14/2/142/pdf

Mayo Clinic. (2017). Post-concussion syndrome. Retrieved from http://www.mayoclinic.org/diseases-conditions/post-concussion-syndrome/basics/definition/con-20032705

McLellan, T.M., Daanen, H.A.M., & Cheung, S.S. (2013). Encapsulated environment. *Comprehensive Physiology, 3*(3), 1363–1391.

Ministry of Labour. (2014). Heat stress. Retrieved from https://www.labour.gov.on.ca/english/hs/pubs/gl_heat.php

National Institute of Arthritis and Musculoskeletal and Skin Diseases (NIAMS). (2017). Sprains and strains. Retrieved from https://www.niams.nih.gov/health_info/sprains_strains/

NIOSH. (2016). NIOSH criteria for a recommended standard: Occupational exposure to heat and hot environments. By B. Jacklitsch, W.J. Williams, K. Musolin, A. Coca, J-H. Kim, & N. Turner. Cincinnati, OH: U.S. Department of Health and Human Services, Centers for Disease Control and Prevention, National Institute for Occupational Safety and Health, DHHS (NIOSH) Publication 2016-106.

Ontario Neurotrauma Foundation. (2016). Four important summits. *Neuromatter Newsletter* Fall 2016. Retrieved from http://onf.org/documents/neuromatters-newsletter/neuromatters-fall-2016/four-important-summits

Parachute. (2017). Canadian guideline on concussion in sport. Retrieved from http://www.parachutecanada.org/injury-topics/item/canadian-guideline-on-concussion-in-sport

Popkin, B.M., D'Anci, K.E., & Rosenberg, I.H. (2010). Water, hydration and health. *Nutrition Reviews, 68*(8), 439–458. Retrieved from http://doi.org/10.1111/j.1753-4887.2010.00304.x

Tator, C.H. (2009). Concussions are brain injuries and should be taken seriously. *Canadian Journal of Neurological Sciences, 36*(3), 269–270

United States (US) Search and Rescue Task Force. (n.d.). Cold water survival. Retrieved from http://www.ussartf.org/cold_water_survival.htm

Weisenthal, B.M., Beck, C.A., Maloney, M.D., DeHaven, K.E., & Giordano, B.D. (2014). Injury rate and patterns among CrossFit athletes. *Orthopaedic Journal of Sports Medicine, 2*(4).

Workplace Safety and Insurance Board (WSIB). (2016). By the numbers. 2016 WSIB Statistical Report. Retrieved from http://www.wsibstatistics.ca

APPENDIX
BFOR PROTOCOLS AND FITNESS STANDARDS

BONA FIDE OCCUPATIONAL REQUIREMENT (BFOR)

The focus of a Bona Fide Occupational Requirement (BFOR) is to determine if the applicant or incumbent has the necessary physical capabilities to safely and efficiently perform the critical on-the-job tasks encountered in a physically demanding occupation (Jamnik, Gumieniak, & Gledhill, 2013). It ensures that individuals have the necessary attributes to efficiently and safely perform the job tasks that are most important and those that are the most frequently physically required. Based on task analysis, these types of job simulations are termed content valid tests (Eid, 2001). A BFOR test legally discriminates for adequate level of skill-related fitness without contravening protected human rights areas like age and gender. These assessments determine whether you can perform the basic physical skills necessary to do the job, based on your level of skill-related fitness, and to ensure safety for the public, yourself, and your partner's well-being.

Prior to doing a BFOR assessment, the individual is required to ensure that they are healthy enough to do the test, understand what the test is about, and understand what may happen during the testing. One of those requirements is to do a pre-exercise clearance, which includes a PAR-Q+ and, if required, the online ePARmed–X+ at www.eparmedx.com (Warburton, Jamnik, Bredin, & Gledhill, 2014). Each person is required to fill out an Informed Consent form and a Consent for Release of Information form. The appraiser will take the individual's blood pressure and heart rate to ensure that he/she meets the requirements to be able to be tested. The appraiser provides time for a demonstration of the test, as well as time to get acquainted with the various equipment used in the test and to answer any questions prior to testing.

The following BFORs are used in Canada by law enforcement agencies.

PHYSICAL READINESS EVALUATION FOR POLICE (PREP) TEST

The PREP test was designed to provide an unbiased and valid occupational requirement that identifies those individuals who possess the physical capabilities needed to meet the rigorous demands of policing in Ontario.

The two components of the PREP test are:

1. pursuit/restraint circuit
2. aerobic fitness test (Léger 20-metre shuttle run)

PURSUIT/RESTRAINT CIRCUIT

The pursuit/restraint circuit (Figure A.1) simulates a police foot chase that includes obstacles (climbing stairs, scaling fences, crawling under barriers), engaging in an altercation to gain control of a person who resists arrest, and then dragging an incapacitated person to a triage area (Gledhill & Jamnik, 2015).

Throughout the pursuit/restraint circuit, you must wear a 4.1-kg (9-lb.) soft belt around your waist and a 4.1-kg (9-lb.) vest, which together simulate the weight of standard police equipment.

The circuit is made up of four laps that are 25 metres each. During the first and third laps of the circuit, you will pull yourself up to look over the far 2-metre (6.5-ft.) fence with a toehold and indicate to the appraiser the number on the floor, climb up and down a set of stairs, and crawl under a barrier of 61 centimetres (24 in.).

During the second and fourth laps, you will scale the near 1.2-metre (4-ft.) fence with no toehold, climb up and down a set of stairs, and crawl under a barrier of 61 centimetres (24 in.).

After completing the second and fourth laps, you will be directed to go to the body-control simulator (force required is 35.5 kg/78 lb.). "Push" or "pull" commands will indicate the action you are required to perform; "right," "centre," and "left" commands will indicate the direction in which you should move. Next, you will proceed to the arm-restraint simulator (grip = 14.5 kg/32 lb.; retraction = 16 kg/35 lb.). Depress the grips and force the arms together, then return them to their starting position.

After completing the second arm restraint, you will be directed over to the victim drag. Using the handle attached to the back of the mannequin's neck, you will drag the 77-kg (170-lb.) mannequin over a resistance mat that requires the same force needed to pull a body out of a car (55 kg/121 lb.). You will continue to pull the mannequin over the floor (resistance of 35 kg/77 lb.), around the pylon, and back until the heels pass the Start marker, a total distance of 6.1 m (20 ft.).

A time of 157 seconds (2 minutes and 37 seconds) or less is required for the successful completion of the pursuit/restraint circuit.

Note: Participants are allowed a 15-minute rest following the pursuit/restraint circuit before beginning the aerobic fitness test.

AEROBIC FITNESS TEST: LÉGER 20-METRE SHUTTLE RUN

The Léger 20-metre shuttle run (Léger & Lambert, 1982), provides an evaluation of necessary aerobic capacity to perform physically demanding tasks during daily activities. In this test, the participant runs back and forth over a 20-metre (66-ft.) course in time with audio signals recorded on a CD. The time permitted to cover the 20-metres initially requires a very slow jog, then the time is made progressively shorter so that the participant runs faster until he or she completes the desired stage, or is no longer able to maintain the required pace.

In each leg of the shuttle run, at least one foot must touch the end line and the warning lines (situated 2 metres (6.6 ft.) from each end of the 20-metre end lines) must be reached before the permitted time elapses. Missing warning lines twice in a row or failing to touch the end line three times will be rated "DOES NOT MEET STANDARD." See Figure A.2.

Candidates who complete stage 7 in the Léger 20-metre shuttle run receive a "MEETS STANDARD" rating in the PREP test.

FIGURE A.1 PREP Test: Pursuit/Restraint Circuit

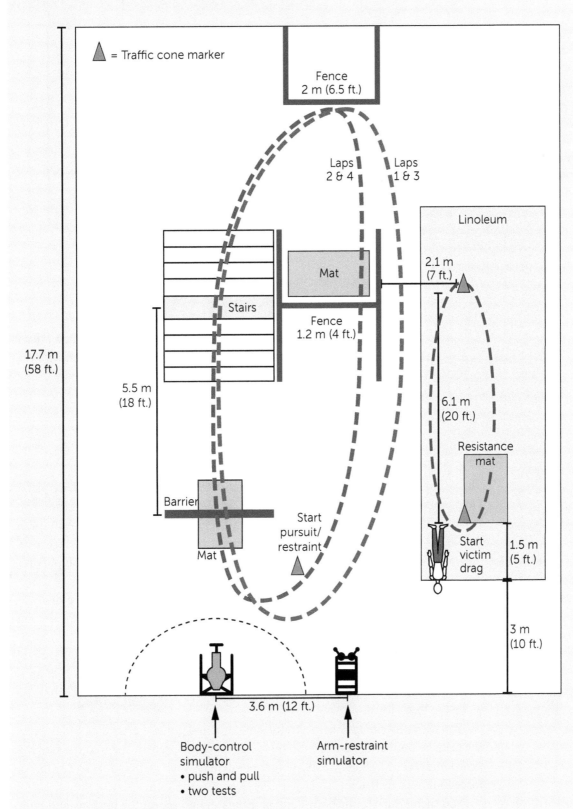

SOURCE: Ministry of Community Safety and Correctional Services, 2015.

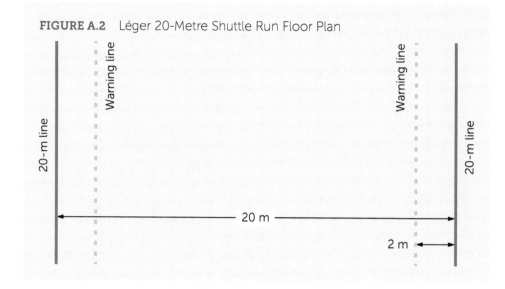

FIGURE A.2 Léger 20-Metre Shuttle Run Floor Plan

ALBERTA PHYSICAL READINESS EVALUATION FOR POLICE (A-PREP)

The A-PREP is designed to simulate a critical incident in which a police officer chases, controls, and restrains a suspect. There are two separate components for the A-PREP (Alberta Solicitor General and Public Safety, 2008):

1. pursuit/restraint circuit
2. aerobic fitness test (Léger 20-metre shuttle run)

PURSUIT/RESTRAINT CIRCUIT

The circuit (Figure A.3) simulates an emergency response in which a police constable pursues an offender a distance of 100 m while scaling four sets of stairs and two fences, engages in a physical altercation to accomplish the control and restraint of a resisting offender, then drags a passive resister or accident victim to a triage area. You will be required to wear a 7.5-kg (16.5-lb.) weighted belt during the pursuit/restraint circuit to simulate the weight of standard police equipment.

In the pursuit phase, you run four laps around a 25-metre circuit as quickly as possible. During each 25-metre circuit, you climb a set of stairs, and on the second and fourth rotation, you scale a 1.5-metre (5-ft.) fence.

Immediately following the 100-metre circuit, you move to the body control simulator and grasp the handles. You are required to move through two 180° arcs, switching back and forth every 90° between pushing and pulling the handle to raise 34 kg (75 lb.).

You then move to the arm restraint simulator and grasp the handles and depress the grips of both arms to force them together and then return them to the starting position. It takes 14.5 kg (32 lb.) of force to depress each grip and 16 kg (35 lb.) of force to retract each arm.

You then return to the body control simulator and repeat the pushing and pulling to raise the 34-kg (75-lb.) weight through two more 180° arcs. Then you return to the arm restraint simulator and repeat the arm retraction exercise.

Lastly, you grasp a 68-kg (150-lb.) mannequin and drag it a distance of 15 metres (50 ft.). You may grasp it by the wrists or ankles.

A time of 130 seconds (2 minutes and 10 seconds) or less is required for the successful completion of the pursuit/restraint circuit.

Note: Participants are allowed a 10-minute rest following the pursuit/restraint circuit before beginning the aerobic fitness test.

FIGURE A.3   A-PREP Pursuit/Restraint Circuit

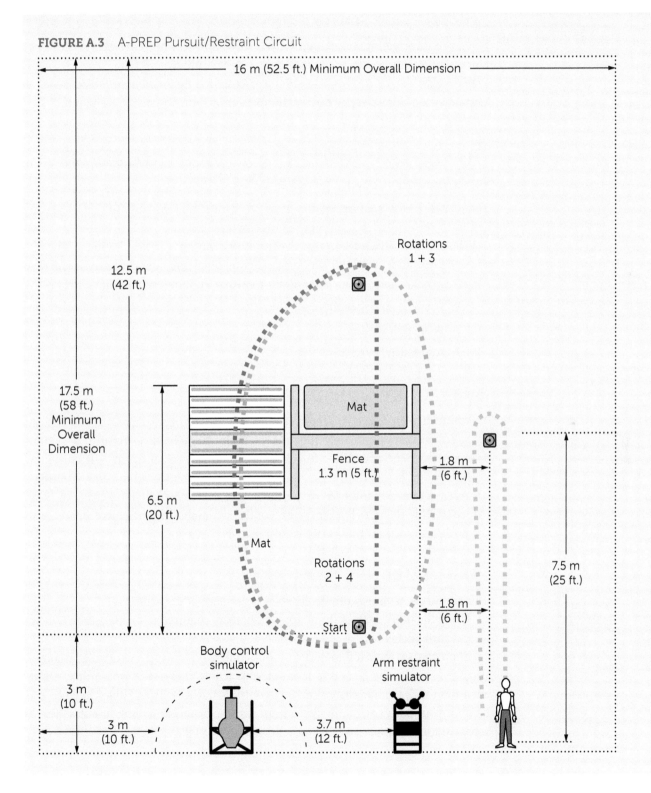

AEROBIC FITNESS TEST: LÉGER 20-METRE SHUTTLE RUN

Refer to the PREP protocol for the explanation of the test. To successfully complete the minimum requirement of the aerobic fitness test, you must achieve stage 7 on the Léger 20-metre shuttle run.

FURTHER RESOURCES

For more information regarding the A-PREP refer to http://www.calgary.ca/cps/Documents/application-forms/fit-to-serve.pdf?noredirect=1 or *Fit to Serve: Preparing for the A-PREP: Alberta Physical Readiness Evaluation for Police* (2008) at https://www.publicsafety.gc.ca/lbrr/archives/cnmcs-plcng/cn31683-eng.pdf.

PHYSICAL ABILITIES REQUIREMENT EVALUATION (PARE) TEST

The RCMP PARE is an occupational test that measures the essential physical capacities to perform satisfactory law enforcement work.

The PARE is divided into three sections simulating a critical incident. The obstacle course and push/pull sections are completed together and are timed. The weight carry section is done after. Refer to Figure A.4 for a schematic of the test.

1. obstacle course section

2. push/pull section

3. weight carry section

OBSTACLE COURSE SECTION

This simulates proceeding to the scene of a problem or occurrence. The total length of the course is approximately 350 m (1150 ft.) long and involves running six laps of a course which includes: direction changes, jumping across a 1.5-m (5-ft.) distance, ascending and descending stairs, jumping over 0.45-m (18-in.) hurdles, vaulting a 0.9-m (3-ft.) barrier, followed by performing a controlled fall and getting back up before starting the next lap. At the end of the sixth lap, the participant proceeds to the push/pull section (body control simulator).

PUSH/PULL SECTION

This simulates having to physically solve a problem or occurrence.

Using the body control simulator, you first are required to push a 32-kg (70-lb.) weight through six 180° arcs.

Then you are required to perform four controlled falls. In a controlled manner, you are to fall to the floor and land on your front. Then stand up without assistance and touch the handle of the body-control simulator. Then fall to the floor and land on your back and stand up without assistance and touch the handles. This is repeated for a total of two falls to the front and two falls to the back.

FIGURE A.4 PARE Test Obstacle Course

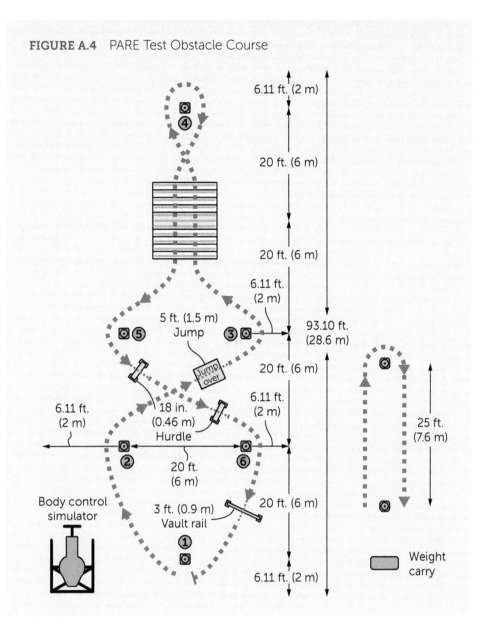

You then are required to pull the weight through six 180° arcs.

Once this section has been completed, the PARE administrator stops the stopwatch and records the time. The timed portion of the PARE is over. A time of 4:45 minutes or less is required for the successful completion by the RCMP for recruit training at Depot during the first two weeks and for applicants with the Canada Border Services. A time of 4:00 minutes or less must be achieved to graduate from Depot or meet incumbent and UN mission standards.

WEIGHT CARRY SECTION

This activity begins within 2 minutes of completing the push/pull section. It simulates having to remove an object or a person from the scene. The torso bag is to be carried over a 15-m (50-ft.) distance. The participant will be given a maximum of three attempts to complete the weight carry section. The weight carry section is not timed.

Participants are allowed to wrap their arms around the bag or grasp the excess material to lift the bag. The bag must be carried in a controlled manner in front of the participant, not over one's shoulders or resting on one's thighs while walking. After the participant has completed the 15-m (50-ft.) distance, they must lower the bag in a controlled manner.

RCMP recruits and Canada Border Services officers are required to carry a 36-kg (80-lb. bag), while RCMP graduates, incumbents, and UN mission officers are required to carry a 45.5-kg (100-lb.) bag.

FURTHER RESOURCES

For more information regarding the RCMP's standards go to http://www.rcmp-grc.gc.ca/en/prepare-for-pare. For more information regarding the Canada Border Services go to http://www.cbsa-asfc.gc.ca/job-emploi/bso-asf/pare-tape-eng .html?wbdisable=true.

POLICE OFFICERS PHYSICAL ABILITIES TEST (POPAT)

The POPAT is a job-related physical abilities test that is designed to simulate a critical incident where a police officer chases, controls, and apprehends a suspect.

There are four stations for the POPAT (Farenholtz & Rhodes, 1986). The first three stations are timed together and consist of the 390-m (426-yard) run, the physical-control simulator, and the modified squat thrust and stand using the vault rail. The fourth station is the torso carry bag.

1. 390-m (426-yard) run
2A. physical control simulator
2B. vault rail
3. torso bag carry

STATION 1: 390-METRE (426-YARD) RUN

The applicant is required to traverse the mobility/agility course six times in order to complete a total of 390 m (426 yards). The mobility/agility run resembles a figure eight (see Figure A.5) and will be marked with brightly coloured traffic cones. In completing six laps of the mobility/agility run, the applicant will be required to change directions, hurdle low barriers, make stride changes, and negotiate stairs.

STATION 2A: PHYSICAL CONTROL SIMULATOR

After completing the mobility/agility run, the applicant will move directly to the pull and push station. The applicant will be required to pull on the rope and hold 36.3 kg (80 lbs.) of weight off the bottom of the body-control simulator and move through an arc of 180°. The applicant will be required to touch a designated line on either side of the machine three times with the left foot and three times with the right foot, for a total of six touches. If at any time during these six 180° arcs the elevated weight stack comes in contact with the bottom of the machine, the applicant will be required to begin the pull portion again.

FIGURE A.5 Police Officers' Physical Abilities Test (POPAT)

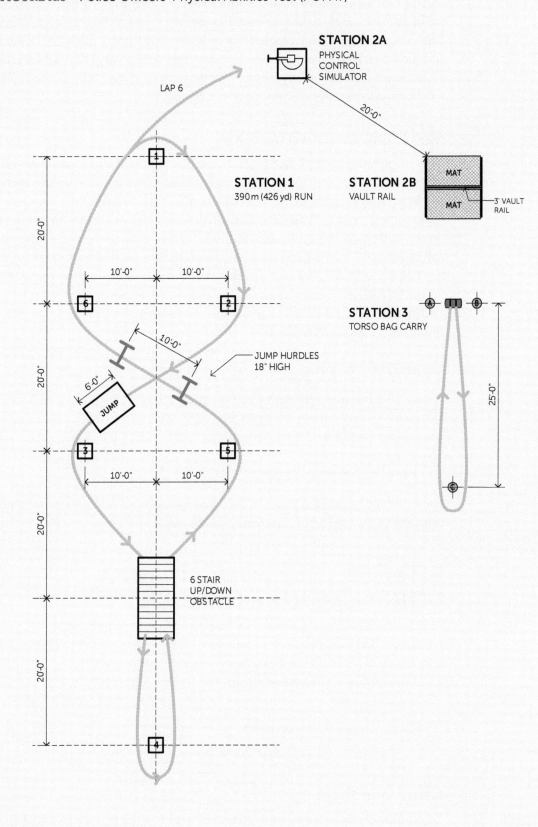

After the sixth arc, the applicant will release the rope and once again raise the 36.3-kg (80-lb.) weight stack off the bottom of the power training machine by pushing on the swing arm of the machine. The applicant must move through another six 180° arcs, touching the designated line on either side three times with the left foot and three times with the right foot. If at any time during these six 180° arcs the elevated weight stack comes in contact with the bottom of the machine, the applicant will be required to begin the push portion again.

STATION 2B: VAULT RAIL

Upon completing the pull and push station, the applicant will proceed directly to the vault rail to perform the modified squat thrust and stand station. The applicant will begin this test lying on his/her chest on the mat adjacent to the rail vault. The applicant will stand and vault over the 3-ft. (0.91-m) high rail to the other side. Once on the other side, the applicant will touch his/her back to the mat. This process will be repeated until the applicant has completed five touches to the chest and five touches to the back. Once the applicant stands for the last time, the running time for the POPAT test is completed.

Note: A time of 4:15 or less to complete stations 1, 2A, and 2B is necessary to successfully pass the POPAT.

STATION 3: TORSO BAG CARRY

Within 30 seconds of completing station three, the applicant will move directly to the torso bag carry station. The applicant will lift and carry a 100-lb. (45.36-kg) torso bag a distance of 25 ft. (7.5 m). This station is not timed but necessary to complete.

FURTHER RESOURCES

For more information on the POPAT test, go to http://deltapolice.ca/joindpd/constable/popat/ or http://www.lepat.com/fit-popat.

FITNESS TEST FOR ONTARIO CORRECTIONAL OFFICER (FITCO)

The Ontario Ministry of Community Safety and Correctional Services' FITCO test was designed to assess whether an individual has the physical abilities necessary for the care, custody, and control of offenders as a correctional officer.

There are three components for this test (Figure A.6) (MCSCS, 2016):

1. cell search
2. emergency response circuit
3. aerobic fitness test (Léger 20-m shuttle run)

CELL SEARCH

To simulate the tasks required to effectively search a cell in a correctional facility, you are required to lift and remove a standard weight mattress from the top bunk of a bed, hold the mattress at arm's length for a time sufficient for a bed search and then are required to find and move four small different coloured blocks of wood from different areas around the bunk for a contraband search.

A time of 120 seconds or less is required for the successful completion of the cell search.

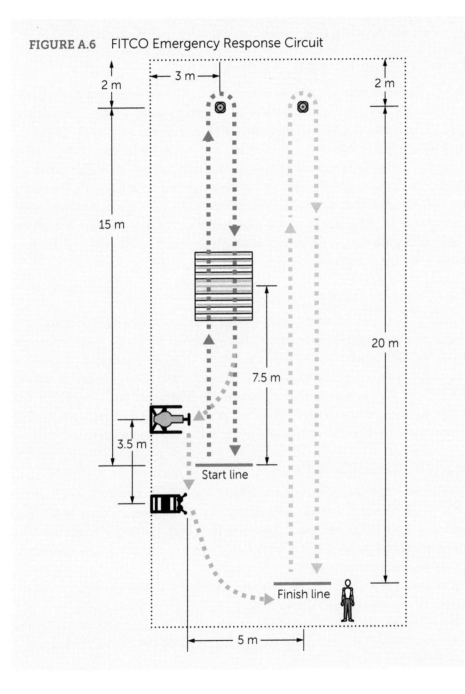

FIGURE A.6 FITCO Emergency Response Circuit

EMERGENCY RESPONSE CIRCUIT

This circuit simulates a typical emergency response in which a correctional officer quickly covers a 60-metre response while scaling four sets of stairs, engages in a physical altercation with a non-compliant inmate (body-control simulator), establishes control for the application of restraints (arm-retraction simulator), then escorts the inmate to segregation at a purposeful walking pace.

60-METRE RESPONSE

On the tester's cue, you will begin by running up and over the stairs (60-metre response)—touching every step on the way up and every step on the way down—then run around the traffic cone and back over the stairs to the starting line. When you reach the starting line, you will turn around and complete the same loop a second time going over the stairs, around the cone, and back over the stairs.

BODY-CONTROL SIMULATOR

Simulating an altercation, start in the centre of the body-control simulator by pushing the handle away and lifting the weight (which requires a force of 38.6 kg or 85 lb.) off the cradle. Release and then pull the handle toward you thereby lifting the weight off the cradle (requiring the same force as the pushing action). While holding the weight up, shuffle step to the right until your foot contacts the wall. Release the weight, then push the handle away lifting the weight off the cradle. While holding the weight up, shuffle step to the centre. Release the weight again, pull the handle toward you and shuffle step to the left until your foot contacts the wall. Release the weight again, push the handle away and shuffle step to the centre. Repeat this process once more to complete two full revolutions.

ARM-RETRACTION SIMULATOR

Simulating the forces required to grip (26 kg/57 lb.) and retract (28.5 kg/62.5 lb.) the arms of a non-compliant inmate, position your feet so that the handle is in line with the midline of your body. Grasp the handle with two hands and squeeze the lever until it is fully depressed without moving your feet. Push the handle toward the middle of the machine so that it passes the indicator line and then return it to the starting position in a controlled manner. After returning the arm to the starting position, move to the other handle and perform the same manoeuvre.

MANNEQUIN ESCORT

You will grasp the mannequin (that weighs 39 kg/86 lb., the equivalent of half the weight of the "average" Ontario male inmate) by the handle and transfer it a total distance of 40 m around the far traffic cone then back across the finish line. The transfer should be completed at a "purposeful walking" pace. It is not necessary to lift the mannequin completely from the ground.

A time of 128 seconds or less is required for the successful completion of the emergency response circuit.

Note: There will be a rest period of a minimum of 10 minutes to a maximum of 20 minutes between the end of the emergency response circuit and the beginning of the Léger 20-metre shuttle run.

AEROBIC FITNESS TEST: LÉGER 20-METRE SHUTTLE RUN

Refer to the PREP protocol for explanation of test.

Candidates who complete stage 5.5 in the Léger 20-m shuttle run receive a "Meets Standard" rating.

CORRECTIONAL OFFICERS' PHYSICAL ABILITIES TEST (COPAT)

The Correctional Officers' Physical Abilities Test (COPAT) was designed to evaluate a potential applicant's physical fitness to ensure they are able to perform the duties of a correctional officer/law enforcement officer. Correctional officers are often required to run short distances during the performance of their duties. Stations 1, 2, and 3 are timed together and station 4 is performed on its own.

STATION 1: STAIR RUN

In station 1, the participant runs 50 ft. (15.24 m). This short run includes two 90° turns. The participant then runs up and down six stairs. This activity is repeated six times consecutively. From the stairs, the participant moves through a 30-m zig-zag course of cones and must jump over three sticks placed 18 in. (45.74 cm) off the ground.

STATION 2: PHYSICAL-CONTROL SIMULATOR

This station involves demonstrating the ability to control 50 lbs. (22.68 kg) or 70 lbs. (31.75 kg) (depending on the province) of resistance while moving through 180° arcs. The first part of this station is the pull. The participant grasps a rope on the body-control simulator and pulls the weight stack off its resting position. While keeping the weight stack off the resting position, the participant moves through six 180° arcs of controlled pulling.

Once the pull is completed successfully, the participant grabs the bar on the body-control simulator and pushes the weight stack off its resting position. With the weight off the resting position, the participant moves through six 180° arcs, as in the push.

STATION 3: VAULT RAIL

This station involves modified squat thrust and stand (STAS) activity followed by jumping over a 0.76 m (2 ft. 6 in.) vault rail. From the pull-push station, the participant moves to station 3 and begins by doing a STAS so that the chest and hips touch the mat. The participant then stands and vaults over the rail, touching the rail with only the hands. Landing on the feet, the participant then does a reverse STAS (to end up on your back) so that the shoulder blades and heels touch the mat. The participant then stands and vaults over the rail and repeats the activity until a total of ten STAS (five to the front, five to the back) and nine vaults are completed. Once the participant finishes the last STAS and stands up in a balanced position, the time is stopped. This ends the timed portion of the test.

All three stations must be completed together, and to pass the COPAT for BC Corrections, the participant must perform all activities as per the defined protocol and complete the timed portion of the test within a set time.

To pass the COPAT, the participant must perform all activities as per the defined protocol and complete the timed portion of the test within 3:20 minutes for Alberta and Nova Scotia and 2:50 minutes for British Columbia Corrections.

FIGURE A.7 Correctional Officer Physical Abilities Test (COPAT) Floor Plan

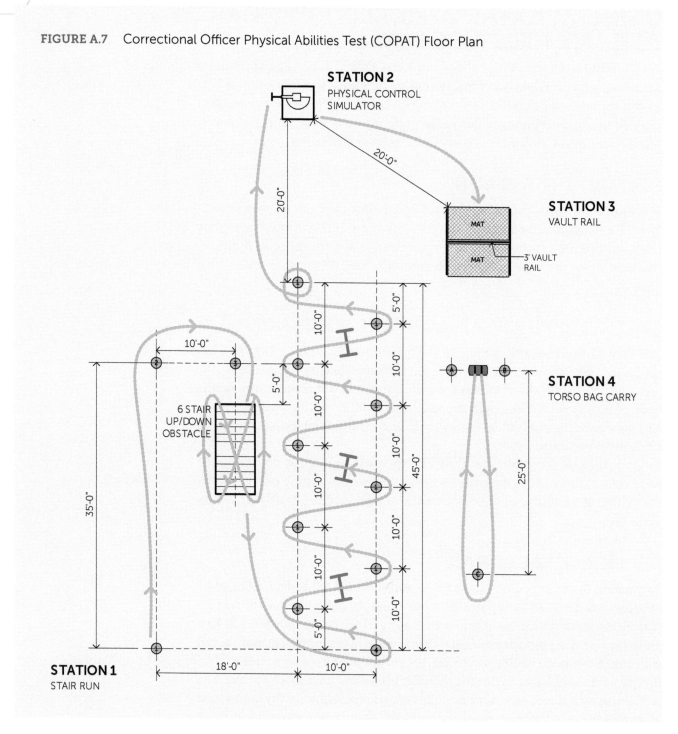

STATION 4: TORSO BAG CARRY

This station is not part of the timed portion of the test, but is necessary to successfully complete the test. A rest period of 30 seconds is given between the end of station 3 and the start of this station.

The participant must pick up a torso bag and carry the bag in front with their hands in a controlled manner for a distance of 50 ft. to meet the standard.

Alberta Corrections requires the participant to lift and carry an 80-lb. (36-kg.) torso bag. Nova Scotia and British Columbia Corrections require the participant to lift and carry a 70-lb. (31.75-kg) torso bag.

FURTHER RESOURCES

For more information regarding the COPAT, go to https://novascotia.ca/just/Corrections/recruitment/copat.asp.

FITNESS FOR OPERATIONAL REQUIREMENTS OF CANADIAN ARMED FORCES EMPLOYMENT (FORCE)

The FORCE Evaluation was designed to incorporate common duties and tasks that Canadian Armed Forces could be called upon to perform. The four tasks that were chosen include:

1. 20-m rushes
2. sandbag lift
3. intermittent loaded shuttles
4. sandbag drag

20-METRE RUSHES

This test simulates escape to cover by assessing an individual's ability to quickly cover short distances while changing body positions every 10 metres. Start by lying on the floor in a prone position with shoulders and hands behind the start line. Lift your hands off the floor. On the start signal, get up off the floor and sprint 10 metres. Your foot must touch on or over the line and then you go into prone position, perpendicular to the line, with shoulders and hands facing forward on or behind the line. Lift your hands, forearms, and elbows off the floor (called a hand release). Then get up and sprint another 10 metres and repeat the hand release protocol. Turn around and repeat until you have performed eight hand releases. On the final hand release (at 80 metres), tap the finish line.

A time of 51 seconds or less is required for the successful completion of the 20-metre rushes. See Figure A.8.

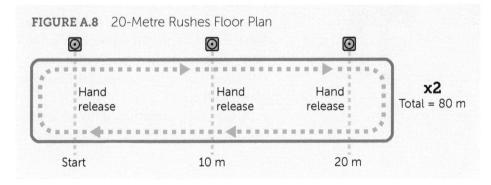

FIGURE A.8 20-Metre Rushes Floor Plan

FIGURE A.9 Sandbag Lift Wall Plan

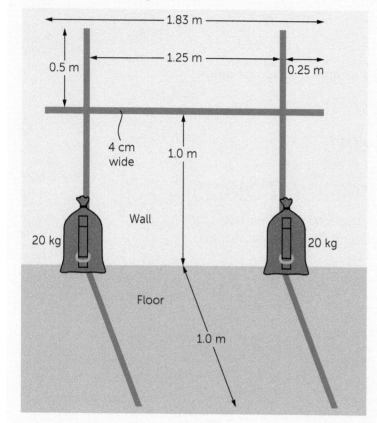

SANDBAG LIFT

This task was designed to simulate self-protection, or protection of others from natural elements or from enemy fire. In an upright position, stand directly behind the sandbag facing the wall. On the command "Go," lift the entire sandbag to touch the midline on or above the intersecting lines at 1 metre above the floor. You can release the sandbag and let it drop to the floor. Shift sideways and position your feet on both sides of the second line. Pick up the second sandbag and touch the midline on or above the intersecting lines on the wall before releasing the bag. Shift sideways to the first and repeat for 30 proper lifts.

A time of 3 minutes 30 seconds or less is required for the successful completion of the sandbag lift. See Figure A.9.

FIGURE A.10 Acceptable Sandbag Safe Techniques

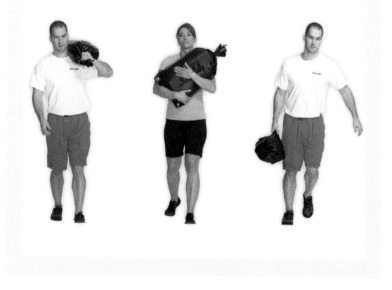

INTERMITTENT LOADED SHUTTLES

This test reflects the shuttling back and forth necessary when transporting equipment. On the cue "Go," you are required to safely pick up the sandbag and, walking with only one foot in contact with the floor, carry the sandbag 20 metres. Go around the cone and return back to the start line placing one foot on or over the start line. Drop the sandbag and complete the second shuttle without weight. You may run during the unloaded trips. You must complete five sets (one loaded and one unloaded shuttle) covering a total distance of 400 metres.

Figure A.10 shows three different options for acceptable sandbag lifting techniques.

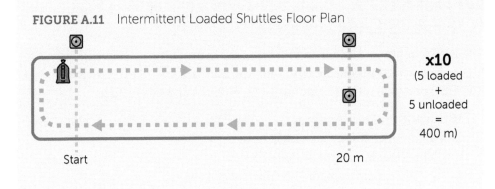

FIGURE A.11 Intermittent Loaded Shuttles Floor Plan

A time of 5 minutes 21 seconds or less is required for the successful completion of the intermittent loaded shuttles. See Figure A.11 above.

SANDBAG DRAG

The Sandbag Drag reflects two common casualty rescue tasks; vehicle extrication and stretcher carry. You are required to pick up the sandbag in a cradle position (hands underneath, fingers laced or crossed) with straps pointing downward and ropes taut. On the signal to go, walk backwards dragging the sandbags to the opposite end. Time will stop when the first row of sandbags cross the 20-metre finish line. Although this is not timed, to be successful you must complete the 20-metre drag without stopping. See Figure A.12.

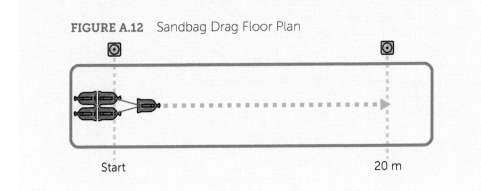

FIGURE A.12 Sandbag Drag Floor Plan

FURTHER RESOURCES

For more information about the FORCE program and training, go to https://www
.cfmws.com/en/AboutUs/PSP/DFIT/Fitness/FORCEprogram/Pages/About-the
-FORCE-Program.aspx.

ONTARIO POLICE FITNESS AWARD (OPFA) STANDARDS

There are four fitness components that are used in the OPFA assessment. They combine to have a maximum score of 100 and you must achieve 75 marks overall to pass. The fitness assessments and grading for the OPFA standards include:

Muscular Endurance (push-ups)	/20
Core Endurance (modified back extension)	/20
Flexibility (trunk forward flexion)	/10
Aerobic Fitness Assessment (1.5-mile/2.4-km run or Léger 20-m shuttle run)	/50
Total Score	/100

Tables and descriptions of the fitness assessments are on the following pages and are adapted from the OPFA standards. Each table provides benchmarks that allow you to score your performance and gauge your improvement as you work toward your goal of meeting law enforcement fitness standards.

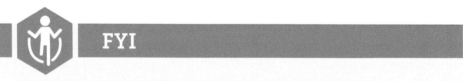

FYI

POLICE FITNESS PERSONNEL OF ONTARIO

In 1986, several individuals got together at the Peel Regional Headquarters for the first meeting of what is now known as the Police Fitness Personnel Ontario (PFPO). They foresaw rapid changes happening in the policing field, the need to present a common philosophy, and the impact such a group could have on management, associations, and the individual police officer.

Projects that the PFPO have undertaken include:

1. the development of fitness standards for entrance and graduation from the Ontario Police College. Since then, the PREP test has become the standard;
2. the development of videos illustrating the proper technique to train for the Ontario Police Fitness Standards;
3. the development of the fitness award program called the Ontario Police Fitness Award (OPFA);
4. the staging of standardized test of fitness workshops, providing official accreditation to fitness evaluators;
5. the staging of a PFPO fitness workshop and two "Fit for Duty" conferences to provide information to assist appraisers around fitness, nutrition, and wellness.

For more information about the Police Fitness Personnel Ontario, go to http://www.pfpo.org.

PUSH-UPS

Push-ups are a test of muscular endurance, which is defined as the ability of a muscle to perform repeated contractions over a period of time. The push-ups are to be performed consecutively and without a time limit. The test is terminated when the participant has completed as many push-ups as possible, or when their form deviates too much from the correct procedure.

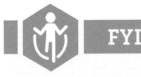 **FYI**

OPFA PROTOCOL: PUSH-UPS

In many cases, lack of compliance with the OPFA protocol (that is, arching the back on a push-up, trying to reach the floor by straining your neck only, not going down far enough, moving hands farther apart, failing to keep the upper body in a straight line, not going to full extension, forcibly straining, or pausing for too long between push-ups) terminates the test. If the person corrects the technique, the inappropriate push-up is not counted, and the participant can continue until he or she deviates in two consecutive repetitions.

It is not acceptable for either females or males to have their feet against a wall or for an additional mat to be placed under the chin.

MALE PROTOCOL

The participant lies on his stomach with legs together. His hands, pointing forward, are positioned under the shoulders. To begin, the participant pushes up from the mat by fully straightening the elbows to full extension, using the toes as the pivotal point. The upper body must be kept in a straight line (Figure A.13). The participant returns to the starting position, chin to the mat. Neither the stomach nor the thighs should touch the mat.

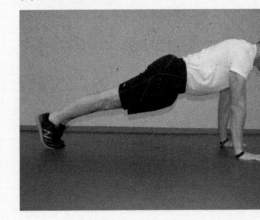

FIGURE A.13 Push-up, Males
(a) Start Position
(b) Full Extension

FEMALE PROTOCOL

The participant lies on her stomach with legs together. Her hands, pointing forward, are positioned under the shoulders. She then pushes up from the mat by fully straightening the elbows, using the knees as the pivot point. Flexing at the elbows, she lowers the body, maintaining a neutral spine (body held in a straight line). The elbow must be flexed to 90° at the bottom of the movement (Figure A.14). The participant returns to the starting position with only the chin to the mat. The stomach and hips cannot touch the mat and the hip should not be flexed. The participant must have the lower leg remain in contact with the mat, ankles plantar-flexed.

Table A.1 shows standard results and scores for males and females.

FIGURE A.14 Push-up, Females

(a) Start Position

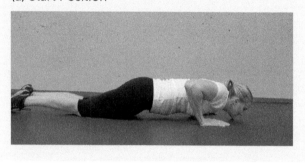

(b) Full Extension

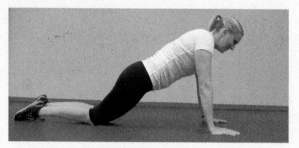

TABLE A.1 Push-ups Results and Scores, Male and Female

| | AGE | | | | | | | | | |
| | 20–29 | | 30–39 | | 40–49 | | 50–59 | | 60+ | |
SCORE	**Male**	**Female**	**Male**	**Female**	**Male**	**Female**	**Male**	**Female**	**Male**	**Female**
20	49+	38+	37+	37+	31+	33+	29+	31+	28+	31+
19	48	37	36	36	30	32	28	30	25–27	30
18	36–47	30–36	30–35	27–35	22–29	24–31	21–27	21–29	18–24	17–29
17	32–35	24–29	25–29	22–26	20–21	20–23	15–20	15–20	13–17	13–16
16	29–31	21–23	22–24	20–21	17–19	15–19	13–14	12–14	11–12	12
15	27–28	20	21	17–19	16	14	12	11	10	10–11
14	25–26	18–19	20	16	15	13	11	10	10	9
12	24	16–17	19	14–15	13–14	12	10	9	9	6–8
10	21–23	14–15	16–18	12–13	12	10–11	9	5–8	7–8	4–5
8	18–20	11–13	14–15	10–11	10–11	7–9	7–8	3–4	6	2–3
6	16–17	9–10	11–13	7–9	8–9	4–6	5–6	1–2	4–5	1
4	11–15	5–8	8–10	4–6	5–7	2–3	4	–	2–3	–
2	10	4	7	3	4	1	3	–	1	–
0	≤9	≤3	≤6	≤2	≤3	0	≤2	0	0	0

SOURCE: PFPO, 2017.

CORE ENDURANCE TEST

This assessment is for those participants who are asymptomatic and pass the pre-screening for having no back problems. The participant must have filled out his or her PAR-Q+ and must have no restrictions.

PRE-SCREENING

The participant lies face down on a mat and performs a straight leg extension with the right leg and then the left, with arms outstretched in front. If there is no pain, then he or she is told to repeat the same movements with the opposing arm outstretched and lifted at the same time (Figure A.15). Then the participant returns to the starting position. If no pain is indicated, he or she proceeds to the test.

FIGURE A.15   Pre-screening for Back Extension

(a) Leg Lift Only

(b) Leg Lift with Opposite Arm

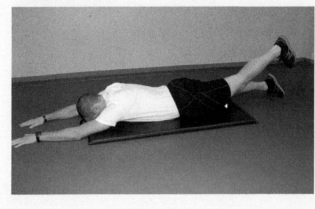
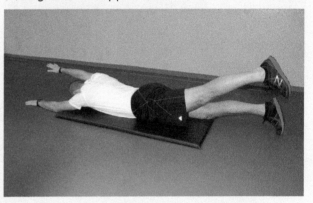

PROTOCOL

The core endurance test is based on the modified Biering-Sorensen back assessment.

FIGURE A.16   Biering-Sorensen Back Assessment Set-up

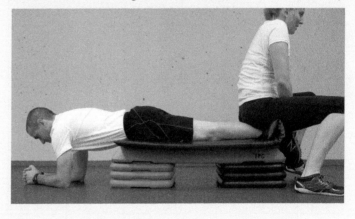

The participant lies face down on top of the bench with the lower body on the bench. The iliac crest is positioned at the edge of the bench (your appraiser will ensure that it is in the right location). The participant needs to be secured by either straps or a partner with their arms supporting their upper body until the test begins (Figure A.16). Before starting the test, the participant is told to use core muscles throughout the test. A towel may be placed under the ankles to add support and keep feet in a neutral position.

Once the participant is secured, he or she is instructed to raise the upper body until it is parallel with the lower body. The participant's arms are placed across their chest with the hands on the opposing shoulders. The participant may not grab on to their shirt or allow their hands to leave their shoulders. The entire body forms one straight line, with no rotation, arching, or lateral shifting. The neck is straight and neutral. The participant stays in this position for as long as possible to a maximum of

180 seconds. Participants are allowed one warning to reposition themselves if they drop below parallel. The test is terminated when the participant puts their hands to the ground, or drops below parallel twice. See Figure A.17.

The score is based on the number of seconds that the test is performed.

FIGURE A.17 Biering-Sorensen Back Assessment

(a) Correct Body Position

(b) Incorrect Body Position (one warning, then test terminated)

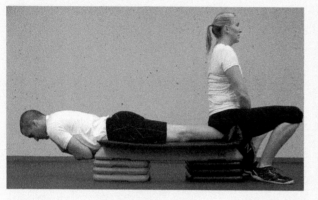

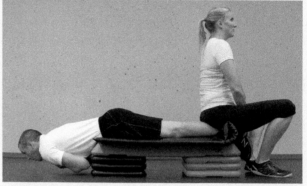

Table A.2 shows standard results and scores for males and females.

TABLE A.2 Biering-Sorensen Back Assessment: Core Endurance Test Results and Scores, Male and Female

	AGE									
	20–29		30–39		40–49		50–59		60+	
SCORE	Male	Female	Male	Female	Male	Female	Male	Female	Male	Female
20	3:00	3:00	3:00	3:00	2:45–3:00	3:00	2:41–3:00	2:36–3:00	2:00–3:00	2:29–3:00
19	2:50–2:59	2:51–2:59	2:43–2:59	2:51–2:59	2:30–2:44	2:46–2:59	2:21–2:40	2:13–2:35	1:53–1:59	2:00–2:28
18	2:40–2:49	2:41–2:50	2:27–2:42	2:43–2:50	2:10–2:29	2:33–2:45	2:00–2:20	1:50–2:12	1:44–1:52	1:31–1:59
17	2:31–2:39	2:32–2:40	2:13–2:26	2:36–2:42	1:55–2:09	2:20–2:32	1:50–1:59	1:38–1:49	1:35–1:43	1:14–1:30
16	2:21–2:30	2:24–2:31	2:01–2:12	2:28–2:35	1:39–1:54	2:07–2:19	1:40–1:49	1:26–1:37	1:26–1:34	0:57–1:13
15	2:12–2:20	2:15–2:23	1:48–2:00	2:20–2:27	1:23–1:38	1:54–2:06	1:27–1:39	1:14–1:25	1:17–1:25	0:39–0:56
14	2:00–2:11	2:04–2:14	1:42–1:47	2:11–2:19	1:19–1:22	1:43–1:53	1:17–1:26	1:06–1:13	1:09–1:16	0:33–0:38
12	1:50–1:59	1:53–2:03	1:36–1:41	2:01–2:10	1:14–1:18	1:32–1:42	1:06–1:16	0:56–1:05	1:01–1:08	0:26–0:32
10	1:39–1:49	1:42–1:52	1:31–1:34	1:52–2:00	1:10–1:13	1:20–1:31	0:54–1:05	0:47–0:55	0:52–1:00	0:19–0:25
8	1:35–1:38	1:30–1:41	1:19–1:30	1:35–1:51	0:59–1:09	1:08–1:19	0:43–0:53	0:37–0:46	0:42–0:51	0:15–0:18
6	1:30–1:34	1:18–1:29	1:07–1:18	1:18–1:34	0:45–0:58	0:55–1:07	0:31–0:42	0:26–0:36	0:30–0:41	0:11–0:14
4	1:26–1:29	1:06–1:17	0:56–1:06	1:01–1:17	0:32–0:44	0:42–0:54	0:20–0:30	0:15–0:25	0:20–0:29	0:06–0:10
2	≤1:25	≤1:05	≤0:55	≤1:00	≤0:31	≤0:41	≤0:19	≤0:14	≤0:19	≤0:05
0	DID NOT ATTEMPT									

SOURCE: PFPO, 2017.

TRUNK FORWARD FLEXION (SIT AND REACH)

The trunk forward flexion test measures the flexibility of the hamstring and lower back muscles. Flexibility depends upon the elasticity of the muscles, tendons, and ligaments, and is the ability to bend without injury. The trunk forward flexion test was chosen as an assessment that could show that restriction in the pelvis and tight hamstring muscles were associated with risk of low back pain.

Participants warm up for this test by performing slow stretching movements before the actual measurements are taken. One of the recommended warm-up stretches includes the modified hurdler stretch (Figure A.18).

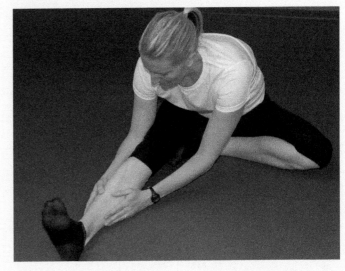

FIGURE A.18   Modified Hurdler Stretch

PROTOCOL

Participants, without shoes, sit with legs fully extended and the soles of the feet placed flat against the flexometer. Keeping the knees fully extended, arms evenly stretched, and palms down, participants bend and reach forward (without bouncing or jerking). The position of maximum flexion must be held for approximately 2 seconds. Participants are advised to lower their head during the motion to maximize the distance reached. Each participant is allowed two attempts, with the higher result scored. See Figure A.19.

FIGURE A.19   Trunk Forward Flexion

(a) Starting Position

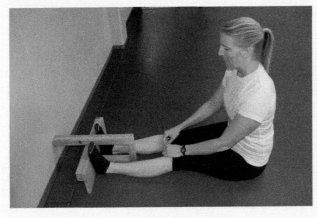

(b) Flexion Position

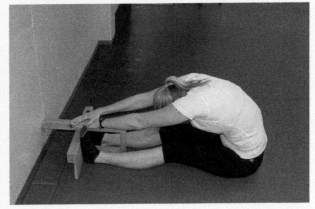

Table A.3 shows standard results and scores for males and females.

TABLE A.3 Trunk Forward Flexion Results and Scores, Male and Female

SCORE	AGE									
	20–29		30–39		40–49		50–59		60+	
	Male	Female	Male	Female	Male	Female	Male	Female	Male	Female
10	45+	46+	44+	46+	41+	44+	42+	44+	45+	41+
9.5	44-44.5	45-45.5	42.5-43.5	45-45.5	39-40.5	42-43.5	40-41.5	42-43.5	40-44.5	39-40.5
9	40-43.5	41-44.5	38-42	41-44.5	37-38.5	40-41.5	37-39.5	40-41.5	36-39.5	37-38.5
8.5	37-39.5	39-40.5	35-37.5	38-40.5	35-36.5	38-39.5	35-36.5	38-39.5	32-35.5	35-36.5
8	34-36.5	37-38.5	33-34.5	36-37.5	32-34.5	36-37.6	33-34.5	36-37.5	29-31.5	33-34.5
7.5	33-33.5	36-36.5	32-32.5	35-35.5	29-31.5	34-35.5	30-32.5	34-35.5	26-28.5	31-32.5
7	32-32.5	35-35.5	31-31.5	34-34.5	27-28.5	32-33.5	27-29.5	32-33.5	24-25.5	29-30.5
6	31-31.5	34-34.5	29-30.5	33-33.5	25-26.5	29-31.5	25-26.5	30-31.5	22-23.5	27-28.5
5	29-30.5	32-33.5	27-28.5	31-32.5	23-24.5	26-28.5	22-24.5	28-2.59	18-21.5	25-26.5
4	26-28.5	29-31.5	24-26.5	28-30.5	20-22.5	24-25.5	18-21.5	25-27.5	16-17.5	23-24.5
3	23-25.5	26-28.5	21-23.5	25-27.5	16-19.5	22-23.5	15-17.5	22-24.5	14-15.5	21-22.5
2	18-22.5	22-25.5	17-20.5	21-24.5	12-15.5	19-21.5	12-14.5	19-21.5	11-13.5	18-20.5
1	≤17	≤21.5	≤16.5	≤20.5	≤11.5	≤18.5	≤11.5	≤18.5	≤10.5	≤17.5
0	DID NOT ATTEMPT									

SOURCE: PFPO, 2017.

1.5-MILE (2.4-KM) RUN

The 1.5-mile (2.4-km) run is a test of aerobic fitness and cardiovascular endurance. It tests the combined efficiency of the lungs, heart, bloodstream, and local muscles in getting oxygen to the muscles and putting them to work. The test is appropriate for those individuals who have engaged in vigorous physical activity within the past six months. Many specialized units use this protocol due to the demands of the job (TRUE, ERT, Canine, etc.).

PROTOCOL

Participants are required to cover an accurately measured 1.5-mile distance in as short a time as possible.

At the start, all participants will line up behind the starting line. On the command "Go" the clock is started and they are asked to begin running at their own pace. The total time to complete the course is recorded and scored. If at any point you can no longer run, you may walk or stop. If you are showing signs of fatigue (such as wobbling, nausea, trouble breathing) you will be encouraged to stop.

Prior to starting, you should complete at least a 5-minute dynamic warm-up which could include a walk or light jog, followed by some basic dynamic stretching exercises. At the completion of the timed run, you will be required to continue a cool-down walk for at least 5 to 10 minutes.

Table A.4 shows the standard results and scores for males and females.

TABLE A.4 1.5-Mile Run Results and Scores, Male and Female

	AGE									
	20–29		30–34		35–39		40–49		50+	
SCORE	Male	Female	Male	Female	Male	Female	Male	Female	Male	Female
50	≤9:00	≤10:35	≤9:20	≤11:00	≤10:06	≤11:53	≤10:54	≤13:04	≤11:59	≤14:22
47.5	9:01–9:30	10:36–11:10	9:21–9:50	11:01–11:35	10:07–10:37	11:54–12:31	10:55–11:41	13:05–13:46	12:00–12:51	14:23–15:08
45	9:31–10:00	11:11–11:52	9:51–10:20	11:36–12:10	10:38–11:10	12:32–13:08	11:42–12:17	13:47–14:27	12:52–13:31	15:09–15:53
42.5	10:01–10:30	11:53–12:34	10:21–10:50	12:11–12:45	11:11–11:42	13:09–13:46	12:18–12:52	14:28–15:08	13:32–14:07	15:54–16:38
40	10:31–10:56	12:35–13:00	10:51–11:20	12:46–13:20	11:43–12:14	13:47–14:24	12:53–13:28	15:09–15:50	14:08–14:49	16:39–17:25
37.5	10:57–11:22	13:01–13:26	11:21–11:50	13:21–13:55	12:15–12:47	14:25–15:02	13:29–14:04	15:51–16:32	14:50–15:28	17:26–18:11
35	11:23–11:46	13:27–13:42	11:51–12:20	13:56–14:30	12:48–13:19	15:03–15:40	14:05–14:39	16:33–17:14	15:29–16:07	18:12–18:57
30	11:47–12:10	13:43–13:57	12:21–12:50	1431–15:05	13:20–13:52	15:41–16:17	14:40–15:15	17:15–17:55	16:08–16:47	18:58–19:42
25	12:11–12:35	13:58–14:12	12:51–13:20	15:06–15:40	13:53–14:24	16:18–16:55	15:16–15:50	17:56–18:21	16:48–17:25	19:43–20:11
20	12:36–12:59	14:13–14:27	13:21–13:50	15:41–16:15	14:25–14:56	16:56–17:33	15:51–16:26	18:22–19:18	17:26–18:05	20:12–21:14
15	13:00–13:30	14:28–14:42	13:51–14:20	16:16–16:50	14:57–15:29	17:34–18:11	16:27–17:02	19:19–20:06	18:06–18:44	21:15–22:00
10	13:31–14:00	14:43–14:57	14:21–14:50	16:51–17:25	15:30–16:01	18:12–18:29	17:03–17:37	20:07–20:41	18:45–19:23	22:01–22:45
5	14:01–14:30	14:58–15:12	14:51–15:20	17:26–18:00	16:02–16:34	18:50–19:26	17:38–18:13	20:42–21:22	19:24–20:02	22:46–23:30
0	DID NOT ATTEMPT OR FAILED TO MEET MINIMUM STANDARD TIME									

SOURCE: PFPO, 2017.

MAXIMAL LÉGER 20-METRE SHUTTLE RUN

The 20-metre shuttle run test is an evaluation of aerobic fitness. This is used both inside (during inclement weather) and outside. A warm-up is included as part of the test and only the last portion of the test may require maximal effort. The objective is to follow the progressively faster pace over a 20-metre course, until you reach your maximal effort.

See PREP protocol for instructions on the 20-m shuttle run. In a maximal effort, the test is completed when the participant:

- stops running due to fatigue/maximal effort
- misses two consecutive warning lines
- commits three faults of failing to touch the end line
- stops by choice

Table A.5 is the scoring results for a maximal 20-metre shuttle run.

TABLE A.5 20-OPFA Result Scores for 20-m Shuttle Run, Male and Female

SCORE	AGE									
	20–29		30–34		35–39		40–49		50+	
	Male	Female	Male	Female	Male	Female	Male	Female	Male	Female
50	≥12	≥9.5	≥11.5	≥9	≥10.5	≥8	≥9	≥6.5	≥7.5	≥5.5
47.5	11.5	9	11	8–8.5	10	7.5	8-8.5	6	7	5
45	11	8–8.5	10.5	7.5	9–9.5	7	7.5	5–5.5	6.5	4.5
42.5	10–10.5	7.5	9.5–10	7	8–8.5	6–6.5	7	4.5	5.5–6	4
40	9–9.5	7	8.5–9	6.5	7.5	5.5	6–6.5	4	5	3.5
37.5	8.5	6.5	8	6	7	5	5.5	3.5	4.5	2.5-3
35	8	6.0	7.5	5	6.5	4.5	5	3	4	2
30	7.5	5.5	7	4.5	6	4	4.5	2.5	3.5	1.5
25	7	5	6.5	4	5.5	3.5	4	2	3	1
20	6.5	4.5	6	3.5	5	3	3.5	1.5	2.5	0.5
15	6	4.0	5.5	3	4.5	2.5	3	1	2	—
10	5.5	3.5	5	2.5	4	2	2.5	0.5	1.5	—
5	5	3	4.5	2	3	1.5	2.0	—	1	—
0	DID NOT ATTEMPT OR FAILED TO MEET MINIMUM SCORE									

SOURCE: PFPO, 2017.

ADDITIONAL FITNESS STANDARDS

Various fitness assessments may provide feedback on the progress of your goals. They can also assist you with key information to help you create or modify your fitness program. The bench press tests upper body strength, the chin-ups test muscular endurance, and the leg press tests leg power. Protocols and standards for the bench press, chin-ups, and leg press have been included below.

BENCH PRESS

The bench press—with standard weights pre-set for a selectorized plate machine—provides an indication of upper-body strength. Based on an old universal machine, this test has been adopted for a Smith machine (for safety and time restraints), although either can be used.

Table A.6 provides the scale from an old universal and the comparison weight on a Smith machine. Each weight is considered a plate on the scoring sheet. Your 100% body weight is the weight closest to your body weight.

TABLE A.6 Comparison of Weight Between Universal Machine (with Pre-determined Weight) and Weights Comparable on Smith Machine

BENCH PRESS SCALE (LB.)	SMITH MACHINE (LB.)
330	330
296	300
279	280
265	265
248	250
231	230
215	215
198	200
182	180
165	165
149	150
132	130
115	115
100	100
80	80
66	65
50	50

SOURCE: Adapted with permission. Marian Reeves. Peel Regional Police Service 2002 recruit standards. 2002 Brampton, Ontario, Peel Regional Police.

The bench press chart in Table A.7 shows the score that you earn when you lift a certain amount of weight. For example, if you lift 5 plates below your body weight, you receive the score of 10; if you lift your full body weight, your score is 20; if you lift 1 plate below your body weight, you score 18; and so on.

TABLE A.7 Scoring for Bench Press

SCORE (/20)	AGE			
	20–29		30–39	
	Male	**Female**	**Male**	**Female**
+1	+4 plates	+3 plates	+4 plates	+3 plates
+1	+2 plates	+2 plates	+2 plates	+1 plates
20	100% body wt.	100% body wt.	100% body wt.	100% body wt.
18	−1 plate	−1 plate	−1 plate	−1 plate
16	−2 plates	−2 plates	−2 plates	−2 plates
14	−3 plates	−3 plates	−3 plates	−3 plates
12	−4 plates	−4 plates	−4 plates	−4 plates
10	−5 plates	−5 plates	−5 plates	−5 plates
8	−6 plates	−6 plates	−6 plates	−6 plates
6	−7 plates	−7 plates	−7 plates	−7 plates
4	−8 plates	−8 plates	−8 plates	−8 plates
2	−9 plates	−9 plates	−9 plates	−9 plates
0	DID NOT ATTEMPT			

SOURCE: Adapted with permission. Marian Reeves. Peel Regional Police Service 2002 recruit standards. 2002 Brampton, Ontario, Peel Regional Police.

PROTOCOL

This test requires the applicant to lie supine on a flat bench with knees bent up and feet flat on the bench or legs bent at the knees such that the feet are in contact with the ground (see Figure A.20). Head and back must maintain contact with the bench. Assistance is given to the applicant to lift the chosen weight until he or she has arms fully extended. When the applicant indicates readiness, he or she will flex the arms, bringing the weight down until an angle of 90° at the elbow is achieved at which time the weight will then be pressed back to the starting position (full extension) (see Figure A.21). Remember not to lift your feet from planted position, lift your head off the bench, or arch your back.

One maximum repetition only is required at the weight chosen by the applicant. You are permitted a total of three repetitions ONLY if you are successful on the previous lift. Do not start at your maximum. Termination happens when you miss one weight. Since you only have a maximum of three attempts, start at a warm-up weight and then move to the weight you believe you can bench.

FIGURE A.20 Bench Press Set-up

(a) Feet Up

(b) Feet Down

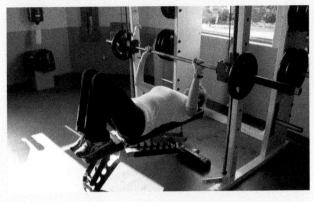 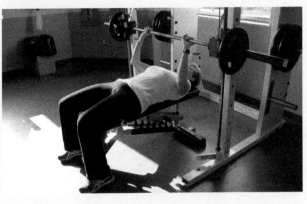

FIGURE A.21 Bench Press

(a) Extension Position

(b) Flexion Position

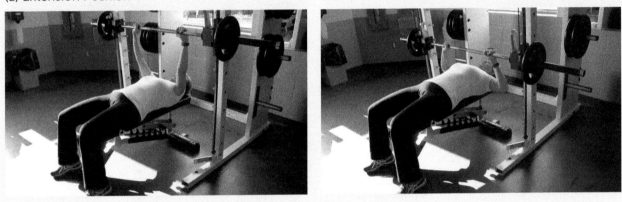

CHIN-UPS

This test requires a functional range of flexibility, good elbow flexor strength, and back shoulder girdle strength.

PROTOCOL

The participant is required to pull him- or herself off the ground by fully flexing the arms. The chin must be brought up above the level of the bar and the body is lowered until the angle at the elbow joint is at least 90°. The hands grip the bar in an underneath grip position while the movement is repeated continually over a period of 30 seconds. See Figure A.22.

FIGURE A.22 Chin-up

(a) Starting Position

(b) 90° Position

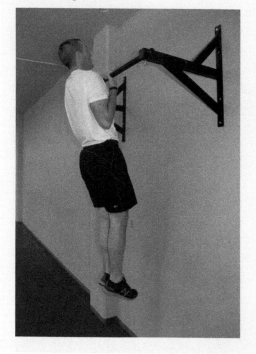

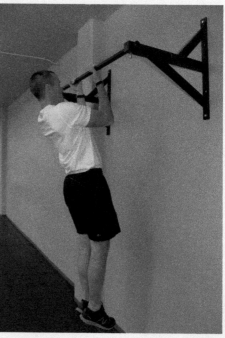

Table A.8 shows the standard results and scores for males and females.

TABLE A.8 Chin-Ups Results and Scores, Male and Female

SCORE (/10)	NUMBER OF CHIN-UPS COMPLETED IN 30 SECONDS			
	AGE 20–29		AGE 30–39	
	Males	Females	Males	Females
+1	30	20	27	16
+1	24	15	22	13
10	18	10	17	10
9	17	9	16	9
8	16	8	15	8
7	15	7	14	7
6	14	6	13	6
5	13	5	12	5
4	12	4	11	4
3	11	3	10	3
2	10	2	9	2
1	9	1	8	1

SOURCE: Adapted with permission from Marian Reeves. Peel Regional Police Service 2002 recruit standards. 2002 Brampton, Ontario: Peel Regional Police.

LEG PRESS

PROTOCOL

Using a universal leg press, you will have three attempts to press your maximum weight as long as you are successful at each attempt (like bench press). Hands grasp the seat's handle with back straight and legs parallel to the floor. Feet are on machine rests with toes pointed slightly outward and the pressure is on the balls and heels of the feet. Extend your legs with knees partially locked. Stop momentarily and then the weight is to be lowered slowly back to the start position. You should not arch or twist your body. See Figure A.23.

FIGURE A.23 Leg Press
(a) Starting Position   (b) Extension Position

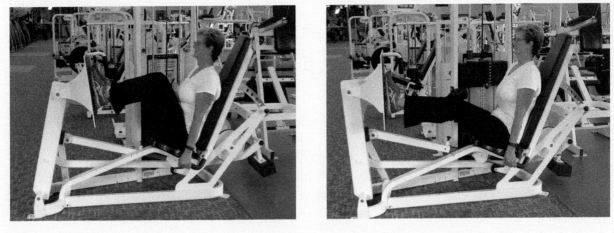

SCORING FOR LEG PRESS

The grading for the 1-RM leg press is based on McArdle, Katch, & Katch (2000) reference values for 1-RM leg press relative to body weight. A perfect score of 20/20 would be a 1-RM leg press that is 2.5 times your body weight.

Take your 1-RM weight from the leg press and *divide it* by 2.5 × *your body weight* and then multiple by *20* for a score out of *20*.

Score = 1-RM / (2.5 × Body Wt.) × 20

So, for example, if you leg press *300 lb.* and you weigh *150 lb.,* your mark would be

Score = 300 / (2.5 × 150) × 20

Score = 300 / 375 × 20

Score = 16/20

PHYSICAL FITNESS LOG

As part of your physical fitness training goals, you may be required to chart your progress throughout the course of your study. To record the results of your workouts or testing, see the running and daily workout logs and result sheets in the *Fit for Duty, Fit for Life* training guide that accompanies this textbook.

FINAL THOUGHTS

At the end of each semester, you may have to change your goals and programs because you have either surpassed them or have not yet obtained them. Remember that the idea is to believe in your abilities, skills, and personal characteristics with a dedicated effort to learn from each experience and develop skills to improve yourself, understanding deficiencies and mistakes, and to develop skills for opportunities for progress. There is always room for growth. Good luck!

REFERENCES

Alberta Solicitor General and Public Safety. (2008). *FIT TO SERVE: Preparing for the A-PREP: Alberta Physical Readiness Evaluation for Police.* Toronto: Queen's Printer of Ontario. Retrieved from http://www.calgary.ca/cps/Documents/application-forms/fit-to-serve.pdf?noredirect=1

Alberta Solicitor General and Public Security. (2008). COPAT Correctional Officer Physical Ability Test. Retrieved from https://www.solgps.alberta.ca/careers/Publications/COPAT Requirements.pdf

CF Morale and Welfare Services. (2016). *FORCE operation manual.* (2nd ed.). April 1, 2016. Retrieved from https://www.cfmws.com/en/AboutUs/PSP/DFIT/Fitness/FORCEprogram/Pages/FORCE-Operations-Manual-2nd-Edition.aspx

Eid, E. (2001). Challenges posed by the Supreme Court of Canada in the Meiorin decision to employers in physically demanding occupations. In N. Gledhill, J. Bonneau, & A. Salmon (Eds.), *Proceedings of the National Forum on Bona Fide Occupational Requirements.* Toronto, ON.

Farenholtz, D.W., & Rhodes, E.C. (1986). Development of physical abilities test for municipal police officers in British Columbia. *Canadian Journal of Applied Sport Sciences, 11*(3), abstract.

Gledhill, N., & Jamnik, R. (2015). *Technical Guide: Physical Readiness Evaluation for Police Constable Applicants (PREP).* Ontario Association of Chiefs of Police Constable Selection System. Toronto: Ontario Ministry of Community Safety and Correctional Services.

Jamnik, V., Gumienak, R., & Gledhill, N. (2013). Developing legally defensible physiological employment standards for prominent physically demanding public safety occupations: A Canadian perspective. *European Journal of Applied Physiology, 113*(10), 2447–2457.

Léger, L.A., & Lambert, J. (1982). A maximal multistage 20-m shuttle run test to predict VO$_2$ max. *European Journal of Applied Physiology, 49,* 1–5.

McArdle, W.D., Katch, F.I., & Katch, V.L. (2000). *Essentials of exercise physiology.*(2nd ed.). Philadelphia: Lippincott Williams & Wilkins.

Ministry of Community Safety and Correctional Services (MCSCS). (2015). *PREP. Fit to Serve. Preparing for the PREP—the Physical Readiness Evaluation for Police.* Retrieved from http://www.applicanttesting.com/images/stories/pdf/FittoServe2015Final.pdf

Ministry of Community Safety & Correctional Services (MCSCS). (2016). Careers in Corrections. Retrieved from http://www.mcscs.jus.gov.on.ca/english/corr_serv/careers_in_corr/careers_corr_about.html

RCMP. (2013). *The RCMP PARE administrator manual and Forms.* Ottawa: Author

Warburton D.E.R, Jamnik, V.K., Bredin, S.S.D., & Gledhill N. (2014). The 2014 Physical Activity Readiness Questionnaire for Everyone (PAR-Q+) and electronic Physical Activity Readiness Medical Examination (ePARmed-X+). *Health & Fitness Journal of Canada, 7*(1), 80–83.

GLOSSARY

absolute strength
maximum amount of force exerted, regardless of body size or weight

acute muscle soreness
reflects simple fatigue caused by a buildup of chemical waste products (lactic acid and hydrogen ions) during or after exercise

aerobic conditioning
an exercise program that incorporates activities that are rhythmic in nature, using large muscle groups at moderate intensities for four to seven days per week

aerobic exercise
exercise that uses oxygen to produce the energy necessary for muscle movement by burning fats and carbohydrates

agonist
a muscle that causes specific movement by contracting

amenorrhea
the cessation of menstrual periods for three or more consecutive cycles

amino acids
the fundamental constituents of proteins; amino acids can be divided into two types— complete (essential) and incomplete

anaerobic exercise
exercise that does not require oxygen to produce energy, and only carbohydrates are burned

anatomy
the study of the structure and parts of the body in relationship to one another

aneurysm
a weak or thin area in a blood vessel that causes it to expand and fill with blood; aneurysms may occur as a result of a disease, an injury, or a congenital abnormality in the vessel

angina
severe chest pains associated with advanced cases of coronary heart disease

anorexia nervosa
an eating disorder in which individuals do not eat enough to maintain a healthy body weight

antagonist
a muscle that acts in opposition to the movement caused by the agonist, returning a limb to its initial position

arrhythmia
irregular heartbeat or rhythm

arteriosclerosis
a blanket term for a group of ischemic cardiovascular diseases characterized by a narrowing or hardening of the arteries

arteriovenous malformation
a malformation of the blood vessels of the brain, usually present at birth; an AVM can increase the risk of stroke

arthritis
a group of conditions in which there is a degeneration of a joint following trauma to the joint (as a result of an infection or aging)

atherosclerosis
a common type of arteriosclerosis; a slow, progressive disease in which arterial blockage results from fatty deposits collecting in the arteries

attitude
value added to one's beliefs

automated external defibrillator (AED)
a portable device the size of a laptop computer that checks the heart's rhythm and can send an electric shock to the heart to try to restore a normal rhythm, aiding in rescuing people having sudden cardiac arrest

ball-and-socket joint
the round head of one bone is held in the cup-like cavity of another bone, allowing movement in all directions

ballistic stretching
a stretching technique that promotes the stretch reflex but increases the risk of injury to muscles and tendons; it requires quick, well-coordinated action–reaction movements that stretch the muscles beyond their normal range of motion

basal metabolic rate (BMR)
the speed at which energy is used by the body

basal metabolism
the amount of energy a body at rest needs to maintain essential functions

belief
acceptance of an idea on the basis of knowledge and conviction

binge eating disorder (BED)
an eating disorder associated with obesity, where the person alternately eats obsessively and then diets and restricts eating; the disorder is diagnosed if the person does not follow the binge eating with compensatory behaviours such as vomiting, excessive exercise, or laxative abuse

blood cholesterol
the cholesterol produced by the liver

body composition
the proportion of lean tissue to fat in the body

body dysmorphic disorder (BDD)
a relatively common disorder where individuals obsess about some aspect of their appearance that they deem to be severely flawed and take exceptional measures to hide or fix it

body mass index (BMI)
a method for assessing body composition, based on weight and height

Bona Fide Occupational Requirement (BFOR)
pre-employment fitness screening based on the quantitative (most frequent) and qualitative (most important) physical demands of the job

Borg scale
a simple method of rating perceived exertion (RPE) and used as a method for determining the intensity of exercise, used as an alternative to heart rate monitoring

bulimia nervosa
an eating disorder in which individuals have an intense fear of being overweight and overfat that causes binge eating followed by self-induced vomiting; in the non-purging type, individuals compensate through fasting or excessive exercise

bursitis
inflammation of a bursa (a sac of fluid near a joint)

cardiac arrest
the heart stops pumping

cardiopulmonary resuscitation (CPR)
an emergency procedure that supports circulation and ventilation through chest compressions and artificial ventilation for a short period of time

cardiorespiratory endurance
heart and respiratory system endurance; the ability to perform prolonged large-muscle activities at moderate to high intensity

cataplexy
a sudden loss in muscle tone and deep tendon reflexes, leading to muscle weakness, temporary paralysis, or a complete postural collapse usually brought on by an emotional outburst

cholesterol
a waxy, fat-like substance important for normal body function that travels through the blood and is linked to atherosclerosis

chronic sleep debt
a pervasive issue and a significant health concern where you begin to feel the cumulative effect of not getting enough sleep (sleep deprivation); it can occur from just a few days of getting less than six hours of sleep

chronic time urgency
a constant state of stress due to putting pressure on yourself to do too much in too little time

chronotype
a person's individual circadian rhythms, including body temperature, cognitive faculties, and eating and sleeping patterns

circadian rhythm
the 24-hour cycle on which the human biological clock is based

circuit training
to perform a number of exercises in succession with little to no rest in between

combat stress
an expected and predictable reaction to combat experiences where you are under constant physiological stress (poor diet, extreme temperatures, poor hygiene, etc.) and psychological stress (concern over explosive devices, snipers, death of service members or civilians, etc.)

concentric contraction
takes place when the muscle actively shortens against the opposing load and the ends of the muscle are drawn closer together

concurrent training
training for either strength or power at the same time as training for endurance

concussion
a type of traumatic brain injury (TBI) caused by a bump, blow, or jolt to the head or by a hit to the body; the impact causes the head and brain to move rapidly back and forth, which causes the brain to bounce around or twist in the skull, creating chemical changes in the brain and sometimes stretching and damaging brain cells

coronary heart disease
a type of ischemic heart disease in which fatty deposits block one or more coronary arteries (arteries supplying the heart)

critical incident or traumatic event
a situation faced by law enforcement that causes them to experience unusually strong emotional reactions that have the potential to interfere with their ability to function at the scene (current stress) or later (residual stress)

DASH diet
a diet that follows Canada's Food Guide in order to reduce sodium, cholesterol, and fat in Canadians' diet

debriefing
the provision of assistance, by a qualified mental health professional, to officers who have been involved in a traumatic incident

degenerative disc disease (DDD)
degeneration of the intervertebral discs, the result of aging and mechanical wear and tear

delayed onset muscle soreness (DOMS)
severe muscle tenderness, stiffness, decreased strength, and decreased range of motion that usually peaks between 24 and 72 hours after a hard workout

diabetes
a chronic disease in which the body cannot properly use glucose for energy

diaphragmatic breathing
deep breathing focusing on the contraction of the diaphragm and expansion of the abdomen rather than the chest

dietary cholesterol
the cholesterol in food

dietary fibre
food components that cannot be digested, found exclusively in plants; the two types of dietary fibre are insoluble and soluble

disordered eating
a broad spectrum of abnormal eating behaviours

distress
a type of stress that results in negative responses both in a person's career and in life

diurnal
awake during the day, asleep at night

dynamic stretching
a stretching technique that involves performing movements within the full range of motion of the joint; it gradually increases reach and range of motion while the limbs are moving

eat the frog
a term that means combatting procrastination by taking on the hardest task first

eccentric contraction
takes place when the muscle actively lengthens as it resists the load and the ends of the muscle are pulled farther apart

embolic stroke
a stroke caused by a blood clot or plaque debris that develops elsewhere in the body and travels through the bloodstream until it becomes stuck in the blood vessel in the brain

eustress
a type of good stress that is caused by the factors that initiate emotional and psychological growth

exercising heart rate
your heart rate when your body is in motion during sustained exercise

extrinsic motivation
motivation to perform a task or goal based on external rewards to avoid negative consequences

fascial stretching
the stretching of the connective tissue that surrounds muscles, bones, joints, and nerves to improve flexibility

fatigue
the state of feeling very tired, weary, or sleepy resulting from insufficient sleep, prolonged mental or physical work, shift work, or extended periods of stress or anxiety

fatty acids
the fundamental constituents of fats; fatty acids can be divided into two types—saturated and unsaturated

female athlete triad
an eating disorder among female athletes that is defined by three conditions: disordered eating, amenorrhea, and osteoporosis

fight-or-flight response
the alarm stage when the body prepares itself to cope with a stressor and you either decide to take on the challenge or back away from it

FITT principle
a guideline to designing a fitness program based on frequency, intensity, time, and type of activity

fixator
a muscle that provides support while movement occurs

flexibility
the ability to move the joints freely through their full range of motion

frostbite
severe condition where both the skin and the underlying tissue (fat, muscle, and bone) are frozen

frostnip
a mild form of frostbite, where only the top layer of skin freezes

functional fitness
training with exercises for a specific task

functional strength
focuses on the amount of strength required for a specific job-related task or sport-related skill

functional training
a program that adapts or develops exercises which allows individuals to perform daily activities, specific sports, or physically demanding jobs more easily and without injury

general adaptation
the process of preparing muscles, joints, tendons, and ligaments for intense training by educating the neuromuscular component so that gains can be seen; characterized by higher repetitions, lower intensities, and short rest periods

general adaptation syndrome (GAS)
the body's reaction to stress

gestational diabetes
a temporary condition in which hormonal changes associated with pregnancy and the growth demands of the fetus increase insulin needs to two to three times the normal level; generally occurs after the 24th week of pregnancy and resolves after delivery

glucose
a simple form of sugar that acts as fuel for the body

glycemic index (GI)
the amount of blood glucose (sugar) levels of certain foods within two hours of digestion

glycemic load (GL)
a measure of how quickly a food is converted into sugar in relation to how much sugar it contains

health
the ability of an individual to function independently in a constantly changing environment

health benefits
improvements to physical, mental, and psychological health

health-related fitness
the components of physical fitness that are related to health status, including cardiovascular fitness, musculoskeletal fitness, body composition, and metabolism

heat cramps
illness caused by a water and sodium deficiency; painful, brief muscle cramps that occur during or after exercise or work in a hot environment

heat exhaustion
excessive heat and dehydration raising the body temperature to 38 to 40 °C (100 to 104 °F) resulting in symptoms that may include heavy sweating and a rapid pulse as a result of your body overheating

heat rash
an irritation of the skin that results from excessive sweating during hot and humid weather

heat stroke
illness caused by failure of the body's heat-regulating mechanism; may lead to permanent disability or death

heavy to light training
decreasing the amount of weight you are lifting as you progress through sets, or even within one set

hemorrhagic stroke
a stroke that occurs when a blood vessel in the brain ruptures and bleeds

herniated disc
the rupture and protrusion of the gelatinous interior through the outer coating of the disc due to sudden pressure

high-density lipoprotein (HDL) cholesterol
"good" cholesterol; it helps clean out undesirable LDL deposits

high-intensity interval training (HIIT)
a form of training designed to increase aerobic performance

hinge joint
the bones are connected in a way that allows movement in one plane only (flexion and extension)

hyperglycemia
high blood sugar (glucose) levels

hyperhydration
water "intoxication," characterized by an abnormal increase in the body's water content

hypertension
high blood pressure—the term "essential hypertension" is used for cases in which the cause is unknown

hypervigilance
an enhanced state of sensory sensitivity along with an exaggerated intensity of behaviours

hypoglycemia
low blood sugar (glucose) levels

hypothermia
a condition occurring when the body's control mechanism can no longer maintain a normal body temperature and the body's temperature drops to an abnormally low level

informed consent
a legal document that ensures that you know about the test protocols and are aware of the stress that they may put you under, and that you have followed appropriate guidelines to affirm that you are able to perform the tasks safely

insomnia
a disorder where an individual has trouble falling or staying asleep

intention
a determination to achieve an aim

interval training
training that is based on the concept that the body's energy systems can make both aerobic and anaerobic gains by training with relatively intense exercises followed by a period of recovery

intervertebral discs
flexible, gelatinous, shock-absorbing pads that separate the vertebrae

intracerebral hemorrhage
bleeding in the brain resulting from the rupture of a blood vessel

intrinsic motivation
motivation to perform a task or goal based on enjoyment of doing the task itself

ischemic heart disease
blockage of the coronary arteries resulting in lack of oxygen, angina, and dyspnea

ischemic stroke
occurs when a blood vessel that supplies the brain becomes blocked or clogged, impairing the blood flow

isokinetic contraction
occurs when muscle length changes, contracting maximally throughout the full range of movement

isometric contraction

occurs when muscle length remains constant, or when contractile force equals resistive force

isotonic contraction

contraction of a muscle in response to a load applied to it; includes concentric and eccentric contractions

jet lag

a disruption to your circadian rhythm based on crossing time zones

kilocalorie (kcal)

a measure of the amount of energy in food; also referred to as a calorie

law enforcement developmental competencies

competencies that can be acquired through training after a person has been hired as a law enforcement officer

law enforcement essential competencies

knowledge, skills, and abilities that are being assessed during the entire selection process; they must be demonstrated to be considered for the position

ligament

strong, fibrous connective tissue that connects bones at joints

light to heavy training

increasing the amount of weight you are lifting as you progress through sets

low-back pain (LBP)

a common disorder involving the muscles, nerves, and bones of the back, resulting in pain

low-density lipoprotein (LDL) cholesterol

"bad" cholesterol; it can build up in the arteries and cause health problems

maximal heart rate (MHR)

your heart rate when your heart beats at maximal effort during a sustained aerobic activity

maximum aerobic capacity (VO2 max or MVO2)

a measure of cardiorespiratory fitness; estimated as the point at which oxygen uptake plateaus and does not increase with further increases in workload

meditation

focusing on the mind while quieting the body

melatonin

a hormone, released in the absence of light, that helps us sleep better by increasing drowsiness and lowering body temperature

Metabolic Equivalent of a Task (MET)

the physiological measure of the ratio of energy expenditure of a physical activity compared to rest

metabolic syndrome

is a cluster of medical conditions that increase the risk of many chronic illnesses including diabetes, hypertension, cardiovascular diseases, chronic kidney disease, and dyslipidemia

metabolism

the chemical processes that occur within a living cell that convert the food we eat into the energy our bodies need to function

micro-sleeping

falling asleep for seconds or milliseconds

mild traumatic brain injury

difficulties with attention, concentration, moodiness, and agitation that an individual may suffer from as a result of physical trauma

mindfulness

a mental state achieved by focusing one's awareness on the present moment, while calmly acknowledging and accepting one's feelings, thoughts, and bodily sensations; used as a therapeutic technique

mission statement

a concise statement of major values and goals that is meant to give direction to the decisions a person will make throughout his or her life

muscular endurance

the ability of a muscle to sustain a prolonged contraction or to contract repeatedly over time

muscular hypertrophy

the growth and increase of size of a muscle characterized by high training volume with moderate training intensity

muscular power

generating as much force as possible, as quickly as possible

muscular strength

the amount of force a muscle can produce with a single maximum effort

musculoskeletal fitness

a combined measure of muscular strength, flexibility, and endurance to provide a measure of health

musculoskeletal injuries

injuries of the muscles, nerves, tendons, ligaments, joints, cartilage, or spinal discs

myocardial infarction

a heart attack

narcolepsy

a disorder that causes brain malfunction, leading to one's falling asleep without warning

neustress

a type of stress where the mind and body are aroused but the stress is neither harmful nor helpful

non-REM sleep

stages of sleep, including N1, N2, and N3, where your body has increasingly slower heart rates, eye movement, and brain wave activity

Ontario Police Fitness Award (OPFA)

a provincial incentive program developed to motivate Ontario police officers and police service employees to remain physically fit throughout their entire careers

operational stress injury (OSI)
a non-medical term that is generally defined as "persistent, psychological difficulties resulting from operational duties" and can include post-traumatic stress injuries and post-traumatic stress disorder

osteoarthritis
arthritic degenerative disorder which causes pain and loss of normal spinal structure and function including vertebrae, facet joints, ligaments, and muscles

osteoporosis
a condition where bones become increasingly soft and porous, thinner, and more brittle, making them susceptible to risk of fracture, particularly of the hip, spine, and wrist

overload
feelings of being burdened by excessive time pressure, excessive responsibility, and excessive expectations to succeed

overtraining
the breakdown of the body from training too hard without sufficient rest

PAR-Q+
the Physical Activity Readiness Questionnaire for Everyone (PAR-Q+), developed to enhance the risk stratification process and reduce the barriers to becoming more physically active for all individuals

performance/skill-related fitness
the degree of fitness required to perform a particular job or sport

periodization
an organized approach to training that involves progressive cycling of various aspects of a training program during a specific period of time

peripheral hallucinations
seeing things out of the corner of your eye that aren't really there

physical activity
all leisure and non-leisure body movement that results in an expenditure of energy

physical fitness
the ability to carry out daily tasks with alertness and vigour, without undue fatigue, and with enough reserve to meet emergencies or to enjoy leisure time pursuits

physiology
the study of function of the human body, or how the parts work and carry out their life-sustaining activities

plyometric training
a method of training that enhances an individual's "explosive" reaction through rapid and powerful muscular contractions through stretch-shortening cycles; a concentric action immediately preceded by an eccentric action

post-concussion syndrome
a complex disorder in which various symptoms—such as headaches and dizziness—last for weeks and sometimes months after the injury that caused the concussion

post-traumatic stress disorder (PTSD)
a mental illness where symptoms evolve in the aftermath of an extreme traumatic stressor that overwhelms the individual's coping capacities

post-traumatic stress injury (PTSI)
a number of mental health issues, including depression, substance abuse, and clinically diagnosed PTSD, within the broad category of operational stress injuries (OSIs)

prediabetes
impaired fasting glucose or impaired glucose tolerance; refers to blood glucose levels that are consistently higher than normal but not over 7.0 mmol/L

principle of diminishing returns
refers to the fact that a person's training gains will reflect his or her prior level of training; people who have had little training make significant gains both in terms of strength and aerobic capacity while those who are fit must work harder to see results

principle of individuality
refers to training programs that are adjusted for personal differences based on abilities, skills, gender, age, experience, motivation, physical condition, the ability to recover after a workout, and susceptibility to injury

principle of progressive overload
refers to training and overloading the muscles that help the body to adapt to more and more stress

principle of recovery
refers to the recuperation time or amount of rest required after a workout

principle of reversibility
refers to all the benefits of exercise that are lost if you stop training

principle of specificity
refers to the ability of the body to adapt to a particular type and amount of stress placed on it

procrastination
the postponement of unpleasant or burdensome tasks

proprioceptive neuromuscular facilitation (PNF)
a stretching technique that involves contracting and relaxing the muscles before stretching

psychosomatic symptoms
physical symptoms resulting from mental conflict

pyramid training
a system that combines the light to heavy and heavy to light approaches for weight training

range of motion
the distance and direction a joint can move to its full potential

rapid-eye movement (REM) sleep
a stage of sleep that allows your body to recover from mental fatigue and helps to store memories and consolidate learning

relative strength
maximum amount of force exerted, related to body size or weight

repetition (rep)
one complete movement of an exercise

resilience
the process of adapting well in the face of adversity, trauma, tragedy, threats, or significant sources of stress

resistance training
the most common form of weight training, which incorporates exercises that result in gains to muscle mass and strength as well as the potential for improved flexibility and range of motion

resting heart rate
your heart rate when you are in a resting state such as sleep

restless legs syndrome (RLS)
a condition characterized by an overwhelming urge to move the legs when they are at rest

rhabdomyolysis
a rapid breakdown, rupture, and death of muscle tissue due to heat stress and prolonged physical exertion, causing irregular heart rhythms, seizures, and kidney damage

rheumatoid arthritis
an autoimmune disease where the body attacks healthy joints, resulting in damage to cartilage, bone, tendons, and ligaments

RICE principle
rest, immobilize, cool, elevate; an immediate, simple treatment for a musculoskeletal injury

sciatica
nerve pain down the leg as a result of nerves being compressed, inflamed, or irritated

seasonal affective disorder (SAD)
a syndrome associated with decreased light due to climate, latitude, and changes in neurotransmitter function as a result of seasonal changes

second impact syndrome
describes rapid swelling of the brain which sometimes can be catastrophic if the person afflicted suffers a second head injury before the symptoms from the first have gone away

self-efficacy
one's ability to take action and perform a specific behaviour

self-esteem
how one feels about oneself and one's characteristics

self-management behavioural strategies
strategies that shift one's attention from barriers toward ideas, feelings, and actions that support change

set
a group of repetitions

seven dimensions of health
an integrated approach that empowers individuals to make positive choices moving away from ideals and specific body types and focusing on healthy eating and participating in physical activity and a variety of exercises to promote overall personal well-being, enhanced quality of life, and better choices in terms of nutrition to maintain a healthy weight

shift work disorder
a circadian rhythm disorder where there is a misalignment or desynchronization in sleep pattern as a result of shift work

shoulder impingement syndrome
squeezing of the rotator cuff (the group of muscles that surrounds the shoulder)

six basic nutrients
the basic nutrients that the body requires to function efficiently: water, carbohydrates, protein, fats, vitamins, and minerals

skinfold measurement
measurement of fat just below the skin surface at five points on the body to determine the percentage of body fat

sleep apnea
a breathing-related sleep disorder in which inappropriate brain signals do not tell the breathing muscles to initiate respiration

sleep-impaired
impaired mental or physical function due to lack of sleep

sleep inertia
when your body feels groggy and sleepy upon waking and motor functions are diminished

SMART goals
goals that are specific, measurable, attainable, relevant and realistic, and time-oriented

social involvement
the support of other people to assist you in achieving your goals

somatotype
there are three somatotypes (body types): ectomorphic, mesomorphic, and endomorphic

spondylosis
a term that refers to the general degeneration of the spine associated with normal wear and tear that occurs in the joints, discs, and bones of the spine as people get older

sprain
a stretching or tearing injury to a ligament

stage of exhaustion
when the body is subjected to continual stress and fatigue for days and weeks and begins to shut down, usually resulting in illness

stage of resistance
when the body actively resists and attempts to cope with the stressor

static stretching
a stretching technique that involves bringing a muscle to a maximum or near-maximum stretch by contracting the opposing muscle and holding the stretch for 20–30 seconds without pain

strain
stretching, pulling, or tearing of a muscle or tendon

stress
a "non-specific response of the body to any demands made upon it"

stressor
any physical, psychological, or environmental event or condition that initiates the stress response

stroke
paralysis and a sudden loss of consciousness caused by an interruption of blood flow to the brain; a thrombotic or thromboembolic stroke occurs when blood flow is interrupted by a blood clot that travels to the brain; a hemorrhagic stroke occurs when very high blood pressure causes a weakened blood vessel near the brain to break

subarachnoid hemorrhage
hemorrhage that occurs when a blood vessel on the surface of the brain bleeds into the space between the brain and the skull

superset training
a system that involves performing two exercises in succession, without rest; often used to exercise opposing muscle groups, it results in increased strength and muscle mass of the targeted muscle group

synergist
a muscle that assists an agonist indirectly in producing a joint's movement

talk test
a method for determining the intensity of exercise, used as an alternative to heart rate monitoring; if a person is breathless and cannot carry on a conversation while exercising, he or she is working too hard

target heart rate (THR) zone
the zone that a person's heart rate must reach during exercise to improve or maintain aerobic fitness

tendinitis
inflammation of a tendon

tendon
fibrous tissue that connects muscles to bones

thrombotic stroke
stroke caused by a blood clot that develops in the blood vessels of the brain

trans fats
unsaturated fatty acids that have been hydrogenated to give them a longer shelf life; diets high in trans fats increase the risk of atherosclerosis and coronary heart disease

transient ischemic attack (TIA)
a temporary interference with the blood supply to the brain

trisets
combining three exercises with little rest in between; can involve working the same muscle group from three different angles, working three different muscle groups, or working different areas of the same muscle from three different angles

type 1 diabetes
diabetes that occurs when the pancreas no longer produces insulin or produces very little

type 2 diabetes
diabetes that occurs when the pancreas cannot produce enough insulin or the body is unable to use the insulin effectively

values
the things that matter most to us and guide our daily behaviour, activities, and decisions

vertebrae
the bones of the spine (singular: vertebra)

visualization
a technique that involves imagining yourself in a quiet and peaceful place; also referred to as guided imagery

waist circumference (WC)
an indicator of health risk associated with abdominal fat around the waist

waist-to-hip ratio (WHR) measurement
a method for assessing body composition, based on the relationship between the girth of the waist and the girth of the hips

wellness
a way of life in which you make decisions and choices to enjoy the highest level of health and well-being possible

wind chill index (WCI)
measure representing how the temperature would feel on your skin if the wind were reduced to a walking pace of 4.8 km/h

Workplace Hazardous Materials Information System (WHMIS)
a system that familiarizes workers with safety information about potentially hazardous products in their workplace

INDEX

1.5-mile run, 442–443

1RM (one rep maximum), 144, 151–152, 163

20-metre rushes, 433

390-metre run, 426, 427

absolute strength, 141, 163

acupuncture, 353

acute muscle soreness, 393, 415

aerobic conditioning, 10, 26

aerobic exercise, 83, 103, 112

aerobic fitness test, 420, 422, 424, 430

agility, 85

agonist muscles, 78–79, 103

Alberta Corrections, 431, 433, *see also* correctional officers

Alberta Physical Readiness Evaluation for Police (A-PREP), 18, 422–424

alcohol, 281

amenorrhea, 187, 188, 189

amino acids, 208, 228–229, 234

anaerobic exercise, 83, 103

anaerobic (lactate) threshold, 126

anatomy and physiology, 70–80
cells, tissues, and organs, 71–72
defined, 103
muscle mechanism, 75–80, 81
number of and major bones and muscles, 72–75

aneurysm, 278, 287

angina, 269, 287

anorexia athletica, 187

anorexia nervosa, 185, 189

antagonist muscles, 78–79, 103

antioxidants, 228

A-PREP (Alberta Physical Readiness Evaluation for Police), 18, 422–424

arrhythmia, 271, 273, 287

arteriosclerosis, 269, 287

arteriovenous malformation, 278, 287

arthritis, 302–304, 319

assignments, organizing, 57–58

atherosclerosis, 269, 287

ATP-PC energy system, 126

atrial fibrillation, 282

attainable goals, 40

attitude, 37, 45, *see also* extrinsic motivation; intrinsic motivation

automated external defibrillator (AED), 274, 287

B vitamins, 228

back health, 293–319
arthritis, 302–304, 319
causes of back pain, 297–298
degenerative disc disease, 300–301, 319
impact of carrying heavy loads on, 295–296
nutrition and, 317–318
posture, 298, 315–317
prevalence of back pain in Canada, 294
preventing back pain, 307–315
repetitive strain injury, 305–306, 319
risk factors for back pain, 295, 298–300
spine, 296–297, 313–315
treating back injuries, 307

balance, 85

ball-and-socket joint, 72, 103

ballistic stretching, 98–99, 103

balloon angioplasty, 272

basal metabolic rate (BMR), 177–178, 189

behavioural change, 32–36, 41–42, 44

belief, 37, 38, 45

bench press, 444–447

between-set rest, 144

BFORs, *see* Bona Fide Occupational Requirements (BFORs)

binge eating disorder (BED), 186, 189

bioelectric impedance, 182

biofeedback, 352

biological and chemical hazards, 413–414

bird-dog, 310

blood cholesterol, 213, 234, 277, 281

blood glucose level, 244, *see also* glycemic index (GI); hyperglycemia; hypoglycemia

blood glucose monitor, 245

blood pressure, 83

bodpod, 182

body composition, 175–189
defined, 84, 103, 175, 189
eating disorders, 183–188
measuring, 178–183
somatotypes, 176–177, 189

body dysmorphic disorder, 175, 186, 189

body mass index (BMI), 178, 189

body positions and movements, 79

body types, 176–177, 189

body weight, 174, 196–198

Bodyweight Training System Manual, 157

Bona Fide Occupational Requirements (BFORs)
defined, 26
history, 13–14
purpose, 419
resistance training and, 139–140
services using, 16–19
tasks used to create, 15–16

bones, 72–73

Borg scale, 119–120, 131

breaks, importance of taking, 379

breathing, 145, 349, 354

British Columbia Corrections, 431, 433, *see also* correctional officers

brittle diabetes, 245

bulimia nervosa, 185–186, 189

bursitis, 398, 415

cadence in running, 123

caffeinated drinks, 230–231

calcium, 228, 317–318

calories, 220–221, 234

Canada Border Services
Agency (CBSA)
functional tasks required
for job at, 140
physical testing for, 425, 426
selection process, 23–24
stressors faced by officers, 331
Canada's Food Guide, 225, 277, 377
*Canadian 24-Hour Movement
Guideline for Children
and Youth,* 118
Canadian Armed Forces,
24, 140, 332–333
Canadian Nuclear Security, 25
Canadian Nuclear Security
Fitness Test (CNSFT), 19
*Canadian Physical Activity
Guidelines,* 85, 90, 120
cancer, 173, 198, 376
carbohydrates, 201–207
cardiac arrest, 270, 273–274, 287
cardiac muscle, 74
cardiopulmonary resuscitation
(CPR), 273, 287
cardiorespiratory fitness, 112–131
assessing, 113–116
benefits, 112–113
creating a program, 121–128
determining training
intensity, 116–121
endurance, 82, 103
importance, 112
weather's impact on
programs, 128–129
cardiovascular disease
(CVD), 263–287
anatomy of the heart, 267–268
arteriosclerosis and
atherosclerosis, 269, 287
coronary heart disease
cardiac arrest, 270,
273–274, 287
defined, 269, 287
heart attack, 269–271, 287
risk factors, 275–277
surgical procedures, 272–273
defined, 264, 268
demographics of people
with, 265–266
diabetes and, 251
Framingham Heart Study, 270

hypertension, 83, 276,
281, 282–284, 287
impact on health-care
system, 264–265
risk factors, 173, 265–266,
275–277, 281–282
risk reduction, 284–286
stroke, 267, 277–282, 287
cardiovascular exercise,
see aerobic exercise
cartilage, 72
cataplexy, 374–375, 383
cat-cow stretch, 313
cell search, 428–429
cells, 71
central cardiorespiratory
fitness, 113–114
central sleep apnea, 375
cervical disc disease, 300
chemical and biological
hazards, 413–414
chin-ups, 447–448
cholesterol
blood cholesterol, 213,
234, 277, 281
defined, 213, 234
function, 211, 213–214
chronic disease, 172–173
chronic sleep debt, 367, 383
chronic stress, 336–337
chronic time urgency, 61, 64
chronotype, 367, 383
circadian rhythm, 367, 370, 383
circuit training, 152–153, 163
circulatory system, 71
cold-related injuries and
illnesses, 411–413, 415
combat stress, 332–333, 354
concentric contraction, 80, 81, 103
concurrent training, 95, 103
concussions, 406–409, 415, *see
also* mild traumatic brain injury
connective tissue, 71
contract–relax (C–R)
stretching, 99
contract–relax–antagonist–
contract (CRAC) stretching, 99
cool-down, 147
coordination, 85
core endurance test, 439–440
coronary (balloon) angioplasty, 272

coronary artery bypass
graft (CABG), 272
coronary heart disease, *see*
cardiovascular disease (CVD):
coronary heart disease
correctional officers, 330–331,
335, 431, 433, *see also* Ontario
Correctional Services
Correctional Services Canada, 23
Corrections Officers'
Physical Abilities Test
(COPAT), 18, 431–433
critical incidents, *see* stress
customs officers, *see* Canada
Border Services Agency (CBSA)

DASH diet, 219, 234, 282
debriefing, 345, 354
degenerative disc disease
(DDD), 300–301, 319
delayed-onset muscle soreness
(DOMS), 82, 103, 393–394, 415
dental problems, 251
depression, 251
detraining, 91
developmental competencies,
20–21, 26
diabetes, 243–257
complications from,
251–253, 255
defined, 244, 257
hiring criteria and, 253–254
prevalence in Canada, 250–251
as risk factor for coronary
heart disease, 276
risk factors for diabetes,
173, 248–249
shift work and, 254–256, 377
symptoms, 247
types, 244–246, 257
diabetic dermopathy, 253
diabetic foot, 253
diabetic nephropathy, 253
diabetic retinopathy, 252
diaphragmatic breathing, 349, 354
dietary cholesterol, 213, 234
dietary fibre, 206–207, 234
diets and dieting, *see also* nutrition
cancer and, 198
DASH, 219, 234, 282
high-protein, low-
carbohydrate, 210

statistics, 184

digestive problems, 251

digestive system, 71

diminishing returns, principle of, 92, 104, 148

dislocated shoulder, 399–400

disordered eating, 187, 188, 189

distress, 327, 354

diurnal, 369, 383

duration of training and stretching, 91, 95, 116

dynamic stretching, 98, 103

eating disorders, 183–188

eating the frog, 56, 64

eccentric contraction, 80, 81, 103

ectomorph, 176–177

Edmonton Obesity Staging System (EOSS), 179

embolic stroke, 278, 287

emergency response circuit, 429–430

emotional and psychological health, 7, 8

employment requirements, *see* hiring criteria; physical testing

endocrine system, 71

endomorph, 176–177

endurance, *see* cardiorespiratory fitness; muscular endurance

environmental health, 7, 8

epithelial tissue, 71

equipment belt, 306

erectile dysfunction (ED), 252

essential activities, 52

essential competencies, 19–21, 26

eustress, 326, 327, 354

exams and tests, 58–60, *see also* physical testing

excretory system, 72

exercise, *see also* cardiorespiratory fitness; physical activity; physical training; resistance training
   aerobic, 83, 103, 112
   arrangement, 147–149
   in cold temperatures, 413
   for a healthy back, 309–315
   principles, 89

exercising heart rate, 117, 131

extrinsic motivation
   benefits and drawbacks, 11, 35, 36
   defined, 11, 26, 35, 45
   importance, 10

eye conditions, 252

family and relationship goals, 39

family and relationships, 334–335, 380–381

fascial stretching, 100, 103

fast-twitch fibres, 77–78

fasting hyperglycemia, 246

fatigue, 365, 383

fats, 210–215

fatty acids, 210, 211, 234

female athlete triad, 187–188, 189

fibre, dietary, 206–207, 234

fight-or-flight response, 327–328, 354

financial goals, 39

fitness, *see also* cardiorespiratory fitness; exercise; physical activity; physical testing; physical training; resistance training
   functional, 93, 103
   health-related, 9, 26, 82–84
   musculoskeletal, 10, 26
   performance/skill-related, 9–10, 26, 84–85
   physical, 9, 26, 70, 103

Fitness for Operational Requirements of Canadian Armed Forces Employment (FORCE) Evaluation, 19, 157–158, 433–435

Fitness Test for Ontario Correctional Officers (FITCO), 16, 18, 157, 428–430

FITT principle, 90, 103, 116

Five Cs of enjoyable physical activity, 43

fixator muscles, 78, 103

flexibility, 84, 97, 103, *see also* stretching

food, *see* nutrition

food labelling, 221–225

four A's of coping with stress, 348

Framingham Heart Study, 270

frequency of training and stretching, 91, 95, 116

frostbite, 411, 412, 415

frostnip, 411, 415

fuelling your body, 158–159, 409

functional fitness, 93, 103

functional strength, 141, 163

functional training, 93, 153–154, 163

general adaptation, 144, 163

general adaptation syndrome (GAS), 327, 354

gestational diabetes, 246, 257

glucose, *see also* hyperglycemia; hypoglycemia
   defined, 257
   food containing, 244
   glycemic index and, 203, 204
   monitor for, 245

glycemic index (GI), 203–204, 205, 234

glycemic load (GL), 204, 234

glycolytic system, 126

goal setting, 31–45
   behavioural change and, 32–36, 41–42, 44
   factors affecting participation in physical activity, 36–38
   importance, 32
   mission statement, 43, 45
   for resistance training, 146–147
   short- and long-term goals, 38–39
   SMART goals, 39–40, 45

gout, 303

grocery shopping, 226, 227

groupwork, 62

hamstring stretch, 314

health, defined, 5, 6–8, 26

Health Belief Model, 33

health benefits, 37, 45, 85–89

health-related fitness, 9, 26, 82–84

heart, anatomy of, 267–268, *see also* cardiovascular disease (CVD): coronary heart disease

heart attack, 269–271, 287

heart rate, 116–119, 120

heat cramps, 410, 415

heat exhaustion, 410, 415

heat loss or gain, 128–129

heat rash, 410, 415

heat-related injuries and illnesses, 129, 131, 409–410, 415

heat stroke, 410, 415

heavy to light training, 153, 163

hemorrhagic stroke, 278, 287

herniated disc, 301, 319

high blood pressure, *see* hypertension

high blood sugar, 244, 246, 247–248, 257

high-density lipoprotein (HDL) cholesterol, 214, 234

high-intensity interval training (HITT)
 defined, 94, 103
 goal of, 94, 122
 for running 5 kilometres, 124
 for shuttle run, 127–128
 upper limit, 126

hinge joint, 72, 103

hip bridge, 311

hiring criteria, *see also* physical testing
 developmental competencies, 20–21, 26
 diabetes and, 253–254
 essential competencies, 19–20, 26
 necessity of meeting, 32
 selection process, 21–25
 seven dimensions of health, 7–8

hydration, 158–159, 409

hydrostatic weighing, 183

hydrotherapy, 353

hyperglycemia, 244, 246, 247–248, 257

hyperhydration, 201, 234

hypertension, 282–284
 defined, 287
 diet for treating, 219, 234, 282
 as risk factor for cardiovascular disease, 83, 276, 281

hypervigilance, 341, 354

hypnosis, 352

hypoglycemia (insulin shock), 244, 247, 248, 257

hypothermia, 411, 413, 415

iliotibial band syndrome, 404

implantable cardioverter defibrillator (ICD), 273

implementation of time management, 55–56

individuality, principle of, 91, 104

inflammation, 392

informed consent, 12, 26

injuries, *see also* musculoskeletal injuries (MSI)
 biological and chemical hazards, 413–414
 cold-related injuries and illnesses, 411–413, 415
 concussions, 406–409, 415
 heat-related injuries and illnesses, 129, 131, 409–410, 415

insomnia, 374, 383

insulin, 203–204

insulin resistance, 246

insulin shock (hypoglycemia), 244, 247, 248, 257

intellectual health, 7, 8

intensity of training and stretching, 90, 101, 116–121

intention, 37, 45

intermittent loaded shuttles, 434–435

Internet, nutritional information on, 231

interval training, 94, 103

intervertebral discs, 297, 319

intracerebral hemorrhage, 278, 287

intrinsic motivation
 benefits and drawbacks, 11, 35, 36
 defined, 11, 26, 35, 45
 importance, 10

iron, 228

ischemic heart disease, 268, 287

ischemic stroke, 278–279, 287

isokinetic contraction, 80, 103

isometric contraction, 80, 81, 103

isotonic contraction, 80, 81, 103

jet lag, 370, 383

joints, 72, 103

kidney disease, 253

kilocalories, 220–221, 234

lactate (anaerobic) threshold, 126

leg press, 449

Léger 20-metre shuttle run, *see* shuttle run

lifestyle goals, 39

ligaments, 72, 74, 103

light to heavy training, 153, 163

low-back pain (LBP), 294, 319

low blood sugar, 244, 247, 248, 257

low-density lipoprotein (LDL) cholesterol, 213–214, 234

lumbago, 300–301

lymphatic system, 71

magnesium, 228

massage, 353

maximal heart rate (MHR), 117, 131

maximum aerobic capacity (VO_2 max or MVO_2), 114–115, 131

measurable goals, 40

meditation, 349–350, 354

melatonin, 370, 383

meniscus, 405–406

mental health and illness, 251, 329, 339–342, 354

mesomorph, 176–177

Metabolic Equivalent of a Task (MET), 120–121, 131

metabolic syndrome (MetS)
 defined, 175, 189, 196, 235
 diabetes and, 245–246, 248
 diagnosis, 196–197

metabolism, 72, 103, 177–178, 189

micro-sleeping, 370, 383

mild sprains, 394

mild traumatic brain injury, 341, 354, *see also* concussions

mindfulness, 347–348, 354

minerals, 216, 218–220, 228, 317–318

Minimum Physical Fitness Standard (MPFS), 19

mission statement, 43, 45

moderate sprains, 394

modified back extensions, 314

modified curl up, 309–310

monounsaturated fats, 211, 212

motivation, *see* extrinsic motivation; intrinsic motivation

muscle dysmorphia, 175, 186

muscle fibres, 75–78
muscle groups, 74–75
muscle soreness, 82
muscle tissue, 71, 73–74
muscles, 73, 78–79, 103, 104
muscular contractions, 80, 81, 103
muscular endurance
    core endurance test, 439–440
    defined, 84, 103, 142, 163
    resistance training
      and, 141, 142
muscular hypertrophy, 143, 163
muscular power, 143, 163
muscular strength, 82–83,
  103, 142, 163
muscular system, 71
musculoskeletal fitness, 10, 26
musculoskeletal injuries
  (MSI), 390–406
    defined, 390, 415
    dislocated shoulder, 399–400
    iliotibial band syndrome, 404
    meniscus, 405–406
    muscle soreness, 393–394
    Osgood-Schlatter disease, 403
    patello-femoral
      syndrome, 400–401
    plantar fasciitis, 402–403
    risk factors, 391
    shin splints, 401–402
    sprains
      defined, 76, 104, 394, 415
      grades, 394–395
      knee, 404–405
      treatment, 396, 405
    strains, 76, 104, 395–396, 415
    tendinitis, 396–398, 415
    treatments, 391–393
music, 352
myocardial infarction,
  269–271, 287
myofibrils, 75, 76
myofilaments, 75–76, 77

narcolepsy, 374, 383
National Defence, 24
nerve tissue, 71
nervous system, 71
neuropathy, 252
neustress, 326, 354

non-REM sleep, 368–369, 383
Nova Scotia Corrections, 431, 433,
  see also correctional officers
nutrient content claims, 223–224
nutrition, 195–235
    back health and, 317–318
    caffeinated drinks, 230–231
    calories, 220–221, 234
    Canada's Food Guide,
      225, 277, 377
    cardiovascular disease and, 277
    finding trustworthy
      information about, 231
    food labelling, 221–225
    grocery shopping, 226, 227
    maintaining a healthy
      weight, 196–198
    serving and portion
      sizes, 225–226, 227
    shift work and, 196,
      228–231, 377–378
    six basic nutrients
      carbohydrates, 201–207
      defined, 199, 235
      fats, 210–215
      minerals, 216, 218–220,
        228, 317–318
      protein, 208–210
      vitamins, 215–216,
        217, 228, 318
      water, 200–201
    snacking, 229–230
    trends in Canada, 196, 197
    wellness initiatives, 232
nutritional aids, 159

obesity
    BMI categorization
      of, 178–179
    issues surrounding, 87,
      172–173, 174, 179
    prevalence, 4, 87–88,
      174, 175, 179, 197
    risk factor for cardiovascular
      disease, 173, 276, 281
    vs. overweight, 175
obstacle course, 424, 425
obstructive sleep apnea, 375
occupational health, 7, 8
omega-3 fatty acids, 213
omega-6 fatty acids, 213

omega-9 fatty acids, 213
one rep maximum (1RM),
  144, 151–152, 163
Ontario Correctional Services,
  23, 140, 254, 428, *see also*
  correctional officers
Ontario police, 15, 21–22, 419
Ontario Police Fitness
  Award (OPFA)
    defined, 14, 26
    purpose, 14–15
    standards, 17, 436–444
      1.5-mile run, 442–443
      core endurance
        test, 439–440
      grading, 436
      Léger 20-metre shuttle
        run, 443–444
      push-ups, 437–438
      trunk forward
        flexion, 441–442
Ontario Provincial
  Police (OPP), 15
Ontario's First Responders Act, 342
operational stress injury
  (OSI), 339, 354
optional activities, 53
organizing, time management
  and, 57–58
organs, 71–72
Osgood-Schlatter disease, 403
osteoarthritis, 302, 319
osteoporosis, 187, 188,
  303–304, 319
overfat, 175
overload, 328, 354
overtraining, 91–92, 103, 152
overweight
    BMI categorization
      of, 178–179
    issues surrounding, 87,
      172–173, 174, 179
    prevalence, 87, 174,
      175, 179, 197
    vs. overfat, 175
oxidative system, 126

pacemaker, 273
PAR-Q+ (Physical Activity
  Readiness Questionnaire for
  Everyone), 11, 12, 26, 419

patello-femoral syndrome, 400–401

performance-enhancing substances, 159–160

performance/skill-related fitness, 9–10, 26, 84–85

periodization, 95–96, 103, 145–146, 163

peripheral cardiorespiratory fitness, 114

peripheral hallucinations, 371, 383

peripheral nerve entrapment disorders, 305

personal goals, 39, 43

pharmacological aids, 159–160

Physical Abilities Requirement Evaluation (PARE), 16, 17–18, 155–156, 424–426

physical activity, see also cardiorespiratory fitness; exercise; resistance training
defined, 9, 26
factors affecting participation in, 36–38
Five C's of enjoyable, 43
guidelines for weekly amount, 10, 85, 90, 118, 120
health benefits, 85–89
impact on preventing cancer, 198
shift work and, 379

physical-control simulator, 426–428, 431, 432

physical fitness, 9, 26, 70, 103

physical fitness log, 12–13, 449

physical health, 6, 8

physical inactivity, 276, 281

Physical Readiness Evaluation for Policing (PREP), 16, 17, 155, 419–422

physical testing, 10–19, see also hiring criteria; Ontario Police Fitness Award (OPFA)
A-PREP, 18, 422–424
assessing cardiorespiratory fitness, 113–116
bench press, 444–447
chin-ups, 447–448
COPAT, 19, 431–433
FITCO, 16, 18, 157, 428–430
FORCE, 19, 157–158, 433–435

history, 13–14
leg press, 449
motivation of law enforcement candidates for, 10–11
PARE, 16, 17–18, 155–156, 424–426
POPAT, 18, 426–428
PREP, 16, 17–18, 155, 419–422
preparation, 11–13
services using BFORs, 16–19
tasks used to create BFORs, 15–16

physical training, see also cardiorespiratory fitness; exercise; high-intensity interval training (HITT); resistance training
as individual process, 81
defined, 80
methods, 93–96, 103
principles of, 89–93

physiological aids, 159

physiology, see anatomy and physiology

phytonutrients, 203

piriformis stretch, 314–315

plank, 310–311

plantar fasciitis, 402–403

plyometric training, 94–95, 103, 143–144, 163

police and policing, see also Ontario Police Fitness Award (OPFA)
functional tasks required for job, 140
in Ontario, 15, 21–22, 419
stressors, 332, 333

Police Fitness Personnel Ontario (PFPO), 14, 17, 82, 436

Police Officer Physical Abilities Test (POPAT), 18, 426–428

polyunsaturated fats, 211, 212–213

portion and serving sizes, 225–226, 227

post-concussion syndrome, 408, 415

post-traumatic stress disorder (PTSD), 339–342, 354

post-traumatic stress injuries (PTSI), 339, 354

postprandial hyperglycemia, 246

posture, 298, 315–317

power, 85, 143, 163

prediabetes, 246, 257

PREP (Physical Readiness Evaluation for Policing), 16, 17, 155, 419–422

principle of diminishing returns, 92, 104, 148

principle of individuality, 91, 104

principle of progressive overload, 89–90, 104, 144

principle of recovery, 92–93, 104

principle of reversibility, 91–92, 104

principle of specificity, 90–91, 104

prioritization, 52–53

private investigators, 25

procrastination, 55–56, 64

professional goals, 39, 43

progressive muscle relaxation, 350

progressive overload, principle of, 89–90, 104, 144

proprioceptive neuromuscular facilitation (PNF), 99, 104

protein, 208–210

protein supplementation, 210

psychosomatic symptoms, 335, 354

pursuit/restraint circuit, 420, 421, 422–423

push/pull section, 424–425

push-ups, 437–438

pyramid training, 153, 163

range of motion, 72, 104

rapid-eye movement (REM) sleep, 368–369, 383

RCMP
functional tasks required for job at, 140
physical testing for, 424, 425, 426
selection process, 22

reaction time, 85

recovery, principle of, 92–93, 104

regular activities, 53

relationships and family, 334–335, 380–381

relative strength, 141, 163

relaxation techniques, 349–353

relevant and realistic goals, 40

repetition (rep), 142, 149–150, 163

repetitive strain injury (RSI), 305–306, 319

reproductive risks of shift work, 376

reproductive system, 71

resilience, 347, 354

resistance training, 137–163
  basic principles, 142–146
  benefits, 140–141
  defined, 94, 104, 141, 163
  fuelling, 158–159
  goal setting, 146–147
  importance, 138–140
  methods, 152–154
  performance-enhancing substances, 159–160
  program design, 147–152
  programs for law enforcement, 154–158
  tips for first-time weight room use, 161–162
  women and strength training, 160–161

respiratory system, 72

resting heart rate, 83, 116–117, 131

restless legs syndrome (RLS), 375, 383

reversibility, principle of, 91–92, 104

rewards, 42

rhabdomyolysis, 129, 131

rheumatoid arthritis (RA), 303, 319

RICE principle, 392–393, 415

running, 123–125, 129–130

sandbag drag, 435

sandbag lift, 434

sarcomeres, 75, 76

sarcopenia, 140

saturated fats, 211–212

scheduling, 53–54, 59–60, 372

sciatica, 301, 319

seasonal affective disorder (SAD), 378, 383

second impact syndrome, 408, 415

security guards, 25, 332, 333

sedentary behaviour, 86–87

selection process for hiring law enforcement officials, 21–25

self-efficacy, 36, 45

self-esteem, 35–36, 45

self-hypnosis, 352

self-management behavioural strategies, 37–38, 41, 45

serving and portion sizes, 225–226, 227

set, 142, 144, 149–150, 163

severe sprains, 394

sexual health, 252

shift work
  coping with, 377–382
  effects, 364, 365, 369–373
  importance of time management in, 50
  medical conditions associated with, 254–256, 374–377
  nutrition and, 196, 228–231, 377–378

shift work disorder, 374, 383

shin splints, 401–402

shoulder impingement syndrome, 397–398, 415

shuttle run
  in A-PREP, 424
  in FITCO, 430
  in OFPA standards, 443–444
  in PREP, 420, 422
  training for, 127–128

side bridge, 311

six basic nutrients, *see* nutrition: six basic nutrients

skeletal muscle, 73, 74

skeletal system, 72

skin infections, 252–253

skinfold measurement, 181, 189

sleep
  effects of shift work on, 364, 365, 369–373
  healthy habits, 378–379, 381–382
  importance, 365–369
  recommended amount of, 366

sleep apnea, 375–376, 383

sleep deprivation, 277, 379

sleep disorders, 374–376

sleep-impaired, 371, 383

sleep inertia, 368, 383

slow-twitch fibres, 77–78

SMART goals, 39–40, 45

smartphones, 58

smoking, 267, 275–276, 281

smooth muscle, 73, 74

snacking, 229–230

social and interpersonal health, 7, 8

social involvement, 42, 45

sodium, 216, 218–220

somatotypes, 176–177, 189

special constables, 24–25

specific goals, 40

specificity, principle of, 90–91, 104

speed, 85

spine, 296–297, 313–315

spiritual health, 7, 8

spondylosis, 300, 319

sprains, *see* musculoskeletal injuries (MSI): sprains

stage of exhaustion, 328, 354

stage of resistance, 328, 354

stair run, 431, 432

Standardized Physical Abilities Test-École Nationale de Police du Québec (SPAT-ENPQ), 18

static stretching, 98, 104

stigma, 347

stir the pot (exercise), 312

strains, 76, 104, 395–396, 415

strength
  absolute, functional, and relative, 141, 163
  muscular, 82–83, 103, 142, 163

strength training, 160–161

stress, 325–354
  coping with
    after critical incidents, 345–346
    four A's, 348
    relaxation techniques, 349–353
    resiliency and mindfulness, 347–348, 354
  critical incidents
    defined, 337, 354
    factors affecting responses to, 338–339
    suicide, 343–345
    symptoms, 339–342
    types, 338
  defined, 326, 354

stress (continued)
   effects, 335–337
   impact on family, 334–335
   response to, 327–328
   risk factor for cardiovascular
    disease, 277, 282
   stressors
    defined, 328, 354
    from workplace health
     and safety hazards, 334
    in daily life, 328–329
    in law enforcement,
     330–333, 335
   types, 326–327
stretching
   benefits, 97–98
   importance for back
    health, 313–315
   safe and effective, 100–101
   techniques, 98–100, 103, 104
stroke, 267, 277–282, 287
subacrachnoid hemorrhage,
   278, 287
sugar
   food and drinks containing,
    201, 202, 244
   glucose defined, 257
   glycemic index and, 203, 204
   monitor for blood glucose, 245
suicide, 343–345
suitcase carry, 312
superset training, 153, 163
synergist muscles, 78, 104

T'ai chi ch'uan, 352–353
talk test, 120, 131
target heart rate (THR)
   zone, 117–119, 120, 131
tendinitis, 396–398, 415

tendon-related disorders, 305
tendons, 73, 74, 104
tests and exams, 58–60, *see
   also* physical testing
thoracic disc disease, 300
thrombotic stroke, 278–279, 287
thyroid disorders, 252
time management, 49–64
   benefits, 50–52
   importance, 50, 63
   stages, 52–56
   strategies for students, 57–62
   time wasters, 51
time (duration) of training and
   stretching, 90, 101, 116
timed goals, 40
tissues, 71
to-do lists, 52–53
torso bag carry, 427, 428, 432–433
training, *see* cardiorespiratory
   fitness; physical training;
   resistance training
trans fats, 211, 214, 235
transient ischemic attack
   (TIA), 278, 287
Transtheoretical Model, 33–34, 35
traumatic events, *see* stress:
   critical incidents
trisets, 153, 163
trunk forward flexion, 441–442
tryptophan, 229
type 1 diabetes, 244–245, 257
type 2 diabetes, 245–246, 257
type of training and stretching (in
   FITT principle), 90, 101, 116
tyrosine, 228–229

underweight, 178–179
unsaturated fats, 211, 212

values, 38, 45
vault rail, 427, 428, 431–432
vegetarianism, 208
vertebrae, 296–297, 319
visualization, 351, 354
vitamins, 215–216, 217, 228, 318
VO$_2$ max (maximum
   aerobic capacity and
   MVO$_2$), 114–115, 131

waist circumference
   (WC), 179–181, 189
waist-to-hip ratio (WHR)
   measurement, 180, 189
warm-up, 147
water, 200–201
websites, nutritional
   information on, 231
weight carry section, 425–426
weight loss, 121, 184, *see
   also* diets and dieting
weight room, 161–162
weights, choosing, 150–152
wellness, 5–6, 26, 232
wind chill index (WCI),
   411–412, 415
Winnipeg Police Service
   Physical Abilities Test
   (WPS-PAT), 18
women and strength
   training, 160–161
Workplace Hazardous
   Materials Information System
   (WHMIS), 413–414, 415
workplace health and
   safety hazards, 334
workspace, 57

yoga, 352

CREDITS

Photos on pages 143, 160, 180–182, 226, 306, 310–315, 437–438, 440–441, 448–450 taken by Heather Gough and Nancy Wisotzki

PART 1

Chapter/part opening photos: Ramsey/iStock

CHAPTER 1

Page 3 (photo): Ramsey/iStock

Page 12 (photo): Reproduced with permission of the Ontario Provincial Police.

Page 15 (Figure 1.1): Reproduced with permission of the Ontario Provincial Police.

CHAPTER 2

Page 31 (photo): Ramsey/iStock

CHAPTER 3

Page 49 (photo): Ramsey/iStock

Page 51 (Figure 3.1): Reprinted with the permission of Gosia Zimniak.

PART 2

Chapter/part opening photos: Martinan/Thinkstock

CHAPTER 4

Page 69 (photo): Martinan/Thinkstock

Page 73 (Figure 4.1): LifeArt

Page 74 (Figure 4.2): blueringmedia/Thinkstock

Page 74 (Figure 4.3): LifeArt

Page 75 (Figure 4.4): LifeArt

Page 76 (Figure 4.5): LifeArt

Page 81 (Figure 4.7): Wikipedia

Page 98 (Figure 4.9): ePainAssist

Page 99 (Figure 4.10): YekophotoStudio/Thinkstock

CHAPTER 5

Page 111 (photo): Martinan/Thinkstock

Page 115 (Figure 5.2): Javier Larrea/age fotostock/Alamy Stock photo

CHAPTER 6

Page 137 (photo): Martinan/Thinkstock

Page 139 (photo): photo Courtesy of Barrie Police Service, 2017.

Page 144 (Figure 6.4): jacoblund/Thinkstock

Page 145 (Table 6.2): Reprinted with the permission of Brian Martin.

Page 155 (Table 6.6): © Queen's Printer for Ontario, 2016. Reproduced with permission.

Page 156 (Table 6.7): Reproduced with the permission of the RCMP.

Page 156 (Table 6.8): Reproduced with the permission of the RCMP.

Page 157 (Table 6.9): Reproduced from *Becoming a Correctional Services Officer: FITCO—Fitness Test for Ontario Correctional Officer Applicants*, 2016. Retrieved from https://www.mcscs.jus.gov.on.ca/english/corr_serv/careers_in_corr/become_corr_off/FITCO/cs_FITCO.html). © Queen's Printer for Ontario, 2016. Reproduced with permission.

Page 158 (Table 6.10): Canadian Forces Morale and Welfare Services. (n.d.). *BodyWeight Training System CF Fitness Anytime, Anywhere*. Retrieved from https://www.cfmws.com/en/AboutUs/PSP/DFIT/Fitness/BTS%20Document%20Library/ENG%20BTS.pdf. Reproduced with permission.

PART 3

Chapter/part opening photos: Purestock/Thinkstock

CHAPTER 7

Page 171 (photo): Purestock/Thinkstock

Page 173 (Table): Reprinted with the permission of the World Health Organization.

Page 176 (Figure 7.2): Granger Historical Picture Archive / Alamy Stock photo

Page 182 (Figure 7.6): CP PHOTO/ Guelph Mercury—Darren Calabrese

CHAPTER 8

Page 195 (photo): Purestock/Thinkstock

Page 198 (Figure 8.1): Reprinted with the permission of World Cancer Research Fund International.

Page 199 (Figure 8.2): a_namenko/Thinkstock

Page 200 (Figure 8.3): Pixabay

Page 207 (Table 8.4): Reprinted with the permission of EatrightOntario.ca.

Page 209 (Figure 8.5): JupiterImages/Thinkstock and Pixabay

Page 211 (Figure 8.6): Pixabay

Page 212 (Figure 8.7): AlexPro9500/Thinkstock

Page 219 (Figure 8.8): Reprinted with permission ©2016 American Heart Association, Inc.

Page 222 (Figure 8.9): © All rights reserved. *Food labelling changes.* Health Canada, 2017. Adapted and reproduced with permission from the Minister of Health, 2017.

Page 222 (Figure 8.10): © All rights reserved. *Food labelling changes.* Health Canada, 2017. Adapted and reproduced with permission from the Minister of Health, 2017.

Page 223 (Figure 8.11): © All rights reserved. *Food labelling changes.* Health Canada, 2017. Adapted and reproduced with permission from the Minister of Health, 2017.

Page 223 (Table 8.8): © All rights reserved. *Nutrient content claims: What they mean.* Health Canada, 2012. Adapted and reproduced with permission from the Minister of Health, 2017.

Page 227 (Table 8.9): © All rights reserved. *Eating Well with Canada's Food Guide.* Health Canada, 2011. Adapted and reproduced with permission from the Minister of Health, 2017.

PART 4

Chapter/part opening photos: Murmakova/iStock

CHAPTER 9

Page 245 (photo): Murmakova/iStock

CHAPTER 10

Page 263 (photo): Murmakova/iStock

Page 268 (Figure 10.2): LifeArt

Page 269 (Figure 10.3): LifeArt

Page 270 (Figure 10.4): LifeArt

Page 272 (Figure 10.6): Solar22/Thinkstock

Page 272 (Figure 10.7): blausen.com staff (2014)/Wikipedia

Page 273 (Figure 10.8): wetcake/iStock

Page 279 (Figure 10.10): ePainAssist

Page 280 (Figure 10.11): ttsz/Thinkstock

Page 283 (Figure 10.12): jauhari1/Thinstock

CHAPTER 11

Page 293 (photo): Murmakova/iStock

Page 296 (Figure 11.1): LifeArt

Page 297 (Figure 11.2): ePainAssist

Page 298 (Figure 11.3): handmadeee3d/Shutterstock

Page 299 (Figure 11.4): Fotosearch

Page 301 (Figure 11.5): ePainAssist

Page 302 (Figure 11.6): stihli/Shutterstock

Page 303 (Figure 11.7): wildpixel/iStock

Page 317 (Figure 11.20): Reprinted with the permission of the Canadian Centre for Occupational Health and Safety (CCOHS).

CHAPTER 12

Page 325 (photo): Murmakova/iStock

Page 328 (Figure 12.2): Wikipedia

Page 337 (Figure 12.3): Pixabay

Page 342 (Figure 12.4): Wilson, S., H. Guliani, & G. Boichev. (2016). "Reviews: On the economics of post-traumatic stress disorder of first responders in Canada." *Journal of Community Safety and Well-Being*. Reprinted with the permission of MultiMed.

Page 343 (Figure 12.5): © All rights reserved. *Suicide in Canada: Infographic*. Public Health Agency of Canada, 2016. Adapted and reproduced with permission from the Minister of Health, 2017.

Page 344 (Table 12.8): Reprinted with permission from The Lifeline Canada Foundation.

Page 348 (Text): Robinson, L., M. Smith, & R. Segal. 2017 *Stress Management. Simple Tips to Get Stress in Check and Regain Control of Your Life*. Retrieved from helpguide.org. Reprinted with permission.

Page 350 (Figure 12.6): Poike/Thinkstock

Page 352 (Figure 12.7): microgen/iStock

CHAPTER 13

Page 363 (photo): Murmakova/iStock

Page 365 (Figure 13.1): monkeybusinessimages/Thinkstock

Page 374 (Figure 13.6): AntiMartina/iStock

Page 374 (Text): National Sleep Foundation. Reprinted with permission.

Page 375 (Text): National Sleep Foundation. Reprinted with permission.

Page 375 (Figure 13.7): creative_outlet/Thinkstock

Page 381 (Figure 13.8): Pixabay

CHAPTER 14

Page 389 (photo): Murmakova/iStock

Page 395 (Figure 14.1): Alila Medical Media/Shutterstock

Page 395 (Figure 14.2): ePainAssist

Page 397 (Figure 14.3): ePainAssist

Page 399 (Figure 14.4): ePainAssist

Page 400 (Figure 14.5): ePainAssist

Page 401 (Figure 14.6): LifeArt

Page 402 (Figure 14.7): Alamy

Page 403 (Figure 14.8): LifeArt

Page 494 (Figure 14.9): ePainAssist

Page 405 (Figure 14.10): LifeArt

Page 406 (Figure 14.11): Wikipedia

Page 407 (Figure 14.12): Reproduced with the permission of Canadian Institute for Health Information.

Page 412 (Table 14.2): © Her Majesty the Queen in Right of Canada, as represented by the Minister of the Environment Canada (2017).

APPENDIX

Page 421 (Figure A.1): Ministry of Community and Safety and Correctional Services, 2015.

Page 425 (Figure A.4): Reprinted with permission from the RCMP.

Page 427 (Figure A.5): Reprinted with permission from Law Enforcement Physical Abilities Testing (LEPAT) Inc.

Page 429 (Figure A.6): Reproduced from Becoming a Correctional Services Officer: FITCO - Fitness Test for Ontario Correctional Officer Applicants, 2016. Retrieved from https://www.mcscs.jus.gov. on.ca/english/corr_serv/careers_in_corr/become_corr_off/FITCO/ cs_FITCO.html). © Queen's Printer for Ontario, 2016. Reproduced with permission.

Page 432 (Figure A.7): Reprinted with permission from Law Enforcement Physical Abilities Testing (LEPAT) Inc.

Page 433 (Figure A.8): Canadian Forces Morale and Welfare Services, 2016.

Page 434 (Figure A.9): Canadian Forces Morale and Welfare Services, 2016.

Page 434 (Figure A.10): Canadian Forces Morale and Welfare Services, 2016.

Page 435 (Figure A.11): Canadian Forces Morale and Welfare Services, 2016.

Page 436 (Figure A.12): Canadian Forces Morale and Welfare Services, 2016.

Page 439 (Table A.1): Reprinted with the permission of Police Fitness Personnel of Ontario.

Page 439 (Figure A.15): Reprinted with the permission of Police Fitness Personnel of Ontario.

Page 441 (Table A.2): Reprinted with the permission of Police Fitness Personnel of Ontario.

Page 443 (Table A.3): Reprinted with the permission of Police Fitness Personnel of Ontario.

Page 444 (Table A.4): Reprinted with the permission of Police Fitness Personnel of Ontario.

Page 445 (Table A.5): Reprinted with the permission of Police Fitness Personnel of Ontario.

Page 446 (Table A.6): Adapted with permission. Marian Reeves. Peel Regional Police Service 2002 recruit standards. 2002 Brampton, Ontario, Peel Regional Police.

Page 447 (Table A.7): Adapted with permission. Marian Reeves. Peel Regional Police Service 2002 recruit standards. 2002 Brampton, Ontario, Peel Regional Police.

Page 449 (Table A.8): Adapted with permission. Marian Reeves. Peel Regional Police Service 2002 recruit standards. 2002 Brampton, Ontario, Peel Regional Police.